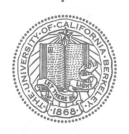

UC Berkeley

THE COMPLETE
HOME WELLNESS
HANDBOOK

THE COMPLETE HOME WELLNESS HANDBOOK

HOME REMEDIES • PREVENTION • SELF-CARE

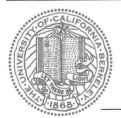

John Edward Swartzberg, M.D., F.A.C.P.,

Sheldon Margen, M.D., and the editors of the

UC Berkeley Wellness Letter

Health Letter Associates

THE UNIVERSITY OF CALIFORNIA, BERKELEY
WELLNESS LETTER

The *Wellness Letter* is a monthly eight-page newsletter that delivers brisk, useful coverage on health, nutrition, and exercise topics in language that is clear, engaging, and nontechnical. It's a unique resource that covers fundamental ways to prevent illness. For information on how to order this award-winning newsletter from the world-famous School of Public Health at the University of California, Berkeley, write to Health Letter Associates, 325 Redding Road, Redding, CT 06896.

Get subscription information online—along with updates on the wellness approach to staying healthy—at our Web site:

www.wellnessletter.com

Library of Congress Cataloging-in-Publication Data

Swartzberg, John Edward, 1945-
   The complete home wellness handbook / John Edward Swartzberg & Sheldon Margen.
      p. cm.
   Includes index.
   ISBN 0-9760152-1-8
      1. Medicine, Popular--Handbooks, manuals, etc. 2. Self-care, Health--Handbooks, manuals, etc. I. Margen, Sheldon. II. Title.

RC81 .S9685 2001
616.02'4—dc21   2001019197

Printed in the United States of America
10 9 8 7 6 5 4 3

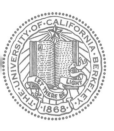

Contents

P romoting good health and preventing disease are the hallmarks of public health. The faculty of the School of Public Health at the University of California, Berkeley are involved in teaching, research, and practice in these areas. As physicians who are members of that faculty, our philosophy is that health promotion and disease prevention are part of good medical care. But we also recognize that, despite our best efforts (and yours), all of us are going to encounter a variety of health problems during our lives. Another aspect of our work, therefore, is to provide information about those ailments, disorders, and complaints that can initially be treated at home, without medical assistance, and also to identify those that always require professional intervention.

The Complete Home Wellness Handbook is our effort to make the best recommendations possible—based on our expertise and that of other researchers and teachers at the School of Public Health. This means you won't find any miracle cures, "magic bullets," or amazing breakthroughs in these pages. Instead, our advice is based on long-term clinical experience and research, and on reviewing and evaluating the best studies available. And while we have great respect for the many medical advances that have helped save lives, we are convinced that the preventive wellness strategies featured in this book are also true life-savers. Chronic illnesses, especially heart disease, cancer, diabetes, emphysema, and stroke, account for nearly 90 percent of all premature deaths in the United States. We think that the incidence of these illnesses can be dramatically reduced with interventions that include such preventive strategies.

We also strongly believe that everyone can benefit from a doctor's expertise (and that everyone is entitled to such expertise). For most people, this will mean choosing a primary-care physician who oversees and coordinates their medical care. Unfortunately, more than 40 million Americans do not currently have access to routine medical advice. Bearing that in mind, we also provide guidelines for choosing and working with a physician when it is essential to do so.

The main section of the book—an A to Z compendium of ailments and disorders—covers virtually every complaint that you can do something about on your own. The entries will also help you convey necessary information to your doctor and ask your doctor useful questions. Obviously, this book is not meant to be a substitute for having a doctor you know and trust. But because the information is presented in a clear, straightforward format, we hope that it will allow you to make informed decisions about your own health (and your family's) and to be an effective partner with your doctor in managing your health and medical care.

JOHN EDWARD SWARTZBERG, M.D., F.A.C.P., an internist with 26 years of clinical experience and a specialist in infectious disease, is a Clinical Professor of Medicine at the University of California, Berkeley and the University of California, San Francisco, and Director of the UCB-UCSF Joint Medical Program at Berkeley's School of Public Health. He also serves as Hospital Epidemiologist and Director of Infection Control at a major hospital in the Bay Area. Dr. Swartzberg is the chair of the Editorial Board of the *University of California, Berkeley Wellness Letter*.

SHELDON MARGEN, M.D., is Professor Emeritus of Public Health and Nutrition in the School of Public Health at the University of California, Berkeley. An internationally respected researcher, he was among the first nutritionists to identify the relationship between diet and chronic disease. Dr. Margen's many professional activities include serving as chair of the Editorial Board of the *UC Berkeley Wellness Letter*—a publication he helped launch in 1984 as part of his effort to make public health information available to a wide audience.

◆　◆　◆

THOMAS DICKEY is a founding editor of the *UC Berkeley Wellness Letter*. He has supervised the creation of several major encyclopedias, including the *UC Berkeley Wellness Encyclopedia* and the *UC Berkeley Wellness Encyclopedia of Food and Nutrition*.

Introduction

This book is divided into six sections. In the first section, "Wellness Strategies," you will find positive, practical tips and guidelines in the areas of nutrition, exercise, alcohol consumption, smoking cessation, weight control, and more. By integrating good health habits into your daily life, you not only increase your chances of preventing serious illness, but you can also fend off many bothersome complaints such as back pain, constipation, and varicose veins. You are also likely to feel younger and more energetic than people who are unaware of habits that are healthy or who simply ignore them.

Even if you are in good health, you need the advice and care of a doctor, who can perform routine tests and examinations that will help you maintain your health. The preventive services you should be aware of, along with guidelines on choosing health-care practitioners, are explained in the second section, "Using the Health-Care System."

Acute medical problems that require a quick response, from bite wounds to heart attack, are covered in the section on "Immediate Care."

Steps you can take for dealing with other health and medical concerns are provided in "Ailments and Disorders," the largest section of the book. To help you find a specific ailment among more than 145 entries arranged alphabetically, we have provided two indexes.

• If you know the name of the ailment, go to the A to Z index on page 138.

• If you're not sure of the ailment, go to page 140, where ailments are arranged by Problem Area and Special Concern. You can then turn to one or more entries for listings of symptoms and detailed explanations, which can help you identify your particular problem. (This information, however, is not intended as a substitute for the advice and expertise of a physician, and you may need to consult a physician to establish a definitive diagnosis.)

You can also consult the general index to look up an ailment, symptom, or remedy.

Entries in the "Ailments and Disorders" section all have the following format.

Symptoms. A listing of the clinical manifestations of the condition.

What Is It? An explanation of the nature of

the condition, what differentiates it from similar ailments, and whom it is most likely to affect.

What Causes It? Established or possible medical causes (such as infections) as well as lifestyle habits and other risk factors that can increase the chances of the condition occurring.

What If You Do Nothing? What to expect if you take no steps to intervene. Some conditions will worsen and/or may develop complications. But many minor health problems resolve on their own without treatment—though you can often speed up healing and alleviate discomfort with self-care measures.

Home Remedies. Self-treatment measures you can try, including over-the-counter medications and other remedies available without a prescription. This part also tells you if home remedies don't work or when they won't suffice. (For some conditions, the first step you should take is to seek medical attention.)

Prevention. Steps to avoid this particular problem (if that is possible) and steps to keep it from getting worse and/or from recurring.

When to Call Your Doctor. Warning signs indicating when you should be evaluated by a doctor—usually a primary-care physician, though for a number of conditions the evaluation should be performed by a specialist, such as a dermatologist.

What Your Doctor Will Do. How the condition will be diagnosed and the most likely modes of treatment.

For More Information. The names of recognized organizations and support groups you can contact for counseling and information about this ailment. Addresses, phone numbers, and Internet sites for these resources are listed in the appendix.

The book's fifth section, called "Your Health," offers an overview of growth and development at different stages of life, along with common health concerns. The information can help make you aware of potential health and developmental problems and how to prevent or manage them.

The final section, "The Drugstore Guide," offers advice on over-the-counter medications, which can play an important role in self-care. Our aim is to help you sort through the hundreds of products you are confronted with on drugstore shelves. As we note, such products must be approved for safety and efficacy by the Food and Drug Administration (FDA). That same rigor, unfortunately, is not applied to dietary and herbal supplements, which are manufactured, promoted, and sold with few restrictions on the claims made for them. Because many people have started using supplements, we offer some general cautionary guidelines along with evaluations of specific remedies.

Considering the overwhelming number of unverified health claims that are passed off as fact these days, we trust it will be a comfort to know you have an authoritative source you can turn to for reliable health information.

Wellness Strategies

for Optimal Health

The first and foremost goal of wellness is preventing illness—in particular, illness that can shorten your life or decrease the quality of life, especially as you get older. Today, in Western societies, the health problems that most significantly affect longevity are chronic diseases such as heart disease and cancer, which are linked in part to lifestyle and behavior patterns that can be modified. This section of the book explains those connections and presents the principal strategies that can reduce health risks and provide a number of other benefits as well.

WHAT IS WELLNESS?

The central tenet of wellness is that advances in medical diagnosis and treatment, while certainly beneficial, are not sufficient to protect and enhance your health. Rather, good health depends upon a wide spectrum of lifestyle habits that can help increase the quality of your life, enabling you to feel better physically and mentally. Equally important, these benefits can help you live longer.

Unlike most of the everyday ailments covered in this book, which initially can be treated at home, the health problems that people in Western societies fear most—chronic diseases that have a major impact on longevity and quality of life—require some form of medical intervention once they develop. But as a growing body of research shows, many such health problems can often be prevented—or the onset of them delayed—through lifestyle changes. Medical researchers still do not completely understand the causes of heart attack, stroke, cancer, or chronic obstructive pulmonary diseases (such as emphysema)—the current leading causes of death—but they have determined some of the principal risk factors that promote these illnesses. That understanding has made it clear that people can take steps to significantly lower their risk of becoming ill from these disorders.

This section provides information on those health measures that constitute the core of wellness—steps you can take that contribute most significantly to a healthy lifestyle. Along with offering details about the benefits of a particular health measure, the following pages will suggest ways of working these changes into your life, in steps that make wellness manageable.

THE BASIS FOR PREVENTION

Today, most Americans are aware that they are bombarded with health advice. Every week, it seems, on television or in the newspaper, a new recommendation is issued by one alleged authoritative source or another about a medication, a vitamin supplement, an exercise regimen, a food to avoid, or a food to be sure to eat—not to mention the fad weight loss diets that appear regularly on the best-seller list. Often this advice is based on new studies that have been released to the media, though sometimes it's based on "evidence" that is anecdotal. And at times the advice, like the results of the studies, can seem confusing, if not contradictory.

Sometimes this is because the reports oversimplify or misstate a study's findings. For example, "Exercise Can Cause Heart Attacks!" was the headline in some media reports a few years ago in the wake of two studies. But the headline was a distortion—the heart attacks occurred only in a few people, nearly all of whom rarely exerted themselves. The true danger for most Americans is lack of exercise.

Sometimes there are flaws in the study. Sometimes health reporters do not have time to read the studies in question, relying only on press releases. Or they may read them but not understand them. And sometimes, of course, the results of a well-executed study do contradict the findings of others—though the reason for the contradictory results may not always be clear.

None of this means that epidemiology—which looks at the distribution of diseases ("epidemics") and the risk factors for those diseases in a human population in an effort to find the determinants of the diseases—doesn't work. One study may not prove anything, but a body of research, in which information accumulates bit by bit, can produce scientifically sound evidence. In any case, changing your daily habits on the basis of a single study is almost never a good idea. Scientific findings should be duplicated by others for validity—and even then there is an element of uncertainty.

Research into human health has made enormous strides. There may be no such thing as a perfect study, but enough research has been done to identify some risk factors with sufficient power to suggest causality—such as smoking and its link to lung cancer. Drawing on hundreds of studies, researchers have compiled considerable evidence showing the extent to which diet, exercise, and the other factors covered in this section influence the risk of disease.

The recommendations on the following pages take into account these findings. The intent is not simply to be current but to provide information that is both practical and likely to remain valid over time. For example, scientists may continue to dispute the details of how plaque forms in coronary arteries, but there is little argument that a diet high in saturated fats contributes to plaque formation, and that you can very likely reduce your risk of heart disease by limiting fat and cholesterol in your diet.

Beyond that, it helps to know which types of food are highest in fat, and if all fatty foods are equally bad for you (they are not). The guidelines presented here, while subject to revision (like information in any field of science), are backed by the consensus of experts as well as by a large body of research showing their value and effectiveness.

KEYS TO LONGEVITY

Earlier in this century, the principal life-shortening diseases—infectious diseases such as typhoid, influenza, diphtheria, and tuberculosis—were aggravated by deficiencies in nutrition, sanitation, and transportation. In Western societies, public health measures as well as new technology (such as refrigeration) resulted in dramatic reductions in mortality from infectious disease. In these societies today, however, the leading fatal disorders are caused or exacerbated by excess. Numerous studies in recent years have shown a correlation between heart disease, cancer, hypertension, stroke, diabetes, and other chronic health problems and the excessive consumption of calories, fat, alcohol, and cholesterol, along with the practice of unhealthy habits, above all smoking (which remains the number-one cause of preventable death in America). And while physical hardship hampered the health of people at the turn of the century, today the problem is a lack of exercise. Complex environmental factors, many of them caused by population shifts, technological innovations, and industrial development, also contribute to disease.

Researchers estimate that three-quarters of all cancers occur mainly as a result of external influences—things people eat, drink, and smoke, as well as other elements in the environment and workplace—and not because of genetic factors. Tobacco use, for example, causes more cancer here and in the rest of the world than does anything else. (Smoking is also a factor in millions of deaths from heart disease.) If all tobacco users in the United States would suddenly quit, and no new customers were recruited, total deaths from cancer would eventually drop by at least a third. Lung cancer would become rare, rather than the major cancer killer of both American

15

men and women that it now is.

Diet causes about one-third of all cancer cases, almost as many as tobacco use, and has also been implicated in two of the three major risk factors in the development of heart disease—high blood cholesterol levels and high blood pressure, or hypertension. There is now a consensus among experts as to which dietary changes individuals must make to reduce their risks of chronic disease. A diet consisting predominantly of fruits and vegetables is the most important factor currently identified in the prevention of cancer (in addition to not smoking). The evidence for this is overwhelming: Study after study has confirmed that people who have the highest intakes of fruits and vegetables have the lowest rates of cancer.

Among other known preventable risk factors for disease, a lack of exercise is one of the most important. Sedentary people who begin a program of regular exercise reduce their risk of a heart attack by 35 to 55 percent. Being active also reduces the risk of stroke substantially, and direct evidence indicates that regular physical activity helps prevent the onset of diabetes. Several studies have suggested that exercise also helps prevent breast and prostate cancer, and there is good evidence that it can prevent colon cancer.

It is tempting, of course, to rely on medical advances, especially new medications, to prevent or postpone disease—for example, to combat a risk factor such as high cholesterol by taking a cholesterol-lowering drug. Certainly, keeping cholesterol in check with drugs is one way to diffuse the risk of coronary artery disease, or CAD, which accounts for over a third of all deaths in the United States—about 460,000 annually. The development and wider use of new, more effective drugs for lowering cholesterol has played an important role in the 28 percent decline in CAD mortality rates during the decade 1988 to 1998—

PREVENTING INJURIES

More than 37 million Americans suffer injuries annually that send them to hospital emergency rooms, and 92,000 die from their injuries—making accidents the fifth leading cause of death in the United States. Automobile accidents, which account for about 45 percent of all injury deaths, lead the toll of accidental deaths among Americans under age 65. Falls, more than half of which occur in the home, take second place overall, but are the leading cause of accidental death for those over 65.

Yet these and other types of accidental deaths are largely avoidable. Many automobile fatalities, for example, could be avoided if both adults and children would use proper safety restraints: according to one estimate, one-half of adult fatalities and 90 percent of the deaths of children under five could be prevented by the use of seat belts and child-restraint seats (see page 526). It is also possible to take precautions that will greatly lessen the likelihood of falls among older people (see page 564).

When accidents do occur, rapid responses can help save lives. A number of common injuries, many of which can occur inside the home, are covered in the section "Immediate Care." Knowing what steps to take will help you cope with these injuries before medical help arrives.

a continuation of a drop in average cholesterol levels (coinciding with a decline in the death rate from CAD) that began in 1960.

Sometimes drugs are necessary to modify a person's risk factors. But medications all have various side effects, and they are also expensive, costing consumers and insurance companies billions of dollars. Moreover, drugs may not be the only answer, or even the most important one. Stopping smoking is the first and most critical measure for preventing CAD, and the other controllable risk factors—which include high blood pressure, obesity, and being sedentary—can often be addressed with changes in diet and exercise habits. (See page 64 for a summary of the steps you can take to prevent a heart attack.)

While these measures are harder to implement than taking a pill, their benefits are greater since they lower the risk of all the major killers, including diabetes, cancer, and stroke, as well as heart disease. Even when medication is appropriate, these lifestyle measures remain necessary. Moreover, although medical technology might rescue you from a serious condition such as heart disease or cancer, your quality of life afterwards may be compromised. Often there is also an increased burden placed on family and friends, not to mention the health-care system.

In truth, the principal benefit of staying well may not be avoiding premature death, but enjoying a better quality of life. Many of the symptoms that we associate with aging, such as weight gain, decreased muscle tone and flexibility, diminished endurance, loss of bone mass, and a slowing of reflexes, are not the inevitable results of growing older; they are more often preventable symptoms of an unhealthy lifestyle. As the following pages make clear, practicing wellness doesn't have to involve radical changes at the out-

set. Indeed, a radical change can backfire, as when someone embarks enthusiastically on a vigorous exercise program, only to drop out after a few days or weeks because of injuries or boredom. Many of the guidelines throughout this section consist of straightforward steps that can make wellness manageable.

EATING A HEALTHY DIET

Many Americans are aware that making some changes in their diet would benefit their health, particularly with regard to lowering their risk of heart disease and cancer. Yet it isn't always clear to them which dietary guidelines are important or how to apply them on a day-to-day basis.

Actually, developing healthy eating habits isn't as confusing or as restrictive as many people believe. The first principle of a healthy diet is simply to eat a wide variety of foods. This is important because different foods provide different nutrients to your body.

Second, fruits, vegetables, grains, and legumes—foods high in complex carbohydrates, fiber, vitamins and minerals, low in fat, and free of cholesterol—should make up the bulk of the calories you consume. The rest should come from low- or nonfat dairy products, lean meats and poultry, and fish.

You should also try to maintain a balance

between calorie intake and calorie expenditure—that is, don't eat more food than your body can use. Otherwise, you will gain weight. Therefore, the more active you are, the more you can eat and still maintain this balance.

A good diet, along with regular exercise, is the pathway to sensible, lifelong weight control and good health. The principles of eating well are essentially the same for all, young and old—though some groups do have some special nutritional needs, as noted in the chart on pages 22-23. (Pregnant women and infants have particular nutritional requirements that are covered in the section "Your Health.")

TWELVE KEYS TO EATING RIGHT

A healthy diet doesn't have to mean eating foods that are bland or unappealing. You can view healthy eating as an opportunity to try different foods—and as long as your overall diet follows these basic guidelines, there is nothing wrong with an occasional rich treat.

1 *Eat a varied diet high in fruits, vegetable, and grains.* Your diet should also include low-fat or nonfat dairy products, nuts, and occasional small servings of meat, poultry, and fish. This is the so-called semivegetarian diet. (A completely vegetarian diet can also be very healthy.) Complex carbohydrates (grains, legumes, and potatoes and other starches) should contribute most of your total daily calories.

Eat five or more servings of vegetables and fruits, and six or more servings of grains or legumes, daily. Whole grains are especially nutritious. These foods will help you obtain the 20 to 30 grams of dietary fiber you need each day and will provide most of the important vitamins and minerals.

You can use the government's food pyramid

ELEMENTS OF A HEALTHY DIET

What do all healthy diets have in common? Plenty of fruits, whole grains, and vegetables, with modest amounts of meats and fish. In other words, a semi-vegetarian diet.

The pyramid recommended by the U. S. Department of Agriculture (USDA) is one example of this: Grains are the foundation of the diet, followed by fruits and vegetables. The daily recommendations also feature only small amounts of fish, poultry, and occasionally red meat, and thus contains little saturated fat and cholesterol.

Studies over the past two decades have shown that vegetarians and semi-vegetarians throughout the world have much lower rates of cancer, heart disease, and other chronic diseases than do those whose diets center around animal products. The rice-based diet in much of China is the most obvious example of this way of eating. So is the traditional Japanese diet, with its emphasis on rice or noodles accompanied by lots of vegetables, seafood, and a wide variety of soy products. (The Japanese have the lowest rate of heart disease in the industrialized world.) And the so-called "Mediterranean diet" consumed in parts of Italy, Greece, and France includes unsaturated fats such as olive oil or canola oil and wine served with meals (which can protect the heart if consumed in moderation).

All of these diets are healthier than the typical American diet, which contains far too much saturated fat and calories from meat, dairy products, and snack foods. Americans need to eat less fat and also different fats. Saturated fat

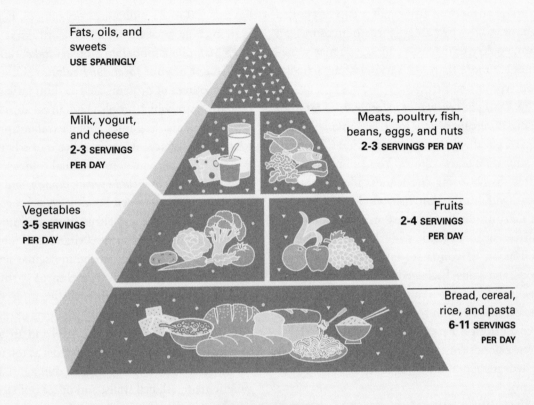

Fats, oils, and sweets
USE SPARINGLY

Milk, yogurt, and cheese
2-3 SERVINGS PER DAY

Meats, poultry, fish, beans, eggs, and nuts
2-3 SERVINGS PER DAY

Vegetables
3-5 SERVINGS PER DAY

Fruits
2-4 SERVINGS PER DAY

Bread, cereal, rice, and pasta
6-11 SERVINGS PER DAY

KEY TO SYMBOLS:

● Fat (naturally occurring and added)   ▼ Sugar (added)

These symbols show that fat and added sugars come mostly from fats, oils, and sweets, but can be part of or added to foods from the other food groups as well.

19

from animal products should be minimal; dairy products should be fat-free or low in fat.

Portion control is important as well. In the food pyramid, serving sizes are small. Examples of one serving are a cup of raw leafy vegetables; ½ cup of chopped, cooked, or canned fruits or vegetables; one medium carrot; one medium-size whole fruit; ¾ cup of juice; ½ cup of cooked beans; 3 ounces of meat, poultry, or fish. The number of servings you need daily from each group depends on your total calorie intake. If you are a woman eating, say, 1,600 calories per day, aim for at least five servings of fruits and/or vegetables. For a very active person consuming 2,800 calories per day, nine servings would be a better goal.

(on page 19) to create a diet weighted toward vegetarian foods. Servings are small: just one slice of bread or piece of fruit; half a cup of cooked rice, pasta, or vegetables; three ounces of lean meat, poultry, or fish. (Of course, you may sometimes eat more than one serving of a particular food type at one sitting.)

2 *Keep your intake of calories from fat at or below 30 percent of your total daily calories.* Some experts put the fat figure even lower—25 percent of your total daily calories. You can reduce your intake by choosing the leanest meats, poultry breast without the skin, fish, and low-fat or nonfat dairy products. Cut back on butter and margarine—or foods made with these products—as well as on mayonnaise, salad dressings, fried foods, and chips. Packaged foods (cookies, cakes, crackers, TV dinners) and fast foods (hamburgers, pizza) are often sources of hidden fats and excess calories. Fats supply more than twice as many calories (nine per gram) as protein or carbohydrates, including sugar (four calories per gram).

3 *Limit your intake of saturated fat to less than 10 percent of total calories.* Choose oils high in monounsaturated and polyunsaturated fats (canola, olive, corn, or peanut oil), but use even these in moderation. Saturated fats, which come chiefly from animal products like fatty meats, whole milk, butter, and cheese, stimulate cholesterol production in the body, as do trans fats, found in the hydrogenated fats in margarine and other processed foods. Keep your intake of saturated and hydrogenated fats to a minimum.

4 *Keep your cholesterol intake at 300 milligrams or less per day.* Cholesterol is found only in animal products, such as meats, poultry, dairy products, and egg yolks. One egg yolk contains about 210 milligrams of cholesterol, or most of your daily allowance. A three-ounce serving of meat, poultry, or fish contains about 60 milligrams (20 to 25 milligrams per ounce). Foods high in cholesterol are not necessarily high in fat.

5 *Maintain a moderate protein intake—about 12 percent of your total daily calories.* Choose nonfat sources of protein, such as skim milk and nonfat yogurt, which are also high in calcium and other nutrients. Legumes are an excellent plant source. The typical American diet is overly rich in protein, particularly from animal sources.

6 *Make sure to include green, orange, and yellow fruits and vegetables.* Foods such as broccoli, carrots, cantaloupe, and citrus fruits are high in antioxidant nutrients such as vitamins C and E and carotenoids. Acting at the molecular level, these antioxidants inactivate a class of particles known as free radicals, highly reactive molecules in the body that are natural by-products of many normal processes at the cellular level and are also created by such environmental factors as tobacco smoke and radiation. They can damage basic genetic material, cell walls, and other cell structures, and in the long run this damage can become irreparable, leading to disease. But antioxidants help mop up these free radicals before they do their dirty work.

A high intake of these substances may be protective against many kinds of cancer. Vitamin E may also lower the risk of heart disease. Vitamins C and E seem to play a protective role against cataracts. Antioxidants may even delay some effects of aging. Researchers are only beginning to understand their importance.

It is better to get antioxidants from foods rather than from supplements. However, some scientists believe that supplements of vitamin E are necessary to achieve a significant effect.

7 *Consume sugary foods only in moderation.*

The only harm that sugar does, in itself, is to contribute to tooth decay. However, sugary foods are often high in calories and little else. Many foods (like cakes, pies, and cookies) that are high in sugar are also high in fat.

8 *Limit your sodium intake to no more than 2,400 milligrams per day.* This is equivalent to the amount of sodium in a little more than a teaspoon of salt. Cut back on your use of salt in cooking and on the table; avoid salty foods, particularly canned soups, cheeses, and pickles. Check food labels for ingredients containing sodium. In some people (the 10 percent of the population that is salt-sensitive), sodium may contribute to high blood pressure. A high salt intake can also promote water retention.

9 *Consume enough calcium.* It builds strong bones and helps maintain bone density and strength through a lifetime. This is especially important for women, whose bone density dramatically declines at menopause.

10 *Get your vitamins and minerals chiefly from foods, not from supplements.* Supplements cannot substitute for a healthy diet, which supplies nutrients and other healthful compounds. Indeed, the cancer-protective elements in foods have only begun to be discovered, and these elements can't be found in pills. Foods also provide the synergy that many nutrients require to be efficiently used in the body—for example, vitamin C helps you utilize iron, and vitamin E helps you use vitamin K. Beta carotene is only one of several beneficial carotenoids in foods and not necessarily the most important one. Scientists believe that each of these compounds plays its own special role in the body and that many work together.

While supplements cannot compensate for poor eating habits, in the context of a healthy diet, certain vitamins and minerals, taken in recommended amounts, may be beneficial (see pages 22-23).

11 *Drink enough fluids.* The body, under average conditions, loses about two to three quarts of fluid daily through perspiration, exhaled moisture, and excretion. You must replace this fluid—hence the rule-of-thumb about consuming the equivalent of at least eight 8-ounce glasses of water daily. Some of the water you need comes from solid foods, especially fruits and vegetables. You get the balance from liquids you consume (juices, milk, soups), which are just as good as water.

12 *If you drink alcohol, do so in moderation.* Experts recommend that men not exceed more than two alcoholic drinks per day, and that women consume fewer than one drink per day. (A drink is defined as 12 ounces of beer, 4 ounces of wine, or 1.5 ounces of 80-proof liquor or spirits.) Excessive consumption of alcohol can lead to a variety of health problems, as explained on pages 115–116. And alcoholic beverages can add many calories to your diet (seven calories per gram) without supplying any vitamins or minerals.

SHOULD YOU TAKE SUPPLEMENTS?

Millions of Americans take vitamin and mineral supplements every day. If you eat a healthy diet, you probably don't need a daily supplement. Conversely, vitamin and mineral supplements cannot completely make up for an unhealthy diet. For example, they will not offset the effects of a high-fat diet or a diet low in fiber.

In certain cases, however, vitamin and mineral supplements can enhance a healthy diet. Even if you eat the right balance of foods, you may not obtain the high levels of certain nutrients (above adequate recommended levels) that many authorities now think you need. In addition, certain groups of people with special needs may benefit

SPECIAL NUTRITIONAL NEEDS: A SUMMARY

VITAMIN OR MINERAL/ FOOD SOURCES	WHAT IT DOES/ POTENTIAL BENEFITS	RECOMMENDED LEVELS
Vitamin A Liver, eggs, fortified milk, fish, and fruits and vegetables that contain beta carotene.	Promotes good vision; helps form and maintain healthy skin and mucous membranes. May protect against some cancers.	800 RE (4,000 IU), women; 1,000 RE (5,000 IU), men. No supplementation recommended, since toxic in high doses.
Beta carotene Carrots, sweet potatoes, cantaloupe, leafy greens, tomatoes, apricots, winter squash, red bell peppers, broccoli, mangoes.	Converted into vitamin A in the intestinal wall. As an antioxidant, it combats adverse effects of free radicals in the body. May reduce the risk of certain cancers as well as coronary artery disease (CAD).	5-6 milligrams (mg). No supplementation recommended. Don't take supplement if you smoke; studies suggest an increased risk of lung cancer in smokers taking beta carotene pills.
Vitamin C (ascorbic acid) Citrus fruits and juices, strawberries, peppers (especially red), broccoli, potatoes, kale, cauliflower, cantaloupe.	Promotes healthy gums and teeth; aids in iron absorption; maintains normal connective tissue; helps in healing of wounds. May reduce the risk of certain cancers, as well as CAD; may prevent or delay cataracts.	90 mg. For supplementation, 250-500 mg a day for anyone not consuming several fruits or vegetables rich in C daily, and for smokers. Larger doses may cause diarrhea.
Vitamin E Nuts, vegetable oils, margarine, wheat germ, leafy greens, seeds, almonds, olives, asparagus.	Helps in formation of red blood cells and utilization of vitamin K. As an antioxidant, it combats adverse effects of free radicals. May reduce the risk of certain cancers, as well as CAD; may prevent or delay cataracts; may improve immune function in the elderly.	8 mg, women; 10 mg, men (12-15 IU). For supplementation, 200-400 IU is recommended to obtain potential antioxidant benefits (see page 25). No serious side effects at these levels, though diarrhea and headaches have been reported.

22

VITAMIN OR MINERAL/ FOOD SOURCES	WHAT IT DOES/ POTENTIAL BENEFITS	RECOMMENDED LEVELS
Folacin A B vitamin, also known as folate or folic acid. Leafy greens, wheat germ, liver, beans, whole grains, broccoli, asparagus, citrus fruit, juices.	Important in normal growth and protein metabolism. Adequate intake reduces the risk of certain birth defects, notably spina bifida. Also appears to reduce the risk of colon and cervical cancer.	400 micrograms (mcg). Women who may become pregnant should obtain at least this amount from supplements and/or foods fortified with folic acid. Good natural food sources include: 1 cup spinach (110 mcg) 1 cup beans (160 to 350 mcg) 1 cup asparagus (180 mcg)
Calcium A quart of milk (nonfat preferred) provides 1,250 milligrams (mg) of calcium; 8 ounces of yogurt, 300 to 450 mg, hard cheeses 200 mg per ounce. Dark green leafy vegetables are very rich in calcium (serving of broccoli has 90 to 100 mg, beet greens 100 mg, kale 133 mg). Herring, salmon, or sardines—if eaten with the small bones.	Builds bone and teeth, maintains bone density and strength. Helps regulate heartbeat muscle contractions. May help prevent hypertension. Adequate intake can help prevent or minimize osteoporosis. Vitamin D (from fortified milk and sun exposure) and lactose (milk sugar) help improve calcium absorption.	1,300 milligrams (mg) daily for adolescents; 1,000 mg for adults to age 50; 1,200 to 1,500 mg daily for women over 50 and men over 65. For those who consume less than the recommended amount from food, supplementation can retard bone loss, especially in conjunction with weight-bearing exercise.
Iron Meat, poultry, fish, eggs, livers, kidneys, peas, beans, nuts, dried fruits, leafy green vegetables, enriched pasta and bread, fortified cereals. Cooking in iron pots adds iron, especially to acidic foods.	Essential to formation of hemoglobin (carries oxygen in the blood) and myoglobin (in muscle). Part of several enzymes and proteins in the body. Heme iron, found in animal products, more easily absorbed by the body than nonheme iron, which comes from plant products. To enhance absorption of nonheme iron, consume foods rich in vitamin C.	15 mg up to age 50 for women; 10 mg afterward. 10 mg for men. Menstruating women, endurance athletes, strict vegetarians, and dieters may be deficient. But consult your doctor before taking iron supplements. Large doses can damage liver, pancreas, and heart.

23

GETTING ENOUGH CALCIUM

If you decide to take calcium supplements (or your doctor recommends them), treat them as something you add to an already balanced diet. Your goal should be to consume at least 1,000 milligrams of calcium a day, or 1,200 to 1,500 milligrams if you are a woman over the age of 50 or a man over 65.

Rely on food, not just supplements. In fact, get as much calcium as you can from foods. Foods contain other important nutrients, some of which promote calcium absorption. The best plan seems to be to get at least 750 milligrams from your diet, then bring your total intake to 1,500 milligrams by taking a 750-milligram supplement.

Examples of good food sources: An 8-ounce serving of plain yogurt has 300 to 400 milligrams of calcium; one-half cup of part-skim ricotta cheese, 337; a cup of milk 300 milligrams (stick to low-fat or nonfat dairy products). A 3-ounce serving of sardines with bones contains 370 milligrams; a cup of kale, 95; and a cup of broccoli, 70.

If you are taking thyroid hormones, corticosteroids, iron pills, or the antibiotic tetracycline, talk with your doctor or pharmacist about calcium supplements, since calcium can interact with these and other drugs.

Take calcium supplements with food. Stomach acid enhances absorption of most calcium supplements, as does the presence of other nutrients (such as vitamin D). Some older people are deficient in stomach acid, but they can take calcium citrate, which doesn't need stomach acid to be absorbed. (It's also good for people with disorders that make them produce less stomach acid—and it's the form of supplement least likely to cause constipation.)

Some kinds of fiber affect absorption—for example, wheat bran may reduce it somewhat—so if you eat bran for breakfast, take your supplement at lunch.

Don't take too much. Don't take more than 500 milligrams at a time. If you're taking 1,000 milligrams a day, divide it into two doses.

Up to 2,500 milligrams daily is considered safe. More and more foods are fortified with calcium today. If you consume those foods, as well as drink milk and take calcium pills, you may be getting too much calcium.

Which form of calcium is best? It makes little or no difference. But be sure to read the labels: check the milligrams of "elemental calcium" you're getting per pill, not the amount of calcium gluconate or calcium citrate or whatever it is. Calcium has to be combined with something else: carbonate, citrate, lactate, phosphate, or gluconate. No pill is pure calcium. All these forms will dissolve reliably if they meet USP standards. (Buy a supplement labeled "USP;" this means that the product meets the U.S. Pharmacopeia's standard for dissolving and for dosage.)

Plain calcium carbonate, as found in antacids, contains the most calcium per pill (40 percent) at the lowest price. If you buy calcium citrate (21 percent calcium per pill) or any of the other forms, you'll have to take more pills, sometimes many more, to get the same amount of calcium. Not only do you need more, they also cost more per pill.

Chewable pills are probably best absorbed. The dissolving process starts in your mouth. Fortified orange juice is also well absorbed.

from taking supplements. These include pregnant women, frequent aspirin takers (such as arthritis sufferers), heavy drinkers (excessive alcohol consumption often depletes B vitamins and vitamin C), and smokers (who appear to use up vitamin C at a faster rate than nonsmokers). If you fall into one of these groups, you should talk to your doctor about supplements (although smokers and heavy drinkers would be better served by quitting their habits).

People over 60 may also be candidates for a basic, inexpensive multivitamin supplement. Many older people develop poor eating habits as a result of problems with chewing or swallowing or because of a loss of interest in food (your senses of taste and smell decline with age). In addition, aging itself makes it more difficult to absorb and use certain nutrients.

Here are some recommendations concerning supplements.

Consider two antioxidant supplements—250 to 500 milligrams of vitamin C daily and 200 to 400 international units (IU) of vitamin E. A large body of basic laboratory research has shown that, as antioxidants, these vitamins help inactivate free radicals—unstable molecules that can damage cells and thereby theoretically lead to chronic diseases. There have been many studies on C and E, and scientists are only beginning to understand how these and other antioxidants work. The evidence is accumulating bit by bit.

That said, some, though not all, members of the Editorial Board of the *UC Berkeley Wellness Letter* have concluded—based on the evidence currently available—that supplemental C and E pose little risk at the levels recommended here, and have substantial potential benefits, including protection against heart disease, certain types of cancer, cataracts, and perhaps other disorders.

If you eat lots of citrus fruits and vegetables and their juices, you may be getting that much vitamin C (a cup of orange juice contains about 100 milligrams), and then you may not need supplemental C. If you do take a supplement, don't pay extra for "natural" forms of vitamin C; natural and synthetic forms are equivalent.

It's difficult, however, to get the recommended amount of vitamin E from food—and most foods that are good sources of vitamin E are high in fat. Vitamin E supplements come in synthetic and natural forms, and any form is worth taking. Most studies showing potential health benefits have used the synthetic form, which is the cheapest and most widely available. However, if you have a choice, buy the natural form of vitamin E, preferably a brand that includes "mixed tocopherols" on the ingredients list.

You may need to supplement your calcium intake. Most nutritionists recommend that, first and foremost, calcium should come from food sources. But many women, especially older women who tend not to eat dairy products, don't get enough calcium. This applies to older men as well. In that case, taking a supplement is better than ignoring calcium altogether; research has clearly demonstrated that supplements can help reduce bone loss, even in older women. (See page 24 for more information on supplements.)

Premenopausal women should be sure to get enough folacin. According to the U.S. Public Health Service, all women capable of becoming pregnant should consume 400 micrograms of folacin daily. Folacin (also called folate or, when used in a supplement or to fortify foods, folic acid) helps protect against spina bifida and other birth defects (see page 541). It may also help protect against cervical cancer, particularly in women at high risk for the disease, as well as colorectal and

25

CHOOSING A MULTIVITAMIN

Multivitamin supplements (multis) generally contain the 13 essential vitamins in amounts that satisfy most minimum daily requirements, along with some key minerals. When shopping for a multivitamin, look for the following:

• Most store-brand and generic products are fine.

• Look for "USP" on the label. This means that the product meets the standards of the U.S. Pharmacopeia, including one for disintegration, and has been tested under controlled laboratory conditions. Generic or store brands are more often labeled USP than brand-name multis, and are cheaper anyway.

• Most important: Look for 100 percent of the Daily Value of the following vitamins: A (some from beta carotene), B1 (thiamin), B2 (riboflavin), B3 (niacin), B6, B12, folic acid, and D.

• Look for up to 100 percent of the Daily Value of the following minerals: copper, zinc, magnesium, iron, iodine, selenium (not more than 200 mcg), and chromium (not more than 200 mcg). Most multis also contain tiny amounts of trace minerals such as boron, manganese, and molybdenum.

• Least important: Most multi products contain some potassium, phosphorus, pantothenic acid, and biotin, but you can ignore these since they are easily found in food.

• Most multis contain 100 percent, or even 200 percent, of the Daily Value of vitamins C and E, but this is not enough to provide the full antioxidant effects and other potential benefits of these vitamins.

We recommend that everyone consume 250 to 500 milligrams of C and 200 to 400 IU of E a day. You'll definitely need a pill to get that much vitamin E.

• Calcium is bulky, so a multi will contain only a small amount of it. Unless you consume enough dairy products, broccoli, and salmon or sardines (with bones), you should take separate calcium supplements (see page 23).

• Premenopausal women should look for 100 percent of the Daily Value of iron. In contrast, people with the genetic disorder hemochromatosis (who absorb too much iron) should avoid supplemental iron.

• More than 100 percent of the Daily Value isn't necessarily better. Up to 200 percent of the B vitamins is okay, but large doses of copper, for instance, can interfere with the absorption of zinc, and vice versa. And large doses of vitamin A or D can be dangerous.

• Take your multi with food. If it contains iron, don't take a calcium supplement at the same time, since iron in the multi interferes with calcium absorption.

• Words you don't need to see listed on the bottle: "stress formula," "sugar-free," "starch-free," "natural," "super-potency," "senior formula," "slow-release," enzymes, hormones, amino acids, PABA, or ginseng and other herbs. These serve no purpose and add to the price.

But keep in mind: Even if you take a multivitamin, you still need to have a balanced, healthy diet. These supplements are not magic bullets. Foods—particularly fruits, vegetables, and whole grains—provide fiber as well as countless beneficial phytochemicals not found in any pill.

lung cancer, among others. In addition, it helps protect against heart disease, as do other B vitamins such as B_6 and B_{12}.

If your diet is rich in leafy greens, beans, and whole grains, and particularly if you eat fortified breakfast cereals, you may already be getting enough folacin. Breads, pasta, grits, cornmeal, and white rice are also fortified, and the folic acid used in fortified foods, as well as in supplements, is much better absorbed than the folacin found naturally in food. But if you can possibly become pregnant, and yet can't be sure that you're obtaining at least 400 micrograms daily from fortified foods, you should take a multivitamin containing at least 400 micrograms of folic acid or a simple 400-microgram folic acid pill.

For many people, and especially those over the age of 60, a basic multivitamin-mineral supplement makes sense. Surveys consistently show that large groups of Americans tend to fall short in a variety of key vitamins and minerals. Many, if most, people over 60 don't get the nutrients they need, for a variety of reasons. For instance, aging itself may make it more difficult to absorb and utilize certain nutrients. The major problem nutrients for older people are vitamins C, D, B_6, B_{12}, and folacin, as well as minerals such as zinc, magnesium, and calcium. All of these can be problem nutrients for older people.

Other people who can benefit from a multivitamin include *premenopausal women* (many of whom don't consume enough iron); *vegans* (who consume no animal products and so may not get enough B_{12}); *people on low-calorie diets, as well as heavy drinkers* (who are likely to have a shortfall of vitamins and minerals); *poor people* (who tend to have the poorest diets); and *anyone else not eating a balanced diet* (who may not be getting enough folacin, B_6, and B_{12}). *Pregnant women* should probably take a multivitamin, but should discuss this with their doctors. (See page 26 for advice on choosing a multivitamin.)

Avoid megadoses. Taking huge doses of most vitamins and minerals isn't wise. Certain vitamins—A and D—are toxic in large doses. Others, like niacin, produce serious side effects in large doses. Excess amounts of water-soluble vitamins (the B vitamins and C) will simply be eliminated by the body.

In planning your diet and in taking supplements, stick with the amounts recommended in the chart on pages 22-23.

STAYING ACTIVE

The benefits of exercise have become increasingly clear: It can improve your cardiovascular fitness and muscular endurance, which translates into an increase in energy; it can dramatically reduce the risk of coronary artery disease; it may also help lower high blood pressure and elevated cholesterol levels, and aid in weight control; it can help delay or prevent the onset of osteoporosis; and it appears to give self-esteem a measurable boost, and in general to improve your sense of well-being.

A lack of exercise, by contrast, is now recognized as a health risk by the American Heart Association, which cited sedentary behavior as one of the important risk factors for cardiovascular disease. And too many Americans have put themselves at risk. As many as 12 percent of all deaths—250,000 per year—in the United States

BEFORE YOU BEGIN

If you are a healthy but sedentary woman over the age of 50 or a man over 40, the American College of Sports Medicine recommends that you consult your physician before beginning an exercise program and have a preexercise medical and physical examination. Your physician may recommend that you take a special exercise stress test.

If you are 35 or older, consult with a physician first if you have any risk factors for heart disease (such as recurrent chest pain, high blood pressure or cholesterol levels, smoking, or obesity). Also, whatever your age, contact your physician if you have cardiovascular or lung disease (or symptoms that might suggest these problems).

may be attributed indirectly to lack of regular physical activity, according to the Centers for Disease Control and Prevention (CDC). Only about 22 percent of adults engage regularly (five times a week for at least 30 minutes) in sustained physical activity of any intensity.

You can derive the benefits of exercise—and of being fit—at any age. Indeed, exercise, or at least staying physically active, appears to be increasingly important the older people get. Many of the problems commonly associated with aging—increased body fat, decreased muscular strength and flexibility, loss of bone mass, lower metabolism, and slower reaction times—are often signs of inactivity that can be minimized or even prevented by exercise.

WHAT IS FITNESS?

During the past two decades, exercising to stay fit has come to be associated with running, cycling, and other aerobic activities, which have been given the most emphasis because they enhance cardiorespiratory endurance—the aspect of fitness that provides the most impressive health benefits. Aerobic exercise will continue to be the cornerstone of fitness programs. Yet many people in long-term aerobic programs may lose muscle mass and flexibility, particularly in their upper bodies.

Physical fitness, as experts in the field have long stressed, actually has the following components.

Cardiorespiratory endurance is reflected in the sustained ability of the heart and blood vessels to carry oxygen to your body's cells.

Muscular fitness consists of both strength and endurance. Muscular strength is the force a muscle produces in one effort—a lift, a jump, a heave—as when you swing a mallet to ring a carnival bell. Muscular endurance refers to the ability to perform repeated muscular contractions in quick succession, as in doing 20 push-ups or sit-ups in a minute. Although muscular endurance requires strength, it is not a single all-out effort.

Flexibility refers to the ability of your joints to move freely and without discomfort through their full range of motion. This varies from person to person and from joint to joint. Good flexibility is thought to protect the muscles against pulls and tears, since short tight muscles may be more likely to be overstretched.

Body composition generally refers to how much of your weight is lean mass (muscle and bone) and how much is fat.

A well-rounded program. Each of these components can be measurably improved with appropriate types of exercise. The American College of Sports Medicine, in its exercise guidelines for healthy adults, recommends a well-rounded program that includes strength training along with aerobics. The emphasis isn't on lifting heavy weights but on resistance training of moderate intensity at least twice a week, in workouts that can take as little as 15 minutes per session. For a sedentary person, strength training and aerobic exercise together will help improve body composition by increasing muscle mass and reducing fat tissue.

While flexibility is not as important to health as cardiorespiratory endurance or muscular fitness, a regular program of stretching can help prevent injuries to muscles, tendons, and ligaments (the connective tissue that binds muscles together or muscles to joints). For sedentary people, stretching also simply provides relief from muscle tension and stiffness.

Variety is a key. Exercise and fitness were once synonymous with exhaustive workouts, running marathons, or "going for the burn." But no longer. Being active is the key to becoming and staying fit, and you can achieve this through a variety of pursuits. Jogging and aerobics classes, once the premier exercise activities, continue to attract participants. But as the nation and its fitness habits mature, people have been shifting to all manner of activities, from fitness walking to ballroom dancing. Two classic low-impact activities, swimming and cycling, continue to gain in popularity. At the same time, others have chosen newer types of sports and recreations, from mountain biking to in-line skating to spinning classes.

No single exercise adequately builds all aspects of fitness equally well, and having more than one activity to turn to keeps exercise from getting monotonous. Studies also show that people tend to continue with activities that are accessible and enjoyable.

HOW MUCH EXERCISE IS ENOUGH?

Numerous studies have shown that exercise helps lower the risk of many major diseases as well as premature death. And studies also suggest that any improvement in physical fitness is beneficial—that it isn't necessary to become an athlete to improve your odds of staying healthy longer.

For years the primary exercise goal of the American College of Sports Medicine (ACSM) has been fairly strenuous: at least 20 minutes of vigorous aerobic exercise (such as running or cycling) at least three times a week in order to strengthen the cardiovascular system. ACSM is the most influential group in this field, and it helps shape the government's official advice. But it's estimated that only 16 percent of Americans meet this strenuous goal, so ACSM modified it in 1998. The goal post was lowered to help get people moving. And several other goals, regarding strength training and stretching, were added.

Here are the latest guidelines from ACSM:

Lower-intensity exercise is good for you. It can lower the risk of heart disease, hypertension, osteoporosis, diabetes, colon cancer, and obesity. The benefits of moderate activity were shown in two studies published in the *Journal of the American Medical Association.* Inactive people can become fitter and healthier by starting with such low-level activity—and they're more likely to stick to it and then eventually increase the intensity. Three out of four Americans are totally or mostly sedentary, and for them the greatest health boost comes simply from getting up and becoming active.

Start by adding a few minutes of increased

29

activity to your day, and work up to 30 minutes most, preferably all, days of the week (for a sample week, see the chart below). All you have to do are the normal things, like walking and taking the stairs, but just more often, a little longer, and/or a little faster.

Short bouts of activity count. During a day, brief exercise sessions have an additive benefit. That

A WEEKLY SCHEDULE

Another way to look at your weekly activity level is by the amount of calories you burn each week in physical exertion—including both conventional exercise and everyday physical activities, such as gardening or housecleaning. The goal should be at least 1,000 calories a week burned in these activities. These findings come largely from several well-known studies of Harvard alumni.

If you are trying to boost your activity level so that you burn about 1,500 calories a week, what would you have to do? The following list is a sample, with caloric expenditure calculated for a body weight of 150 pounds. It's not a tough schedule, and it would put you fairly high on the fitness ladder. Spreading the exercise over fewer days would be okay; so would doing different things.

ACTIVITY	CALORIES
Monday	
Walking to and from work, 30 minutes total	140
Stair climbing, 5 minutes	35
Tuesday	
Weight training, 20 minutes	135
Cycling, stationary, 20 minutes (10 mph)	195
Wednesday	
Walking to and from work, 30 minutes total	140
Thursday	
Housecleaning, 30 minutes	120
Friday	
Swimming or basketball, 20 minutes	180
Saturday	
Stair climbing, 10 minutes	70
Weight training, 20 minutes	135
Running, treadmill, 10 minutes	95
Washing car, 20 minutes	65
Sunday	
Walking, 15 minutes	70
Gardening, 20 minutes	110
Grand total (about 4 hours)	1,490

is, three 10-minute periods of exertion can be almost as beneficial as one 30-minute session.

So does more intense exercise. For additional cardiovascular benefits and to boost HDL ("good") cholesterol significantly, however, more intense workouts (such as brisk walking, cycling, or running) lasting at least 20 minutes at least three times a week are necessary. Cardiovascular benefits increase with the length and intensity of your workouts. The optimal intensity will depend on your age and physical condition.

Strength training is recommended for everyone. Two or three sessions per week should be the minimum. Start with light weights or low settings on weight machines. One set of 8 to 15 repetitions of each exercise can improve muscle strength and endurance nearly as much as the traditional three sets, at least for beginners.

Add stretching. A stretching routine to build flexibility should be done for 10 to 20 minutes at least two or three times a week.

The bottom line is simple: some exercise is good, and more is better than some.

FOR YOUR HEART: AEROBIC EXERCISE

Aerobic exercise utilizes oxygen for energy production for long periods, thereby working your heart and lungs to promote cardiovascular fitness. The best aerobic exercises are brisk walking, distance running, swimming, cycling, aerobic movement, cross-country skiing, rowing, and jumping rope. In addition to helping build cardiorespiratory endurance, these activities help make muscles stronger and more limber. Most of these are outdoor activities, but if exercising outdoors is not convenient, fitness machines can allow you to perform most outdoor activities indoors. You can also take up these activities at

any age and continue them for a lifetime.

Based on guidelines from the ACSM, here are recommendations concerning three key factors—frequency, duration, and intensity—in aerobic exercise.

How often, how long. If you are below average in cardiovascular fitness, you should aim at three exercise sessions per week, for 20 to 30 minutes per session, preferably on alternate days. After six to eight weeks, if you wish to continue improving your cardiovascular fitness, you can increase the frequency and duration of your sessions. This is also necessary if you want to lose body fat. The optimal schedule is four weekly sessions of 40 minutes each (not including the warm-up and cool-down). Exercising more than this will not improve your fitness significantly, and it can increase your risk of injury if you are exercising at a high intensity.

How hard. To achieve an aerobic training effect, the ACSM suggests that you exercise at a level of intensity called your target heart rate. The easiest way to calculate this rate is to subtract your age from 220—a person's theoretical maximum heart rate—then take 60 percent and 80 percent of that number (multiply the number by 0.6 and by 0.8). The results are the upper and lower end of your target heart-rate zone.

While you exercise, your heart rate per minute should fall somewhere between these two numbers: for example, a 40-year-old has a target heart rate of 108 to 144 beats per minute. (If you take medication for your heart or blood pressure, your target heart rate may be lower than determined by this calculation.) Exercising in the low to middle range of the target heart rate zone is best for most people, especially those who are not in peak condition.

Once you learn how it feels to work out at your

31

NINE EXERCISE GUIDELINES

People who have been relatively inactive often take up exercise enthusiastically—so much so that it's easy for them to be carried away by the joy of the moment and to forget, or skip, certain measures that can reduce the risk of injury. Even veteran exercisers may neglect certain basic precautions that can help minimize aches and pains. The following guidelines and tips can protect you from injury and will make exercise itself more enjoyable.

1 **Set realistic exercise goals.** Set goals that you know you can achieve and that are specific, not vague. ("I'll cycle 20 miles this week," not "I really should get more exercise this week.")

2 **Whatever activity you pursue, don't overdo it.** Studies show that the most common cause of injury is exercising too aggressively— the "too much, too soon" syndrome. Even if you consider yourself in good shape, start any new exercise at a relatively low intensity and gradually increase your level of exertion over a number of weeks. In an exercise class, don't feel compelled to do any set number of repetitions or to lift a predetermined amount of weight. You don't have to keep up with an instructor or other exercisers. If a class includes an exercise that is too difficult for you, substitute something easier.

3 **"No pain, no gain" is a myth.** Exercise should require some effort, but discomfort isn't necessary. If you are in an exercise class, beware of any instructor who says that exercise must hurt (or "burn") to do any good. Indeed, pain is a warning sign you are foolish to ignore. If you have continuing pain during an exercise, stop and don't do it again unless you can do so painlessly. (If the pain occurs in the chest or neck area, you should see a doctor immediately.)

General muscle soreness that comes after exercise is another matter: it usually indicates that you are not warming up sufficiently or that you are working too long or too hard. Sore muscles need not make you stop exercising, but they should make you slow down.

4 **Use adequate footwear.** Wearing improper or worn-out shoes places added stress on your hips, knees, ankles, and feet— the sites of up to 90 percent of all sports injuries. Select shoes suitable for your activity and replace them before they appear worn out; with frequent use, athletic shoes can lose one-third or more of their shock-absorbing ability in a matter of months. Loss of cushioning in the shock-absorbent midsole occurs long before the outer sole or upper shoe shows wear.

5 **Control your movements—if you can't, slow down.** Rapid, jerky movement can set the stage for injury. Flailing your arms or legs can overstress joints. Instead, as you move your limbs, keep the muscles contracted and move them as if you are pushing against some resistance—for instance, squeezing a beach ball or pushing a weight.

6 **Watch your form and posture.** In most activities, stress can result from poor form, whether it's landing on the balls of your feet (instead of your heels) when running, or constantly cycling in the highest gears. Keep your back aligned (abdominal muscles contracted, buttocks tucked in, and knees aligned over feet). This is particularly important when jumping or reaching overhead.

7 **Don't bounce while stretching.** Ballistic stretching, in which you stretch to your limit

and perform quick, pulsing movements, actually shortens muscles and increases the chance of muscle tears and soreness. Instead, do static stretches, which call for gradually stretching through a muscle's full range of movement until you feel resistance. This gradually loosens muscles without straining them.

8 Warm up and cool down. Slowly jog for five minutes before your workout to gradually increase your heart rate and core temperature. Cool down after exercising with five minutes of slower movement. This prevents an abrupt drop in blood pressure and helps alleviate potential muscle stiffness.

9 Replace fluids lost through sweating. This is particularly important in hot weather, when you can easily lose more than a quart of water in an hour. Neglecting to compensate for fluid loss can cause lethargy and nausea, interfering with your performance. Even if you don't feel thirsty, it's important to drink at regular intervals when exercising. (Thirst is satisfied long before you have replenished lost fluids.)

• In hot weather, drink at least 16 to 20 ounces of fluid two hours before exercising and another 8 ounces 15 to 30 minutes before beginning. While you exercise, drink 4 to 8 ounces every 10 to 20 minutes.

• After exercising, drink enough fluid to replace the fluid you've sweated off. In hot weather, weigh yourself before and after working out; drink one pint for each pound lost, and eat normally.

• While heat buildup may be slower when you exercise in cold weather or in water, you still lose fluid from sweating. Therefore, it's important to replace fluids just as regularly when you swim or work out in the cold as you do in the heat.

target heart rate, you may be able to estimate your heart rate just by focusing on how you feel—for instance, you notice how hard you are breathing, how much you are sweating, and how your heart is pumping. Experts call this the "rate of perceived exertion." At the same time, don't focus too much on your heart rate. All this really means is that exercise is good for your heart and overall health.

If one of the factors in your exercise program is low, compensate by increasing the others. For example, if you exercise only for short periods, increase the frequency of the activity—five times a week instead of three. Or increase the intensity of the exercise (but only do this gradually).

CONTROLLING YOUR WEIGHT

For most people, *overweight* and *obese* are not scientific terms, but loaded words that trigger anxiety and frustration. In our culture, weight gain is often noticed and generally perceived as an important change—in an adult, usually for the worse. Yet, although these two terms are often used interchangeably, they do not mean the same thing. Obesity is a medical term for the storage of excess fat in the body—but no single measure of excess fat is generally accepted in determining obesity. It is often defined as being 20 percent heavier than your "healthy weight"— but according to what standard? A 250-pound football player may be overweight according to government weight tables, but may actually have a below-average amount of body fat. Conversely, a person in a normal weight range who is out of shape could have small muscle mass and from the perspective of body fat be classified as obese.

The line between desirable weight and overweight, and between overweight and obese, is not clear-cut, even for experts. Both *overweight* and *obesity* must be measured against some arbitrary standard, and the definition must take into account the amount of muscle mass a person has and where the fat is distributed on the body (excess abdominal fat is more of a health risk than fat on the hips).

By virtually any standard a great many of us have been getting fatter—not only in the United States, but around the world. A report published in 1999 in the *Journal of the American Medical Association (JAMA),* which analyzed data from a national survey conducted by the Centers for Disease Control and Prevention (CDC), found that the prevalence of obesity among Americans rose by nearly a third—from 12 percent to nearly 18 percent—between 1991 and 1998. For this survey, obesity was defined as a body mass index, or BMI, of 30 or higher. Obesity increased in every state, in both sexes, and across all age groups, races, and educational levels. Another report, based on the Third National Health and Nutrition Examination Survey (known as HANES III), used a lower cutoff point for overweight—a BMI of 25 or higher—and concluded that more than half of adults in the United States are overweight or obese.

HEALTH RISKS

Doctors have observed for many years that overweight and obesity are associated with disease.

Studies also show that the risk for disease rises with increasing weight.

Coronary artery disease (CAD). Obesity is associated with an increased risk for developing, and dying from, CAD because it may raise LDL (low-density lipoprotein, or "bad") cholesterol and lower HDL (high-density lipoprotein, or "good") cholesterol. Hypertension and diabetes, also associated with obesity, are contributing factors to heart disease mortality.

Hypertension. On average, overweight adults have a risk of hypertension three times greater than for normal-weight people.

Diabetes. Type 2 (non-insulin-dependent) diabetes can be delayed or averted by weight control. Diabetes is three times more common in people who are overweight.

Cancer. Studies have shown that certain cancers (of the colon and prostate in men, of the breast in postmenopausal women, and of the uterus in all women) are more prevalent in the obese than in the nonobese. One large, long-term study conducted by the American Cancer Society revealed that women who were 40 percent heavier than average had a 55 percent higher overall cancer risk than normal-weight women; for obese men, the cancer risk was about one-third higher than for normal-weight men.

CAUSES OF WEIGHT GAIN

Why do some people get fat and others don't? The possibility of a genetic determinant was raised in press reports when researchers at Rockefeller University announced several years ago that they had mapped and cloned an obesity gene in mice. The ob gene, as it is called, apparently produces a hormone that is secreted by fat cells and controls body weight. The researchers quickly cautioned that more investigation was needed, and that a fat gene in mice doesn't necessarily mean that human beings are similarly encoded.

Certainly behavioral factors—overeating and being sedentary—are at work in causing people to be overweight. But other factors are involved as well. These include race, gender, and economic status as well as genetics. African-American men between the ages of 35 and 55 are more likely to be overweight than white men in the same age group, and African-American women 35 to 55 are almost twice as likely to be overweight as their white counterparts. For reasons not well understood, those who live below the poverty line, particularly women, are more likely to be overweight than people at the top of the economic heap.

The tendency to be overweight also appears to run in families—though no one is certain to what extent this is a matter of eating habits or heredity. But a study some years ago in the *New England Journal of Medicine* by Dr. Albert Stunkard and his colleagues concluded, "Genetic influences have an important role in determining human fatness in adults, whereas the family environment alone has no important effect."

Dr. Stunkard studied 540 middle-aged adults who had been adopted as children. Their body mass index (see below), which many experts consider the best method to define overweight, bore little relation to their adoptive parents' index; instead, the daughters tended strongly to follow the pattern of their biological parents, particularly of their mothers, although the sons showed

CALCULATING BODY MASS INDEX

The body mass index, or BMI, is another method of evaluating body weight according to height—one that many experts think provides reasonable guidelines for defining overweight. But the measurement isn't simply a ratio of your weight to height. You must divide your weight by your height *squared*—and this has to be done in kilograms and meters.

Here's a short formula: multiply your weight (in pounds) by 705; divide the result by your height (in inches); then divide *again* by your height. That will give you your BMI.

A "healthy" BMI range is between 19 and 25. That corresponds to the numbers on the U.S. government's weight table. Between 25 and 29 is considered moderately overweight, and above 29, seriously overweight (or obese). For a man or woman five feet six inches tall,

that works out to a healthy range of 118 to 155 pounds, with severe overweight starting at 179. The Canadian guidelines for healthy weight mark the upper cutoff at a BMI of 27, the point at which there's a high risk of serious health problems.

Bear in mind that the BMIs, weight tables, and other indices only serve as an approximate guide to what you should weigh. Many factors must be considered. BMIs don't make allowance for your bone structure and gender; consequently, you should. Because women tend to have less muscle and bone than men and are generally shorter, they should probably be at the lower end of the "healthy" BMI ranges, while large-boned, muscular men will probably fall at the higher end of the ranges.

no such relationship to either set of parents. This again emphasizes the complex relationship of genetics and environment to obesity.

Heredity is not destiny. A genetic tendency toward being overweight does not doom a person to be fat—any more than a familial tendency in the other direction guarantees thinness. Studies have shown that rats bred for thinness can still get fat on a diet of snack foods; animals genetically prone to be fat will get fatter on the same diet. But both groups lose weight if returned to a normal maintenance diet. Furthermore, even fat-prone rats can be saved from obesity if their physical activity is increased.

If you know that being overweight runs in your family, you can use the knowledge preventively. Because Americans, as a whole, live relatively sedentary lives and have plenty of food available to them, those looking to lose weight must make an effort to keep active and to eat a low-fat, high-carbohydrate diet that is moderate in calories.

WHAT IS A HEALTHY WEIGHT?

Clearly, medical science has more work to do on this whole vexing and confusing subject. Even the most famous weight table, which is based on the actuarial tables of the Metropolitan Life Insurance Company, may be misleading. Actuarial tables do show who lives the longest—no argument there—but only among people who buy life insurance. In this country only a select group can afford to carry life insurance and thereby show up on the actuarial tables in the first place.

The question "What is a healthy weight?" has no easy answer. Being obese is undeniably laden with risk. On the other hand, a study published in the *International Journal of Obesity* analyzed 19 other studies of mortality and body weight

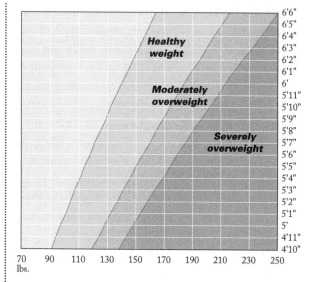

and concluded that being moderately overweight was not associated with increased mortality from all causes. It appears likely, then, that the health risks of carrying a few extra pounds may have been exaggerated. But where does *overweight* end and *obesity* begin?

Weight tables and other indices can only serve as an approximate guide to what you should weigh. The chart above, from the U. S. government, maps out the general weight ranges, plus two categories of overweight. If you take the government's guidelines seriously, the permitted ranges may seem extremely wide. You do have to make some allowance for your bone structure and gender: though this single chart covers all people, women tend to have less muscle and bone than men and are generally shorter, so they should stick to the lower end of the ranges, while large-boned men will need to aim at the higher end.

Waist size and body shape. Another indicator of weight-related health problems is waist size. A Dutch study published in 1998 found that this simple measurement may be as effective as more complex measures of obesity such as the body mass index. The study found that for women, a waist measurement of 34.5 inches signals a serious risk. For men, the cut-off point is 40 inches. People with apple-shaped figures (fattest in the abdominal area) have lower HDL ("good") cholesterol and higher LDL ("bad") cholesterol than their thinner counterparts. They are at increased risk for heart disease, as well as stroke, hypertension, and diabetes.

SUCCESSFUL WEIGHT CONTROL

Many people who lose weight regain it later. About 40 percent of men and 25 percent of women are on a diet at any given moment, and it's estimated that within a few years 90 percent of them will regain most or all of the weight they lose. Studies indicate that this scenario of repeatedly losing weight and then regaining it—sometimes referred to as yo-yo dieting—is not necessarily fraught with health hazards, as was once thought. In fact, given the serious proven risks of obesity, *it is better to have repeatedly lost and regained weight than never to have lost any weight at all.* But maintaining a stable, healthy weight is obviously preferable.

Even modest weight loss is beneficial. If you are obese or seriously overweight, don't let worries about yo-yo dieting or fears that you won't be able to shed enough pounds deter you from trying to lose weight. According to a report in the *American Journal of Public Health,* even a modest weight loss—10 percent of total weight—for those with mild-to-severe obesity can bring impressive health benefits. These include a reduction in the years of life spent with hypertension, diabetes, and especially heart disease—if the weight loss is maintained.

Your goal should be to commit yourself to life-long changes—notably, increasing physical activity and cutting your caloric intake by decreasing your consumption of meats, sweets, and fats and substituting fruits, vegetables, and grains. As with any attempt at changing habits, you may have to go through several cycles of success and relapse to finally succeed.

If you are not seriously overweight, avoid special weight-loss diets. Popular weight-loss programs typically emphasize a particular food or food group. While severely restricting fat intake or consuming a low-carbohydrate/high-protein diet can produce a short-term drop of pounds, such a program almost invariably can't sustain permanent weight loss. A report in 2001 from the U.S. Department of Agriculture confirmed that, while most popular diets help people drop pounds initially, only a balanced moderate-fat, high-carbohydrate eating regimen (such as that shown in the food pyramid on page 19) is likely to keep the weight off. This type of diet was also found to produce some of the best improvements in controlling levels of blood cholesterol, blood sugars, and blood pressure.

Eat fewer calories, not just less fat. Many people assume that if they eat a low-fat diet, as they have been repeatedly told to do, they will lose weight. While a low-fat diet by itself helps lower blood cholesterol and thus reduces the risk of heart disease, it won't necessarily make you lose weight. Most low-fat diets are low in calories, but not all are.

Calories do count—and so it simply isn't true (as some nutrition gurus preach) that you can eat whatever you want, in any quantities whatsoever, as long as you stick to low-fat foods. A low-fat diet can be high in calories if you depend too much on some of the new low-fat or nonfat

37

DIET DRUGS: CAVEAT EMPTOR

Most "diet drugs" decrease appetite by altering chemicals in the brain. Many, if not most, have proven to be dangerous and are thus reluctantly prescribed or have been withdrawn from the market by the Food and Drug Administration (FDA). For instance, dexfenfluramine (brand name Redux) and fenfluramine (Pondamin) were withdrawn because they may promote heart disease and other serious side effects in some people.

The FDA has approved another appetite-suppressant, Meridia, but it can cause increases in blood pressure and pulse rate that may be dangerous for some people. Another real drawback of these drugs: Nobody can take them forever, and you gain back lost weight when you stop using them.

A Newer Diet Pill

A different option is the prescription drug orlistat (Xenical), which works by blocking the absorption of fat calories. When taken before, during, or after a meal, orlistat prevents the absorption of about 30 percent of the fat in that meal. The fat then passes through the gastrointestinal tract and is excreted.

But orlistat is far from a miracle drug. Only truly obese people (defined as those with a body mass index, or BMI, of at least 30) are candidates. And studies show that the actual weight loss orlistat produces is small—in one study, those taking the drug three times a day for a year lost only about six extra pounds. After eight months, subjects started to regain weight and continued to regain on a "maintenance diet," with or without orlistat. The drug must be combined with a balanced, low-fat diet to be effective. There are also side effects, including excess gas, and the drug may block some important fat-soluble nutrients. It can also interact with other medications, such as the anticoagulant Coumadin.

For most obese people, the drug may be more trouble than it's worth, and it certainly should not be taken by people who are only moderately overweight.

Herbal and OTC Concoctions

Do-it-yourself weight-loss products are even more questionable. Recently, over-the-counter products containing phenylpropanolamine (PPA), a widely-used ingredient in appetite suppressants and decongestants, were taken off the market following a safety warning from the FDA). A number of herbal remedies that are on the market for weight loss also pose health risks. Some contain laxative herbs, which should always to be avoided as diet aids. Another key ingredient in many preparations is ephedra, also called ma huang, an amphetamine-like substance that has been linked to dozens of deaths over the years.

Ephedrine, the active ingredient of ephedra, is used in many over-the-counter decongestants and asthma drugs, but with clear warning labels about possible side effects and drug interactions. In supplements, you have no idea how much you're getting. The FDA has proposed restrictions on the use of ephedra and recently funded a study which concluded that dietary supplements containing ephedra are clearly dangerous for some people, particularly those who already have high blood pressure or a heart condition (as many obese people do).

cakes, cookies, ice creams, and other products that contain lots of sugar and calories but few nutrients and little fiber. A diet rich in fruits, vegetables, and grains (especially whole grains), which are high in complex carbohydrates and fiber, is very unlikely to be high in calories.

Set realistic goals for slow, steady weight loss—no more than one pound per week. Your ultimate goal should be to maintain a stable weight. If you find yourself steadily gaining or regaining weight, that should send up a red flag to reevaluate what you're doing.

Exercise is a key. Exercise is sometimes overrated as a weight-control tool. But adding a program of regular exercise to a lower-calorie diet will help you shave off more weight by expending more calories. Exercise also helps prevent the loss of muscle and the drop in metabolic rate that usually accompany dieting. And it is an excellent way to maintain weight loss and prevent future weight gain.

QUITTING SMOKING

More than 430,000 premature deaths a year in the United States—or about one in five of the total deaths—are attributed to the smoking habit. Up to age 65, people who smoke a pack a day or more die at almost twice the rate of nonsmokers in the same age group. The deadliest risks from smoking are cancer of the lungs, throat, and mouth. (About 90 percent of lung cancer cases are directly attributable to smoking.) Smoking is also the main

cause by far of chronic obstructive pulmonary disease (COPD)—a progressive blockage of airflow into and out of the lungs due to chronic bronchitis and emphysema. COPD affects some 14 million Americans, 80 percent of whom have significant exposure to tobacco smoke. Smoking is a major risk factor in heart attacks. Almost one-fifth of the nearly one million deaths annually from cardiovascular disease are attributed to smoking—many more than the number of smoking-related deaths from cancer and COPD. Also, mounting evidence indicates that smoking may place young women at risk for cervical cancer.

Besides greatly increasing your risk for life-threatening diseases, smoking has many smaller disadvantages. Long-term smokers are four times more likely to turn gray prematurely. Men who smoke are twice as likely to be bald or balding as nonsmokers. Smokers are also more likely to develop serious premature wrinkling and are twice as likely to lose their teeth, since smoking leads to periodontal disease, regardless of how well smokers take care of their teeth.

Low-tar-and-nicotine brands of cigarettes haven't helped. Even though tar and nicotine levels of cigarettes have declined substantially since 1955, American smokers (especially women) now smoke more cigarettes, inhale them more deeply, and start at earlier ages. Thus, smoking-related mortality rates are much higher today than they were 40 years ago.

Of the estimated 48 million Americans who smoke, 70 percent want to quit, and 34 percent try to quit each year. Unfortunately, fewer than 3 percent of those who try to quit succeed. Despite campaigns against smoking—which have had some notable victories—the smoking rate among American adults did not continue to drop during the 1990s. Most heavy smokers continue

39

to smoke. And each year some one million young people (ages 11 to 20) take up the habit—at least 3,000 each day, of whom an estimated one-third will eventually die from tobacco-related illnesses. Many statistics show sharp increases in teenage smoking in recent years. (Smokers have their first cigarette, on average, at age 13, and become daily smokers within a few years.)

On the other hand, about 1.3 million Americans become former smokers each year. In all, nearly 45 million have succeeded in quitting—a sure sign that you can choose not to smoke. The great majority of those former smokers quit on their own—the simplest method and the one most likely to work. But there are a number of effective strategies you can draw on to help break the habit.

WHY QUITTING IS TOUGH

Psychology and physiology play complex roles in the smoking habit. Nicotine is a psychoactive, addictive drug that causes marked alterations in body chemistry. It acts through specialized cell formations in the brain and muscles, but unlike alcohol or other psychoactive drugs, it does not produce dramatic evidence of intoxication, and thus people underestimate its power. (Tobacco companies have long recognized the addictive power of nicotine and have purposely manipulated its concentration in tobacco.)

Inhaled nicotine goes almost immediately to the brain, rapidly producing a sense of euphoria, particularly if you are smoking the first cigarette (or pipe or cigar) of the day. By taking more or fewer puffs, inhaling more or less deeply, and pacing your cigarettes, you unconsciously try to recreate this feeling again and again. What appears to be casual and random behavior is instead highly controlled.

Nicotine directly affects blood pressure, heart rate, skin temperature, hormone production, muscle tension, and pain sensitivity. It also alters mood. You are not merely imagining that smoking a cigarette enhances your powers of concentration or soothes your anxiety. Yet the tense, uptight feeling that a cigarette supposedly relieves can itself be caused by nicotine. It's a vicious cycle.

Smoking and sex appeal. Smoking is not just a matter of nicotine. Nearly all smokers start at age 18 or younger, and typically, an adolescent takes up smoking to gain peer approval, to express rebelliousness, or simply to satisfy a curiosity. What psychologists call modeling is a strong factor. If the people you admire smoke, you may emulate them. As you begin to smoke, you learn that just handling cigarettes can be a pleasurable activity. You learn to associate them with such pleasures as mealtime, or the end of classes or work, or with the relief of tension. And if you go by the ads, the brand of cigarette you choose confirms your masculinity or your femininity, or identifies you as avant-garde or as a lean adventurer. The charming, healthy young men and women in ads (who mostly aren't shown smoking) are swimming or playing tennis or sailing. Who wouldn't wish to be part of their world?

Cigar smoking—and trendy cigar bars—have been growing in popularity, especially among educated people who don't smoke cigarettes. Though cigars may be less damaging than cigarettes, they are far from harmless. Cigar smoking increases the risk of emphysema and cancers of the mouth, throat, and lungs. Smoking five or more cigars a day increases the risk of oral cancer by a factor of six, compared with nonsmokers. Drinking alcohol with cigars appears to worsen the health risks.

Intermittent "pack-a-week" smokers. Social

restrictions on smoking have resulted in a growing class of occasional or intermittent smokers, who sneak in a few cigarettes a day or every other day. Some used to be heavy smokers, some are new smokers. According to estimates from the Centers for Disease Control and Prevention (CDC), about 6 percent of smokers, or three million, fall into this category.

Although research into intermittent smoking is virtually nonexistent, studies on light daily smoking indicate that the more you smoke, the greater the damage. One study showed that men who smoked anywhere from one to nine cigarettes daily had nearly five times greater risk of dying from lung cancer than nonsmokers. There is also some evidence that how long you have smoked may be an even greater risk factor for lung cancer than the amount you smoke.

KEYS TO QUITTING

Nearly every method—no matter how odd—has worked for somebody. If you know former smokers, talk to them. Chances are you'll find some "go-it-aloners," others who joined a group, and even one or two who swear by hypnosis or acupuncture. The important thing is to find a method that suits your needs. A previous failure is nothing to be ashamed of. If you've tried and failed and are now trying again, that simply indicates the strength of your motivation. Abandoning tobacco is a learning process—so don't give up. Like learning to ride a bike, it may take more than one try.

Finding a substitute. The best way to quit smoking varies according to what kind of smoker you are, what you think you get out of smoking, and what it seems to do for you. Knowing why you smoke will help you find substitutes for smoking. For example:

• If you smoke for stimulation or a lift, find a healthy substitute, such as a brisk walk or moderate exercise.

• If you smoke for pleasurable relaxation or to relieve tension (sometimes it's hard to discern the difference), physical exertion, social activity, a new hobby, or deep breathing can serve as a partial substitute.

• If you feel as though you can't start the day without a cigarette, you are likely smoking because of the physiological effects of nicotine. Going cold turkey may be the only way to combat this. First, try switching to a brand you dislike in order to decrease your nicotine intake and thereby alleviate later withdrawal symptoms. To work up to quitting, set a final date, then smoke too much for a day or two.

• Some people have quit by switching to low-tar, low-nicotine cigarettes for a week or two, then quitting completely. Others have found help in nicotine chewing gum or patches (see page 42). The only catch is that the nicotine in these devices can also be addictive.

• If the habitual factor is strongest, work to alter your daily patterns. Cut down gradually—eliminate a certain number of cigarettes each day. Form the habit of asking yourself if you really want the cigarette you are about to light. You may be surprised at how often you say no.

• If handling the cigarettes is important, try doodling or keeping some small object in your fingers. Take up cooking or a craft such as embroidery that supplies tactile sensations.

QUITTING ON YOUR OWN

If you decide to quit on your own, choose a weekend (but not a holiday) or some time when you are under the least possible outside stress and you have some time to devote to yourself.

• Throw out any cigarettes in the house along

with matches, lighters, and ashtrays.

• Visit the dentist and have the tobacco stains removed from your teeth. Steer clear of friends and family members who smoke. Plan a number of activities for the day you quit.

• Go places where smoking is not permitted—museums, stores, theaters. Take public transportation. Swim, jog, ride a bike, or play tennis.

• Try to avoid any activity that you associate strongly with smoking.

• Be especially watchful when you drink alcohol. Researchers have long known that drinkers tend to smoke more and that drinking often serves as a cue to smoke simply out of habit, but a study at Purdue University showed that, in smokers, alcohol also actually increases the craving to smoke.

It is realistic to expect unpleasant or even severe withdrawal symptoms, which may include headaches, constipation, productive coughing, drowsiness, a sore mouth, impaired concentration, irritability, "the crazies," "the munchies," and depression. However intense your symptoms may be, they are temporary and in no way threatening to your health and well-being. The worst symptoms should subside after a week or two. Intense cigarette cravings usually last only three to five minutes.

When you feel the craving, take a break or a walk. Have something to eat or drink. Brush your teeth often, and use a tasty mouthwash. Breathe deeply or do stretching exercises.

DRUGS THAT CAN HELP

Health professionals now believe that smokers must choose their own route. In recent years pharmaceutical aids—in the form of nicotine replacement devices, as well as antidepressant drugs—have come on the market. If you can quit cold-turkey, that's the safest way. But if you can't, one or more of these may be worth considering.

Nicotine replacement devices, which put nicotine (the addictive drug in cigarette smoke) in your blood, can buffer withdrawal symptoms. If you have heart disease, particularly angina or arrhythmias, talk to your doctor before trying nicotine replacement. Nicotine gums and patches pose some risk, though not as much as continuing to smoke.

Here is what is available:

Nicotine gum. Sold over the counter, nicotine gum is convenient and supplies nicotine faster than a patch. There are two formulations: 4 milligrams (for very dependent smokers) and 2 milligrams (for average smokers). Most people chew 10 to 15 pieces a day and settle at half that amount after the first couple of weeks. You can't eat or drink within 15 minutes after chewing the gum, because that reduces its effectiveness. You chew the gum slowly until you experience a peppery taste, then park it between your gums and cheek, continuing the process for about half an hour. Ten pieces (about one day's supply) of the stronger version costs about $7, and the 2-milligram formulation about 50 cents less.

Drawbacks: You may not like to be seen chewing gum. It may cause indigestion. And it's hard for some people to give up the gum. You should wean yourself off it after you've quit smoking, but chewing the gum long term is less harmful than cigarettes.

The nicotine patch. This device, sold over the counter, can take two to four hours to deliver nicotine. But it's less obtrusive than gum, and provides a steady blood level of nicotine. It's also less likely to result in addiction. If you weigh under 110 pounds or smoke fewer than 10 cigarettes daily, you should use a lower-dose patch.

After a couple of months, most people are able to switch to lower doses and finally taper off. The patch can be combined with other forms of nicotine replacement—for example, with an inhaler. This may be recommended if you've failed to quit with other methods, but talk to your doctor before combining nicotine products. The patch costs about $4 a day.

Drawbacks: Possible skin irritation. You shouldn't smoke while using the patch, since that can cause a heart attack.

The nicotine inhaler. Available by prescription only, the inhaler looks like a cigarette (it has a mouthpiece and a porous plug containing a nicotine cartridge) and may help people who miss the act of smoking as much as the nicotine. You may need from 6 to 16 cartridges a day, for up to six months. You are supposed to taper off during the last three months. As with gum, you must not eat or drink within 15 minutes after using the inhaler. It is expensive—about $11 for 10 cartridges.

Drawback: Possible throat and mouth irritation, coughing.

Nicotine nasal spray. This prescription-only device is the fastest nicotine-delivery system. You use about two doses an hour for the first eight weeks, then reduce the dose and daily frequency for the next four to six weeks. Cost: $5.40 for 12 doses. Like the inhaler, this can be costly.

Drawbacks: Possible nose and throat irritation, sneezing, coughing, and watery eyes—but most people develop a tolerance. Also, some people find it embarrassing to use the spray in public.

Antidepressant therapy. Certain prescription antidepressant medications can help some smokers quit, particularly when combined with some type of nicotine replacement. The only drug approved by the FDA for this use is Zyban, the quit-smoking version of the antidepressant Wellbutrin (generic name: bupropion hydrochloride).

Zyban alters brain chemistry to reduce cravings and depression. Combined with nicotine replacement, it has the highest quit rate in studies—and the combination is more effective than either method alone. It's not a magic bullet, but it can help.

If you decide you want to try Zyban, talk with your doctor. This is important if you also plan to use the patch, since the combination can raise your blood pressure. You'll need to plan a quit date, then begin taking the drug one or two weeks beforehand, continuing for 7 to 12 weeks. If you have a history of eating disorders, are a heavy drinker, or are taking other antidepressants, you should not take Zyban. It poses a slight risk of seizures. Pregnant and nursing women should avoid it. Cost: about $3.50 a day. Medical insurance often does not pay for it.

Drawbacks: Possible dry mouth and insomnia. You'll need to have your blood pressure checked periodically. While Zyban is the best drug treatment, it doesn't work for everyone. In case it doesn't work for you, your doctor may want you to try an older antidepressant, Pamelor. It's less expensive, but has not been approved by the FDA as a quit-smoking aid. Clonodine, used to treat high blood pressure, may also work as a quit-smoking aid, but also is not approved for this purpose. Your doctor must closely monitor you if you take this drug because its side effects can be significant.

THE REWARDS OF QUITTING

All the experts suggest plenty of self-congratulation in the first few days. According to an article in *American Family Practice*, "Smokers who give themselves a pat on the back when they try

43

to quit smoking have a better chance of success than smokers with 'Kick me if I smoke again' mind-sets."

As part of treating yourself well, add up the costs of smoking—just the short-term costs of tobacco and paraphernalia, throwing in a calculation for accidental damage to clothing and furniture. After a week or two, buy yourself a present with the money saved. Or calculate your savings for a month or a year (plus interest) and see what reward you will be able to give yourself or your family.

As your withdrawal pangs subside, the rewards will begin to accumulate. Nothing you do for your health—not even dieting and exercise—so quickly pays so many satisfying dividends as giving up smoking. After only a week your body will be free of nicotine. You will notice that your senses of smell and taste are a keen source of pleasure. Your food, breath, body, and clothing will smell better. Your cough will go away. Breathing will be easier. You won't have to go to the trouble of buying tobacco.

Newly created nonsmokers are also pleased with the sense of mastery and accomplishment that accrues. Most important, you will add healthy years to your life. Within two years of quitting, much of your risk of heart disease will have disappeared. Within 15 years, your risk will approach that of those who have never smoked. The risk of lung cancer and other malignancies begins to decrease steadily after you quit—and is cut in half within five years. After 15 years your risk is almost as low as that of nonsmokers—even if you've smoked for years. As an added benefit, nonsmokers have stronger bones and less chance of getting osteoporosis.

QUITTING AND WEIGHT GAIN

Many smokers, women in particular, fear that giving up cigarettes inevitably results in weight gain. Not all quitters do put on weight, but in a review some years ago of a number of studies of smoking cessation, the Surgeon General's Office calculated that about 79 percent of quitters do gain. This news was somewhat softened by the

SMOKING AND ATTITUDE

Giving up smoking is a complex process. The quitter must end the physiological addiction to nicotine as well as correct a pattern of personal habits and associations. Maybe the hardest part is acquiring new attitudes, because smokers really do see things differently from ex-smokers and nonsmokers.

A study of smokers and ex-smokers in Australia published in the *American Journal of Public Health* found that "fewer smokers than ex-smokers accept that smoking causes disease, and smokers also maintain more self-

exempting beliefs." Twice as many smokers as ex-smokers agreed with the statement, "most people smoke." And five times as many smokers as ex-smokers went along with the idea that many smokers live to a ripe old age and thus cigarettes can't be so bad.

Smokers also clung to the belief that most lung cancer is caused by air pollution, or that once you've smoked for years it's too late to quit anyway. Shedding such beliefs, the researchers concluded, is an important part of the quitting process.

fact that more than half of those who continued to smoke also gained weight. A recent study of 4,000 adults published in the *Journal of Consulting and Clinical Psychology* confirmed that smoking does not keep people thin. Over the course of seven years, weight gain was common (averaging more than a pound a year), whether the subjects smoked or not. Weight control is not a benefit of smoking.

Nevertheless, a government study of over 5,000 adults age 35 and older found that giving up cigarettes was accompanied by weight gain—an average of about 9 pounds for men and 10 pounds for women. But other studies have come up with lower figures. Putting on lots of weight (20 pounds or more) is rare.

Why does weight gain occur? Nobody knows, but there are many ideas. Some researchers think cigarette smoking boosts metabolism, burning extra calories. Thus, when you quit, these extra calories catch up with you. Others have accused ex-smokers of binge eating, although this is probably unfair. A review of research by Kenneth Perkins of the University of Pittsburgh School of Medicine found that metabolic differences between smokers and nonsmokers are, in fact, slight. However, Perkins thinks that smoking produces a feeling of postmeal satiety that makes it easier for smokers not to snack.

No one is sure whether it's the nicotine or one of the other 4,000 chemicals in cigarette smoke that affects metabolism and appetite. A clearer understanding of this problem might lead to more effective ways of beating the cigarette habit. Maybe it's just that when smokers quit, they put food in their mouths instead of cigarettes.

Meanwhile, prospective quitters may find it helpful to be realistic about the possibility of gaining a few pounds. If you dread weight gain,

remember that the health risks of gaining 10 pounds don't begin to approach those of continuing to smoke. You'd have to gain 80 to 90 pounds to put the same strain on your heart as a pack-a-day habit. Fortunately, studies have shown that the tendency to gain weight after smoking may be only temporary—that is, you'll be able to take control fairly soon.

Furthermore, if you exercise while you're quitting—even if all you do is walk a mile every day—it can burn 100 calories and offset weight gain as well as keep your mind off cigarettes. If snack attacks overwhelm you, try munching raw carrots or other vegetables in lieu of, say, potato chips or candy, since the former contain fewer calories as well as better nutrition.

One thing at a time. Quitting smoking is so difficult that you probably shouldn't combine it immediately with a weight loss program. Two studies published in the *American Journal of Public Health* cautioned against tackling both problems at once. In one study, quitters who simultaneously quit and went on a weight loss program did succeed in giving up cigarettes—but gained as much weight as the control group (which wasn't trying to lose). In the other study, weight loss programs added to a standard smoking cessation program seemed to increase the risk of smoking relapse.

The best idea may be to deal with one thing at a time—quit smoking first, since that's the most important single thing you can do for your health. Then turn your attention to exercise, improving your diet, and controlling your caloric intake.

CESSATION PROGRAMS

If you want a group program, the local chapter of the American Cancer Society can supply information and so can most public libraries. The Yel-

45

low Pages (look under "Smoker's Information and Treatment Centers") will also tell you what's available nearby. There are live-in programs and five-day plans. You will probably find a list of counselors, clinics, hypnotists, acupuncturists, and other self-proclaimed experts in behavior modification.

Remember that there is no scientific evidence that hypnosis, acupuncture, or "total immersion" are effective. Whatever method you choose, ask in advance what the costs will be, what the dropout rate is, what percentage of people in the program succeed in quitting for an entire year, and whether there is any follow-up. Also, remember that no program will work unless you are strongly motivated to quit—and that even with the help of a program, successfully quitting may require more than one attempt.

PASSIVE SMOKING

Virtually every health organization, from the National Academy of Sciences to the American Medical Association (AMA), has concluded that exposure to secondhand smoke—which comprises the smoke that is exhaled by smokers as well as smoke that comes off the burning end of a cigarette—is responsible for the deaths of tens of thousands of nonsmoking Americans each year, mostly from heart disease. It also sickens hundreds of thousands of children.

According to a major government report, passive smoking is responsible for 35,000 to 62,000 heart attack death annually and 3,000 lung cancer deaths. Among children, as many as 26,000 new cases of asthma and 300,000 cases of bronchitis are due to passive smoking.

All the compounds in mainstream smoke that damage the heart have been found in secondhand smoke as well. In fact, compared to the inhaled smoke, the smoke coming off the end of a cigarette actually contains higher amounts of the compounds that tend to cause heart disease and lung cancer. Although this smoke is more diluted, these compounds occur in smaller particles, and even though the passive smoker breathes in less smoke, the small particles tend to settle deep in the lungs, where it takes longer for them to clear. (Of course, active smokers inhale both kinds of smoke.)

According to a study of nearly 11,000 people published in the *Journal of the American Medical Association,* repeated exposure to secondhand cigarette smoke increases the risk of damage to coronary arteries (atherosclerosis) by 20 percent. The study suggests that passive smoking causes one-third as much arterial damage as active smoking. This effect of passive smoking is particularly dangerous for those with other risk factors for cardiovascular disease, such as diabetes or high blood pressure.

If you live, work, or socialize with smokers, take the following measures to protect yourself from exposure to secondhand smoke.

• Don't rely on air filters and "smokeless" ashtrays. They won't filter out the toxins in smoke.

• Set aside a smoke-free zone in your home and persuade household smokers to respect it.

• Needless to say, it's better to be polite, but don't be afraid to speak up. "Please don't smoke" is always a valid request.

DRINKING ALCOHOL: BENEFITS AND RISKS

Every month, it seems, another study shows that "moderate" amounts of alcohol help protect against heart attacks. Yet the studies often disagree about what type of beverage is beneficial, what the optimal intake is, and who will benefit.

The U.S. government, in its official dietary guidelines, as well as the American Heart Association, have confirmed the coronary benefits of "moderate" drinking. Yet the American Cancer Society, in its guidelines, has recommended limiting alcohol consumption or abstaining from it, since even a moderate intake may increase the risk of cancer in some people.

It is clear that while heart disease is the nation's leading cause of death, alcohol's benefits can certainly be offset by its hazards:

• Alcohol is associated with about 100,000 deaths from diseases and injuries in the United States each year.

• Alcohol may prevent 80,000 deaths from coronary artery disease (CAD) each year, according to one report from the American Heart Association. But that's merely the mean point of a wide range of estimates (anywhere from 12,000 to 136,000) based on data from a dozen studies.

In fact, both these figures are only rough estimates. It's hard to say exactly how many Americans die as a result of alcohol consumption. It's even harder to figure out how many deaths from heart disease may be prevented by moderate drinking. Moreover, such a weighing of the beneficial and adverse effects of alcohol doesn't take into consideration the big differences between the two groups involved. While most alcohol-related deaths occur in relatively young people, the deaths prevented by alcohol are generally in older age groups—those with high rates of cardiovascular disease.

So what is the real bottom line on alcohol? Should you start drinking—or cut down or even quit?

WHICH BEVERAGES ARE PROTECTIVE?

Studies have consistently found that a regular consumption of moderate amounts of alcohol helps prevent heart attacks in middle-aged or older men and women by 30 to 50 percent. Red wine has gotten the most publicity, but some studies have found that white wine also helps, and other studies have found that wine, beer, and liquor are all equally effective. Though wine and other beverages contain various antioxidant phytochemicals that may help protect against heart disease and cancer, the crucial element is the alcohol itself.

Scientists estimate that about half of the protective effect comes from alcohol's ability to boost HDL cholesterol, the "good" kind that removes plaque from the arterial wall. Thus alcohol may reduce atherosclerosis, the hardening and narrowing of the arteries leading to the heart, which can cause a blockage and heart attack. Alcohol also reduces the stickiness of the blood and interferes with the formation of clots.

Wine may seem healthier than other drinks

47

because wine drinkers tend to be better educated and more affluent than other drinkers, which may account for other traits (such as a better diet or better health care) that help keep them healthy. Two studies published in 1999—one from England, the other from Denmark—found that wine drinkers have healthier habits (better diets, less likely to smoke) than other drinkers.

Wine also tends to be consumed with meals, which may be preferable. Food slows the absorption of alcohol, prolonging the potentially beneficial effects on the blood (especially important after a fatty meal) and moderating blood alcohol levels. In addition, people who drink only with meals tend to do so in moderation. Those who drink excessively tend to drink mostly outside of meals.

WHAT IS "MODERATE"?

This is the tricky part. Most experts say that moderation means no more than *one drink per day for women and two drinks for men.* A standard drink is 12 ounces of beer (the most common size of a bottle or can of beer), 4 to 5 ounces of wine (a smallish glass), or 1.5 ounces of 80-proof liquor (the amount in a not-quite-full shot glass); all of these supply about the same amount of pure alcohol. In most studies, people who drink that much have the lowest overall mortality rates, especially from heart disease—lower than teetotalers, occasional drinkers, and heavier drinkers.

However, not all studies have agreed with those numbers. A few studies have found that higher intakes can also be beneficial overall. Other studies suggest that "light" drinking (not even one drink a day, but two to six drinks a week) is better than a "moderate" intake.

A study from Harvard University followed 22,000 male physicians for 11 years and found

that those who had two to six drinks a week had the lowest overall death rates. The men who averaged two drinks or more a day had the highest death rate, because of an increase in deaths from cancer, primarily lung cancer. But this was an unusual study, in that the men (partly because they were doctors) were quite healthy, and relatively few died from heart disease.

Moreover, only 3 percent of them fell into the "two or more drinks a day" category. Because the study lumped together moderate and excessive drinkers in this highest open-ended category, it couldn't determine the risks faced by men who consumed only two drinks a day, nor could it define where the real danger begins. Also, the results can't be extended to women.

In general, problems arise with how drinking levels and patterns are categorized in virtually all the studies. For example, the studies rarely measure when and how alcohol is consumed: 10 drinks a week could mean a beer or two with dinner or two five-martini binges, which would have very different effects in the body. And for various reasons, people may not report their alcohol intake accurately.

Men and women. Alcohol affects men and women differently. A woman will get more intoxicated than a man from the same amount. Women tend to be smaller than men and to have proportionately more fatty tissue and less body water than men. Alcohol is distributed through body water and is more soluble in water than in fat, so the blood alcohol concentration from a given intake will be greater for a woman. Moreover, the stomach enzyme that breaks down alcohol before it reaches the bloodstream is less active in women than in men, so that more alcohol enters the bloodstream from the stomach.

Thus, excessive drinking tends to have more

48

serious long-term consequences for women. They are more likely to develop damage to the liver, heart muscle, and brain at lower levels of alcohol intake than men. Alcohol may also put them at increased risk for osteoporosis and possibly breast cancer. Studies also suggest that alcohol has a greater effect on driving skills in women—and at a given blood alcohol concentration, women have a higher risk than men of dying in a crash.

ALCOHOL AND CANCER

Several widely publicized studies have suggested that alcohol increases the risk of breast cancer. But other studies have found no increased risk— or found it confined to specific groups: those who consumed more than two drinks a day, or only premenopausal women, or only postmenopausal women. One 1993 study did show that when premenopausal women drink, they have higher levels of estrogen in their blood, which might explain an increased risk of breast cancer, if there is one. On the other hand, a more recent study suggested that a compound found in wine may counteract the effect of estrogen in the body. In 1999, research from the ongoing large-scale Framingham study found that alcohol does not increase the risk of breast cancer.

This has resulted in confusion for women, who wonder whether to drink moderately to protect against heart disease or to abstain because of alcohol's potential effect on breast cancer risk. Remember, however, that heart disease kills 10 times as many middle-aged and older women as breast cancer—and that questions still remain about the link between alcohol and breast cancer. If you're a woman who has a drink a day, there's no health reason to quit, unless you are pregnant or nursing—or possibly if you are at

49

DRINKING: DO YOU HAVE A PROBLEM?

Alcohol problems occur at all educational and social levels and in every age group. Although no objective definition exists for problem drinking, there are general guidelines to indicate whether someone is having trouble controlling his or her alcohol intake. Ask yourself the following questions. If the answer to any of them is yes, you need to reexamine how alcohol is affecting your health, safety, and relationships with others.

• When under pressure at your job, do you calm down with a drink at lunch?

• Do you ever have hangovers?

• Do family quarrels most often occur after you have had a drink or two?

• Does your family think you drink too much?

• Have you ever injured yourself or another person after drinking?

• Are you often on—and off—the wagon?

• If you drink regularly, do you know how much you spend at the liquor store or in restaurants, or do you avoid the calculation?

• Do you avoid situations where you think it would be impossible for you to get a drink if you wanted one?

• When pouring yourself a second or third glass of wine or beer, or mixing the additional highball, do you reassure yourself that you deserve it?

• If you know that you have to drive home in an hour, do you go ahead and have another drink anyway?

high risk for breast cancer or are on hormone replacement therapy.

Alcohol has been linked to several kinds of cancer. The recent Harvard study found an increased risk of lung, esophageal, gastric, pancreatic, urinary tract, and several other cancers. But studies have yielded inconsistent results about precisely which cancers are affected. One thing is certain: smoking and drinking act together to increase the risk of several cancers.

OTHER RISKS
LINKED TO ALCOHOL

After tobacco, alcohol is the leading overall cause of premature death in this country—and many of these deaths occur in young adults. Long-term, heavy drinking (three or more drinks a day) increases the risk of liver disease, damage to the brain and pancreas, high blood pressure, and hemorrhagic stroke. It can also cause heart disease by damaging the heart muscle. Even moderate drinking during pregnancy increases the risk of fetal alcohol syndrome, which can result in mental retardation and birth defects.

People with type 2 diabetes, who are at high risk for heart disease, may lower their risk by consuming a drink a day. But the well-known risks posed by alcohol, such as interactions with drugs, or falls and accidents, may be particularly dangerous (so be sure to discuss this issue with your doctor if you have type 2 diabetes).

Drinking alcohol also increases the risk of accidental injury and death in a number of settings. A seemingly small amount of alcohol can impair judgment, concentration, and reaction time. In many states a blood alcohol level of 0.10 is defined as legal intoxication. (Some states have lowered this level to 0.08.) Although many factors—such as whether alcohol is consumed with food and how fast it is consumed—affect blood alcohol levels, on average a 170-pound man would reach a blood alcohol level of 0.10 by having four or five drinks in an hour, a 137-pound woman three drinks.

In 1998, nearly 16,000 people died and more than 305,000 were injured in vehicular crashes where police reported alcohol as a factor. This works out to an average of one person injured every two minutes. Thanks to lowered speeding limits, the wider use of seat belts, and the raising of minimum-age drinking laws in all states to 21, the number of fatalities has decreased by 33 percent since 1988. Still, 38 percent of total traffic fatalities in 1998 were alcohol-related. The injured people included not only drivers but also pedestrians, motorcyclists, and bicyclists who had been drinking. (More than one-third of the pedestrians 16 years of age or older who were killed by cars had elevated blood alcohol levels.)

In addition to vehicle and cycling accidents, alcohol takes a toll in workplace and firearms injuries, as well as homicides and suicides. Moreover, alcohol abuse alters judgment and creates unhealthy family dynamics, contributing to domestic violence and child abuse.

SHOULD NONDRINKERS START?

Few if any medical experts advise nondrinkers to start drinking for health reasons. Alcohol probably kills more people than it saves—but the beneficial and adverse effects of alcohol occur with different levels of intake and largely in different groups. Most alcohol-related deaths occur in relatively young people, while deaths prevented by alcohol are generally in older age groups—those with high rates of cardiovascular disease.

If you abstain for religious or personal reasons, or simply don't like the taste or effects of alcohol, you shouldn't feel pressured to drink.

If you don't drink (and don't fall into one of the groups listed below) and are considering starting—or if you do drink and think you shouldn't—talk to your doctor about alcohol's risks and benefits for you, considering your age, sex, risk factors for various diseases, and family history. In general, men over the age of 45 and women over 55 statistically have a much greater chance of developing heart disease than cancer; if you are in one of these groups, moderate drinking may improve your odds of staying healthy. However, there are even better ways to improve your odds of warding off a heart attack: lose weight if you're overweight, stop smoking, eat a low-fat diet, and start exercising if you are sedentary. And if you have a tendency to drink too much or drive after drinking, don't drink at all.

WHO SHOULD AVOID ALCOHOL?

There are several groups of people who should consume no alcohol at all.

Do not drink

• if you are pregnant, are trying to conceive, or are nursing. No safe level of alcohol consumption during pregnancy or breast-feeding has been determined, but recent studies suggest that even a small amount of alcohol can inhibit motor development in an infant.Women trying to conceive can improve their chances if they give up alcohol.

• if you can't restrict your drinking to moderate levels (a special concern for recovering alcoholics and those with a family history of alcohol abuse).

• if you are taking certain medications.

• if you have very high triglyceride levels in your blood.

• if you have uncontrolled hypertension, liver disease, abnormal heart rhythms, peptic ulcers, sleep apnea, or certain other disorders.

Finally, don't drink if you plan to drive or take part in an activity that requires attention or skill.

TAKING CARE OF YOUR TEETH

Dentistry has made enormous strides. Fluoridated drinking water and fluoridated toothpastes, along with dental sealants, have made cavities and fillings almost a thing of the past, while improved preventive care and therapy for periodontal disease may eventually do the same for toothlessness. Through root canal therapy and restorative dentistry, severely decayed teeth can be saved, and even lost teeth can sometimes be successfully replaced with implants.

Perhaps the greatest gain has been in self-care: the role that people can play in their own dental health has become clearer. Brushing is very important for maintaining healthy teeth. Flossing and regular dental checkups are equally important. But knowing these facts isn't always the same as acting on them. Only half of all Americans see a dentist twice a year, and 29 percent don't even go once a year. While 80 percent say that flossing is important, only 36 percent actually do floss daily.

Most people would say they don't have periodontal disease, but 75 percent of those over 35 have symptoms of it. (The first sign is gums that bleed when you brush your teeth and red swollen gums, which usually indicates gingivitis). In an age when cavities are preventable, periodontal disease persists. It isn't usually painful in itself, but it is the leading cause of tooth loss in adults. Bad as that may be, periodontal disease may have other consequences, too. Several recent studies have even suggested a link between gum disease and heart disease. This is still under investigation, but it may be that the bacteria that cause gum disease can enter the bloodstream and promote blood clots or damage the heart muscle. It's also now known that if a woman develops severe periodontal disease during pregnancy, she is more likely to give birth to a low-birth-weight infant.

Periodontal disease is preventable and can be successfully treated. The most important factor, however, is you, and the care you take of your teeth.

BASICS OF DENTAL CARE

Your first line of defense is brushing thoroughly at least twice a day and flossing once a day. *Spend a minimum of five minutes each day* to clean all tooth surfaces, especially those between the teeth. Rinsing well is important—plain water is fine. Mouthwash is unnecessary, unless for some reason you use a nonfluoridated toothpaste and thus need a fluoridated mouthwash.

The right way to brush. After applying paste to the bristles, start with the brush at a 45-degree angle against the tooth at the gum line, catching the biting edge under the outside row of bristles. You can use a circular brushing motion or a straight-downward one.

Brush the gum line as well as the teeth. Be sure you brush all chewing surfaces thoroughly: Hold the brush vertically to reach the inside surfaces of the front teeth. Be sure the head of the brush is not too large to fit into the back of the mouth.

Don't overbrush, however. At least 10 percent of people brush too hard, which can cause "toothbrush abrasion" and lead to sensitive teeth, receding gums, and wear around the roots. If you clench or grind your teeth, they are even more vulnerable to overbrushing. A brush with bristles that are too stiff is often the problem. Dentists recommend soft-bristled brushes, yet many brushes sold in the United States have medium or hard bristles. Use a gentle grip (not a fist) when brushing and don't press hard.

The right toothbrush. The most important feature of a toothbrush is the bristles, which should be soft, so that vigorous brushing won't injure the gums. The toothbrush should also be new enough to clean teeth and gums effectively. Choose any size or shape brush head that best allows you to get at hard-to-reach places in your mouth. Some people find a child-size toothbrush does the job best. Others like a bigger model.

There's no evidence that rippled bristles or tapered heads or other innovative toothbrush designs are more effective than conventional toothbrushes in keeping your teeth clean. Handle design doesn't matter. And buy by price: An inexpensive brush can do as good a job as a costly one.

If you have some condition that limits your dexterity, or if you particularly like high-tech gadgets, or if you are trying to motivate a child to brush, you might want to invest in an electronic or sonic toothbrush.

Discard your old brush at least every three months or whenever the bristles begin to look worn. Keep a supply of brushes in the house so you can change frequently.

The right toothpaste. Toothpaste isn't essential for cleaning your teeth—it's the brushing action, not the paste itself, that removes plaque and

52

cleans the teeth. Mild abrasives in toothpaste also help with the cleaning. But the biggest advantage a toothpaste offers is that if it contains fluoride, it gives you proven protection against cavities. Always buy a fluoridated toothpaste that bears the seal of the American Dental Association, or ADA. This means that it has been evaluated as safe and effective at preventing tooth decay. (Parents should always supervise small children to make sure they don't swallow toothpaste, since fluoride in large amounts can be toxic to children.)

A tartar-control paste may be a good choice, though no paste controls tartar below the gum line. Brushing with any toothpaste (or even without paste) will help control tartar, but eventually you'll need a professional cleaning.

Baking soda toothpastes are as good as any other toothpaste so long as they contain fluoride. The same is true of plain baking soda—a good tooth cleaner, but you should probably use a fluoride rinse along with it.

An anti-gingivitis toothpaste containing a disinfectant called triclosan (Colgate's Total) has been shown to reduce both plaque *and* gingivitis (the first stage of periodontal disease).

Desensitizing toothpastes contain strontium chloride or potassium nitrate to block pain transmission and can help if your teeth are sensitive to heat or cold. But check with your dentist to make sure that you have no underlying problem. It may take two or three weeks for the desensitizing effect to begin.

Whitening toothpastes contain various agents

YOUR DENTAL CHECKUP

A dental checkup is the cornerstone of good dental care. See your dentist twice a year for evaluation, cleaning, and polishing, or more often if you have a problem that needs attention. The dentist should carefully evaluate the state of your teeth and gums. Periodic x-rays, taken once every 18 to 36 months depending on your oral health, are essential, and the dental exam should include some probing of the gums. Full-mouth x-rays are not necessary unless signs or symptoms of dental problems appear. (The radiation exposure from today's dental x-rays is very small, but there's no point in getting x-rays you don't really need.)

Your dentist or hygienist should cover you with a lead apron and collar during the x-ray procedure. Pregnant women should postpone x-rays if possible, and children under five years of age should not have them.

Your dentist or the dental hygienist should scale and plane your teeth: this usually includes scraping the tartar off your teeth at and below the gum line with a sharp metal instrument. The dentist may also use an ultrasonic or sonic scaler with a vibrating tip to dislodge tartar. This may be followed by cleaning with a mild abrasive.

If you need an anesthetic, procaine hydrochloride (Novocain) is the best and most common local anesthetic for dental work. It's safe, effective, and has almost no side effects. Laughing gas (nitrous oxide) also has a good safety record, but it can cause nausea and vomiting. Laughing gas should be reserved for people with high levels of anxiety about having dental work performed.

that may remove some stain. But none of these pastes will whiten your teeth significantly. If you serious discoloration, see your dentist.

Toothpastes with "natural" ingredients are okay, too, as long as they have fluoride and the ADA seal. In spite of their claims, they offer no special benefits for dental hygiene.

A new toothpaste called Enamelion claims to reduce tooth decay by "remineralizing" teeth—using calcium and phosphate along with fluoride to not only prevent cavities, but repair tiny lesions on tooth surfaces before they become visible. How effectively it works on healthy people hasn't been established by clinical trials. But the paste has been shown to to reduce cavities in people at high risk for tooth decay (for example, those undergoing radiation therapy). A remineralizing paste could be helpful for those at high risk for cavities or with sensitive teeth. But it is not a substitute for thorough brushing and flossing.

The right way to floss. Think of floss as an extension of the brush, a means of cleaning surfaces that the brush can't reach. Take a length of floss and wind the ends around your index fingers, so you can hold it taut, unwinding and winding as you go, in order to have a clean section of floss for each tooth. Slip the thread gently between the teeth and under the gum line.

Remember you're after the plaque on the side of the tooth. When you reach the gum line, curve the floss into a C shape and slide it carefully between tooth and gum until you feel a resistance. Pull the floss vertically along the side of one tooth, pull it out, then reinsert it for the side of the adjacent tooth. Avoid pulling it back and forth. Go between all the teeth, and don't forget the backs of your molars.

Though few people like to do it, flossing should be painless. It does require practice if you aren't accustomed to it. If your gums bleed at first, keep on flossing—the bleeding should subside as your gums get used to the procedure. If you have sharp edges or other problems that make it difficult to floss, ask your dentist to smooth over the sharp spots and check to see if any fillings are cracked.

The right floss. Use any kind you prefer—waxed or unwaxed, flavored or unflavored. There's no evidence unwaxed floss does a better job. Waxed floss slips more easily between teeth and is less likely to fray or break. If your teeth are tightly spaced, you might like a brand such as Glide or Precision, made of a teflonlike, shredproof material. Either of these is less likely to fray and may thus be worth the higher price.

Sugar and teeth. Limit the amount of sweets you consume, or at least brush as soon as possible after eating them. This is particularly important for older people, whose roots may be exposed. Sugar is particularly hard on dental enamel.

Mouthwash. You can use a mouthwash if you wish or if your dentist has directed you to do so, but the great majority of nonprescription mouth rinses are simply temporary breath fresheners. They have little effect against plaque (the thin film on teeth where decay-causing bacteria live), and they don't prevent gingivitis. Fluoride, which prevents tooth decay, can be effectively delivered in a mouthwash, but fluoride does not prevent gingivitis.

No mouthwash can take the place of regular brushing and flossing. If you want to temporarily freshen your breath or because you like the taste, any mouthwash will do. The only over-the-counter mouthwash with the ADA seal in the battle against plaque and gingivitis is Listerine. If you have periodontal disease, your dentist may prescribe Peridex or Periogard mouthwashes, which contain an antibacterial ingredient.

Dental appliances. You'll find a huge range of products for sale to help you with home dental care, including stimulators, rubber tips, interdental brushes, floss holders, toothpick holders, irrigators, and electric toothbrushes. If any of these appeal to you or solve specific problems, or if you have been advised by your dentist to purchase and use any of these items, they are fine. Before using rubber tips and stimulators, or any item that poses a risk of gum injury if improperly used, ask your dentist or hygienist for instructions. However, none of these things can take the place of regular brushing and flossing—and regular professional dental care.

PROTECTION FROM THE SUN

Spending too much time in the sun is damaging to your skin—even if you gradually tan over several weeks, rather than get a sunburn. Though a suntan may protect you against sunburn, it does not protect you against accumulated radiation. All exposure to ultraviolet (UV) rays is cumulative. Thus, the sun exposure you get at age 10 can affect you adversely at age 35.

There are two types of UV radiation. UVA, or ultraviolet A, is long-wave radiation that's part of the ultraviolet spectrum. It penetrates more deeply than UVB, or ultraviolet B, and causes wrinkling and leathering, damages connective tissue, and promotes tanning, although it is less likely to cause an immediate burn. It may be crucial in the development of melanoma, the most deadly of skin cancers. (Tanning lamps emit mostly UVA rays.)

UVB is short-wave radiation. It reddens and burns the skin and causes tanning. It also promotes basal and squamous cell carcinoma and may worsen the effects of UVA.

Next time you're out in the sun, bear in mind what the UV radiation is doing to your body. The amount of damage depends on your genetic factors, race, and ethnicity, as well as your complexion. Damage occurs the following ways:

• ***Suntan.*** A tan is a sign that your skin has been injured by the sun. It results from UV rays penetrating to the skin's inner layer to produce more melanin pigment. A tan may protect against sunburn but does *not* protect the skin from other damage.

• ***Aging skin.*** Many of the skin changes that people associate with the aging process are largely caused by long-term sun exposure. Photodamage from excessive solar radiation results in dry, wrinkled, thickened (leathery) skin. Cumulative exposure damages connective tissue, including collagen, resulting in less elastic—that is, sagging—skin. Blood vessels in the skin can also be damaged, leading to purple blotches. Freckles, white (depigmented) spots, and "liver spots" may also form, as well as other discoloration.

• ***Actinic keratoses.*** These are red or gray scaly patches that are precursors of certain kinds of skin cancer.

• ***Immune system.*** The skin is a major part of the immune system and contains special cells (Langerhans) that detect foreign threats to the body and initiate immune responses to them. Animal studies show that UV rays weaken the

55

function of these cells. At the same time, UV rays activate white blood cells (suppressor T cells) that interfere with the immune response. By thus undermining the body's defenses against tumors, UV exposure may promote skin cancer and other diseases. This may be especially dangerous in people who are already immunocompromised, such as those with leukemia or AIDS. However, the sun's effects on the immune system are complex and not fully understood.

• *DNA damage.* UV rays may promote skin cancer by causing genetic mutations that lead to abnormal cell division.

• *Skin photosensitivity or allergic reactions.* Some people develop allergic reactions—hives, bumps, or rashes—every time they are in the sun. Other reactions are due to certain common medications (oral or topical) or cosmetics that increase skin sensitivity.

• *Other health problems.* Sun exposure can worsen some medical conditions. These include cold sores (herpes simplex), lupus, erythematosus, and certain other skin diseases.

• *Cataract risk.* Though advancing age is the single greatest risk factor for cataracts, lifelong exposure to UV light appears to be a primary cause in promoting them.

BEING SUN SMART

When you're spending any amount of time in the sun, take these steps to protect your skin.

Avoid long sun exposure, even if you are wearing a sunscreen. Minimize sun exposure between 10 AM and 4 PM, when the sun is strongest. If your shadow is shorter than your height, you'll know the sun is strong enough to burn.

Wear protective clothing and a hat. Wear garments with a tight weave. (If you hold a shirt up to a lightbulb and it allows a lot of light to pass through, the weave is probably too loose to guard against ultraviolet radiation.) A hat with a three-inch brim all around offers the best protection. At the beach, lie under a beach umbrella.

If you are very sensitive to the sun, look for special UV-protective garments. These are usually treated with a chemical that helps block the rays, without making material stiff or bulky.

Use a broad-spectrum sunscreen rated SPF 15 or higher. Be sure to apply a generous amount, and put it on half an hour before you go outside.

If you're fair-skinned or will be outdoors for hours, use a sunscreen with a higher SPF (sun protection factor), and protect your lips, nose, and other sensitive areas with an opaque sun block, such as one containing zinc oxide.

The slightly greater protection offered by higher SPF ratings may be needed for children, for very long exposure, in extreme climates (high altitudes or southern latitudes), or for people who are very fair-skinned, who've had skin cancer, or who have lupus.

For more information on choosing and using a sunscreen, see page 605.

Never use a sunlamp or tanning parlor. Artificial tanning beds emit UVA and UVB rays, which can cause serious skin damage. UVA is now linked to the skin cancer melanoma.

Examine your skin on a regular basis. Any mole that changes shape, color, or size, any sore that doesn't heal, any persistent patch of irritated skin, or any small growth may be a sign of cancer and needs professional evaluation (see page 60).

Don't let teenagers off the hook. They may be reluctant to listen, but keep preaching about the dangers of suntanning and especially sunburns. *On average, half of a person's lifetime sun exposure occurs before age 18.*

Protect all infants from the sun. Infants six

months old and younger should never be exposed to the sun for extended periods because the melanin in their skin will not yet protect them significantly. When you go outside, cover the baby in a tightly woven long-sleeved shirt, long-legged pants, and a wide-brimmed sunbonnet.

PREVENTING STDS

Sexually transmitted diseases, or STDs, are among the most prevalent kinds of infections in the United States, with millions of new cases reported every year. In recent years, AIDS and HIV (the virus that causes AIDS) have received far more attention than any other STDs. Yet researchers have identified more than twenty sexually transmitted diseases, and the most common ones affect an estimated one out of four Americans. (The index on pages 138-139 lists the specific diseases that are covered in detail in this book.)

Incidences of some STDs have climbed dramatically. The rate for chlamydia has risen to 264 per 100,000 since 1984, when it was only 6.6 per 100,000. Genital herpes and genital warts are also extremely widespread. Syphilis and gonorrhea, on the other hand, have declined during much of the 1990s—though the incidence of gonorrhea rose 9 percent between 1997 and 1999. According to the Centers for Disease Control and Prevention (CDC), every year 15 million Americans become infected with an STD (excluding HIV).

All of these diseases are called STDs because they are transmitted by sexual contact, usually sexual intercourse. Syphilis and hepatitis B and C, like AIDS, can also be spread by infected blood. The herpes virus, if mouth sores exist, can be transmitted by kissing. STDs are *not* transmitted by toilet seats, towels, dishes, or other objects; by ordinary contact such as shaking hands, sharing meals, or using the same telephone; or by mosquitoes or other insects. Organisms that cause sexually transmitted diseases usually die within minutes outside the body.

If you have been in a mutually monogamous sexual relationship, sexually transmitted diseases are very likely not something you need to worry about. But anyone who has had multiple sexual partners, or has a relationship with someone who has multiple partners, may be at risk.

Virtually all of the STDs covered in this book are preventable with proper use of a latex condom. (The exception is human papilloma virus, or HPV, which causes genital warts). Most are also treatable. Syphilis, gonorrhea, and chlamydia can be cured with antibiotics. Genital herpes, genital warts, and AIDS cannot be cured, but they can be treated or managed. However, no sexually transmitted disease can be accurately diagnosed and treated without professional help. There are no home remedies, so see a doctor or another health-care professional if you are infected or suspect you have become infected.

KEYS TO PREVENTION

Apart from abstinence, the most reliable preventive is long-term monogamy with a monogamous partner. If you're healthy and have a long-term monogamous relationship with a healthy partner, you're at no risk. If you have not had a long-standing monogamous relationship, take the following protective measures.

57

CHOOSING AND USING A CONDOM

Here's how to buy and use a condom properly to enhance its effectiveness:

• Use recently manufactured latex condoms—no more than a few years old. Lambskin condoms are not recommended: they are more porous than latex, and while they block sperm and so protect against pregnancy, some viruses, such as HIV, can get through. Polyurethane condoms have a much higher breakage rate and slippage rate than latex.

• Use a water-based lubricant, such as K-Y Jelly. This lessens the chance of breakage. The condom can be prelubricated, or you can apply the lubricant before intercourse. Avoid oil-based products, such as petroleum jelly, mineral oil, or baby oil, which can cause latex to deteriorate quickly.

• Find a condom that fits. Condom width varies, as does length. A condom that is too tight can break, while a loose one can slip off.

• Handle a condom carefully. Fingernails and rings can damage it. Don't unroll it until you are ready to put it on.

• Put on the condom before any genital contact occurs. Place the condom against the head of the erect penis. Squeeze out the air from the reservoir end or the space you've left at the tip. Unroll the condom to the base of the penis. (If it doesn't unroll easily, it may be inside-out; if so, discard and use a new one.)

• Immediately after ejaculation (and before the penis becomes flaccid), hold the condom's rim to the base of the penis while withdrawing so the condom doesn't leak or slip off.

• Unless you are in a long-term monogamous relationship, use a condom every time you have intercourse, whatever your age. Even if you or your partner has been sterilized so that pregnancy is not a concern, you should still use one to protect yourself.

• Don't reuse condoms. Use a new condom for every act of intercourse. If a condom breaks or falls off during intercourse, stop and put on a new one.

Use latex condoms. When used correctly and consistently, latex condoms provide highly effective (though not infallible) protection against infection. Condoms made from natural membrane (lamb skin) cannot be relied upon to block the transmission of HIV and other sexually transmitted viruses.

According to the CDC, no data exist to indicate that condoms lubricated with spermicide are more effective than other lubricated condoms in protecting against the transmission of HIV and other STDs. Spermicides used alone without condoms are not effective for preventing infection. Recently, some researchers have begun to suspect that nonoxynol-9, the most common active ingredient in spermicides, might even facilitate transmission of HIV by causing inflammation in vaginal tissue. It's also thought that nonoxynol-9 may increase the risk of urinary tract infections. Thus the CDC does not recommend using spermicides alone, either for contraception or protection from STDs. Whether a condom should be lubricated with nonoxynol-9 is uncertain—risks may outweigh benefits, but some authorities still recommend it, especially for men who have sex with men. A condom with nonoxynol-9 is better than no condom.

Remember that nonbarrier forms of birth control (oral contraceptives, IUDs) offer no protection against sexually transmitted diseases. While a diaphragm and cervical cap protect against pregnancy, they are not reliable against infection; use a condom as well.

Note: Condoms may not offer adequate protection against genital warts (HPV infection).

Know who your partner is. It's risky to have sexual intercourse with someone you've just met or someone you won't be able to locate later.

Be observant. Don't have sexual contact with anyone who has genital or anal sores, a visible rash, a discharge, or any other sign of venereal disease. But being observant is not a substitute for knowing your partner.

Be informed. Recognize the symptoms of STDs and seek medical treatment at once if you notice them in yourself. A lesion, blister, sore, discharge, or rash in the genital or anal area should be a signal to seek medical help. If you're at risk for STDs, persistent unexplained flulike symptoms and abdominal pain are other signals to see your doctor.

Be responsible. If you think you may have been exposed to a sexually transmitted disease, don't have sex again until you've seen a doctor and been diagnosed and, if necessary, treated. If you are infected, inform your partner or partners and advise them to seek medical help.

Remember, no STD confers immunity: You can be reinfected with the same disease. Refrain from all sexual activity (even if you have no symptoms) until your doctor tells you you're cured (or in the case of genital herpes and genital warts, until you can manage the condition)—and until your partner has sought treatment and been given the same assurance.

Syphilis and hepatitis B and C, like HIV, can be transmitted by contaminated needles. Make sure such instruments used in tattooing, acupuncture, and even ear piercing are sterile (or, better yet, disposable). Of course, injectable drug users should never share needles.

Get vaccinated against hepatitis B. This will protect you against contracting the disease.

Inform others. If you have adolescent children, make sure they understand what STDs are and how they can be contracted and prevented. If they are not sexually active now, don't assume they'll remain inactive. Sex education classes in school can help, but don't rely on them exclusively. There's no substitute for parent-child discussions about sexuality.

It bears repeating that STDS are transmitted by sexual contact, primarily, and by contaminated needles (with regard to hepatitis B and C, syphilis, and HIV). Two possible exceptions: A person with fever blisters (caused by the herpes virus) can spread the disease by kissing, and a carrier of hepatitis B can spread the virus by sharing personal items (such as razors, toothbrushes, and washcloths) with blood or saliva on them.

SELF-EXAMS

Although many diagnostic tests are performed in a doctor's office, you can do certain examinations at home to check for cancer. In fact, individuals—not doctors—more often find their own cancers. Therefore, regular self-examination is one of the best preventive measures you can take to significantly increase your chances of detecting cancer at an early stage.

MONITORING MOLES

The American Academy of Dermatology has devised an acronym for discovering melanoma—ABCD—which has proved to increase detection (see illustration). "A" stands for asymmetry. Unlike normal moles, melanomas cannot be evenly divided. "B" stands for border. Melanomas tend to have notched, irregular borders that may blend into surrounding skin. "C" is for color. Melanomas almost always appear in shades of black, brown, or tan, and may be multicolored. "D" is for diameter. Melanomas are usually larger than the size of a pencil eraser. They often develop in moles, which can be flat and mistaken for freckles.

If you develop a growth that doesn't appear normal, your doctor (or a dermatologist) may perform a biopsy—that is, remove all or part of the growth. To check for cancer, this sample of tissue is examined under a microscope to detect cancerous cells. If cancer is found, the doctor will determine what stage it is in and suggest treatment options. (For more information, see page 443).

Asymmetrical shape

Border irregularity

Color variance

Diameter
greater than 6 mm

SKIN EXAM

More than half of all adults never examine their skin, but doing so could be lifesaving. Skin cancer is one of the most prevalent forms of cancer, and it can be deadly (see page 443). Fortunately, it is also one of the easiest types to detect and treat. Examining your skin is primarily up to you, since most doctors do not perform an overall check of patients' skin regularly. A skin exam is a simple process that should take no more than 15 minutes, and should be performed monthly.

When you examine your skin, you are looking for any change from what's normal for you. Spend some time looking at your skin, noticing where you have moles or birthmarks along with their color, shape, and size. Then each month perform the following steps:

❶ Undress completely, and look at yourself in a full-length mirror in a well-lighted room. Scan your skin overall (use a hand mirror to check places you can't easily see; you may also wish to have a friend or spouse help you examine these areas). Look for any changes in color, size, or shape of moles and birthmarks, or the appearance of new ones; any rough or waxy-looking patches; or any sores or scabs that are crusting, oozing, or bleeding or have not healed within a week or two. Pay special attention to areas where you have been sunburned in the past.

❷ Begin a head-to-toe examination of your skin. Run your fingers over your scalp feeling for any bumps or rough or scaly spots. Lift your hair and visually examine the skin underneath. Pay special attention to bald spots.

3 Closely examine your face and the front of your neck in the mirror. Be sure to check your ears and the skin below your jaw line and chin. Men with facial hair should be sure to check the skin underneath. These areas are very susceptible to damage from the sun.

4 Look at your hands and arms, turning them over so that you can examine the skin on each side. Look for dark spots under your fingernails, which may be an early sign of melanoma. Run your hands across your arms and shoulders to feel for any rough spots you cannot see. These are also high-risk areas.

5 Use a hand mirror to examine the back of your neck and shoulders, also areas that are susceptible to sun damage.

6 Examine your back, buttocks, and the backs of your legs with a hand mirror.

7 Examine your chest and your abdomen in the mirror.

8 Look carefully at the fronts of your thighs, legs, and feet. Be sure to check the bottoms of your feet and between your toes. As with your fingernails, check for any dark spots under your toenails.

BREAST SELF-EXAM

One out of every nine women will get breast cancer in her life—it's the second leading cause of death in women after lung cancer, and it kills more women in their 40s than any other illness. But if breast cancer is diagnosed early enough, women have a much greater chance of recovery.

Since about 90 percent of palpable breast masses are discovered by women themselves, it's a good idea to develop the habit of breast self-examination. The key is being able to detect changes in your breasts. Regular examination is necessary to familiarize yourself with what your breasts are normally like.

Keep in mind that self-exams are not a substitute for regular examinations by your physician and regular mammograms (breast x-rays). *Mammograms are still the most effective method for the early detection of breast cancer (see page 76).*

Monthly self-exams are recommended; doing it more often can be confusing, since your breasts change throughout the month. Do the exam at the same time each month—within a week after your menstrual period, since that is the time when breast swelling is at a minimum. Follow these steps:

1 Begin with a visual exam. Stand in front of the mirror with your arms at your sides. Familiarize yourself with the appearance of your breasts and nipples, including their shape, texture, and any normal asymmetry. Lean over to see breast contour in that position. After learning what's usual for you, look for any of these changes: bulging or flattening in one breast but not the other; puckering or redness of the skin; or reddening, crustiness, or unusual hardening or inversion of the nipples.

2 Raise your arms over your head and check for the same signs. Inspect your breasts while pressing your palms together over your head, and then again with your hands on your hips. Both of these positions contract chest muscles and may make it easier to spot any changes in your breasts.

3 Gently squeeze each nipple to check for any blood-tinged discharge.

4 The next part of the exam—feeling, or palpation—can be done while lying down, or in the shower or bath. Water and soap make it easier to slide your fingers over your breasts, but to examine the lower half of them, you should be lying flat. Lie down on your back with your right hand under your head. You can put a small pillow under your shoulder to help flatten your breast against your chest. Using the flat part of the fingers of

61

A SKIN GUIDE

When you examine your skin, you may notice a variety of spots and growths. The ones described below, which are usually associated with aging, are benign and nothing to worry about—everybody can expect to have one or more of them. Some are annoying or unsightly, but most can be treated.

Some changes on your skin do call for medical attention, however, because they may be signs of skin cancer. These include

- moles that change their shape, size, or color,
- a reddish patch that hurts or crusts over,
- a sore that won't heal,
- bleeding or ulceration.

If you have had skin cancer, you should be sure to have your skin checked regularly.

Skin tags, or cutaneous tags. Small protrusions (less than half an inch) on a narrow stalk, usually flesh-colored or darker, and usually on the neck or upper body; harmless, painless, and of unknown cause. No treatment is necessary. A doctor can remove a tag by freezing (cryotherapy) or burning (electrotherapy) if it is unsightly or subject to constant friction from clothing (like a shirt collar or bra strap).

Cherry spots, ruby spots, or cherry (or strawberry) angiomas. Bright red spots (flat or raised slightly), ranging from pinhead size up to a quarter inch in diameter, usually on the trunk, arms, or legs. They are formed by clumps of dilated capillaries and are harmless, painless, and of unknown cause. They can bleed heavily if punctured. No treatment is necessary. They can be removed by cryotherapy or electrotherapy, if you wish.

Liver spots, or age spots. Both terms are misnomers, since liver disorders don't cause these spots and they often appear around age 40, well before old age. They are usually located on the back of your hands or on your face, and may be yellow, tan, or brown in color, and round, oval, or irregular in shape. Flat and up to an inch in diameter, with a clearly defined border, the spots are caused by exposure to sunlight (but are not precancerous). They are painless and harmless. Bleaching creams won't remove them. (If liver spots change significantly in color, size, or shape, have a doctor check them.)

Senile purpura. Dark purple, irregularly shaped patches caused by small hemorrhages in sun-damaged connective tissue in exposed areas such as the face, back of the hands, and forearms. They are painless and harmless, and often quite mild in older people. No treatment is required except for cosmetic reasons. The patches tend to fade within a few weeks.

Seborrheic keratoses. Wartlike, waxy, scaly growths, usually on the face, chest, shoulders, or back, seen chiefly on light-skinned people. Yellow, dark brown, or black in color, these growths may start small and grow to over an inch in diameter. The causes are unknown, but seborrheic keratoses seem to run in families. Painless, harmless, and not precancerous, they can be removed with cryotherapy or surgery.

Moles. Pigmented growths (flesh-colored, black, or brown), usually small. Almost universal: Adults typically have 10 to 40. In most cases they are harmless and painless. Some moles can become dysplastic—that is, they begin to grow abnormally and, if untreated, can develop into malignant melanoma. These moles are asymmetrical and irregularly shaped and may contain different shades of brown, mixed with other colors.

your left hand, start pressing the right breast lightly against the rib cage. Begin at the outside edge of the breast and rotate in a spiral toward the nipple, without lifting your fingers, until you have covered the entire area of the breast.

5 Next, move your arm down to your side and feel the upper and inner part of your armpit, the area between your armpit and your nipple, and finally between the outer lower part of your breast and the nipple.

6 Repeat these steps for your other breast, using the opposite hand to examine it.

7 Expect to feel many normal lumps and textures; try to get to know these so you can detect any changes, such as thickening or hardening of tissue, or pea- to grape-size lumps. At first you may want to make a chart recording where normal gland tissue is found. Any changes should be reported to your doctor, but they don't necessarily mean you have breast cancer. Studies indicate that 80 to 90 percent of all breast lumps are benign.

Men can get breast cancer, too. Although they get it much less frequently than women, it's fatal more often, since this type of cancer in men is not usually detected until it's in an advanced stage. So it's a good idea for men to examine themselves occasionally.

TESTICULAR EXAM

Many men don't know about testicular cancer, even though it's the leading form of cancer in men between the ages of 20 and 35 (see page 548). Even fewer know how they can detect it.

A monthly self-exam is the best way to detect it in its earliest stages. After a warm bath or shower, when the scrotal skin is relaxed, gently roll each testicle between the thumb and fingers of both hands. Make sure you cover the entire area of each testicle. Feel for lumps, nodules, swelling, or a change in consistency. Be sure to examine the ropelike part at the back of the testicles called the epididymis.

Each man is different, and it may take a few examinations to know what is normal for you, but if you feel anything unusual, consult your physician right away—even though the odds are that it's not cancer. Symptoms of testicular cancer include a slight enlargement of one of the testes and a change in its consistency. Pain is usually not experienced, but often there's a dull ache in the lower abdomen and groin area.

Men with an undescended or partially undescended testicle have a greater risk of developing testicular cancer. Normally, the testes descend soon after birth; male infants should be checked to make sure the testes have descended properly. An undescended testicle is easily corrected; boys or men with this condition should be checked by a physician.

PROTECTING YOUR HEART

Nearly 60 million Americans suffer from cardiovascular disease—multiple ailments that affect the coronary arteries and the blood vessels of the heart, the brain, and extremities. Of all the chronic diseases that affect the health of Americans, these disorders have the greatest impact.

Coronary artery disease, or CAD, is the most life-threatening of these ailments. In most people,

63

the underlying cause of CAD is atherosclerosis, a narrowing of the arteries caused by the formation of plaques—a mixture of fatty substances, cholesterol, and cellular elements. Atherosclerosis occurs gradually over many years. Eventually, the plaque may accumulate to the point at which it begins to obstruct the flow of blood, limiting the amount of blood and oxygen reaching that part of the heart muscle supplied by that artery. If the obstruction becomes so large that it completely blocks a coronary artery, or if it promotes the formation of a blood clot in the artery, the heart muscle is deprived of oxygen, resulting in a heart attack, or myocardial infarction. *(For the warning signs of a heart attack, and what to do, see page 117.)*

The myth that a heart attack is something that happens only to men—especially stressed-out business executives—is on its way to oblivion. Although women under age 50 suffer from CAD far less than men, after 50 they begin to develop the disease at an increasing rate. By the time they reach 60, the rate is the same as for men at age 50. At age 65 as many women die of heart disease as of cancer, and after age 75 heart disease is the chief killer of women.

All told, CAD alone accounts for more than 450,000 deaths annually. (By comparison, deaths from all forms of cancer total 560,000.)

The good news: scientists now know far more about the major risk factors for CAD than for most other diseases. A risk factor increases the probability that you will develop CAD; it doesn't guarantee that you will develop it, nor does its absence (or even the absence of all risk factors) guarantee that you won't have a heart attack. Some of these—like getting older, being a man, or having a family history of heart attack—you can't do anything about. *But you can modify, control, or treat most risk factors to reduce your risk of a heart attack.*

Many of the wellness strategies discussed in this section of the book will have a heart-protective benefit. Here is a summary of nine steps that have been shown to help modify the risk factors for CAD in healthy people. (Each of these steps is covered in detail elsewhere.)

1 *If you smoke, quit.* This is perhaps the single most effective step you can take. Anywhere from 20 to 40 percent of all CAD deaths in the United States are directly attributable to smoking. It more than doubles your chance of eventually having a heart attack and increases the chance of dying from it by 70 percent; it is also the leading cause of sudden cardiac death. The good news: quitting smoking quickly reduces your CAD risk; within five to ten years of quitting, your risk of heart attack declines to a level close to that of people who never smoked, regardless of how long you smoked.

2 *Eat right.* Base your diet on fruits, vegetables, whole grains, nonfat or low-fat dairy products. Eat fish twice a week, and consume only small portions of trimmed, low-fat cuts of meat and poultry. Keep animal fats to a minimum. Eat a small amount of nuts a few times a week. Replace saturated fats with polyunsaturates and monunsaturates (for example, use canola oil and/or olive oil instead of butter). All of these dietary measures clearly play a role in many of the other measures listed here, such as controlling cholesterol, blood pressure, and body weight.

3 *Stay active.* Exercise protects against CAD by helping the heart work more efficiently, reducing blood pressure, raising HDL cholesterol, decreasing the tendency of blood to form clots, moderating stress, helping the body use insulin, and helping people maintain a healthy weight.

Sedentary people who begin to exercise regularly reduce their risk of a heart attack by 35 to 55 percent. Low-intensity activities, such as gardening or walking, if done regularly and over the long term, can decrease the risk of heart attack.

④ ***Maintain a healthy weight***. Roughly one in two American adults can be considered overweight or obese (weighing at least 20 percent above the "suggested" weight for their height), which doubles their risk for CAD at a given age. Obesity also increases the risk for diabetes, hypertension, and high blood cholesterol, which further worsen the risk for CAD.

⑤ ***Know your blood cholesterol levels and keep them under control.*** For every 1 percent reduction in high blood cholesterol (above 200 milligrams per deciliter), there is a 2 to 3 percent decline in the risk of heart attack. Often, cholesterol levels can be controlled through diet and exercise. Some people require cholesterol-lowering medication.

⑥ ***Avoid or control hypertension.*** High blood pressure, or hypertension, is a risk factor for stroke and heart attack. For every one-point reduction in diastolic blood pressure that is above 80 mm Hg, there is a 2 to 3 percent decline in the risk of heart attack. If you can reduce your blood pressure by making the appropriate lifestyle changes outlined on pages 334-335, the coronary benefits are likely to be particularly great. You may also benefit from medication.

⑦ ***Avoid or control diabetes.*** Type 2 diabetes (non-insulin-dependent), which afflicts more than 16 million Americans, is an important risk factor for both CAD and hypertension. Diabetic men have two to three times the risk of having coronary heart disease than those without diabetes. Weight control and exercise can improve the utilization of blood sugar and prevent or slow down the onset of diabetes—and reduce the incidence of heart disease.

⑧ ***Consider a drink a day.*** There is a growing consensus that light to moderate alcohol consumption—that is, two drinks or less a day for a man, one drink for a woman (a drink is defined as 12 ounces of beer, 4 ounces of wine, or 1.5 ounces of 80-proof spirits) can help prevent heart attacks. However, drinking more than that can increase the risk of heart attack and stroke, as well as cirrhosis, cancer, and accidents.

⑨ ***Consider low-dose aspirin.*** The recommended regimen—a baby aspirin (81 milligrams) daily or half a regular aspirin (160 milligrams) very other day—can lower the risk of heart attack by about one-third by reducing the ability of platelets in the blood to stick together and thus form a clot. It is particularly advisable if you have an elevated risk of CAD. Aspirin can have side effects and isn't right for everyone, so be sure to consult with your physician first.

A note on vitamin supplements. There is some evidence suggesting that the antioxidant vitamins C and E help reduce the risk of CAD. Vitamin C helps tiny blood vessels dilate, which may lower heart attack risk. And vitamin E reduces the tendency of blood to clot (though in a different way from aspirin—so you may benefit from taking both, though always discuss aspirin therapy with your doctor before starting it). Vitamin E may also protect the heart by decreasing the oxidation of LDL ("bad") cholesterol. Because most people do not obtain the amounts of C and E needed for a maximum heart protective benefit through diet alone, especially in the case of vitamin E, we recommend you consider taking supplements: 250 to 500 milligrams of vitamin C and 200 to 400 IU of vitamin E. Please see page 25 for further discussion.

PREVENTING A STROKE

Like a heart attack, a stroke is caused by blockage of an artery—but the artery is supplying blood to the brain. There are two types of stroke: ischemic (the most common), in which a clot forms and blocks blood flow to the brain; and hemorrhagic, which involves bleeding from a vessel into the brain.

About 160,000 Americans die of a stroke each year. Only cancer and heart disease kill more Americans, and nothing is more disabling. Yet it's estimated that more than half of all strokes could be averted if more people took the right preventive steps. (For the symptoms of a stroke, and what to do, see page 134.)

Some factors that affect the risk of stroke are beyond your control. These include age and gender. The incidence of ischemic stroke more than doubles with each decade after the age of 55. And men are about 30 percent more likely than women to have a stroke (though after age 55, a woman's risk of stroke begins to catch up to a man's).

But other risk factors you can control. *Most of the steps for reducing stroke risk are identical to those for preventing heart disease:* controlling high blood pressure (the single most important risk factor for stroke); not smoking; drinking alcohol moderately (if you drink at all); keeping your cholesterol in check; getting regular exercise; and controlling diabetes.

Here are two other steps specific to preventing stroke:

Get checked for atrial fibrillation. About 15 percent of people who have a stroke have a heart disorder called atrial fibrillation, or AF. The condition is a type of heart rhythm abnormality in which the atria (the two upper chambers of the heart) beat rapidly and irregularly and allow blood to pool in the heart. When blood pools, it tends to form clots, which can escape from the heart, travel to the brain, and cause a stroke. The prevalence of AF increases with age. It can be treated with an anticoagulant drug, such as warfarin (Coumadin), to prevent clot formation.

Get checked for circulatory disorders. A number of problems involving vessels that supply blood to the brain can cause strokes. These include heart disease, severe anemia, and sickle cell disease, which are generally treatable with medication or, in some instances, surgery.

A note on diet: There are no standard dietary prescriptions for preventing stroke. But eating a healthful low-fat diet helps prevent a number of risk factors associated with stroke, such as high blood pressure and diabetes.

In addition, a study published in the *Journal of the American Medical Association* found that people who ate at least five servings of fruits and vegetables a day had a 30 percent lower risk of ischemic stroke compared to those who ate little produce. Each daily serving reduced the risk of stroke by 6 percent. The most protective choices were cruciferous foods such as broccoli and cabbage; green leafy vegetables; and citrus fruits and juices.

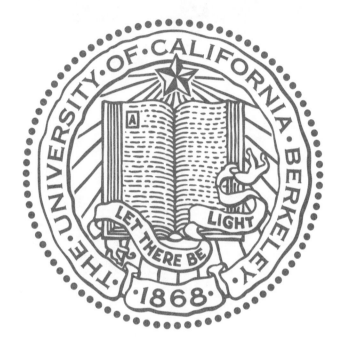

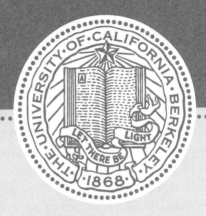

Using the Health-Care System

No matter how much attention you pay to to your health, there are times when you can benefit from professional advice. This section will help you understand and evaluate important resources available in the health-care system—beginning with preventive screening tests you should receive based on age, gender, and personal risk factors. It also points out what to look for in choosing a doctor, how to become more of a working partner with your doctor, and the services that doctors and other types of health-care professionals can provide.

PREVENTIVE SCREENING TESTS

Medical experts disagree about a lot of things, but one thing they all agree on is that the good health of Americans today and in the next century will depend largely on improved access to and increased use of clinical preventive services— that is, immunizations, screening tests for early detection of disease, and education about healthful habits and injury prevention. It's estimated that today only 1 to 3 percent of the country's annual health care bill goes for such preventive services. If everybody knows that an ounce of prevention is worth a pound of cure, why does that precious "ounce" so often go undelivered?

Part of the problem is contradictory recommendations and thus confusion—among patients, doctors, and public-health officials. What should a medical checkup consist of? Should you get a checkup every so often, even though you're feeling fine? How regularly should you be screened for various diseases? Which screening tests are truly effective? Should all adults be routinely tested for glaucoma? For diabetes? Should they be examined for cancer?

It used to seem simple: people were advised to undergo a standardized annual or biennial "complete physical." That head-to-toe physical exam has now been discarded for seemingly healthy people, since it yielded too few benefits for its cost. Over the long run it didn't pay off in terms of better health and longer life.

Some preventive or early-detection tests that once were routinely done, such as chest x-rays, electrocardiograms (EKGs), urine tests, and complete blood counts, are generally no longer recommended for healthy adults. Such tests are still important, but they are reserved for people with symptoms or risk factors—in other words, they are not general screening tests and are not done routinely.

But there's little or no argument that some screening tests, such as mammography, Pap smears, blood pressure checks, and blood cholesterol measurement, along with a variety of immunizations, are essential as preventive tools for healthy people.

TASK FORCE RECOMMENDATIONS

In the 1980s, at the request of the government, an independent committee of physicians known as the U.S. Preventive Services Task Force reviewed the available evidence about preventing illness, evaluated the balance of benefits and drawbacks of common screening tests, and came up with recommendations. The task force concluded that it's pointless for all people to have the same battery of screening tests.

In 1996 the task force released an update of its conclusions, after reviewing thousands of studies and consulting hundreds of scientific reviewers. Based on the degree of evidence for the benefits, the task force gave each test one of five ratings: (A) good evidence for the test, (B) fair evidence for it, (C) insufficient evidence to recommend for or against it, (D) fair evidence to exclude it, and (E) good evidence to exclude it. Since many of the recommendations fall into category C, it isn't surprising that disagreements among various medical-specialty groups and the

WHO PAYS FOR SCREENINGS?

One obvious reason why many Americans miss out on preventive care is financial: millions can't afford it and either have no health insurance or none that covers preventive tests. Even Medicare seldom pays for early detection and preventive care. Why?

Insurance companies base their business on the idea of cushioning the impact of unpredictable and potentially catastrophic events—that is, acute illness. Thus health insurers have resisted paying for checkups, most immunizations, mammograms, and Pap tests. After all, they reason, you know in advance if you need an annual mammogram, so you can budget for it. Yet many people put off or neglect to get services that aren't covered by insurance.

Health care with health maintenance organizations (HMOs) is pre-paid, which means that an HMO contracts with doctors, hospitals, and laboratories for care at agreed-upon fees. Patients go only to physicians who are members of the plan and need only pay a small fee for each visit. But you aren't necessarily likely to obtain preventive services more easily or cheaply from an HMO than you are from a preferred provider organization (PPO) or traditional insurer. Some HMOs will cover preventive services, but they don't publicize this fact to their members. Others don't cover preventive services at all. If you are with an HMO, be sure to ask what tests and screenings you are entitled to.

In a PPO, a panel of hospitals and doctors also contracts to provide care to members under a negotiated fee schedule, usually at a discount—similar to some HMOs. Fewer PPOs and still fewer traditional insurers cover preventive services. Some may pay only a small percentage of the fees (though some do cover the full cost).

The preventive services recommended in this book are well worth budgeting for and paying for out of your own pocket if your insurance policy doesn't cover them or reimburses you for only a small percentage of the fee. If more people demand coverage for preventive services, insurance companies may be more willing to offer these benefits.

task force often arise about which tests are essential, who should get them, and how often.

In 2000 the task force again began updating recommendations and evaluating additional new topics related to disease prevention—an ongoing process that is expected to take several years. Reviews and recommendations for this most recent update, as well as all recommendations released in 1996, can be viewed on the Internet at www.ahcpr.gov/clinic/prevenix.htm.

The guidelines arrived at by the authors of this book, along with the Editorial Board of the *University of California, Berkeley Wellness Letter*, largely—but not completely—reflect the findings of the task force. But controversies continue to surround some of these tests. For instance, widespread debate continues about the PSA test for detecting prostate cancer, which the task force recommended against, at least as a routine procedure for asymptomatic men (see page 80). Recommendations concerning common screening tests are summarized in the chart on pages 72-73. (The recommendations are also shown—by age group—in the section "Your Health" that

GUIDE TO PREVENTIVE SERVICES FOR HEALTHY ADULTS

These are the major screening tests (that is, routine tests for people without symptoms) and adult immunizations. The advice is based in part on recommendations of the U.S. Preventive Services Task Force.* Infants, children, and pregnant women need other kinds of professional preventive care not covered in this chart. For routine childhood vaccinations, see page 522.

SERVICE	WHO NEEDS	HOW OFTEN
Blood pressure measurement (to detect hypertension)	All adults.	Periodic screening. Optimally once every 2 years for those with normal blood pressure. (Those with elevated blood pressure need to be tested at least once a year.)
Cholesterol measurement	All adults. The task force and some other experts have recommended screening only men age 35-65 and women age 45-65, but we advise screening all adults.	At least once every 5 years, but more frequently if your total number is elevated, your HDL is low (below 35 mg/dl), and/or you have cardiac risk factors such as hypertension, a family history of heart disease, or cigarette smoking.
Pap smear (for early detection of cervical cancer)	All women with a cervix, starting at age 18, or earlier if sexually active.	Every 3 years. Possibly more often, depending on risk factors such as smoking or multiple sex partners. Some experts advise that women who have never had an abnormal result can stop being screened after age 65.
Breast cancer screening (mammogram and clinical breast exam)	All women age 50 and over; those 40–49 should discuss their risk factors with their doctors (see page 76).	Annually.
Colorectal cancer screening (fecal occult blood test and sigmoidoscopy or colonoscopy)	Everyone age 50 and over; earlier in those at high risk. A digital rectal exam (DRE) should also be done.	Occult blood test and DRE annually; sigmoidoscopy or colonoscopy every 5 to 10 years, on professional advice (see page 78).

*The American Diabetes Association, with the support of federal authorities, recommends a routine screening to test for type 2 diabetes for everyone age 45 and older (see page 82).

SERVICE	WHO NEEDS	HOW OFTEN
Prostate cancer screening (Prostate specific antigen, or PSA test, and digital rectal exam)	Men age 50 and over, especially those who are African-American or who have a family history of prostate cancer.	On professional advice. Usefulness of PSA test remains controversial (see page 80). All men age 50 and over should have an annual DRE.
Thyroid disease screening	People over 50, especially women, should discuss this test with their doctors (see page 84).	On professional advice.
Glaucoma screening	People at high risk: those over 65, very nearsighted, or who have diabetes; African-Americans over 40; people with a family history. Many eye specialists advise testing all adults starting at age 40 or 50.	On professional advice of eye specialist (see page 289).
Dental checkup (should include cleaning)	All adults.	On professional advice. Typically every 6 months for cleaning.
Tetanus/diphtheria booster	All adults. People over 50 are least likely to be adequately immunized.	Every 10 years.
Influenza vaccine	Everyone age 50 and over, people with lung or heart disease or cancer, and others at high risk. Even healthy younger adults can benefit and should consider getting the shot.	Annually, in autumn.
Pneumococcal vaccine	Everyone age 65 and over, and others at high risk for complications.	At least once. Effective against most strains of pneumonia bacteria; lasts at least 5 years.
Rubella vaccine	All women of child-bearing age. Not recommended during pregnancy.	Once.
Hepatitis B vaccine	All adolescents, as well as all adults at high risk (see page 326).	On professional advice.

starts on page 506.) In addition, the following pages offer helpful details about certain tests, controversies over screening guidelines, and recommendations on what to do.

SCREENING FOR CERVICAL CANCER: THE PAP TEST AND HPV TEST

Universal, regular use of the Pap test could virtually wipe out death from cervical cancer—which remains the major cancer killer of women in countries where the test is not routinely used. The Pap smear was developed by Dr. George Papanicolaou in the 1940s, and its subsequent widespread use has proved to be a highly effective way to prevent deaths from cancer of the cervix. About 2 percent of all women over the age of 40 will develop cervical cancer, but the cure rate nears 100 percent if the cancer is detected early. This is because cervical cancer generally develops far more slowly than most other cancers, progressing through a long preinvasive stage of 10 to 15 years, during which it grows but does not invade healthy tissue.

The test has reduced deaths from cervical cancer by at least 70 percent over the past 50 years, saving millions of lives. In countries where the Pap test is in widespread use, deaths from cervical cancer are relatively rare. These days women who die of the disease typically haven't had a Pap in five years or have never had one.

Obtaining a Pap smear is simple, painless, and inexpensive; most insurance plans cover at least part of the cost. A woman can be tested by a physician, nurse, or any health-care professional trained in taking a cervical smear. Holding the walls of the vagina open with a speculum, the clinician uses a small wooden spatula and a tiny soft-bristled brush to collect cells from the cervix.

The cells are then put on a slide and sent to a lab for analysis.

How often should you be tested? Most medical authorities, including the American College of Obstetricians and Gynecologists (ACOG), the American Cancer Society, and the National Cancer Institute, agree that every woman should have the test starting at age 18 or when she begins sexual activity, whichever occurs first. After the first Pap test, you should have three more tests at yearly intervals.

If no abnormalities are found, you can drop back to a once-every-three-year schedule. However, if you have certain risk factors for cervical cancer, you should be tested more often. Risks include multiple sex partners, early sexual activity, cigarette smoking, and evidence of infection with the human papilloma virus. You should tell your doctor if you have any of the above risk factors and follow your doctor's recommendation on how frequently to have Pap smears.

Being tested at regular intervals means that precancerous cells can be detected in time to prevent them from going further (cervical cancer is slow to develop). Regular testing can also compensate for occasional errors in getting a good cervical sample or for mistakes at the lab. (However, new technologies and new regulations have made Pap testing more accurate than ever, and women who get tested on schedule don't need to worry.)

Women who have had a hysterectomy in which the cervix was removed do not require Pap testing, unless the hysterectomy was performed because of cervical cancer or its precursors.

You should continue to be tested throughout your life. This is true even if you have had a hysterectomy, so long as you have retained your cervix. Some doctors think a woman can discontinue testing after age 65. You should discuss this matter with your physician or nurse-practitioner. But the risk of cervical cancer does not decline with age, and both authors of this book recommend that you should continue to be tested at three-year intervals after age 65, particularly if you are sexually active. We also recommend that older women who have never been tested (now a declining percentage of the population) should get their first test.

Should you be tested for HPV? Cervical cancer is one disease whose "necessary cause" (meaning that the disease will not develop unless this factor is present) can be pinpointed. It is a virus known as human papilloma virus, or HPV. Now there is a test—known as the Digene Capture II HPV test, recently approved by the FDA—to identify this virus.

HPV is a huge family of viruses, 77 types of which have been identified. They are very common and have an affinity for the skin and mucous membranes. Some cause warts on the fingers or the genitals. Out of the whole family, 13 are known to be associated with cancer. Without the presence of one of these 13, cervical cancer will almost never develop, no matter what other risk factors a woman may have. Though not a lot of fanfare has greeted this advance in scientific knowledge, cervical cancer is the only cancer so far to be so well understood.

Some experts have suggested making the HPV test routine, but it's too early to recommend this. No one yet knows how accurate the test will ultimately prove to be when used for thousands of women. Eventually, a home test kit could be important for women with limited access to health care. But for now a woman can remain in good health without ever being tested for HPV, so long as she gets regular Pap tests. You need only consider the HPV test if the results of your Pap test aren't normal.

What to do if your test results are abnormal. What the Pap test does so well is to detect precancerous cells at various stages. But an abnormal result doesn't mean you have cancer. In fact, less than 10 percent of atypical cells will ever progress to cancer. Benign conditions such as hormonal changes, infections, or the effects of birth control pills or pregnancy can produce atypical cells. The cells most often return to normal by themselves. Usually, all you'll need to do is have another Pap test in six months, or whenever your physician advises.

If suspicious-looking cells are still present, or if you have had abnormal results at some earlier time, then an HPV test may be in order. It, too, is a simple and painless smear, and the cost, though somewhat higher than a Pap, is usually covered by insurance.

If cancer-causing viruses are present, this will serve as an alert that close follow-up is necessary. But don't be unduly alarmed: HPV usually disappears by itself. And remember, *the great majority of women infected with HPV don't develop cervical cancer.*

Can you trust your test results? Like any test, the Pap is subject to human error, and lawsuits have been filed against labs for misreading results. Even if you are tested on a regular basis, you may still doubt whether you can trust your health-care provider and/or the laboratory to provide accurate results. You may also wonder if you should pay more for a lab that utilizes computerized techniques, rather than relying on human technicians.

All women should be assured that a conventional test, with the sample properly collected and evaluated by human beings rather than machines, is still very reliable. No test, of course, is ever 100 percent reliable. But because of recent improvements in the overseeing of lab work, you can be more confident that a "normal" reading is normal. Government regulations require that cytotechnologists (the people who read the slides) must pass a rigorous national exam and must have medical training in addition to a college degree. And every lab now has safeguards against a poor sample. If the slide is inadequate or cannot be read, a repeat of the test is requested.

Because cervical cancer is slow to develop, an error, if one should occur, will not put you at risk for disastrous consequences unless you skip the test for several years. *So it's important to have regularly scheduled tests.*

What you can do. For 24 hours before the test, abstain from sexual intercourse and avoid using vaginal creams, spermicides, medications, tampons, or talcum powder. Do not douche before the test (we advise against douching in any case). Schedule the test at the midpoint of your menstrual cycle, if possible.

By all means talk to your physician, nurse-practitioner, or whoever does your test. Ask about the methods of obtaining cells. Ask how the lab was chosen. The cost of a test should run about $20. Medicare now pays for the test every three years (though if you have had abnormal results it may cover annual testing). Your HMO or doctor should not be selecting a lab only on the basis of price.

Remember that the greatest risk of dying of cervical cancer comes not from poor lab work, but from not getting your Pap test in the first place. Be sure you find out the results: phone the office if no report comes by mail or by phone.

SCREENING FOR BREAST CANCER: MAMMOGRAMS

Growing older is the most important risk factor for developing breast cancer. Screening does not reduce the chances of getting breast cancer, but it does reduce the chances of dying from it. The mammogram, which is an x-ray of the breast done to detect breast cancer, is one of the most valuable diagnostic tests available. This procedure is a highly reliable way to detect breast cancer in its earliest, most treatable stage—long before tumors can be felt during a clinical breast examination.

But many women aren't sure when to have a first mammogram. The American Cancer Society, the National Cancer Institute, and many other authorities now recommend age 40. Other experts disagree, suggesting 50 as the starting point for most women. Most studies have found a 30 percent reduced death rate from breast cancer in women over 50 who get screened annually. The procedure is credited with the recent marked drop in deaths from breast cancer in this country, Canada, and elsewhere. The benefits are not so clear for women in their forties.

But many women under 50 fear breast cancer and feel that by not having mammograms they are being denied a benefit that could save their lives. The forties is the decade when breast cancer risk begins to rise markedly. If you're in your forties and want to start having mammograms, it's important for you to understand the risks as well as the benefits of mammography before 50. A well-informed and sympathetic physician should be able to help you make up your mind.

What you should consider. Some studies actually have shown that regular screening with mammograms can prevent breast cancer deaths among women in their forties, reducing mortality rates

GETTING THE BEST MAMMOGRAM

When you turn 40, discuss your risk factors for breast cancer with a physician. On that basis, decide whether it's advisable to begin mammography. In any case, begin having annual professional breast exams and mammograms at 50, and perform monthly self-exams.

A mammogram can be expensive ($150 or more, usually paid on the spot), but many insurance plans cover at least part of the cost. Medicare also provides partial payment for a screening mammogram. Low-cost and even free screening is available in some communities. Phone your local health department, public library, or chapter of the American Cancer Society for more information.

Your physician or radiologist should keep all your films on file, so that each new mammogram can be compared with previous ones. (You may need to carry your films from the doctor's office to the radiologist and back again.) You are entitled to copies if you want them (there may be a charge); the films must be accessible for at least five years. If you move or switch doctors or radiologists, remember to take your films with you or have them sent to your new doctor.

Other Tips and Facts

• If possible, go to a comprehensive breast center for screening; in any case, make sure the site is certified by the FDA. (The Mammography Quality Standards Act, passed in 1994, requires that all facilities be government certified and inspected.) If possible, choose a center accredited by the American College of Radiology, which sets strict qualifying standards. If there is not one near you, at least ask if the facility uses up-to-date, dedicated machines. You can get a list of centers in your area by calling your local chapter of the American Cancer Society or the National Cancer Institute at 800-4-CANCER.

• If you go to a new center, request copies of your past mammograms and bring them with you.

• At an accredited center, a breast exam is usually part of getting a mammogram. If not, you should get a professional exam elsewhere. Yearly professional breast exams are also essential. And monthly self-examinations of your breasts are a good idea.

• The day you go, it's more convenient to wear a two-piece outfit. That way you won't have to undress completely. Don't use an antiperspirant that morning. The aluminum in these products can make your film hard to read. You may have to wash and repeat the procedure. Talcum powder can also interfere with an accurate picture.

by 16 to 18 percent (saving one or two lives per 1,000 women per year). The problem is that mammograms don't work as well in premenopausal women, since breast tissue is denser at that time of life. Thus X-ray results are harder to interpret accurately, and false positives occur more often.

Indeed, nearly one-third of women in their forties having annual mammograms will have a false-positive result, leading to unnecessary biopsies and/or other kinds of testing. This is not only expensive but stressful. About 80 percent of women in their forties undergoing surgical biopsies turn out not to have cancer.

Risk factors in your forties. You also need to think about the factors that can put you at higher risk for breast cancer. If one of your close relatives (mother, sister, aunt) has had the disease, you should consider having mammograms before 50. Other risk factors include:

• early onset of menstruation (before 12).

• having your first child in your mid-thirties or later, or not having had children.

• being African-American.

• a suspicious finding in a professional breast exam.

Any of these factors may lead you to begin yearly or bi-annual (every other year) screening before 50. Potential benefits from mammography rise as you approach 50, so you might start in your late forties if you have risk factors.

Is radiation a worry if you start early? Over the years the amount of radiation delivered by mammograms has been reduced and is considered minimal when done by today's "dedicated" machines. Any increase in breast cancer risk would be so small as to be theoretical, and would be far outweighed by the lifesaving benefits of mammography.

While the mammogram remains the "gold standard" of testing for now, simpler and more reliable tests may soon be in the offing. Blood tests for breast cancer are on the horizon, though not in use yet. Other improvements, such as computer-assisted diagnosis, are already in use and are on the verge of being standard. Digital mammography allows the radiologist to enhance X-ray images for more accurate reading and to store them on disk. Ultrasound, while not a substitute for X-rays, is a useful adjunct.

SCREENING FOR COLON CANCER

Colorectal cancer kills more people in the United States and Canada every year than any other cancer except lung cancer. Yet this disease, which includes cancers of the colon (large intestine) and rectum, is highly preventable or curable if polyps are detected early. (The cancer shows up first as one or more small polyps—growths of soft tissue—in the intestinal lining.) The polyps don't always turn cancerous, and people may have no idea the polyps are there, though sometimes these do cause symptoms such as bleeding, constipation, diarrhea, or cramps.

Starting at age 50 everyone should undergo some kind of colorectal screening. Insurance will pay for some of the tests. But about 60 percent of eligible people have never had any kind of test. Many things discourage people from getting screened—embarrassment, for example, because the screening tests require a direct examination of the bowels or stool. But not least is the confusion about which test to take. Doctors, too, are divided about which test to use.

Some researchers have reported that one test—colonoscopy—was more reliable for routine screening than the others. But this test is invasive and expensive. Insurance may not pay for it. What should you do to protect yourself against colon cancer? This list will help you review the options:

Digital rectal exam. Because it is a quick, simple test, it is routine in most physicals (where it is also used to examine the prostate gland). But it can detect only about 10 percent of tumors.

Fecal occult blood test (FOBT). This is the simplest and cheapest test, except for digital rectal exam. Since many cancers of the colon and rectum bleed, FOBT is designed to detect hidden ("occult") blood in a stool sample. At home, you smear small samples on a card over several days and then mail it to a lab or doctor's office for analysis. If blood is detected, further diagnostic testing will be done.

Besides the difficulty some people have collecting the samples properly, this test will miss many precancerous polyps and some cancers, and it produces some false-positives because many other factors besides cancer (such as hemorrhoids, ulcers, or taking aspirin) can result in traces of blood in stool. Certain foods and other substances can also yield a false positive. But the stool test is still recommended by most authorities as a first step, and it has been shown to save lives. Insurance covers it.

X-ray with barium enema. Following a positive FOBT, your doctor may order this test, which examines the entire colon. First, a barium enema is administered, then the colon is inflated with air and X-rayed. It is useful but may miss smaller polyps. As a screening test, it is covered by insurance every 5 to 10 years for those 50 and older.

Flexible sigmoidoscopy. In this test, a flexible, lighted tube is used to examine the rectum and lower portion of the colon. The test is very accurate, as far as it goes—only about one-third (two feet) of the colon's length (a portion known as the sigmoid colon). Although a sigmoidoscopy may be uncomfortable, it should not be painful. It can be done in a doctor's office (the process takes 15 minutes to a half hour). You take a laxative and/or enema in preparation and you will probably be asked to follow a special diet for a day or two before the test. Sedation is not needed, but you can request a mild tranquilizer.

A sigmoidoscopy can detect and remove polyps; a biopsy can then be done to see if they are precancerous or cancerous. As a screening test, it is covered by insurance starting at age 50 and every five years thereafter, which is the recommended frequency. But surprisingly few doctors offer the test to patients. If your doctor doesn't suggest it and you are 50 or older, you should ask about the test.

Colonoscopy. As the name implies, colonoscopy is a visual exam of the entire colon, via a flexible scope monitored on a video screen. It must be performed by a specially trained physician. You must take laxatives and eat no solid foods the day before, and you usually need sedation, as well as a few hours to recover. A highly accurate and valuable tool, colonoscopy can remove polyps that it detects. Complications, including perforation of the colon and hemorrhage, are rare but not unknown.

The test is very expensive—up to $1,500. Most insurance covers colonoscopy only for people who have symptoms, a strong family history, or inflammatory bowel disease (not to be confused with irritable bowel syndrome), or who have had abnormalities detected by the previously mentioned tests. Strong family history is defined as colorectal cancer or polyps in your mother, father, sister, or brother under age 60; or in two of these close relatives at any age. (Recently, Congress passed legislation to expand Medicare coverage of screening colonoscopy. It allows any beneficiary who qualifies for a fecal occult blood test or sigmoidoscopy to choose a colonoscopy instead. But unless you are considered at high risk for colon cancer, Medicare will cover the cost of a second colonoscopy only after 10 years, or 4 years after a sigmoidoscopy).

The test is also highly accurate. Two well-designed studies published in the *New England Journal of Medicine* in 2000 found that about half of people diagnosed with cancer of the upper colon via colonoscopy showed no sign of it in the

79

lower colon. Sigmoidoscopy would not have found these cancers.

Something called virtual colonoscopy is on the horizon. It's done via CT scans or MRI (magnetic resonance imaging). The colon has to be inflated for the procedure; it's less invasive than an actual colonoscopy, and may prove effective and less expensive. If anything shows up, you will have to undergo an actual colonoscopy.

One problem with colonoscopies: practitioners performing them are specialists who need to be well-trained. If most people over 50, or even over 65, wanted the procedure, there would not be enough specialists to perform them.

What you should do. If you are at high risk for colon cancer (that is, if you have a strong family history, inflammatory bowel disease, or have had precancerous polyps removed already), you should undergo colonoscopy periodically according to your physician's advice. Insurance will cover colonoscopies for people considered at high risk, but "high-risk" may not include everyone with a family history.

If your only known risk factor is being over 50 and you have no symptoms, where does this leave you? About 75 percent of colon cancers occur in people who are not at high risk. If no one in your family has had the disease, that doesn't mean you won't get it.

All of the tests are worth doing—they not only are able to detect colon cancer early, when it can be successfully treated, but often are even able to prevent it.

At a minimum, ask your doctor for a fecal blood test annually and a sigmoidoscopy every four to five years. Together, these methods will detect most colon cancers: they offer substantial protection and save thousands of lives. Insurance covers both tests.

Also talk with your doctor about colonoscopy. It requires more preparation and a longer recovery time than sigmoidoscopy, and poses a greater risk of complications. If you can afford to pay for a colonoscopy, you may decide that the added benefit is worth the money and risk. You need it only once every 10 years if the results are normal—so if it costs $1,500, that works out to $150 a year. If you can't afford that, the combination of fecal blood test and sigmoidoscopy is still an excellent option.

SCREENING FOR PROSTATE CANCER: THE PSA TEST

Prostate cancer, a phrase once uttered in whispers, is now in the news almost daily. Thousands of men, including public figures whose prostate cancer has received daily coverage, have had their cancers diagnosed with the help of a PSA test.

What the test shows. PSA stands for "prostate specific antigen," a protein produced in the prostate gland and released into the blood. (The prostate, a small gland behind the bladder, produces seminal fluid.) PSA levels are normally very low, but rise when prostate disorders—such as infection, benign enlargement, or cancer—occur. Digital rectal exam (DRE), usually done at the same time as PSA testing, also helps detect some cancers, but not as many as the blood test.

The controversy over PSA testing. The problem is that nobody has ever been able to show that PSA testing actually saves lives. Do men live longer if they discover their cancers early and undergo treatment? There is still no definite proof, via a clinical trial, but the good news has been slowly accumulating. It now appears that the death rate from prostate cancer has declined since testing began.

For example, a study by National Cancer Institute researchers found that for white men, the death rate from prostate cancer had declined below levels of 14 years ago, when PSA testing was first approved. (The death rate among African-Americans has also begun to decline, but not as much.) Among men aged 60 to 79, the death rate was even lower than that—lower than 50 years ago. Some researchers attribute this to PSA testing, but others disagree.

Currently, some official organizations, such as the American Urological Association, recommend regular PSA testing for all men over 50. But other experts are less sure of the benefits and do not recommend routine PSA testing. What's behind these differences of opinion is a complicated story.

Prostate cancer is quite common. Autopsies have shown that 30 percent of men over 50 and 70 percent at age 80 have small prostate cancers that haven't spread or caused symptoms. But only 3 percent of men die from it. In many men the disease does not spread and has few symptoms, or none. On the other hand, it can be deadly—it kills more men (32,000 in the United States each year) than any other cancer except lung cancer. And though this is typically an older man's disease, it sometimes strikes men in their fifties or even younger. For reasons not wholly understood, African-American men are more likely to have prostate cancer—and also more likely to die from it than other men.

The downside of PSA testing. A simple blood test that can help detect cancer might sound like a dream come true, but in fact the PSA test detects only high levels of PSA, not cancer. The only way to tell which men have cancer and which have some benign disorder is through a surgical biopsy—an expensive and unpleasant procedure. It's estimated that only about one-third of men with high PSAs turn out to have cancer. However, researchers at the Washington University School of Medicine in St. Louis reported that of some 1,500 men undergoing surgical biopsies, only 165 turned out to have cancer. That is just over 10 percent, which is not very many, considering the expense, particularly the psychological expense for the men undergoing testing.

Other problems: There is no way to predict for sure which cancers (detected by biopsies) will be aggressive and which will stay confined to the prostate and cause few or no symptoms.

It is also possible to have a low PSA and still have prostate cancer. Indeed, one in five men with prostate cancer do not have an elevated PSA. Moreover, as noted, a high PSA can arise from other disorders or be elevated for no apparent reason.

Even if you're diagnosed with prostate cancer, there is no one best treatment. Surgery to remove the prostate and/or radiation are standard; but both treatments often produce such complications as impotence and urinary incontinence. For older men "watchful waiting" rather than treatment is sometimes best. This means frequent visits to the doctor for retesting and examination, with an eye to beginning therapy if the cancer progresses. Trials are underway to determine whether "watchful waiting" is better than immediate surgery.

The benefits of testing. In spite of all the drawbacks, millions of men are currently being tested, and death rates from prostate cancer appear to be declining markedly. In a report to the American Urological Society, researchers from Italy and Austria reported a big decline in prostate cancer deaths in the Austrian state of Tyrol, where PSA screening was offered free to men

81

aged 45 to 75 beginning in 1993. Two-thirds of all males were screened, and the death rate plummeted—41 percent below expected levels in 1998. (This study has received a lot of publicity but has not been published, and there could be many questions about this result.) There are currently two large studies in progress, one in the United States and one in Europe. They are specifically designed to determine whether PSA screening decreases mortality. Results from this research will be available beginning in 2006.

What you should do. Given the advantages and disadvantages of this test, a man should discuss the issues thoroughly with his physician before being tested. Here is our advice:

• If you are under 50 and have no symptoms of prostate cancer, and no family history of it, you need not be tested.

• If you are African-American or have a family history of prostate cancer, begin screening at age 50. Some doctors say you should begin at age 40.

• If you are 50 to 75 with no family history or other risk factors, you may choose not to be screened.

• If you are over 75, and symptom-free, you may choose not to be screened.

• If your PSA level turns out to be high, get retested before having a biopsy.

• If you are taking any drug (such as Proscar) or herbal product (saw palmetto) for prostate problems, be sure to tell your doctor before your test, since these products may affect PSA levels.

• If you are 50 or older, Medicare will now cover the cost of annual testing.

SCREENING FOR DIABETES

The American Diabetes Association (ADA), backed by federal health authorities, has called for routine screening of all Americans starting at age 45, using a simple, inexpensive test to detect more cases earlier of diabetes—specifically, type 2 diabetes. This form of diabetes, previously called non-insulin-dependent or adult-onset diabetes, accounts for 90 to 95 percent of cases of the disorder. Until now, the disease has generally been diagnosed when people develop symptoms, such as unusual thirst or frequent urination, or when people at high risk for the disease (such as those with a family history of it) are tested for it. Now blood sugar testing may become as routine as blood pressure screening.

The association has also issued new guidelines that lower the cutoff points between normal, borderline, and high (diabetic) levels of blood sugar (see chart opposite). These guidelines, combined with widespread screening, are expected to identify an additional 2 million Americans who have diabetes. It's estimated that the number of Americans with diabetes totals 16 million, but one third to one half have not been diagnosed with the illness. The rest typically had the disease for seven years before it was diagnosed.

Benefits of early detection. It is hoped that early detection will identify cases when they are still mild. It's expected that this way, before symptoms develop, people can take steps to minimize the subtle damage to organs and blood vessels caused by years of high blood sugar levels, thus avoiding later complications of diabetes such as heart disease, stroke, and diseases of the eyes, nerves, and kidneys, which often lead to premature death. The incidence of type 2 diabetes is on the rise, largely because the United States population is aging and getting heavier.

DIABETES TEST: THE NEW GUIDELINES

• If you are 45 or over, you should be tested every three years.

• You should be tested earlier and more frequently if you

— are obese (more than 20 percent above healthy body weight). The number of obese Americans has risen dramatically during the past two decades and now constitutes one-third of the population.

— have a parent or sibling with diabetes.

— are African-American, Hispanic, or Native American, or belong to another high-risk ethnic group.

— gave birth to a baby weighing more than nine pounds, or developed gestational diabetes during pregnancy.

— have high blood pressure (140/90 or higher).

— have an HDL ("good") cholesterol level of 35 or below and/or a blood triglyceride level of 250 or higher.

• The ADA recommends the fasting plasma glucose test (no food for eight hours before blood is taken) because it is simplest, cheapest (about $10), and most likely to be utilized on a regular basis. The same vial of blood drawn for the test can also be used to measure cholesterol and for other standard blood work, if needed.

• A result of 126 mg/dl (milligrams of glucose in one-tenth liter of blood), repeated at least once, means you have diabetes. The former guidelines set the cutoff at 140. Researchers now believe that serious problems linked to diabetes begin with test results in the mid-120s.

BLOOD SUGAR (MG/DL)	DIAGNOSIS
Less than 110	Normal
110-125	Impaired fasting glucose
126 and above (in two tests)	Diabetes

If you are diagnosed with diabetes in its early stages, you'll be advised to lose weight if you're overweight, exercise more, improve your diet (choose the same low-fat, semivegetarian diet that is known to lower the risk of heart disease and some cancers), and quit smoking if you smoke. The goal of early detection is to avoid diabetes medications, or at least postpone or minimize their use, not to merely start drug therapy earlier.

If your result is between 110 and 125, you fall into a new category called "impaired fasting glucose," sort of a danger zone or borderline area. This means that you should take the same steps as outlined above, since blood sugar levels tend to rise with age. Here is where it may truly be possible to prevent diabetes.

Unfortunately, there's no clear evidence that earlier treatment with drugs will reduce the long-term complications of type 2 diabetes (though it does for type 1). In any case, if screening for diabetes serves as an additional incentive for people to make lifestyle changes (such as losing weight and exercising), that can only be beneficial.

SCREENING FOR THYROID PROBLEMS

An important gland located in your neck just below the Adam's apple, the thyroid produces a hormone affecting many bodily functions, including heart rate, respiration, the central nervous system, and the reproductive system. This hormone also helps control the metabolic rate of the body—that is, the rate at which your body burns energy. So if the thyroid isn't functioning normally, a lot can go wrong. There are two main abnormalities, with generally opposite symptoms:

Hypothyroidism (underactive thyroid): With too little hormone, you may experience fatigue, weight gain, memory problems, hair loss, depression, insomnia, difficulty swallowing, mood swings, enlarged thyroid gland (also known as goiter), dry skin, intolerance to cold, and/or high cholesterol levels.

Hyperthyroidism (overactive thyroid, including Graves' disease): With *too much* hormone, you may experience irritability, nervousness, muscle weakness, tremors, irregular menstrual periods, weight loss, sleep disturbances, goiter, vision problems, palpitations, heat intolerance, and/or impaired fertility.

Women are at much higher risk than men for thyroid disorders. Hypothyroidism is more common than hyperthyroidism, especially among older women. It's estimated that up to 12 percent of Americans have thyroid disorders, according to a study of nearly 26,000 people. The risk increases with age: about 6 percent of 40-year-old women have hypothyroidism, for instance, but 21 percent of those over 75. More than half of all cases have not been diagnosed. Hypothyroidism is treated with oral doses of synthetic hormone.

Unlike most other chronic diseases, thyroid problems are not caused by diet, lack of exercise, smoking, or other factors you can change. Thyroid disease caused by iodine deficiency, which was common a century ago, is no longer a significant problem, since iodine is now widely dispersed in the American food supply.

Detecting thyroid problems. Symptoms for thyroid disorders—which include weight gain, fatigue, cold sensitivity, depression, hair loss, and decreased sex drive—can also be caused by a variety of other common ailments, and this frequently leads to misdiagnosis. Beginning around 1960 many doctors readily prescribed thyroid hormones for general symptoms, often without measuring hormone levels. But thyroid hormones have no benefits unless you really are deficient. And since they can have serious side effects, such as bone loss, you don't want to take them unless you really need them.

Fortunately, there is a reliable, inexpensive blood test to screen for thyroid disease—the TSH (thyroid stimulating hormone) test, which measures TSH levels in the blood.

The cholesterol/thyroid connection. Lack of thyroid hormone decreases the liver's ability to clear cholesterol from the blood: thus, people with hypothyroidism tend to have elevated blood levels of total cholesterol, LDL ("bad") cholesterol, and triglycerides. Moreover, a large Dutch study of women over age 55 found that those with low levels of thyroid hormone (11 percent of the group) had about double the risk of atherosclerosis and heart attack.

If you have high blood cholesterol, your doctor should check to see if an underactive thyroid is responsible, especially if you are an older woman. If so, it makes more sense to treat the thyroid condition first than to try to lower cholesterol via diet or medication, which will have little effect. Treating the thyroid problem typically results in a 20 to 30 percent reduction in cholesterol. If cholesterol levels remain high, other treatments should be tried.

What to do. Routine screening—that is, testing all people, even if they have no symptoms or risk factors—for thyroid problems remains controversial. However, thyroid testing should certainly be done if

• You have a family history of thyroid problems, since there seems to be a genetic element.

• You have symptoms that may be related to a thyroid disorder.

• You have high cholesterol levels.

• You have had radiation to the neck, have diabetes or pernicious anemia, or have taken lithium for psychiatric disorders. If you fall into any of these categories, you are at high risk for thyroid problems.

Even if you don't fall into one of these categories, if you are a woman over 50 talk to your doctor about thyroid testing. Be sure to report any symptoms you have. According to the American Association of Clinical Endocrinologists, disorders of the thyroid are underdiagnosed in Americans, especially in older women, who are at greatest risk for thyroid disease. Some authorities recommend testing every five years.

If you do need thyroid hormones, you must be carefully monitored to make sure your dosage is correct. The good news is that hypothyroidism responds very well to treatment.

YOU AND YOUR DOCTOR

Taking care of yourself—in terms of your health and your medical needs—is something you should do in partnership with your doctor. Studies consistently show that "patient activation" leads to better outcomes in the treatment of a wide range of disorders. The more you and your doctor work as partners, the more you are likely to feel in control, tolerate symptoms, and take the necessary steps to get well.

LESS FREEDOM TO CHOOSE

Americans want the freedom to choose their own doctors, according to virtually every survey on the subject. Yet until recently, few have taken full advantage of the freedom to search for a physician. They have simply used the same one they have always used—the one their parents used or friends recommended—and have almost felt married, for better or worse, to that doctor ever since.

But with the growth of Health Maintenance Organizations (HMOs) and other managed-care plans, more and more Americans are being asked to find a new doctor. Usually this doctor will be a primary-care physician—a family practitioner or internist who will consider all aspects of your personal and medical history when making a diagnosis and who can refer you to a specialist if you need one. Even if you have ties to a specialist, such as a gynecologist or a cardiologist, most managed-care organizations insist that you first see a primary-care physician before you consult a specialist. (In response to a backlash by con-

85

A GLOSSARY OF SPECIALISTS

The following are some of the most common types of medical specialists. (Mental health practitioners are described on page 94).

Anesthesiologist. Decides which type of anesthesia will be used during surgery, administers it, and monitors its effects after surgery.

Cardiologist. Specializes in diagnosing and treating abnormalities of the heart and the blood vessels.

Dermatologist. Diagnoses and treats disorders of the skin, hair, and nails.

Emergency medicine physician. Deals with a broad range of problems, including life-threatening conditions, that require immediate medical treatment.

Gastroenterologist. Diagnoses and treats disorders of the digestive system and liver.

Geneticist. Specializes in diagnosing and predicting inherited disorders, such as cystic fibrosis, hemophilia, some forms of mental retardation, and many metabolic disorders.

Hematologist. Diagnoses and treats disorders of the blood and blood-forming organs.

Infectious disease specialist. Diagnoses and treats disorders caused by microorganisms.

Neurologist. Diagnoses and treats disorders of the brain and nervous system.

Neurosurgeon. Operates on disorders of the brain and the blood vessels that supply the brain, the spinal cord, and the peripheral nerves.

Obstetrician/gynecologist. Specializes in the health of the reproductive systems of women. A gynecologist can treat diseases of the reproductive organs with or without surgery. An obstetrician specializes in the treatment of pregnant women and delivering babies.

Oncologist. Diagnoses and treats cancer. Many oncologists specialize in a particular type of cancer.

Orthopedist. Treats injuries to any part of the musculoskeletal system; some specialize in athletic injuries.

Otorhinolaryngologist (Ear, Nose, and Throat, or ENT). Specializes in medical and surgical

---

sumers, many HMOs are now allowing a patient to go directly to specialists on the patient's panel without going through the "gateway" of the primary-care doctor. Whether or not this will continue, and how pervasive it will be, is unclear.)

Having a primary-care physician is one of the most important ways you can take charge of your own health care. In addition to treating you when you're sick, he or she can help you keep healthy in the first place.

If you belong to an HMO, you will probably have to choose a primary-care physician from a list of doctors who participate in the plan. In some instances, the physician who is your first choice will not be accepting new patients, so you will have to select another one (or be assigned to one by the HMO). You may feel limited in your choice, though most HMOs are flexible about allowing you to change your primary-care physician to another (who must be a member of that plan) if you are not satisfied.

As difficult as this shake-up may be, it can be an opportunity for patients to take some control of their medical care if they can obtain information about the doctors available to them. One way to do this is by getting referrals from people you trust and respect—coworkers, friends, or other health-care professionals. Hospitals are treatment of disorders of the head and neck (but excluding the brain, eyes, and spinal cord).

Physiatrist. Specializes in physical medicine and rehabilitation.

Physical therapist. Administers techniques to enhance recovery, from massage to rehabilitative exercises. A therapist typically has a degree in physical therapy and is licensed by the state as a registered physical therapist (RPT). Seeing a therapist requires a doctor's referral in most states.

Podiatrist. Deals with foot and foot-related problems, which are among the most common sports-related injuries. Though not MDs, podiatrists receive special training and are licensed by the state.

Psychiatrist. Treats mental illnesses and emotional and behavioral problems. Psychiatrists often use psychotherapy in helping patients, but as medical doctors they are also able to prescribe medications.

Radiologist. A diagnostic radiologist uses imaging techniques such as x-rays and ultrasound radiation to diagnose medical problems. Interventional radiologists use imaging techniques to perform invasive procedures (for example, lung biopsies).

Radiation therapist. Skilled in the application of radiation for the treatment of pathologies, usually certain forms of cancer.

Rheumatologist. Diagnoses and treats nonsurgical disorders of the musculoskeletal system (such as arthritis and rheumatism) and autommimune diseases.

Surgeon. Specializes in the diagnosis and the surgical treatment of a wide range of diseases. A general surgeon may choose to specialize further, choosing, for example, to be a thoracic and cardiovascular, pediatric, colon and rectal, or plastic surgeon.

Urologist. Diagnoses and treats (with medications or surgical procedures) disorders of the urinary tract and, in men, problems in the reproductive system.

another source. Many have referral services that can recommend doctors who are on staff or who have admitting privileges; they can also provide information about each doctor's training. City or county health departments should also have the names and specialties of doctors practicing in your area, though this information will say little or nothing about the level of care you can expect from a physician.

Surveys have shown that many people are dissatisfied with their physicians, not so much with their medical expertise as with their manner. The most common complaints are that doctors seem uncaring and hurried, don't listen to what the patient says, don't remember their medical history, and don't take the time to help the patient understand what's going on. What do people look for in a doctor? The best medical care, of course, but also a willingness to answer questions and respond to concerns in a manner that makes them comfortable.

With that in mind as a foundation, here are guidelines for selecting and working with a primary-care doctor and for seeking out a specialist. (Information on alternative treatment practices and practitioners starts on page 97.)

BASIC TYPES OF PRIMARY-CARE DOCTORS

A primary-care physician ought to be competent to recognize and handle the full range of problems that individuals usually encounter. There are four basic types of primary-care physicians from which to choose:

General practitioners. At the turn of the century most doctors were general practitioners—able to deliver a baby, set a broken bone, and even perform surgery. Then the age of specialization arrived, and the number of general practitioners (GPs) fell dramatically. Yet there are still some general practitioners in business—usually older men who went into practice after only a year of postgraduate training and who often make up in clinical experience what they lack in formal education.

General practitioners still treat the full range of medical problems, though they usually refer patients to specialists for consultation and sometimes ongoing care for such conditions as heart disease, diabetes, arthritis, asthma, cancer, and most surgical procedures. They are usually associated with community hospitals.

Family practitioners. Because of the decline in the number of general practitioners, the American Medical Association (AMA) in 1969 recognized family practice as a specialty. To qualify, a physician must complete a three-year residency that covers certain aspects of internal medicine, pediatrics, obstetrics, and orthopedics and then must pass a comprehensive exam.

Family practitioners handle a wide range of problems for people of all ages, treating most acute and chronic illnesses, and even offering psychological counseling for family problems like alcoholism. For complicated disorders, they refer individuals to appropriate specialists.

Internists. These doctors specialize in adult medical problems. Internists must take a three-year residency after medical school and must pass a rigorous examination to receive specialty certification. They have more advanced training in the diagnosis and management of such common medical problems as heart disease, diabetes, arthritis, and cancer.

Some internists will take further training in a medical subspecialty (for example, cardiology or gastroenterology). A general internist may refer a patient to a subspecialist for evaluation but will usually continue to see the patient for supervision of treatment.

Pediatricians. These doctors specialize in the care of infants, children, and adolescents. Like internists, pediatricians may become subspecialists—for example, in pediatric oncology or pediatric cardiology.

WHEN YOU NEED A SPECIALIST

Primary-care physicians (except GPs) are, in effect, specialists. But since the science of medicine has become so complex, many doctors specialize even further. Common specialties are briefly described in the box on pages 86-87.

Specialties in medicine can range from the broad—for example, an obstetrician, who provides care during pregnancy and delivers babies—to the very narrow, such as a gynecological oncologist, who treats cancers of the female reproductive system. When you have a specific problem or condition that your primary-care physician is not equipped to handle, a specialist's experience and knowledge in that area can be invaluable.

How do you know if you need a specialist? The best way is to ask your primary-care physician. If he or she says that you have a particular medical problem, ask if anyone specializes in that area and if you would benefit from a consultation. Many health-care plans require that you get prior authorization before consulting a specialist.

How narrowly focused the specialist should be depends on the nature of your problem. It's important to remember that many insurance companies will not completely cover the cost of visits to very specialized physicians.

If you've determined that you need to see a specialist, remember that any doctor can legally use the title specialist without completing any official training or gaining certification from the American Board of Medical Specialties. (Certification guarantees minimum competence and shows that the physician has had the requisite training.) Therefore, you should ask for a referral from your primary-care physician.

Other good sources include local hospitals and professional organizations. Every specialty has at least one leading organization, such as the American College of Obstetricians and Gynecologists or the American Academy of Dermatology, that can supply names of practitioners. The reference department of a local public library or the library of a large hospital or medical school should have a copy of either the AMA Directory of Physicians (which lists all licensed doctors and indicates if they are board-certified) or the Marquis Directory of Medical Specialists (which lists only board-certified physicians).

MAKING A DECISION

Whether you're choosing a primary-care physician or a specialist, you should do some investigating before selecting one. In making your choice, you will want to consider the following:

Is the physician competent? The most difficult—and yet most important—task is to make some judgment of a physician's technical abilities. Check educational background and professional associations, including hospital privileges and board certification. Ask if the doctor is certified by one of the recognized boards. Family doctors are certified by the American Board of Family Practice, internists are certified by the American Board of Internal Medicine, and pediatricians are certified by the American Board of Pediatrics. If possible, look for a physician who teaches at a university medical center.

Is the physician easily available? If you have an emergency, he or she (or the doctor's associates) should be able to make time to see you the day you call, as well as be available to talk to you by phone and to return your calls promptly.

Is the doctor in a solo or group practice? If solo, are other doctors available who will cover when your doctor is away—and who will have access to your medical records? If the doctor is part of a group practice, do you have confidence in the associates as well?

What is the physician's typical response? Does he or she listen carefully and weigh each problem you present? Is there a tendency to dismiss all your problems—or to prescribe medication every time you have a complaint?

What kind of payment is required? Do you have to pay the fee directly, or will the doctor's office bill the insurance company or accept Medicare or Medicaid?

Do you trust the physician? That is, do you feel you can confide in the doctor completely, and can you expect an informed and considered opinion?

IMPROVING COMMUNICATION

Competence, knowledge, and expertise are important qualities in a physician, but the rapport between doctor and patient also plays a crucial role in the quality and effectiveness of treatment. Many doctors, of course, are overworked or are brusque by nature. Some truly believe the centuries-old authoritarian approach is best. But there is evidence it may not be.

• Studies consistently show that "patient activation" leads to better outcomes in the treatment of a wide range of chronic disorders, from hypertension to diabetes. If your doctor treats you as a partner, you're more likely to feel in control, tolerate symptoms, and take the necessary steps to get well.

• The spoken word is the most essential tool in medicine, so doctor-patient communication is crucial. An analysis by the American Society of Internal Medicine estimated that 70 percent of correct diagnoses depend solely on what patients communicate to the doctor.

• Realizing that physician-patient communication is important to patient welfare and can enhance the outcome of treatment, experts are now recommending an empathetic or affiliative communication style for doctors, rather than an authoritarian approach. Affiliative is a ten-dollar word for "friendly, interested, and respectful." Patients, certainly, are better satisfied with this approach, whatever the outcome of the treatment, and a satisfied patient is more likely to comply with medical advice as well as to be honest about symptoms and personal habits.

• Poor interpersonal skills can hurt the doctor, as well as the patient. Several studies concluded that patients are more likely to sue for malpractice if they feel that a doctor is uncaring—that is, doesn't listen to them, rushes them, and fails to inform them adequately. Several insurance companies have offered discounts on liability premiums to doctors who take a brief course on physician-patient communication.

• Recognizing all this, medical schools (and medical groups) now stress interpersonal skills and try to train doctors to be good listeners and to be more compassionate.

GETTING THE MOST FROM YOUR DOCTOR

Patients, too, need training in effective communication and "physician management"—but such training is hard to come by.

The time to establish a relationship with a doctor is before you need treatment. Opening lines of communication isn't easy with someone you see infrequently and usually only in times of stress. Keep these guidelines in mind:

Prepare for your appointment. Doctors often work under great pressure, so keep your remarks to the point. Before you go, give some thought to your concerns. Be as detailed and specific as possible when describing your condition—jot down your symptoms and concerns if it will help you.

If it's your first visit to a doctor, be well versed in your own and your family's medical history. Bring along any medications you are taking, and mention any treatments you are undergoing. Try not to leave anything out; what you think is a minor detail could be important. If you have a symptom you're uneasy about, don't put off mentioning it.

Ask your doctor questions. There are no "dumb" questions. You're entitled to a diagnosis given in terms you understand. You should also get a full explanation of treatments and expected outcomes, as well as the risks and benefits of the various options. One of your rights as a patient is access to information, including your medical records.

Your doctor should encourage you to make an informed decision about your treatment. If you want details about your condition, ask the doctor to recommend reading material. If there is a medical school nearby, you can do research in their library.

Take part in your own health care. Your doctor's advice can only help if you follow it. Listen attentively to instructions and don't hesitate to ask for them to be written down. Ask for a convenient time to call if you have additional questions. If lab tests or x-rays are required, have them done promptly, and be sure the doctor reports the results to you—by telephone, mail, or in person.

You may decide to put up with a crusty manner if the physician is truly skilled. But if a physician is rude, dismissive, or intimidating, you are justified in looking for another. Don't stay with a doctor just to protect his or her feelings, or because you were referred to the doctor and think you can't make the decision to switch on your own. Make sure your records, including x-rays and lab work, are forwarded to your new doctor.

WHEN TO SEEK A SECOND OPINION

A second opinion may be a good idea when you are facing a less-than-straightforward medical problem and you are presented with several options for treatments and/or procedures. A second opinion is especially common for patients who are facing surgery. Many insurance plans now require you to get a confirming opinion before some kinds of elective surgery—for example, surgical repair of a hernia or removal of tonsils, uterus, gallbladder, or enlarged prostate. Medicare and Medicaid may require a confirming opinion, too.

There are many strong arguments for seeking a second opinion. Even though the second surgeon may only confirm the opinion of the first

one, the patient can benefit. Sometimes it's the only way a person can be reconciled to having surgery, and someone who is more confident that a medical procedure is appropriate will be a better patient and more likely to comply with instructions.

Finally, although it may be rare for the second surgeon to disagree with the first, it does happen, and thus some unnecessary surgery can be avoided. If this occurs, you'll be happy you took that extra step.

Keep in mind the following points:

• Consultation has always been part of good medical practice, and no competent doctor should be insulted if you decide to get a second opinion, even if your insurance company does not require you to do so. Nonetheless, be tactful about it.

• Seek out the most highly qualified consultant available. At the very least, make sure that the second physician has been certified by the American Board of Medical Specialties. If you are uncomfortable asking direct questions about a doctor's qualifications when you make the appointment, ask your family doctor, a local medical society, or the surgical department of your nearest medical school.

• A consultation allows you to compare medical opinions about how a treatment, procedure, or operation is likely to affect your quality of life, the risks involved, and other options that might be available. It gives you a chance to ask additional questions that might occur to you. Perhaps the most important reason to seek a second opinion is that it puts the final decision in your hands.

YOUR MEDICAL RECORDS

In the past, many doctors and health-care providers argued against patients' right of access to medical records, since these files are often highly technical—and possibly confusing and alarming. However, in recent years, thanks in large part to lobbying by consumers' groups, many states now guarantee access to medical (and often mental health) records.

To obtain a copy of your records, simply contact your doctor's office or the hospital where tests or procedures were done. Even in states without full guaranteed access, most doctors and hospitals will honor requests for copies. You may be charged for photocopying and mailing. A good way to keep records up to date is to regularly request copies of test results and notes from your doctor after each visit.

EMERGENCY ROOMS

In case of accident or sudden illness, most people don't call a doctor. Instead, they go to the nearest emergency room.

It makes sense to know when it's appropriate to use an emergency room (see page 104). For that reason, it also makes sense to investigate emergency rooms in your area beforehand, particularly if you have small children in the house or anyone with a chronic condition that might require attention in a hurry.

In some emergencies (if you or the person you are caring for has chest pain, severe bleeding, or some other condition that rules out driving), you'll need to call your local paramedics, who may not be able to allow you a choice of facilities. You may want to keep the number of a private ambulance service close to your telephone, so that you can be taken to the hospital of your choice. But in any life-threatening situation, you should, of course, go to the nearest hospital. (If you're not satisfied, you can always arrange a transfer later.)

You can't always judge the quality of an emer-gency room by the reputation of a hospital. A certain hospital in your area may have a good reputation, but it doesn't necessarily follow that its emergency room is the best, since many emergency rooms are operated on a contract basis. Obviously, if there's a fine hospital nearby, you should investigate its emergency services as part of your research. For starters, it's a good idea to ask your doctor and your neighbors about local emergency rooms. You can also write or phone the local health department. Consider the following criteria in your investigation:

Location. Pick a nearby facility and check how long it takes you to get there by car or taxi. If you are driving, notice where the entrance is and where you can park. Go inside the hospital and look around.

Service. By phone or in person, find out what the hours are, whether a physician is always on duty, and whether a surgical team is available to treat severe injuries.

Payment. You should also find out about billing and payment procedures. Is the hospital willing to bill you or do they want immediate payment? Will they bill your insurance company? Will they accept a credit card? Will the physician's bill be included in the emergency-room fee, or should you expect a separate charge? (Note that emergency rooms are obligated by federal law to see anyone who seeks treatment, regardless of the patient's insurance status or ability to pay. However, the hospital will bill for the treatment, and will make an effort to collect payment.)

MENTAL HEALTH PRACTITIONERS

Many kinds of problems can lead people to search for mental health care for themselves, a family member, or a friend. The range is quite wide and may include grief (which is normal but sometimes unmanageable) over a death in the family or another traumatic event; difficulty communicating; anxiety or chronic depression that seems to have no immediate cause; and drug or alcohol addiction. Other reasons include phobias and panic disorders, compulsive behavior, eating disorders, neuroses, psychoses, a suicide attempt, or what is sometimes called a "nervous breakdown," characterized by marked personality changes, fits of weeping, or sudden aggressive behavior.

Unfortunately, many people deny the need for help. To admit that a problem exists is often the first step in solving it. No form of therapy is a guaranteed cure—indeed, emotional difficulties may not be curable in the same sense that strep throat is curable. But the very act of seeking help may be a form of therapy in itself.

THE THERAPEUTIC PALETTE

93

Psychotherapy, the general term for face-to-face discussions and other treatments that try to resolve psychological problems, takes place in many settings and in many forms. It may consist of analysis that goes on for years or short-term individual counseling. Sometimes methods overlap. For example, individual therapy may be combined with group therapy or self-help groups.

One-on-one therapy. Most forms of therapy have their roots in psychoanalysis, which is designed not only to deal with immediate problems but also to uncover underlying causes in the past. Many approaches have evolved; there's little data to indicate that one kind of therapy is superior to another.

Group therapy. This differs from a self-help group in that it has a paid, professionally trained leader—a psychiatrist, a psychologist, or another trained and licensed mental health professional. The leader's approach may vary from highly directive to passive.

Family therapy. This may involve the entire family or different combinations of family members. Marriage counseling focuses on the couple. Psychiatrists, psychologists, and social workers may all use family therapy as a tool.

Self-help groups. These are informal support groups that meet to discuss shared problems, such as a mental or physical illness, addictions, personal crises and life changes, and the problems of single parents. Studies of such groups show that the recently bereaved, cancer patients, and others often benefit from participation in a group. Members may pay dues, but there is usually no paid leader. Members try to guide one another. Alcoholics Anonymous is the oldest and best-known group. People in crisis may need a professional therapist in addition to a support group.

WHO THEY ARE

It's easy to be confused about the training and licensing of mental health professionals.

Psychiatrists. These are doctors of medicine (MDs) with several years of postgraduate training in the diagnosis and treatment of emotional and mental disorders using various forms of psychotherapy and medications. They can prescribe drugs and hospitalize patients. They may treat a range of problems, from severe psychoses to milder emotional disorders, and may use many types of psychotherapy, from short-term therapy to long-term psychoanalysis. They may specialize in child, adolescent, or geriatric psychiatry, or in drug and other abuse problems.

Psychoanalysts. Most are MDs with 6 to 10 years of postgraduate psychoanalytic training, but there are also "lay" analysts who train and practice without the MD degree. Only those who are MDs can prescribe drugs and hospitalize patients. Though conventional psychoanalysis is a long-term form of treatment that can continue for years, many analysts see clients for short-term psychotherapy. Members of the American Psychoanalytic Association have received rigorous training in psychoanalytic institutes approved by the association. However, other institutes also train analysts, and almost anybody can legally call himself a "psychoanalyst."

Psychologists. Clinical psychologists may conduct psychotherapy with single patients (as medically trained psychoanalysts and psychiatrists do) or may work as counselors in businesses, schools, mental health centers, and hospitals. Requirements for licensing vary from state to state; practicing psychologists usually must have a doctorate plus postdoctoral training.

Social workers. The single largest group of professionals in the mental health field, social workers may direct clinics or have private practices and are often active in community programs, such as drug-abuse treatment. *Clinical social workers* have a master's degree and can offer psychotherapy or counseling and a range of diagnostic services. Health insurance in some states will not cover private treatment from social workers.

Marriage and family therapists. Many states also license counselors who specialize in marital problems and child-parent problems, though they can also treat individual problems such as anxiety and depression. The emphasis in treatment is on short-term therapy. Therapists undergo about the same amount of training as social workers.

Psychiatric nurses. This special area of nursing is concerned with the prevention and treatment of emotional and mental disorders. These registered nurses with advanced degrees may conduct individual and group therapy in or out of hospitals.

Psychotherapists. If you choose someone who practices under this title, ask about his or her training and background. Virtually anyone can use this title, so psychotherapists may or may not be trained, licensed, and qualified. If you are uncertain about credentials, check with the appropriate local professional associations.

HOW TO FIND HELP

When you're looking for a practitioner, educational and licensing qualifications are important, but you should consider other factors as well. What kind of therapist and what kind of therapy do you need? There is no simple answer, but there are certain guidelines.

If you or a family member suffers from psychosis, you'll need a practitioner who is an MD, because hospitalization and psychotherapeutic drugs may be necessary in addition to psy-

94

MENTAL HEALTH RESOURCES

If you are seeking help for emotional problems, potential sources of referrals for therapy and counseling include teaching hospitals, university departments of psychology and social work, and local self-help (support) groups. Increasingly, employee assistance programs are offering confidential counseling and referral. You can also check the Yellow Pages.

Many organizations provide information about mental health issues. These national organizations can be very helpful:

•**The Knowledge Exchange Network (KEN),** part of the federal government's Center for Mental Health Services, can direct anyone to federal, state, and local organizations that treat and prevent mental health problems. You can also gain access to more than 200 publications. Write to KEN, P.O. Box 42490, Washington, DC 20015. Telephone: 800-789-2647. Fax: 301-984-8796.

Web site: www.mentalhealth.org

•**The National Mental Health Association (NMHA)** can provide brochures and fact sheets on a variety of mental health topics as well as referrals for local treatment services. Write to them at 1021 Prince Street, Alexandria, VA 22314. Telephone: 800-969-NMHA [6642] or 703-684-7722. Fax: 703-684-5968. Web site: www.nmha.org

•**The National Mental Health Consumers' Self-Help Clearinghouse** helps connect individuals to self-help and advocacy resources for dealing with mental health issues. Write to them at 1211 Chestnut Street, Suite 1207, Philadelphia, PA 19107. Telephone: 800 553-4KEY [4539] or 215 751-1810. Fax: 215 636-6312. Web site: www.mhselfhelp.org

Professional Organizations

•**The American Psychiatric Association** offers pamphlets on mental disorders, substance abuse, and choosing a psychiatrist. Write to the APA Division of Public Affairs, Department KEN-97, 1400 K Street NW, Washington, DC 20005. Telephone: 202-682-6000 or 202-682-6325. Web site: www.psych.org

•**The American Psychological Association** also publishes pamphlets on mental health problems, as well as lists of psychological associations in your area. Write to the APA, Office of Public Affairs, 750 First Street NE, Washington, DC 20002-4242. Telephone: 800 964-2000 or 202 336-5700. Web site: www.helping.apa.org

•**The National Association of Social Workers (NASW)** publishes the Register of Clinical Social Workers, which provides a listing of clinical social workers who have met the national standards for education, credentials, and experience established by the association. The NASW Register can be purchased as a book or a CD-ROM, or it can be searched on the organization's Web site.

Contact the organization at 750 First Street NE, Suite 700, Washington DC 20002-4241. Telephone: 202-408-8600. Web site: www.naswdc.org

•**The American Association of Marriage and Family Therapy** provides tapes and brochures on topics affecting couples and families, including "A Consumer's Guide to Marriage and Family Therapy." It also provides listings of licensed counselors in the United States and Canada. Write to them at 1133 15th Street NW, Suite 300 Washington, DC 20005-2710. Telephone: 800-374-2638 or 202-452-0109. Fax: 202-223-2329. Web site: www.aamft.org

chotherapy. If you are dealing with less severe emotional difficulties (problems in your job, loneliness, marital tensions, or a divorce), you may do just as well with a trained and qualified therapist who is not an MD.

Maybe all you need is some sympathetic advice, or just somebody to listen to you and reassure you. Short-term therapy may be appropriate and is growing in availability. Indeed, one of the strongest trends of recent years has been toward a varied menu of therapies—everything from years of psychoanalysis to single sessions to self-help groups. It is important to find out how your therapist works and how you feel about the process.

If you're trying to help a child or adolescent, schools may have a list of recommended therapists and counselors. Whatever form of therapy you opt for, shop around before making a commitment. Find out what's available and what it costs. Talk with several therapists, if you wish, and compare approaches. Some people feel more comfortable with a therapist of the same sex. Most people will want to be sure that the therapist is comfortable with them, too—that he or she can treat emotional and sexual problems without prejudice. You'll be charged for trial visits to most therapists. Some therapists may be willing to discuss their methods over the telephone without charging.

EVALUATING THE CARE YOU GET

A therapist's credentials and reputation are important, but so are your own feelings. You should ask yourself if you feel comfortable with your therapist, and if you believe this person can help you. According to guidelines issued by the National Institute of Mental Health, you should be able to express your concerns openly with your therapist. If you don't "click" with one therapist, you should consider finding another. What professionals call "a positive therapeutic alliance" is important to making progress—which means, essentially, that you need to see your therapist as understanding and helpful. Be sure that both you and your therapist or group leader understand your goals—even if your goal is as vague as simply feeling less miserable. If you have doubts, express them to your therapist.

Do expect the same courtesy and level of professionalism, including confidentiality, from a therapist that you would from any doctor. Harsh criticism from a therapist is not appropriate, nor is group therapy that involves intimidation or verbal abuse. A sexual relationship or any out-of-the-office close personal relationship between a therapist and a patient is unethical and potentially damaging to the patient.

PAYING FOR CARE

A self-help group is usually free, which is an advantage. But self-help may not meet your needs. Psychoanalysis, on the other hand, can cost thousands of dollars annually. Drugs, if you require them, may be expensive. Short-term care is obviously less costly. Many doctors and clinics have fee scales and try to charge what their patients can afford.

Think twice before counting on your health insurance policy. Most insurance policies pay for "ambulatory" mental health care only in part. Some policies exclude psychiatric treatment altogether. Even more unfairly, if you've ever gone on record as having had psychiatric treatment, you may be turned down if you apply later for life insurance or other health insurance. Insurance companies classify mental health problems as "chronic diseases." Thus you may be penalized for undergoing any kind of therapy—and if you apply for reimbursement, it's part of your permanent medical record. Thus your future insurability may be jeopardized.

ALTERNATIVE THERAPIES AND PRACTITIONERS

If you have a chronic disorder or are suffering from persistent pain and your doctor can't help you, you can hardly be blamed for seeking relief through alternative forms of treatment. A variety of therapies and practitioners are considered part of alternative or complementary medicine—that is, they are not an integral part of conventional medicine as practiced by physicians with MD degrees and other health-care professionals who typically work with medical doctors.

Alternative therapies include traditional systems of medicine developed in other cultures (such as Chinese acupuncture or the Indian system of Ayurvedic medicine); Western treatment systems such as homeopathy; mind-body therapies such as meditation or hypnosis; remedies based on herbal or dietary supplements; therapies consisting of body movement and manipulation (chiropractic and massage, for example); and energy-based therapies such as Reiki (a Japanese-derived treatment based on channeling spiritual energy through the practitioner). Each therapy has its advocates and critics among patients, physicians, and researchers. One aspect all these therapies share is that their effectiveness has been difficult to demonstrate in controlled studies; evidence about them is frequently based on anecdotes from people who have gotten relief.

Therefore, it is safest to think of alternative treatments as adjunct therapy. In other words, don't substitute one or more of them for your regular medical care. Talk to your physician about any new approaches you're considering, and make sure he or she continues to keep an eye on your condition. There is little potential harm in trying an alternative treatment for pain relief, unless it keeps you from getting a correct diagnosis of a treatable or curable condition.

Be skeptical of treatments that claim to cure everything from depression to fatigue to cancer. Also beware of practitioners who are unlicensed or unregulated—and be wary of their products as well. For example, although there are a handful of medical doctors who practice homeopathy in the United States, in most states anybody can set up shop as a homeopath. A homeopathic practitioner will almost certainly sell you remedies that are made up of extremely diluted natural products and often contain nothing more than water or alcohol. (Homeopathic remedies are also easily purchased without a practitioner's advice—including remedies that claim to cure such diseases as arthritis, high blood pressure, and cancer.) It's true that these solutions are not likely to harm you—but can they do you any good?

What follows are descriptions of four types of practitioners who may be helpful for some conditions in some people. Still, when considering these alternatives to conventional medicine, stop and think: Are you certain of your diagnosis? Have you sought a second or even third opinion? Does your health insurance plan provide coverage? (An increasing number of plans are beginning to cover the cost of some alternative treatments, but many still do not. Be sure to check your plan.)

ACUPUNCTURISTS

Practiced in China for some 2,000 years, acupuncture has become one of the most popular alternative treatments in the United States. The theory of acupuncture is that by penetrating the skin with thin metal needles at specific anatomical locations, called acupuncture points, the flow-patterns of energy (called "Qi") will be altered healthfully or therapeutically. Sometimes the acupuncturist inserts the needles and leaves them in place for a period of time. Sometimes he or she manipulates them or applies electricity. Scientific medicine, of course, cannot show that Qi exists, cannot measure it, and cannot show that it is produced by any structure or process in the body—let alone find out whether inserting needles beneath the skin would alter it. Acupuncture needles should be inserted where Qi comes to the surface, but it is hard to ascertain where this is.

A panel of experts convened by the National Institutes of Health (NIH) to review studies of acupuncture concluded that it may be helpful for some conditions. The panel stated that biological responses have been demonstrated in people having acupuncture. That is, their bodies react chemically. It may be that needle-sticks at various points stimulate the body to produce pain-relieving and mood-lifting chemicals (such as endorphins and serotonin) or anti-inflammatory substances. Skeptics say that wishful thinking may also play a role—that acupuncture is possibly an example of the placebo effect: if you think it can help, it will.

What acupuncturists provide. Acupuncture has been used to treat a variety of kinds of pain—from backaches and headaches to dental problems. In China it's even used as anesthesia for some patients undergoing surgery. It appears to be effective as a short-term treatment; few studies have looked at its long-term effectiveness. Some researchers have reported that acupuncture can be effective even for animals in pain.

According to the NIH panel, there is clear evi-

CERTIFICATION FOR ACUPUNCTURISTS

If your prospective acupuncturist is a physician, check to see if he or she belongs to the American Academy of Medical Acupuncturists (AAMA) or was trained in an accredited acupuncture school. The AAMA group requires 200 hours of competency training as well as practical experience. Telephone: 800-521-2262; Web site: www.medicalacupuncture.org

If your acupuncturist is not licensed, another credential to check for is certification from the National Certification Commission for Acupuncture and Oriental Medicine (NCCAOM). To receive a Diplomate of Acupuncture, or Dipl.Ac., the acupuncturist must pass a written and practical exam and have a reasonable level of training.

Telephone: 703-548-9004.

Both organizations will also help you locate acupuncturists in your area.

dence that acupuncture is useful to treat the following: adult nausea and vomiting resulting from surgery or chemotherapy; morning sickness in pregnancy; and postoperative dental pain. It might be helpful as an adjunct or alternative therapy for conditions such as the following, although the evidence is not clear: menstrual cramps, addictions (such as smoking), muscle pain (as in conditions like fibromyalgia), tendinitis (tennis elbow), carpal tunnel syndrome, headache, low-back pain, asthma, and stroke rehabilitation.

Special risks. When performed by a trained practitioner who always uses sterile needles, acupuncture presents few risks. Incorrectly inserted needles can cause tissue swelling. If the needles are not sterilized and the skin not adequately cleaned, local infection or bloodborne diseases such as infection with HIV (the virus that causes AIDS) or hepatitis may result. Because of the risk of AIDS and hepatitis, disposable needles are recommended; some states require that acupuncturists use disposable needles. Electric stimulation, either from needles or from a transcutaneous electrical nerve stimulation (TENS) device, should not be used on a person with a pacemaker, a fever, or an irregular heartbeat.

Choosing an acupuncturist. Approximately 7,000 nonphysician acupuncturists currently use acupuncture to help control pain and to treat addictions, depression, insomnia, and other health problems. Also, an estimated 3,000 medical doctors and osteopaths have studied and use acupuncture in their medical practice.

Keep these points in mind when choosing an acupuncturist:

• In the United States, acupuncture can be legally performed in all states. Some states permit only physicians to perform it, while others allow supervised or unsupervised laypeople to practice. In choosing an acupuncturist, you should be aware of the licensing regulations in your state. The majority of states (and the District of Columbia) license nonphysician acupuncturists. However, not all states require competency exams or extensive training.

• If you are in a state that licenses acupuncturists, choose a state-licensed, board-certified practitioner (see page 98).

• Make sure the practitioner attended an accredited U.S. acupuncture college or a reputable overseas school. (Most American-trained acupuncturists now receive four years of education in accredited schools.)

CHIROPRACTORS

According to one estimate, about 5 percent of Americans see chiropractors regularly, and the majority like what they get. Yet many laypeople and physicians think chiropractic is worthless, fanciful, or even harmful. Indeed, chiropractors and the medical profession have waged verbal and economic war on one another for many years.

Chiropractic (a noun derived from the Greek *cheir*, meaning hand, and *praktikos*, meaning practical) was founded in 1895—about the same time that modern medical schools came into being. Chiropractic was based on the theory that subluxations (that is, minute misalignments of the vertebrae) are the source of illness, and that spinal manipulation can therefore prevent or cure illness. However, many chiropractors no longer endorse this "single source" theory or base their practice on it.

What chiropractors provide. One problem in sorting out the claims and counterclaims about chiropractic is that chiropractors now represent such a wide range of practices and treatments.

99

Within the profession, there are the "straights," or old-line practitioners, whose theoretical base is subluxation and who may obtain frequent x-rays and perform manipulations. The "mixers" may adopt other approaches. Some promote health fads like iridology and hair analysis, as well as prescribe and then sell vitamin supplements and "glandular" treatments of dubious value. Some look upon themselves as family doctors—and as the only health provider you'll ever need. Others work with medical doctors, referring patients and taking referrals.

Some newer-minded chiropractors have voiced criticisms of older theories and practices. The most progressive group, the National Association for Chiropractic Medicine (NACM), has disavowed the subluxation theory. NACM members limit themselves to treating low-back pain and are likely to work in tandem with medical doctors—considering themselves partners of the medical profession rather than competitors.

Recently, the RAND Corporation reviewed all existing scientific evidence and found that chiropractic can be effective in treating acute back pain when no serious neurological symptoms are present. But these findings were limited—in the RAND study, for example, only patients with acute low-back pain did better with chiropractic treatment. Those with chronic low-back pain, sciatica, or neurologic involvement did not do so well. Another review, published in the *British Medical Journal*, found that evidence supporting chiropractic treatment was not conclusive.

Evaluating practitioners. Chiropractic, like other professions, is evolving. One reason people like chiropractors is that they seem to take more time with patients, and the treatment is usually hands-on.

If you have acute low-back pain and wish to see a chiropractor, take these precautions:

• Be wary of any chiropractor who claims that subluxations are the root of most illnesses. Similarly, be wary of practitioners—and there are many—who claim to cure everything from bed-wetting, chronic fatigue syndrome, and migraines to menstrual cramps, cancer, and heart disease. A recent promotional piece from one New York chiropractor, for instance, claims that by "correcting spinal nerve stress" he can "turn on your inner doctor" and cure any of these ailments and more. The ad goes on to say, though, that chiropractors don't "treat disease." This is double talk.

• Be wary of any chiropractor who sells you the supplements and nutritional treatments he prescribes. State laws generally prohibit physicians, except in special circumstances, from selling the medicines they prescribe to their patients, and for good reason: such regulations were designed to protect patients from being exploited.

• Avoid any manipulation involving the neck, as this can be very dangerous.

• Don't agree to full-spine or full-body x-rays. According to the chiropractors who now work with the National Council Against Health Fraud (a California-based physician group), full-spine x-rays have little or no diagnostic value and expose patients to unnecessary and potentially dangerous amounts of radiation.

• When dealing with a chiropractor, as with any practitioner, it pays to be well informed and to protect yourself. As you would with a medical doctor, question a chiropractor about treatments. Don't believe anybody who promises miracles or who asks you to sign a "treatment contract" obligating you to show up every week or every month to "maintain" your health.

• The National Association for Chiropractic Medicine, whose members confine chiropractic treatment to management of neuromusculoskeletal disorders, offers assistance to consumers in finding member practitioners. For consumer information send a self-addressed stamped envelope to NACM, 15427 Baybrook Drive, Houston, TX 77062. You can also visit their Web site: www.chiromed.org

MASSAGE THERAPY

Massage (the word comes from the Arabic massa, to stroke) is one of the oldest hands-on therapies, but modern medical researchers have paid it little attention. Few controlled studies of the physical effects of massage have ever been attempted. What massage therapy can accomplish, however, is to relax muscles, relieve muscle spasms and pain, increase blood flow in the skin and muscles, ease mental stress, and induce relaxation. It can also be useful in increasing the range of motion of joints after injuries.

What massage therapists provide. Massage can be done to the entire body or restricted to the back, neck, shoulders, or feet. It typically involves kneading and stroking of the skin, and the application of pressure on tense muscles. The most common technique in America is known as "effleurage," or Swedish massage, a gentle stroking and kneading, sometimes with tapping, clapping, or similar percussive movements with the hands. Acupressure and shiatsu (finger pressure) are other massage systems that can be used along with or instead of stroking and kneading. There are many other massage techniques involving manipulating and pressing joints, bones, and soft tissues.

To do you good, massage should feel good. When tense muscles are massaged, you may feel discomfort or even brief pain. But a good massage should not be painful and should leave you feeling relaxed—not tense and certainly not sore.

Though you can massage your own body, massage is most relaxing when someone else does it for you. Many health professionals practice massage—physical therapists, athletic trainers, nurses, chiropractors, and, of course, qualified massage therapists.

Massage can be comforting and helpful, but it is not a substitute for the medical treatment of an injury. If you have an acute injury such as a sprain, tendinitis, or a swollen joint, get a physician's advice. Injuries should not be massaged directly. Because it is relaxing and stimulates blood flow, massage can be helpful for injured or sick people, especially if they are confined to bed.

Choosing a massage therapist. A number of states have agencies that regulate massage practice and require professional training for licensing (usually a minimum of 500 classroom hours). If you are looking for a masseur or masseuse in one of these states, seek a licensed therapist.

Elsewhere, find a member of the American Massage Therapy Association (AMTA); telephone: 847-864-0123. The association also has a Web site: www.amtamassage.org

Members have to graduate from an approved study program and pass an exam. Many doctors can refer you to a qualified massage therapist.

OSTEOPATHIC PHYSICIANS

Osteopathic medicine occupies a unique niche. Though osteopathy once stood very much outside the conventional medical establishment, its practitioners have moved increasingly toward the practice of mainstream medicine. Doctors of osteopathic medicine, or DOs, receive training akin to that of MDs. They complete a four-year program of basic medical education at an osteopathic medical college, then typically serve an

101

internship where they gain experience in internal medicine, family practice, pediatrics, and obstetrics. Many DOs then take a residency program in a medical specialty. Indeed, DOs practice in all branches of medicine, from psychiatry to obstetrics to emergency medicine, though most function as primary-care practitioners rather than as specialists. And they are licensed in all 50 states to deliver the same kinds of services—from prescribing drugs to delivering babies and performing surgery—that MDs can.

Osteopathic medicine was developed in the late 1800s by Dr. Andrew Still, who believed that manual manipulation of the musculoskeletal system was useful in stimulating the body's ability to fight disease and restore health. But as medical science developed, osteopaths, unlike chiropractors, incorporated many of modern medicine's techniques, and today's practitioners typically utilize standard diagnostic tests, medication, and surgery. Still, many (though by no means all) DOs have continued to place an emphasis on the musculoskeletal system as the key to understanding and treating many health problems. Some DOs also incorporate other modes of alternative medicine such as homeopathy and craniosacral therapy (manipulating the skull bones to relieve pain) into their treatment. Currently, there is much debate within the osteopathic community over the role of manipulation therapies and other alternative treatments.

What osteopaths provide. Osteopaths, especially those in general or family practice, treat a wide range of conditions, from colds and flu to asthma, migraines, high blood pressure, gynecological problems, sinusitis—virtually any health problem an MD will deal with. Typically, a DO will evaluate your condition using blood and urine testing, x-rays, and other medical diagnostic tools—but will also touch your back and limbs and check your joints, muscles, and ligaments for tenderness, pain, and signs of injury or impairment. Once a problem has been diagnosed, treatment may entail a combination of osteopathic and conventional methods. In treating, say, an attack of sinusitis, a DO might employ manipulation to help drain sinuses and relieve pain, but will also prescribe an antibiotic to combat the infection.

Back pain and other musculoskeletal problems are still among the most common complaints that initially send people to an osteopath. Few studies have been done assessing the effectiveness of osteopathic manual therapy for treating back pain. But one study published in the *New England Journal of Medicine* found that patients treated by DOs for low-back pain that had lasted three weeks to six months had as good an outcome as patients treated by MDs—and the DO-treated patients recovered with less reliance on medication. Of course, the effect of any treatment for low-back pain is difficult to measure, since most cases of back pain will eventually improve without any treatment.

As osteopathy has moved closer to mainstream medicine, it's often not clear what a DO offers that is truly distinctive from the services of an MD. Some osteopaths claim that their form of medicine focuses on preventive care and treating the "whole person"—but in recent years, MDs have paid increasing attention to disease prevention and wellness, further blurring the line between the two professions. In a parallel trend, one survey of osteopaths found that younger DOs are less likely than their older colleagues to use osteopathic manipulation in treating patients.

Two distinctions are worth considering. A greater percentage of DOs than MDs work in rural communities underserved by MDs—and DOs are more likely than MDs to end up as primary-care and family practitioners. Hence, in some communities, gaining access to a DO may be easier than obtaining care from an MD. DOs may also charge less than MDs.

Choosing an Osteopath. There are about 40,000 DOs in practice in the United States (they make up about 5 percent of American physicians). DOs are licensed by state boards, just as MDs are, for the full practice of medicine and surgery. In some states, the same tests are given to DOs and MDs; other states administer separate licensing exams. Increasingly, medical insurance covers services from a DO.

You can locate a licensed DO in your area by contacting the American Osteopathic Association at 142 East Ontario Street, Chicago, IL 60611. Telephone: 800 621-1773; Fax: 312 202-8200; Web site: www.am-osteo-assn.org

In addition to listing practitioners, the association also has information on osteopathic services and training and provides listings of accredited colleges and osteopathic organizations in different states (which can also provide names of DOs in your area). The association does not represent all DOs, and it embraces many of the benefits attributed to osteopathic manipulation.

If you decide to turn to a DO for primary care, choose one who has trained as a medical resident. Ask about his or her philosophy of diagnosis and treatment—and opt for a practitioner who does not promote osteopathic manipulation either as a general therapy or as the primary treatment for health problems other than back pain.

When It's a Medical Emergency

Most health complaints aren't emergencies. But some problems demand urgent care—which means either calling your local Emergency Medical Service or getting to the nearest emergency room. You shouldn't attempt to treat the problem yourself unless you are trained in emergency first aid. Symptoms and warning signals that doctors generally consider emergencies are shown below in blue.

However, emergency rooms should not be used for nonemergency situations or in place of routine medical care. In fact, going to an emergency room for routine medical care is usually a mistake. Emergency rooms will not have access to your medical records and are, in any case, oriented to handle emergencies rather than ordinary medical problems (like most of those described in this book). In addition, many insurance companies will not pay for nonessential visits to emergency rooms.

- severe chest pain
- difficulty breathing or shortness of breath
- severe abdominal pain
- slurring or loss of speech
- convulsions
- unconsciousness
- uncontrollable bleeding
- bullet or stab wounds
- broken bones
- head injuries
- eye injuries, sudden loss of vision, or foreign substances in the eyes

- poisoning
- drug overdose
- choking
- smoke inhalation
- gaseous fume inhalation
- heat stroke or dehydration
- hypothermia
- prolonged vomiting or diarrhea
- snake or animal bites
- insect stings resulting in shortness of breath

The following are not good reasons to go to an emergency room, but consider calling your doctor.
- colds, coughs, sore throat, flu
- rashes
- moderate to high fever
- earache
- possible sprain
- small cut or superficial dog bite
- conjunctivitis (pinkeye)
- bladder infection

Immediate Care

Bite Wounds • Bruises • Burns • Choking • Cuts, Scrapes, and Wounds • Frostbite • Heart Attack • Heat Exhaustion and Heat Stroke • Hypothermia (Cold Exposure) • Knocked-Out Tooth • Nosebleeds • Poison Ivy, Oak, Sumac • Poisoning • Snake Bites • Spider Bites • Stings from Insects • Stings from Marine Animals • Stroke • Tick and Chigger Bites

▶ BITE WOUNDS

Any bite wound is a cause for concern, since animals harbor a multitude of microorganisms in the mouth—and bite wounds that break the skin therefore carry a risk of infection that includes *Staphylococcus, Streptococcus, Pasteurella multocida* (bacterial infections of the skin), and tetanus (a disease of the central nervous system caused by infection of a wound with spores of the bacterium *Clostridium tetani).*

The most worrisome concern after an animal bite is rabies, a viral brain disease that is almost always fatal if not treated promptly (see page 108). However, if the bite hasn't come from a wild animal, infection from rabies is unlikely, since most rabies in the United States—over 90 percent—is carried by wild animals. In addition, depending on the depth and extent of the wound, there is a possibility of damage to bone, tendons, and other underlying tissues.

Dog and Cat Bites

The great majority of bites come from dogs and cats. Over the past few years dog bites have become a significant problem—first and foremost for children, who are most vulnerable to serious injury from dogs. Dogs bite more than four million people in the United States each year, and the number of dog bites needing medical attention jumped from 585,000 in 1986 to about 800,000 annually by the mid-1990s—a period when the dog population did not increase by much.

According to data from the National Center for Health Statistics, the median age of patients bitten was 15 years, with children, especially boys aged five to nine, having the highest incident rate. Young children in particular were also more likely than adults to get bitten in the head, neck, and face area.

Though they may seem less serious, cat bites are actually more likely to lead to infection than dog bites—30 to 50 percent of cat bites become infected compared with 5 to 10 percent of dog bites. This is because cats have sharp teeth that can penetrate deep into the skin and reach the muscle, tendons, and bone underneath.

Immediate Care for Bites

Animal bites should always be treated promptly, no matter how minor they seem. But the treatment varies depending on how severe the bite is and whether or not the animal is a household pet or an unfamiliar or wild animal, as explained below.

• *For a superficial bite or nip from a household pet that has been vaccinated,* wash the bite and any scratches thoroughly with plenty of soap and running water. This can reduce exposure to infectious agents. You can also apply a small bandage.

• *Be sure that tetanus immunization for you, or for a child who has been bitten, is up to date.* If you haven't had a tetanus shot within 10 years, you may need one.

• *For a deeper bite, or a bite from a wild animal or an unfamiliar domestic animal,* washing the bite area is the most valuable first step. After washing thoroughly, elevate the injury and apply ice. Then call your doctor or go to the emergency room of a hospital.

Prevention Tips

The people most likely to suffer bite wounds are children. Moreover, most bites are caused by a person's own pet or by an animal the person is familiar with. About 5 percent of bites come from rodents and other wild and domestic animals.

Bites from both domestic and wild animals are highly preventable.

• *Be a responsible dog owner.* You can significantly reduce the chance that your dog will bite you or anyone else by properly training your pet.

• *Obey leash and licensing laws*—they protect dogs as well as people. Keep vaccinations up to date, and provide good health care for your dog.

• *Don't assume that even the gentlest dog will behave with children,* unless the animal is accustomed to children's ways and has been socialized. Infants and toddlers are the most frequent victims of dog attacks—and the attacker is most often a family pet. Even a small dog can severely injure or kill a small child. Provide supervision, and teach your children how to interact with dogs.

• *Approach a strange dog with caution, and tell kids not to approach a dog on their own.* When entering a house where there's a dog, let the owner introduce you and any child in your care. Speak to the dog, offer a hand (fist closed) to be sniffed. Let the dog warm up to you first. If it appears reluctant or uninterested, let it be.

• *Never beat, kick, jerk, tease, or torment a cat or dog.* Gentleness is the watchword.

• *Never goad a dog to attack.* Don't play rough games with a dog, such as wrestling or tail pulling.

• *Don't bother a dog* that is eating, sleeping, or caring for puppies. To wake a dog, call it rather than touching it.

• *If you encounter a strange dog off the leash, stay still.* Don't run or scream. Dogs, like wolves, will instinctively chase and attack a fleeing target. If a dog growls, bristles, or stands stiff-legged, it may be about to attack.

• *If you are attacked by a dog, protect your face, arms, hands, and legs.* Roll up on the ground with your back in the air.

• *Observe wild animals from a distance.* In particular, don't try to make a pet of a raccoon, squirrel, or other wild animal. Be particularly cautious

107

HUMAN BITES

After dog and cat bites, human bites are the most common mammalian bite. If a bite breaks the skin, the chance of infection is 10 to 50 percent. Up to 42 species of bacteria have been isolated from the human mouth, and human bites are generally more likely to produce infection than dog bites. It's also possible for a human bite to transmit herpes viruses or hepatitis B and C.

People, particularly children, may bite others during fights; some serious bites occur during sexual activity. Dentists get bitten, and sometimes people having seizures inadvertently bite those trying to help them.

• The most common human bites are called "simple"—meaning that teeth sink into the skin. If the bite is superficial, just breaking the skin, simply wash the wound well with soap and water and apply a small bandage. But a deep bite wound should not be neglected. Before you leave for the emergency room or the doctor's office, wash the wound thoroughly with soap and water—always the first line of defense against infection.

• Less common and much more serious is the so-called "clenched fist injury," occurring when one person punches another in the mouth and the knuckles are lacerated. These injuries are most likely to result in infection; bones are often broken as well, or fingers dislocated. Such wounds require medical attention as soon as possible.

about wild animals that appear tame or lethargic, or that are fearless or aggressive. Also beware of any ordinarily nocturnal animal that is out in daylight. Such odd behavior might be a sign of rabies.

Minimizing the Risk of Rabies

Rabies is a viral disease transmitted by the saliva of infected animals. Any warm-blooded animal can carry it, but it is mostly found in raccoons, foxes, skunks, and bats. (Being bitten by an infected animal is almost the only way that humans are exposed to the disease, though airborne transmission is possible in a heavily infested bat cave.)

Animals that do not carry rabies include small rodents such as mice (though squirrels can carry the disease) and reptiles such as lizards and snakes.

Symptoms of rabies may include fever, pain at the site of the bite, aggressive behavior, hallucinations, extreme weakness, throat spasms that prevent swallowing, and thirst. Rabies may occur months or even years after the animal bite (another reason why all bites require prompt medical attention).

If left untreated until symptoms appear, rabies is usually fatal, but it can be caught and stopped if treatment is begun within 10 days after exposure. A series of five injections—using a version of the rabies vaccination discovered a century ago by Louis Pasteur—is very effective in combating the virus.

The treatment is expensive but less painful and less drawn out than it was years ago. Every year about 20,000 Americans get these shots. Serious side effects from the vaccine are quite rare.

Raccoons, which thrive in great numbers as suburban scavengers, are now the chief source of rabies, and while rabid raccoons seldom attack people, they do attack dogs and cats. Vaccination

of pets, practiced since the 1940s, almost wiped out rabies in domestic animals. In the 1950s skunks and foxes became reservoirs of the disease in the wild, later to be outpaced by bats and then, in the 1970s, by raccoons, so that unvaccinated pets are now at greater risk of exposure.

No human deaths have been attributed so far to raccoon rabies, but unvaccinated dogs and cats have died. To minimize the likelihood that you or your pet will be exposed to rabies, follow these steps:

- *Vaccinate your pets regularly,* as recommended by your veterinarian.
- *Don't let pets roam outdoors at night,* when they are more likely to come into contact with wild animals.
- *Keep outdoor garbage cans tightly sealed* to discourage animal scavengers.

For More Information

- American Academy of Dermatology
- Medlineplus (National Institutes of Health)

▶ BRUISES

A bruise is a discoloration of the skin that appears shortly after an impact injury caused by a blow or a fall, for example. Such an injury causes damage to blood vessels and subsequent bleeding into the skin. Bruises can also arise from taking certain medications that interfere with blood clotting (including aspirin), thereby causing more bleeding into the skin and tissues.

Bruises typically start out as reddish tinges, but change to black-and-blue or purplish hues before finally turning greenish-yellow as the body reabsorbs the blood. The discoloration that appears on the skin is actually blood that has settled in the area just below the skin surface or above the muscle.

Immediate Care for Bruises

Most bruises will heal by themselves in a week or so. But you can speed healing and get some pain relief with the following measures.

• **Reduce swelling**. Apply an ice pack to the area as soon as possible . The cold constricts the blood vessels and thereby stops the bleeding. The more blood that collects after an injury, the more pronounced the bruise will be and the longer it will take to disappear.

Put the ice pack over a clean towel and place it directly on the injury site. Hold it there for about 20 minutes. Depending on the size and severity of the bruise, repeat every two or three waking hours for the first 24 to 48 hours to minimize swelling.

• **Switch to heat**. After 48 hours, apply heat to the area for 15-minute increments, three times a day. A warm bath or shower, a warm washcloth, a heating pad on a low or medium setting, or a whirlpool all work well to open the surrounding blood vessels and speed up healing.

• **Minimize pain**. For minor discomfort, take acetaminophen according to label directions. Avoid NSAIDs such as aspirin and ibuprofen because of their tendency to thin the blood and possibly cause additional swelling and bruising.

• **Elevate**. If possible, keep the damaged area raised above the level of the heart. This will allow blood to flow away from the injured area, helping to decrease bleeding and swelling.

When To Seek Medical Help

Contact your physician if bruises appear on the body for no apparent reason. They may be symptomatic of different diseases, including leukemia, hemophilia, and aplastic anemia.

Bruises that appear under the fingernails may be a warning sign of an early melanoma (the most dangerous form of skin cancer), and so should be evaluated by a physician.

Contact your ophthalmologist if you are struck in the eye and develop a black eye. The colorful bruising of the skin around the eye is typical after impact, but the impact itself may be damaging to the eye and should be evaluated.

Also see a doctor if a bruise doesn't appear to be healing after two or three days.

For More Information

• American Academy of Dermatology

▶ BURNS

A burn is damage to the skin from a heat source, a corrosive chemical, or electricity. Chemical burns, which can range from mild to severe, result from contact with acids or alkalis (such as lye). Electrical burns occur when someone touches faulty or uninsulated wiring (or when a child chews through the wiring).

Types of Burns

Burns are classified according to their degree of severity and the amount of skin involved.

First-degree burns damage only the epidermis (the outer skin layer). They cause reddening of the skin, tenderness, possibly some swelling. This type of burn is not dangerous but can be extremely painful. Such a burn is usually the result of some minor household accident, such as grabbing the handle of a pan that's too hot, touching a hot iron, or scalding yourself with hot water or steam. Mild sunburn is also classified as first degree.

Second-degree burns damage the epidermis and part of the dermis (the underlying skin layer). They cause pain, blistering, redness, mild to moderate swelling. Because of fluid leaking from damaged blood vessels, the layers separate from one another, which causes blisters to form. Although very painful, second-degree burns are generally not critical unless they are quite large or become infected.

Third-degree burns destroy all skin layers and cause damage to muscle, bone, blood vessels, and nerves beneath the skin. The skin may turn white, red, brown, tan, or black (charred) in color. There is no blistering, but extensive swelling occurs. Because of nerve damage, there is often little or no immediate pain and generally no bleeding.

Third-degree burns, which often leave scars when they heal, are serious; they can be fatal (because the skin can no longer insulate the body from microorganisms that cause disease), and they should always be treated as a medical emergency.

Immediate Care for Minor Burns

Most minor burns—which include first-degree burns and second-degree burns that are small and haven't occurred in sensitive areas such as the genitals, face, or soles of the feet—will usually heal without treatment. However, applying cold water right away to a burn will help minimize damage, speed healing, and reduce the chance of potential infection. More severe burns require medical attention.

The best way to treat a minor burn is not, as many people believe, with butter; butter won't relieve pain and may cause infection if blisters form and then break. The following measures provide relief and speed healing.

• *Rinse the burned area in cold water.* Cold water is by far the most effective first-aid treatment; it eases the pain as it cleanses. If you burn yourself, immerse the burn in cold water (or ice water), or hold it under cold running water for 15 minutes. Continually applying fresh cold-water compresses will help if it's not practical to immerse the burned area, or use ice wrapped in a towel.

For chemical burns, immediately rinse the skin with a steady flow of water from a spigot, shower, or hose for 10 to 15 minutes.

• *Bandage the burn.* After applying cold water or compresses to a burn, you can bandage it with sterile gauze pads held on by tape if you wish. However, if blisters appear, try not to burst them. Dry the burn carefully before bandaging. You can apply a light dressing of an over-the-counter antibiotic cream (such as Polysporin or Neosporin), which will soothe the area, keep the skin moist, and protect it from infection.

• *Don't apply burn ointments.* Like butter (or mayonnaise), these ointments, usually oil-based, won't relieve pain but instead will trap heat, slow down healing, and increase the risk of infection.

• *Leave small blisters alone.* Blisters smaller than a dime that appear soon after the burn will usually shrink within a day or two and be reabsorbed by the body.

• *Contact your doctor if a burn site becomes infected.* Signs of infection include redness and pain that grow worse over a few days, pus that forms in blisters, an offensive odor at the burn site, and/or fever. After examining the burn to assess its severity, your doctor will clean and dress the injury and may also prescribe oral antibiotics to ward off infections.

Immediate Care for Major Burns

Seek medical attention right away if there are signs of a third-degree burn (lack of immediate pain, whiteness, and charring) or for a second-degree burn that covers an area larger than your hand or is on the face, hands, genitals, or other sensitive areas.

In the meantime, cover the area with sterile gauze, if possible.

For an electrical burn, get medical help even if it appears superficial, since damage from electrical burns is usually deeper and more serious than the surface burn indicates.

It's also usually advisable to contact your doctor for bad sunburn if the pain is especially intense or there is severe blistering.

Prevention Tips

Burns are often caused by accidents that are preventable. In addition to commonsense care when cooking or ironing, take these steps:

• *Be sure to secure any containers of corrosive chemicals,* repair loose wiring, and—if you have small children in your home—place covers over any unused electrical outlets.

• *Wear protective clothing and glasses* when working with chemicals.

• *Have working smoke detectors* on each floor of your home and a fire extinguisher in the kitchen.

For More Information

• Medlineplus (National Institutes of Health)

▶ CHOKING

Upper-airway obstructions account for about 3,000 deaths in the United States each year. Slapping someone on the back is not as effective as abdominal thrusts, sometimes called the Heimlich maneuver. Most people have probably seen this maneuver illustrated on posters in restaurants, and ideally everyone should know how to do it. It is best to learn it in a first aid or CPR class. Classes are offered by the American Heart Association and the American Red Cross.

Immediate Care for Choking

In general terms, here is what you should do if someone is choking. If he can still breathe and speak, wait a moment to see if he can dislodge the obstruction on his own. If he can't breathe (or only with difficulty), speak, or cough (or only weakly) and is clutching his throat, do the following while someone else calls 911 or the Emergency Medical Service.

• *Stand behind the choking person and wrap your arms around his or her waist.* Tip the person forward slightly.

• *Make a fist with one hand.* Place your fist with the thumb against the abdomen between the breastbone and navel, slightly above the person's navel.

• *Grab the fist with the other hand and thrust quickly and firmly upward into the abdomen.* Repeat until the food or object is dislodged.

The above maneuver should not be used for babies less than a year old. Instead, do the following:

• *Hold the baby along your forearm or arm,* positioning the body so that the head is lower than the feet.

• *With the heel of your hand, deliver four firm blows* between the baby's shoulder blades.

• *If this doesn't stop the choking, turn the baby over* and use your forefinger to deliver four quick upward thrusts to the chest.

• *If the baby is still choking, open the mouth* and move the jaw and tongue to look for an object in the throat. If you can see the object, try to gently remove it using a sweeping motion with your little finger. (Only do this if you can see the object;

otherwise, inserting your finger in the child's throat may push the object further in or trigger a gag reflex.)

Keep repeating all of the above steps until the object is dislodged. If the baby doesn't begin to breathe at that point, apply mouth-to-mouth resuscitation.

Performing Heimlich on Yourself

The do-it-yourself Heimlich maneuver is a good thing for everyone to know, in case choking occurs when no one is around. Make a fist and place the thumb side against your abdomen, slightly above the navel. With the other hand, grasp the fist and press it in and upward with quick, sharp thrusts.

Another method: press your abdomen forcefully against the back of a chair, table, sink, or railing. Repeat until air is forced through the airway and the food is expelled.

For More Information
- American Red Cross
- American Heart Association

▶ CUTS, SCRAPES, AND WOUNDS

At some time in your life, you are bound to suffer an accident in which you scrape, cut, or puncture your skin—injuries in which the outer skin barrier has been penetrated. Symptoms range from narrow tears in the skin (cuts) to superficial abrasions (scrapes) to deep holes (punctures). Usually bleeding occurs, though some puncture wounds may bleed only slightly. Because any such injury leaves you prone to infection, the damage needs to be dealt with immediately.

Types of Injuries

A cut is typically caused by a sharp implement with an edge that may be smooth (a knife or a razor blade, for example) or jagged (a piece of broken glass). If the cut is deep, it will bleed profusely, and there may be damage to underlying muscle, tendons, and nerves.

A scrape results from skin being rubbed against a rough surface like pavement. The outer skin layer may not be completely broken, but because small blood vessels are ruptured, the skin may ooze blood.

A puncture wound is caused by a nail, pin, or other sharp object with a penetrating point.

Immediate Care for Cuts and Scrapes

Most minor cuts and scrapes will heal on their own. However, skin is a barrier against germs and infections, so ignoring cuts and scrapes, no matter how minor, can leave you vulnerable to infection. Deep cuts or puncture wounds require medical attention.

Many remedies—from hydrogen peroxide to Mercurochrome to antiseptic sprays and ointments—have enjoyed popularity over the years. The truth is, most small wounds can be attended to without much doctoring and will heal in a week to 10 days.

• *First, stop the bleeding*—if there's any amount of it—by applying pressure with a clean cloth or tissue. Since blood takes a while to clot, you may need to press down for as long as 10 minutes.

If blood soaks through the cloth or tissue, don't remove it. Instead, apply another cloth on top of what you have in place and apply more pressure. If possible, elevate the wounded part above heart level to slow blood flow. (Exception: a puncture wound, from a nail or needle or similar long, sharp object, should be encouraged to bleed as part of the cleansing process.)

• **Second, avoid infection.** This is the main concern with any small wound. You can best accomplish this by cleaning the wound and keeping it clean. Cleanse a scrape or cut by swabbing gently with a clean wet cloth or by holding the injured part under cold running water. Use a mild soap in the area, but try to keep it out of the wound *per se* because it can cause irritation. If there are dirt particles clinging to a scrape or cut, remove them with tweezers (wash the tweezers first and dip the tips in alcohol before using).

• **If you can't wash the wound, lick it.** Licking a wound is a time-honored practice that may actually help disinfect it and promote healing, according to a small study in *The Lancet*. Researchers found that nitrites in saliva react with the skin to make nitric oxide, a chemical that can kill bacteria. Saliva also contains other substances that can help in healing.

• **Apply a bandage.** If the wound is likely to get dirty, if the area needs protection from further injury, or if you would just feel more comfortable, a homemade or store-bought adhesive bandage is in order. Change the bandage at least once daily to keep the wound clean.

• **Don't pick.** It's a good idea to keep small wounds dry and expose them to air as soon as possible. While scabs may not be desirable for large or surgical wounds, they protect against infection in small wounds. Don't pick a scab off—allow it to fall off after the skin has healed.

• **Don't apply antiseptics.** Contrary to myth, hydrogen peroxide does not cleanse wounds, but can irritate the skin and retard healing. Antisep-

BANDAGES: OFTEN NOT NECESSARY

For most small wounds, keeping the wound dry and exposed to air will make it heal faster. A scab helps protect the area from infection and shouldn't be removed until the wound has healed. But for temporary protection of a minor wound, ready-made bandage strips are fine. These come in a variety of shapes and styles for different small injuries.

Do buy: A generic-name bandage, since it is as good as any brand name, provided you can get the size and type you like. Waterproof bandages can be worth the extra cost if the wound is constantly exposed to water.

Don't buy: Bandages with antiseptics (applying antiseptics to a wound isn't a good idea anyway, as explained above); bandages with antibiotic creams (which can irritate the skin or induce allergic reactions, and offer few benefits); bandages with aloe or vitamin E on the pad (these aren't worth paying extra for, since they will have little effect on a wound—and topically applied vitamin E may cause rashes in some people).

For certain large serious wounds, some studies have shown that moisture can aid healing. Flexible, transparent, waterproof bandages called occlusive bandages are designed to retain moisture around a wound and protect it from dirt and bacteria. Hospitals use occlusive bandages, but you can also find them in drugstores. However, if you have a wound serious enough for an occlusive bandage (which has to be changed at intervals if the wound is draining), you probably need medical advice.

tic solutions—rubbing alcohol, iodine, and hexyl-resorcinol—kill some microorganisms and the Food and Drug Administration (FDA) permits them to be sold for cleaning small wounds. But they really are not needed and in fact can be damaging. (Iodine can actually burn your skin under a tight bandage.)

Such solutions as Mercurochrome and Merthiolate (once medicine cabinet staples) contain mercury, which is highly toxic, and are not judged safe or effective by the FDA.

For cuts and scrapes that are hard to keep clean, try Betadine (povidone iodine) ointment.

• *Antibiotic ointments are unnecessary for small wounds.* These products offer no benefits for helping a wound to heal. If you want an ointment to keep a bandage from sticking to the wound, use petroleum jelly.

Immediate Care for Puncture Wounds

• *Help the bleeding.* A puncture wound often doesn't bleed freely, so bacteria, instead of washing away, may be sealed in. If such a wound is not bleeding enough, press gently around the wound to encourage bleeding.

• *Clean the wound.* Examine the wound and remove any dirt particles or other foreign objects from it with tweezers. (Wash the tweezers first and dip in rubbing alcohol before using.) Clean the wound with soap and cool running water and cover it with a sterile dressing.

• *Reduce the risk of infection.* A deep puncture wound on the hand may lead to an infection that is hard to combat; preventive antibiotic treatment may be advisable for such a wound. If the wound is deep or was made with a dirty object and you haven't had a tetanus shot within 10 years, contact your doctor about tetanus immunization.

When To Seek Medical Help

In any of the following situations, call your doctor or go straight to the emergency room:

• If bleeding comes in spurts. This indicates that an artery may have been cut and that you might not be able to stop the bleeding. Cover the wound with a large, soft cloth, and if possible elevate it above heart level. Press directly on the wound to help stop blood flow; apply an additional compress on top of the first, if necessary. Don't use a tourniquet, which can damage nerves.

• If a cut looks very deep, or if the edges of the wound gap open. A jagged cut, particularly from broken glass, is likely to need medical attention. If you need stitches, you should not wait more than six hours to get them.

• If a scrape is very large (for example, the whole length of your arm or leg) and there are bits of debris in it.

• If your face is cut. You may need plastic surgery to avoid scarring.

• If you have a deep puncture wound, especially if it was made with a dirty object (for example, a gardening tool), and if you haven't had a tetanus booster within the past 10 years. If more time has passed or you don't remember when you last had one, arrange to have a tetanus immunization as soon as possible.

• If you have a puncture wound of the head, chest, or abdomen—particularly if you experience numbness or tingling, which may indicate nerve damage.

• If you think a wound has hidden dirt or debris in it.

• If any sign of infection develops. Signs include redness, swelling, or discharge; fever; red streaks spreading from the wound site. You may need to soak the wound to keep the puncture open and encourage draining.

After a careful examination a physician may administer a local anesthetic, and if you have a deep abrasion, the area will be cleaned completely. If necessary, deep cuts will be closed with stitches to eliminate the risk of infection and ensure proper healing. To reduce visible scarring due to cuts on the face, consult a plastic surgeon as soon as possible.

Tetanus

Tetanus is a serious, potentially fatal infection you can get from a wound. You should get a tetanus booster shot every 10 years. If it's been more than 10 years since your last inoculation, your doctor will give you a booster shot. For a severe, dirty, or contaminated wound, a booster shot is advised if it's been more than five years since your last booster.

For More Information

- American Red Cross
- Centers for Disease Control and Prevention

▶ FROSTBITE

Frostbite occurs from exposure to cold weather. Temperature and length of exposure determine how quickly frostbite occurs, and the wind-chill factor is also critical. At 30°F, with no wind, exposed hands would only become frostbitten after prolonged exposure. But at the same temperature in a 40-mile-an-hour wind, the wind-chill equivalent is 4°F, and frostbite becomes a real risk.

Risk of frostbite also increases if you are wearing damp clothing, have consumed alcohol, have a below-average percentage of body fat, or have a previous history of frostbite.

Signs of Frostbite

Frostbite can be insidious—if you've been out in the cold a while and your skin and extremities already feel cold and numb, you may not notice that it has set in. One it has set in, symptoms can progress from mild to serious, designated by the following categories:

Frostnip. The first hint of frostnip is numbness, followed by a whitening of the tissue—a change that can take place very quickly. Skin may also start to harden. Frostnip usually affects the nose, ears, hands, or feet.

Superficial frostbite. If frostnip progresses to superficial frostbite, the area will appear very white and waxy and will feel hard on the surface, yet will have its normal resilience in the lower layers.

Deep frostbite. At this stage, the tissues can turn blotchy or blue and will be very hard, without any underlying resilience. Blistering may also occur.

115

Immediate Care for Frostbite

If you do not get out of the cold, frostnip will progress to frostbite—and at that point, medical attention is required to avoid severe damage to skin. *If you suspect symptoms of either superficial or deep frostbite, contact the nearest doctor or hospital emergency room.*

Treatment for each type of frostbite varies. But until medical aid is available, several guidelines apply to all three types:

- Never massage or rub frostbitten areas (with or without snow).
- Do not apply any ointments.
- Get out of the cold, if possible.
- Don't drink alcoholic beverages.
- When checking any frostbitten part of the body, press very gently. Be careful not to hit, bump, or rub the area.

• **For frostnip,** apply warmth directly. Blow on the areas, or get someone else to do so; if your nose is frostnipped, apply your warm hands. If it's your hands that are freezing, put them in your warm armpits. Your skin will probably burn and tingle as it warms, but there should be no lasting injury.

• **For superficial frostbite,** warm the affected areas. Superficial frostbite requires medical attention, but there are some steps you should take first. Once you've gotten out of the cold, warm the area, preferably by immersion in warm water (100°F to 105°F—a temperature that should feel comfortably warm, but not hot, to undamaged skin). The warming process may be painful. Keep adding warm water as necessary, but take care that the water doesn't get too hot.

Avoid dry heat or uncontrolled heat sources such as campfires. Also, don't try to walk on frostbitten feet, and avoid the temptation to rub frostbitten hands or fingers. On the way to the emergency room or doctor, keep the area warm.

• **For deep frostbite,** get to an emergency room. Don't try to administer first aid or thaw the tissue. Wrap the frozen area in a blanket or other soft material to prevent bruising, and keep it elevated on the way to the hospital.

Prevention Tips

Proper clothing and some commonsense precautions are the key to preventing frostbite.

• **Be careful when temperatures dip below 20°F.** The risk of frostbite is much higher, so plan carefully before going outside. A cold wind will accentuate the chilling of tissue, and altitude is also a factor: it's generally colder at higher elevations.

• **Use skin moisturizer before going outside.** This will slow the loss of body heat. Apply it to your hands, face, and any other body part that may become exposed to the cold.

• **Dress appropriately for the conditions.** Dress in layers (see page 122); make sure that the outer layer is windproof and waterproof. Footwear should be watertight. Make sure ears, nose, and face are adequately covered. For extra protection, wear a face mask.

• **Wear heavy mittens instead of gloves.** When the fingers are together in the mitten, their collective body heat keeps the hand warm.

• **Don't drink alcoholic beverages.** Although alcohol gives the illusion of warmth, in addition to causing heat loss by widening the blood vessels, alcohol may also cause you to ignore critical frostbite signals.

• **Don't smoke.** Nicotine impairs blood flow by constricting small arteries in the skin and the extremities.

• **Never touch very cold metal with your bare hands.** Moisture on the skin will cause it to stick to the metal and become damaged.

• **Be careful at the gas pump.** Gasoline splashed on exposed skin in freezing temperatures lowers skin temperature, making it more susceptible to frostbite.

• **Equip your car.** When traveling during the winter, keep a blanket or sleeping bag in your car at all times. If weather conditions force you to pull over to the side of the road, use the covers or bag to keep warm. Unless you're properly dressed, don't leave the car in frigid weather; you put yourself at high risk.

For More Information

• Centers for Disease Control and Prevention

116

▶ HEART ATTACK

Most of us know that chest pain or pressure is a key symptom of a heart attack. But studies show that many people don't recognize other symptoms or don't seek emergency help right away—perhaps out of denial or because they are embarrassed—that the problem will turn out not to be serious. There are also differences between how men and women experience, and respond to, heart attack symptoms.

A heart attack is one situation where it's critical to get the right help—fast. Receiving medications or surgery to relieve a blocked artery within two hours after the onset of symptoms greatly increases not only your chances of surviving the heart attack, but of recovering with little or no damage to the heart muscle.

Signs of Heart Attack

Chest pain that feels crushing or spreading is the most common symptom of heart attack for both women and men. It's not wise to try to explain it away. *Shortness of breath, in particular, and radiating pain in one or both arms are other symptoms to take seriously.* Additional warning signs include:

- nausea and vomiting.
- heavy sweating.
- pain in the jaw, head or shoulders.
- a feeling of intense anxiety or malaise.

Women and Heart Attack Symptoms

Women having a heart attack are somewhat more likely to experience nausea, pain in the jaw, neck, shoulder, back, or ear, and a feeling of intense anxiety. Surprisingly, a recent study found that one-third of people having a heart attack, including women, don't have chest pain.

More than one study has shown that women are less likely to identify their own heart attack symptoms and thus may postpone seeking help. A study conducted at the University of Washington and the Fred Hutchinson Cancer Research Center in Seattle showed that women are in danger of mislabeling their symptoms—perhaps passing them off as indigestion, food poisoning, or the onset of flu. Few women (36 percent) knew that nausea and shortness of breath might signal a heart attack.

Amazingly, only about one-quarter of the women with common symptoms said that they'd call 911 or go to the hospital. The typical response was to do nothing or to try to call a doctor—both of which can seriously or even fatally delay treatment.

Most women have not been educated about the less common symptoms of a heart attack. And even if they have chest pain and other classic symptoms, they may believe that heart attacks are a man's disease. They see breast cancer as their biggest enemy—and this misperception may contribute to misinterpreting heart attack symptoms ("not me, I'm a woman").

Yet heart disease is still the leading cause of death for both women and men in the United States and Canada, and women's risk of heart attack rises sharply after menopause.

Immediate Care for Heart Attack

For men and women—or anybody assisting a person with chest pain—the first goal is to get expert medical help as fast as possible. Don't panic. Do the following:

- *Call 911* (or have someone else call) and report that you are having a heart attack.
- *Chew and swallow an aspirin (full size).* This will help dissolve the blood clot if there is one.
- *Don't drive yourself to the hospital.* But if you

are helping someone else and are sure you can get to the emergency room faster than if you wait for the ambulance—without speeding or running red lights—do drive.

Fortunately, there are many steps you can take to prevent a heart attack. For a summary of all the strategies that can dramatically lower your risk, see pages 63–65.

▶ HEAT EXHAUSTION AND HEAT STROKE

Exposure to heat and humidity can pose a serious health problem, especially during summer months when the temperature is regularly above 70°F and the humidity is often greater than 70 percent. When relative humidity increases, the air becomes saturated with water vapor, reducing the effectiveness of sweat evaporation to cool you down. At 100 percent relative humidity, evaporation stops completely. The accumulation of sweat on your skin may also close your sweat ducts, thus allowing your skin to become hot and dry. Without sweat evaporation, your body temperature starts to increase.

Heat Exhaustion

Also known as heat prostration or hyperthermia, heat exhaustion is the excessive loss of body fluids and salt, combined with a sharp rise in body temperature (up to 103°F). The condition is generally temporary and rarely fatal. Unless the case is severe or the person has a heart condition, it is often possible to relieve symptoms without calling your doctor.

Contributing to hyperthermia is the fact that thirst is satisfied long before you have replenished lost fluids. If, after prolonged exercise, you replace fluids only when you are thirsty, it can take several days to reestablish your body's fluid balance.

Heat-related problems can occur in dry climates, where sweat can evaporate so rapidly that you may lose a tremendous amount of fluid before you realize it. Dehydration can occur in a short time or develop over several days. If you exercise under these conditions and don't drink fluids, your body will not be able to produce enough sweat to cool itself.

In extremely hot weather, heat exhaustion can develop into heat stroke, a life-threatening medical emergency caused by the complete breakdown of the body's heat-sensing mechanism followed by the onset of severe internal overheating. Heat stroke requires immediate medical attention.

Signs of Heat Exhaustion

Any of the following can indicate heat exhaustion: profuse sweating; pale, moist, clammy skin; weakness and fatigue; headache; dizziness; muscle cramps; intense thirst; darkened urine; nausea and vomiting.

Immediate Care for Heat Exhaustion

If heat exhaustion is allowed to persist and too much fluid is lost through perspiration, heat exhaustion can rapidly become heat stroke, an emergency condition that can lead to death if not quickly treated.

• ***Stop whatever you're doing.*** Once you feel overheated, stop your activity. Continuing to push yourself will worsen the situation, and it may escalate to heat stroke. Instead, go to a cool place, lie down, and elevate your feet slightly so that more blood will flow to the brain.

- **Drink plenty of fluids.** You need to drink enough to replace the fluid you've sweated off. Plain water is best. Start by drinking 16 to 20 ounces of fluid. If you feel dizzy, sip the drink or, alternatively, suck on ice cubes.
- **Cool yourself.** Take a tepid bath or shower. If you have air conditioning or a fan, use it. The cool environment will help to lower your body temperature and speed recovery.

When To Seek Medical Help

Contact your physician if heat exhaustion causes you to vomit, faint, or become nauseated. Also contact your doctor if the home remedies listed here fail to relieve symptoms or if your symptoms worsen.

If you are found to be suffering from extreme heat exhaustion, your physician may administer intravenous fluids to rehydrate you.

Seek immediate medical attention if heat exhaustion leads to heat stroke (see below).

Signs of Heat Stroke

Heat stroke is usually preceded by heat exhaustion and its symptoms. It typically affects the elderly, people who are chronically ill, and those taking certain prescription medications that interfere with the ability to dissipate heat.

In addition to a body temperature of 104° F or higher, the following symptoms can occur: hot dry skin; extreme irritability; shallow breathing but rapid pulse; slurred speech and/or hallucinations; loss of consciousness.

Immediate Care for Heat Stroke

If you suspect someone has heat stroke, call for emergency medical help right away. Also take the following first-aid measures:

- **Move the person quickly to a cool spot**—either a shaded area or, better, an air-conditioned environment.
- **Cool the individual** by pouring cold water on the skin, by sponging the skin with cold water, or wrapping the person in sheets soaked in cool water.
- **Do not give the person anything to eat or drink.** Any mental confusion the person may be experiencing could cause food or fluids to be aspirated (drawn into the lungs).

Prevention Tips

There are plenty of steps you can take to avoid heat exhaustion:

- **Dress properly.** To permit maximum evaporation of perspiration in hot weather, wear light, loose-fitting clothing that "breathes" and allows as much skin exposure as possible.
- **Hydrate yourself.** The most important thing is to drink—even if you don't feel thirsty. Thirst is satisfied long before you have replenished all the lost fluids, so continue to drink. When you are planning to exercise in the heat, be sure to drink at least 16 to 20 ounces of fluid two hours prior to your workout, and another 8 ounces 15 to 30 minutes before you begin the workout. While you exercise, drink 4 to 8 ounces every 10 to 20 minutes.
- **Restrict your outdoor activities.** When the weather is hot and humid, try to schedule your more vigorous activities for the early morning or late evening, if possible. Also, consider indoor exercise as an alternative. (The table on page 120 lists the "apparent temperature"—how hot it feels—at various combinations of heat and humidity, along with the dangers posed by physical activity and/or prolonged exposure.)
- **Acclimate yourself.** If you must compete in an athletic event or perform strenuous work when

119

the temperature and humidity are high, slowly acclimate yourself to the weather. Allow yourself 10 to 14 days of daily work in hot weather to adjust, gradually spending more time in the heat.

• *Don't take salt tablets.* You lose proportionately more water than sodium when you sweat in the heat. Extra salt is unnecessary—you already get enough from your daily diet. It is also potentially dangerous because it causes water to be drawn from the tissues into the stomach in order to help dilute the increased sodium from the tablets. This can quickly lead to dehydration.

• *Limit caffeine and alcohol.* Caffeine, found in coffee, tea, and soft drinks, is a diuretic and can cause excessive water loss through increased urination; the same is true for alcoholic beverages.

• *Weigh yourself daily.* During hot weather, weigh yourself every morning after going to the bathroom. If your body weight is two pounds lower than the previous day, you may be dehydrated. You need to drink more water before being active outside again.

• *Don't skip any meals.* Eating helps keep you hydrated. Food contains water, and it also increases the concentration of sugars and salt in the blood, thereby activating thirst.

• *Be prepared in cold conditions as well as in the heat.* While heat buildup may be slower when you exercise in cold weather or in water, you still lose fluid from sweating. Therefore, it's important to replace fluids just as regularly when you swim or exercise in the cold as you do in the heat.

120

HEAT AND HUMIDITY INDEX

	AIR TEMPERATURE (F°)									
	70°	75°	80°	85°	90°	95°	100°	105°	110°	115°
RELATIVE HUMIDITY					APPARENT TEMPERATURE					
0%	64°	69°	73°	78°	83°	87°	91°	95°	99°	103°
10%	65°	70°	75°	80°	85°	90°	95°	100°	105°	111°
20%	66°	72°	77°	82°	87°	93°	99°	105°	112°	120°
30%	67°	73°	78°	84°	90°	96°	104°	113°	123°	135°
40%	68°	74°	79°	86°	93°	101°	110°	123°	137°	
50%	69°	75°	81°	88°	96°	107°	120°	135°	150°	
60%	70°	76°	82°	90°	100°	114°	132°	149°		
70%	70°	77°	85°	93°	106°	124°	144°			
80%	71°	78°	86°	97°	113°	136°	157°			
90%	71°	79°	88°	102°	122°	150°	170°			
100%	72°	80°	91°	108°	133°	166°				

APPARENT TEMPERATURE	RISKS WITH PHYSICAL ACTIVITY AND/OR PROLONGED EXPOSURE
90°–104°	Heat cramps or heat exhaustion *possible*.
105°–129°	Heat cramps or heat exhaustion *likely*. Heat stroke *possible*.
130° and up	Heat stroke *likely*.

- **Consult your physician if you're on medication.** If you are taking antihistamines, beta-blockers, calcium channel blockers, anticholinergic drugs, diuretics, antidepressants, or antiparkinsonian drugs, speak to your doctor before undertaking activities in the heat. Some drugs can cause dehydration.

For More Information

- Centers for Disease Control and Prevention

▶ HYPOTHERMIA (COLD EXPOSURE)

Hypothermia occurs when your body loses heat rapidly, to the point where there is a drop in core body temperature below 95°F—three to four degrees below what is normal in most people. This generally happens whenever your body is exposed to cold temperatures for an extended period—from several hours to several days—or when your skin becomes both chilled and damp. (You can develop hypothermia even at temperatures of 50°F if the weather is especially windy or wet.) Often a person who slips into hypothermia is overwhelmed by drowsiness and may fall asleep, at which point there is a risk of freezing to death.

What Puts You At Risk

Hypothermia is generally caused by a combination of inadequate clothing protection and exposure to cool or cold outdoor temperatures, especially when combined with wind and/or rain. Hypothermia can also occur when a person stays in cold water for too long.

Although it is mostly associated with cold outdoor winter weather, hypothermia can also occur indoors during the winter months. Elderly adults may be especially susceptible, particularly if they keep their thermostats set low to save on heating costs. Older people are often less able to shiver effectively, which is one of the ways your body increases heat production to stay warm.

Various medications taken by older people can also contribute to the onset of hypothermia by interfering with the body's natural heat-regulating mechanism in the brain. The more common drugs that can have this effect include barbiturates, tricyclic antidepressants, and benzodiazepines.

Being slender can make a person more prone to hypothermia. A slender person usually has a comparatively low level of body fat and therefore less natural insulation from the cold, so body heat is lost more rapidly.

Signs of Hypothermia

Any of the following can indicate hypothermia: numbness; excessive shivering, or no shivering; cold skin; fatigue or sleepiness; faint or slow pulse; loss of coordination; slurred speech.

A drastic drop in pulse and breathing rate, or loss of consciousness, are emergency symptoms that require emergency medical care.

Immediate Care for Hypothermia

Contact a doctor or medical facility as soon as possible if you suspect someone you are with has hypothermia. If not dealt with promptly, hypothermia can quickly become a medical emergency. A hypothermic person is at risk of developing frostbite, and, more seriously, can slip into a coma if body temperature is not restored to normal.

In extreme cases, where breathing has slowed or stopped, call 911 or get to a hospital emergency room immediately.

If severe hypothermia is diagnosed, the person will be gradually rewarmed over a period of time.

121

This will prevent the rapid enlargement of blood vessels at the skin's surface, which could affect blood flow and severely impair the functioning of the inner organs.

Take the following steps until professional help is available:

• **Warm up.** Get the person out of the cold and into a warm room. Remove all wet clothing. If possible, get the person into warm, dry clothing and wrap him or her in blankets to prevent further loss of body heat. (Be sure to wrap the head and neck.)

• **Carefully check for frostbite** and take appropriate steps to treat it (see page 115).

• **Supply warm fluids.** Have the person drink warm fluids like soup, coffee, or tea (but not if he or she is too drowsy to drink without choking or regurgitating). Absolutely avoid alcoholic beverages: they will dilate blood vessels under the skin and accelerate the loss of body temperature.

• **Preserve wakefulness.** If a hypothermic person is losing consciousness, do whatever you can to keep the person awake, including talking, jostling, playing music, or using some other noise.

Prevention Tips

Being properly dressed is the most important step for preventing hypothermia. Wear protective water- and windproof outer garments when going outside in cold and wet weather for any length of time. Dress in layers to best trap valuable body heat and insulate yourself. Put on a first layer of thermal undergarments; a middle layer of a synthetic or fleece jacket, or a wool or synthetic sweater; and, for an outer layer, a jacket that's waterproof, wind-resistant, and breathable, so that moisture isn't trapped inside.

Mittens are warmer than gloves, since they keep your fingers together. Be sure to wear a hat:

it will trap body heat and keep it from escaping through your head.

The following measures are also protective against cold.

• **Eat something.** Be sure to eat and drink before heading outside in frigid, cold, damp, and windy weather. This ensures that your body will have the necessary fuel it needs to keep going and stay warm. Keep nibbling on high-energy snacks during extended outdoor stays to help maintain body heat.

• **Avoid alcohol.** Alcoholic beverages interfere with the body's ability to regulate temperature.

• **Keep warm.** Make sure your indoor home temperature is in the 70°F range and that you wear adequate clothing at all times.

• **Stay inside during severe winter storms.** Don't put yourself at risk in extremes of temperature, no matter how well you're dressed.

• **Get out of wet clothing immediately.** Water speeds the loss of body heat and is a major contributor to hypothermia.

• **Be prepared.** Make sure you have emergency provisions in your car during winter weather. Also, take along emergency equipment whenever hiking or camping in cold, damp weather, and be sure your clothing and sleeping gear are sufficiently protective for the nighttime temperatures you'll be coping with.

• **Check on those at risk.** Drop by or telephone elderly relatives and friends regularly during the cold winter months to see how they are doing.

For More Information

• Centers for Disease Control and Prevention

▶ KNOCKED-OUT TOOTH

It's not uncommon for a tooth to be knocked out because of an accident, fight, sports injury, or rough play. A hard blow to the tooth is enough to dislodge it or shear it off. This happens to as many as three million Americans annually. Failing to take immediate action can result in the loss of the tooth.

Immediate Care for a Knocked-Out Tooth

If dealt with promptly and calmly, a dislodged permanent tooth, in most cases, can be successfully reattached and retained for life. (Baby teeth, however, can rarely be saved, and replanting them may damage the underlying tooth bud. Contact your dentist for advice.)

If you or a child of yours knocks out a tooth, pick it up, rinse it off if you can, replace it in the socket if possible, call your dentist, and get to his or her office as soon as you can. Research shows that you have a 50 percent chance of a successful replantation if you get to the dentist within 30 minutes.

Accomplishing this may not sound difficult, but don't underestimate the trauma of the situation: blood and confusion may delay you. Try to remain calm and rational—saving a tooth is definitely worth the effort. Even if more than 30 minutes elapse, take the tooth to the dentist anyway and let him decide what to do.

In the meantime, follow this step-by-step postaccident procedure.

• *Rinse the tooth.* The primary reason adult teeth cannot be replanted is that the cells on the root have been allowed to dry out. After finding the tooth, rinse it gently in tepid tap water, holding it by the crown (nonroot) surface. Don't scrub the tooth—this could injure the surface root tissue needed for successful replantation.

• *Try to insert the tooth.* Call the dentist to inform him of your imminent visit. Unless he tells you not to, gently insert the tooth in the socket. To seat the tooth properly, bite down firmly on a clean handkerchief or piece of cloth for at least five minutes; keep biting down with moderate pressure until you get to the dentist's office.

• *Keep the tooth moist.* If reinsertion at the scene of the accident isn't possible, place the tooth, bathed in saliva, under your tongue or inside your cheek until you get to the dentist's office. If a child is so young that he or she may swallow the tooth, transport it in a plastic cup or bag filled with milk or tap water and a pinch of salt.

Your dentist will assess the situation and readjust the tooth in the socket. The tooth will then be fastened with wire or bonding material. It may take up to eight weeks to determine whether the tooth will reattach itself. Once the tooth does reattach, a root canal procedure may be in order because the nerve often dies as a result of the trauma.

Prevention Tips

According to the American Dental Association, wearing a sport mouthguard can prevent a great number of tooth injuries by cushioning the teeth and providing a buffer between teeth and lips. Sports where mouthguards should be worn include soccer, volleyball, basketball, baseball, softball, in-line skating, skateboarding, martial arts, boxing, hockey, and mountain biking. Local sporting goods stores carry a wide variety of models. You can also talk to your dentist about a custom-made model.

When To Seek Medical Help

If the accident victim shows any sign of head injury, unconsciousness, nausea, or persistent head pain, he or she first needs to be evaluated for head injury by a physician. Once a head injury has been ruled out, contact your dentist immediately concerning tooth replantation or else go directly to a local hospital emergency room for treatment.

For More Information
- American Dental Association

▶ NOSEBLEEDS

Nosebleeds are very common, and unless you've had a blow to the nose, a nosebleed usually starts and stops spontaneously. The septum (nose partition) is the most common site of bleeding from the nose. The forward part of the nose has fragile membranes that crack easily, and it doesn't take much to damage blood vessels that lie just beneath their surface. These thin membranes offer little supporting tissue, especially as they grow more delicate with age.

Nosebleed Triggers

The dry air of wintertime can be a major factor, as can the low humidity of an airplane cabin. Both conditions can cause nasal membranes to dry out and crack. Inflammation from a cold, an allergy, or sinusitis can also weaken the nasal tissue.

Picking your nose or blowing your nose hard can set off a nosebleed; so can hard rubbing of your nose and, of course, a bump or blow.

A nosebleed doesn't herald a stroke, nor does it necessarily signal hypertension, as some people believe. Of course, those with hypertension who take aspirin or other blood-thinning drugs may have more frequent episodes of nosebleed.

In people past middle age, nosebleeds sometimes start farther back in the nose, beyond the fleshy area. A blow to the nose can also result in bleeding farther back in the nose (posterior bleeding). This type of nosebleed is harder to stop; it can cause significant blood loss and requires medical assistance if it doesn't cease within a few minutes.

Immediate Care for Nosebleeds

Most nosebleeds will stop spontaneously or with the application of simple remedies. The following measures usually stop a nosebleed quickly.

- *Sit up.* This allows gravity to lower pressure in the veins. To keep blood from running back into the throat, tilt your head forward a little.

- *Pinch the fleshy part of the nose.* This is the part between the bridge and the nostril. Pinch with your thumb and index finger for 5 to 10 minutes, breathing through your mouth. Applying ice probably won't help, since it's really pressure, not temperature, that stops the bleeding.

- *Be careful how you blow your nose once the bleeding stops.* Don't blow your nose too hard or too often. Sneeze through an open mouth, and avoid strenuous sports for a few days. Apply a little petroleum jelly inside the nostrils several times a day for a few weeks to keep the membranes moist.

Prevention Tips

- *Humidify at home.* If you have a history of nosebleeds, it may help to use a home humidifier to keep the air from becoming too dry.

- *Use petroleum jelly.* In very dry air, keep membranes moist by applying a little petroleum jelly with your fingertip or a small cotton swab just inside the nostrils. If your nose bleeds on plane trips, try using petroleum jelly before you depart.

- *Avoid repeated rubbing or picking.*
- *Blow gently.* You can give yourself a bloody nose if you blow hard enough. And if you are suffering from an upper respiratory infection and have nasal discharge, forcefully blowing your nose may send bacteria from the nose to your ears and so contribute to an ear infection.

When To Seek Medical Help

If the bleeding lasts longer than 20 minutes after applying home treatment, or if blood is continuing to drain down the throat from the back of the nose, contact your doctor or seek help from an emergency room. A nurse or doctor will try to stop the bleeding by compressing the nostrils (even if you have tried this yourself). If this fails, he or she may then try to locate the bleeding point and cauterize it (apply a heated instrument to tissue to halt bleeding).

Another option is to pack the site with gauze in order to apply pressure to ruptured blood vessels.

Also contact your doctor if nosebleeds recur frequently.

For More Information

- American Academy of Otolaryngology-Head and Neck Surgery

▶ POISON IVY, OAK, SUMAC

The itching and the rash associated with poison ivy, oak, or sumac are immune-system reactions that result from either touching the plants directly or coming in contact with clothing, garden tools, or pets that have been exposed to the plants (which are scattered around most of the United States and Canada).

Signs of a Reaction

A red, bumpy, itching rash will develop at the site of exposure. Often the rash is followed by small blisters and localized swelling of the skin. About 85 percent of the population will develop symptoms, which may take one to two weeks to develop on first contact. After any subsequent exposure, a rash can appear after only two or three days.

The source of this allergic reaction is urushiol (you-ROO-she-all), a colorless or sometimes slightly yellow oil that occurs in the sap of the plant genus Rhus. Poison ivy, oak, and sumac all belong to this genus (cashews and mangos are close relatives).

Just one billionth of a gram of urushiol is enough to make allergic people itch incessantly. The chemical is also very durable—if you don't wash it off clothing, shoes, or tools, it will still be there many months hence and can cause a reaction.

125

Immediate Care for Poison Ivy

Sensitivity to poison ivy varies from person to person, with individual sensitivity diminishing as one gets older (though at any age the first bout of poison ivy can be quite severe). Once contracted, poison ivy rash, blisters, and itch will normally disappear in 14 to 20 days without any treatment. But most people will need relief from the intense itch; some may require prescription medication.

If you think you have come in contact with any of the poison plants, here's what to do.

- *Wash your exposed skin immediately.* Wash with soap and lots of water within 5 to 10 minutes if possible. The longer you wait, the less effective washing becomes. If you're out in the woods, use water from a lake or stream, or even beer from a picnic basket if you have any.
- *Apply rubbing alcohol.* This inactivates any remaining urushiol. Don't use a washcloth; this

can spread urushiol. Instead, dab your skin with alcohol-soaked cotton balls.

• *Clean your clothing and anything else exposed to the plants.* Urushiol can spread from clothing to you, so be extremely careful when undressing. Wear rubber gloves while handling clothes and other items, and then discard the gloves. Wash the contaminated clothes (separately from other clothes) in strong detergent.

Shoes, tools, and other items that may have been in contact with urushiol need to be wiped off with alcohol and water.

• *Try not to scratch.* Scratching can lead to infection. However, contrary to popular myth, scratching the rash (and breaking the blisters) won't cause the rash to spread, since the water inside the blisters does not contain urushiol. In fact, once the rash appears, the urushiol is gone from that area—which is why the rash won't spread elsewhere on you or from you to someone who might come in contact with it.

• *Try calamine lotion.* For mild cases that afflict small areas, this popular lotion cools the skin and causes the blood vessels to constrict. The lotion leaves a powdery residue that absorbs the oozing and develops a crust that keeps it from sticking to your clothing. Apply it to the itchy areas every three to four hours. Discontinue after the oozing stops.

• *Nonprescription creams can also help.* For mild itching, 1 percent cortisone creams—twice the strength of the old 0.5 percent formulations—can provide relief. However, over-the-counter cortisone creams won't help if you have severe itching.

• *Have a milk soak.* A compress with cold milk helps dry the rash and soothe the itch. Just soak milk in gauze and apply to your skin for 5 to 10 minutes.

• *Soak in the tub.* A tepid tub bath, two to six

times daily, with colloidal oatmeal (Aveeno) added, may be soothing. Since the oatmeal makes the tub slick, be sure to have a nonskid bath mat in place.

• *Rub on baking soda.* If your rash is weeping or blistering, make a paste of water and baking soda and apply it to your skin. This helps dry up the oozing blisters.

• *Ice it.* The cheapest remedy for the itch of poison ivy is to apply an ice cube to the affected area for about a minute. If you don't have an ice cube, run cold water over the area.

Prevention Tips

Being able to recognize these poisonous plants is the key to avoiding them and the rash that they trigger. The old adage "Leaflets three, let it be" is accurate. But the poisonous plants vary tremendously—which is why many people don't recognize them and end up in misery each year. They can grow as woody vines or shrubs. The leaves can be dull or glossy, from one to five inches long, and have edges that are saw-toothed, lobed, or smooth. Though usually green, in autumn they can turn yellow; in spring they often bear small green or white flowers that mature into berries in late summer.

Poison ivy grows in every state but California, which is where one type of poison oak is concentrated. Another type of poison oak grows in the southeastern states. In damp areas like swamps or bogs, you may encounter poison sumac, a small tree or shrub related to poison ivy that has seven to eight leaflets on each stem.

• *Dress for the occasion.* If you hike in woods known to have the itch-causing plants, wear gloves as well as clothing that will cover your arms and legs.

• *Buy protection.* To help prevent another

attack, an effective Food and Drug Administration (FDA) approved lotion is available over the counter that protects against poison ivy. Applied at least 15 minutes before exposure to poison ivy, Ivy Block (bentoquatam), which is sold in most pharmacies, binds to the urushiol and prevents it from being absorbed through the skin, or at least reduces a rash's severity. Ivy Block has not been tested on children under six, but it may be useful for those who work and play outdoors and can't avoid the poison plants.

• **Bathe your pet**. Animals pick up plant secretions on their fur and bring it home. Wash your cat or dog (carefully, wearing gloves) if you suspect that the animal has been through poison ivy.

When To Seek Medical Help

Contact your physician if symptoms grow worse, if the rash spreads to your mouth, eyes, or genitals, if it covers more than 20 percent of your body, or if you have had severe reactions to poison ivy (or poison oak or sumac) in the past.

To control the rash and itching, your physician will probably prescribe a topical corticosteroid or an oral antihistamine, or both. If your face, hands, or an extensive area of your body is afflicted, oral steroidal medication will be prescribed.

For More Information

• American Academy of Dermatology

▶ POISONING

Poisons are substances that interfere with the normal functioning of the body. With some substances, a minute dose can be fatal; other substances, such as certain medications, are non-toxic in small amounts, but dangerous when taken in large doses. Many common household items can be toxic. These include insecticides, mothballs, paint, pesticides, fuels, polishes, soaps, and solvents. Hundreds of plants are also poisonous.

The key to dealing with poisoning is to call your local poison control center. Poison control centers exist in every state, and emergency personnel can give immediate instructions on how to proceed in the event of poisoning. The control centers can also answer questions about the toxicity of specific products and plants.

Find the number of your regional center and keep it near your phone before you need it.

Immediate Care for Poisoning

If you or someone in your household or workplace has swallowed a poisonous substance, call your poison control center immediately—unless the person is unconscious or having convulsions; in that case, call 911 or your local emergency number.

Be ready to provide the following information: the age and weight of the person, what was ingested (have the bottle or container with you), when it was ingested, how much was taken, how the victim is feeling or acting at that moment, and your name and phone number.

If you are instructed to go to a hospital emergency room, bring the container of the poison or a sample of the substance with you.

You should keep a bottle of syrup of ipecac on hand to induce vomiting—it is available without a prescription at pharmacies. But you should not use it unless instructed to do so by the poison control center or a physician. Some corrosive chemicals, such as bleach, and petroleum products, such as gasoline, can cause more harm if they are brought up.

(For illness related to food poisoning, see page 267.)

▶ SNAKE BITES

Compared with other risks, such as injuries on the highway, getting bitten by a snake is a pretty remote possibility, unless you handle snakes regularly or camp out for long periods. Still, about 45,000 snake bites are reported every year in the United States; of these, about 8,000 are venomous.

The bite of a poisonous snake can be painful and even fatal, and often requires hospitalization and treatment. Most poisonous snake bites are highly treatable, however—fewer than 20 people die each year. The great majority of venomous bites occur in the southern states and in the Southwest, including California.

Rattlesnakes are responsible for two-thirds of the bites and almost all the deaths. Copperheads and cottonmouths (which, along with rattlesnakes, are known as pit vipers), imported snakes (kept by collectors), and the occasional coral snake account for the rest of the bites.

Signs of Snake Bite

A bite from a poisonous snake will leave a pattern of tooth marks topped by two fang puncture wounds. Symptoms of venom from a pit viper include pain and rapid swelling at the bitten area; dizziness; nausea; sweating; and numbness around the mouth.

Symptoms of venom from a coral snake include pain at the bite site; drowsiness; slurred speech; double vision; nausea; sweating; and delirium.

Immediate Care for Snake Bite

It's important to get medical help at once if you've been bitten by a snake, even if the bite seems minor.

If you are certain the snake that bit you was nonvenomous, the bite can be treated like any other animal bite (see page 106). This may include a tetanus shot. Fortunately, you don't have to be concerned about rabies from a snake bite.

If you've been bitten by a poisonous snake, or if you're not sure what kind it was, get to the nearest emergency room, preferably with a companion, since you may quickly begin to experience pain and weakness if the snake did inject you with venom. A doctor will want a description of the snake. After ascertaining the severity of the bite, the condition of the patient will be assessed to determine the treatment, including the use of antivenin injections to counteract the venom. (Most hospitals in areas where snakebites are common are equipped with these medications.)

If you're caring for a snake bite victim, keep the person warm and try to keep him or her calm. Remember that the most important task is finding medical assistance.

Before you reach an emergency room, follow these steps.

• ***Never try to capture or kill the snake and take it along.*** That only wastes valuable time and puts you at risk of being bitten again.

• ***Immobilize the bitten body part and keep it below heart level.*** If your foot or leg has been bitten, it's a good idea to be carried, if there's any way to arrange this. Try not to panic—antivenins are available and effective.

• ***Remove rings and other constricting items.*** Most snake bite wounds will cause swelling, so rings, watches, or other items worn on the hand, arm, or foot can cause pain and/or impede blood flow. The items also become difficult to remove as swelling worsens.

• ***Cleanse the wound, if possible.*** Use soap and water and cover the wound with sterile gauze or another clean dressing.

• ***Do not apply ice.*** This can actually drive the venom deeper as well as damage tissue if it is left in place too long. Nor should you apply a tourniquet that shuts off the flow of arterial blood, as this can result in loss of the limb.

• *Use a constricting band only in very special circumstances.* If medical help is more than half an hour away, and if not more than five minutes have elapsed since the bite, use a constricting band around a bitten arm or leg. Apply it two to three inches above the bite and tighten it so that you can still slip two fingers under the band. Check for a pulse below the band to make sure the blood is still circulating, and keep checking periodically. (Pulse points can be felt in the wrist and on the top of the foot above the instep.)

• *When to suck on a wound.* Cutting a wound and sucking out the poison, once thought essential, should be considered only in extreme situations (for example, if you are hours away from any medical care). It should be done only if you have a suction cup, can start treatment within five minutes, and have had some training in the procedure. And no matter what old-timers do in the movies, don't give a snake bite victim a shot of whiskey or alcohol in any form.

Prevention Tips

Preventive steps are by far the best "treatment" for snake bite.

• *Learn how to handle pets.* If you or an acquaintance keeps snakes as pets, don't handle them until you've had proper training. Never tease or hurt a snake.

• *Outdoors, stay back.* If you see a snake outdoors, keep away from it. Remember that snakes try to avoid people.

• *Dress smart.* If you're out in the wilderness, wear long pants and footgear that covers your ankles. Thick gloves are practical, too, if you're gathering firewood.

• *Be cautious when turning over a rock or fallen branch.* Don't reach or step into dark places, such as heavy underbrush. Make sure you can see what you're getting into. Don't put your hand into rocky crevices while climbing.

• *Stay in the clear.* Camp in an open space—and never gather firewood at night.

For More Information

• Centers for Disease Control and Prevention

▶ SPIDER BITES

For most of us, spider bites are not much of a threat. Of the more than 100,000 species of arachnids (which include spiders, scorpions, ticks, and mites), most are harmless. In spite of their horrific reputation, spiders are reclusive and unlikely to sit down beside us. But a few species bite, and in rare cases the bite, if untreated, can be serious or even fatal.

Signs of a Spider Bite

Reactions to a spider bite usually peak within two to three hours, then begin to subside. They can include muscle pain and swelling around the bite site; itching and/or burning; sweating, nausea, vomiting; and severe headache.

Types of Spider Bites

Two kinds of spiders were responsible for almost half of the spider bites reported to poison-control centers in the United States in the mid-1990s (the most recent period for which the Centers for Disease Control and Prevention has national figures): the black widow and the brown recluse. The female black widow is about half an inch long with a shiny black body and a red hourglass-shaped

129

mark on its underside. The brown recluse is smaller and has a violin-shaped mark on its upper body. Both types tend to dwell in dry, dark surroundings such as under porches or in woodpiles.

Another troublesome arachnid, the hobo spider, common in the Pacific Northwest, is thought to have inflicted many of the 5,300 other bites classified as "other/unknown," and possibly some of those blamed on the brown recluse. Indeed, spider bites are more often reported in the Pacific Northwest (Oregon, Washington, Idaho) than in any other areas.

Tarantulas, a kind of large, hairy spider found mostly in the Southwest, racked up 82 bites. Some 15,000 insect bites are reported annually—but most people don't know what kind of insect or spider bit them. If a spider bites you and you kill it, it may help if you take the spider along with you to a physician.

Immediate Care for Spider Bites

Most spider bites don't require medical attention, but it's important not to break the skin or lance the bite, which can lead to a secondary infection. For milder bites, which should heal in a day or two, cold compresses on the bite are helpful.

When To Seek Medical Attention

If a bite causes a severe reaction—which can include symptoms such as intense pain, muscle spasms, fever, chills, difficulty breathing, and/or convulsions—try to get medical help right away.

Also seek medical help for children under three or adults older than 70. This is especially important if the bite is from a black widow or brown recluse; bites from these spiders can be fatal for children or the elderly without treatment.

If a bite seems to be getting worse, it's a good idea to seek medical attention.

For a serious bite, you may need a tetanus shot and wound care. Antivenins (antivenom drugs) are available for black widow bites, but because of concern about adverse reactions, they are used only for severe cases.

Prevention Tips

Protecting yourself from bites is the best policy. If you're working in a crawl space, working outdoors where brush is piled up, or gathering wood for a campfire, it's always a good idea to wear gloves and other protective clothing. If you have to use an outdoor privy, look before you sit. Inspect your shoes before putting them on when you're out camping—or if you're putting on boots or shoes that you haven't worn in some time.

For More Information

- Centers for Disease Control and Prevention

▶ STINGS FROM INSECTS/ ANAPHYLACTIC SHOCK

Stings from bees, yellow jackets, hornets, wasps, and fire ants are a common occurrence during the summer months (and year-round in warm climates). For most people the reaction to a sting is harmless (albeit potentially painful). However, some people—about 3 percent of the population—are so sensitive to the venom that even one sting can provoke their immune system to overreact drastically. This is known as anaphylactic shock (from the Greek *ana*, meaning excessive, and *phylaxis*, meaning protection). About 50 Americans die each year as a result of being stung by bees, wasps, or hornets. No other venomous animal, even snakes, kills that many. And this figure may be too low: experts suggest that an unknown number of deaths attributed to heart failure may actually be caused by stings.

Signs of Insect Bites and Stings

The venom of stinging insects contains toxins that produce fierce burning and swelling at the site of the sting. Reactions can also include redness and sometimes welts and itching in the area around the sting.

Allergic Reactions

The cause of more severe allergic reactions to stings is not well understood. Anyone who has experienced any symptoms of anaphylactic shock or any systemic reactions after being stung should know that reactions usually become increasingly severe with successive stings. Life-threatening reactions most often occur in people over the age of 30.

These reactions include rapid swelling of the lips, tongue, throat, and eyes; nausea and vomiting; irregular heartbeat; difficulty breathing; loss of consciousness. (Multiple stings can also produce the same symptoms.)

Immediate Care for Insect Stings

In most people the pain and swelling from a single sting disappears after a few hours. If you are allergic, however, you should seek medical help, even if the reaction appears to be mild. Multiple stings can also produce a toxic reaction that requires immediate treatment.

For pain and swelling at the site of the sting, the following measures can help. (If you're hypersensitive to stings, you should have an emergency kit containing adrenaline whenever you're outdoors, as noted in the box at right. Also consider desensitization shots, especially if you spend a good deal of time outdoors in areas populated by bees.)

• ***Start with soap and water.*** The best way to treat a sting is to wash it with soap and water. Applying an ice pack or flushing with cold water can also help relieve pain and reduce swelling.

• ***Try tenderizer.*** You may also obtain some relief by applying calamine lotion or a paste made by mixing baking soda or unseasoned meat tenderizer and water. (The tenderizer contains papain, an enzyme that breaks down toxins in the venom.) Aspirin or another over-the-counter anti-inflammatory drug such as ibuprofen can also help alleviate pain.

• ***Remove bee stingers at once.*** Conventional wisdom says that pulling a stinger from the skin with tweezers or fingers is a bad idea because it tends to inject more venom. Thus, standard advice has been to scrape the protruding venom sac away with a sharp blade and then remove the stinger (and to leave the stinger in until you can do this).

131

AN EMERGENCY TREATMENT KIT

If you know you are highly allergic to bee stings, a dose of epinephrine (adrenaline) can arrest the attack that occurs during the initial moments of a serious reaction. An emergency kit, prescribed by your doctor, includes a syringe and epinephrine, or an EpiPen, which comes with a spring-loaded mechanism that automatically triggers the injection of epinephrine when pressed against the skin.

Take the kit with you whenever you go outdoors in bee season. If you get stung, remove the stinger as soon as possible, using your fingers to pull it out. Once you inject yourself, rub the site vigorously in order to increase the absorption rate.

However, in a study published in the *The Lancet*, bee stings swelled less and hurt less when the stinger was removed immediately by whatever method—including pinching the stinger. (Beekeepers have known this for centuries, it seems.) If you are among the small percentage of people subject to anaphylactic shock, removing the stinger quickly can help save your life.

• *If you're near a hive, retreat.* As it stings, a honeybee releases a chemical that identifies you and draws other bees. So if you've been stung close to a hive, hurry to a safe place.

Prevention Tips

You can avoid being stung by taking a few preventive measures:

• *Dress for protection.* Wear shoes and socks outdoors; don't go barefoot. When gardening, wear a long-sleeved shirt, long pants, and gloves. Bees can mistake you for flowers, so avoid brightly colored clothes and floral prints.

• *Spray yourself.* There are dozens of products with DEET (N, N-deiethyltoluamide), which works well and has an excellent safety record when used according to directions. For ordinary purposes, don't use a product on your skin that has more than a 30 percent concentration. It helps to apply insect repellent on exposed skin (but not on broken skin or over cuts) and also on trouser and sleeve cuffs, and on shirt fronts.

Avoid wearing sweetly scented perfumes, soaps, or lotions.

• *Be cautious about eating outside.* Bees are particularly attracted to sweet, drippy foods like ice cream or watermelon.

• *Don't try to fight.* If an insect is annoying you, don't swat it—either walk away or, if attacked by a swarm, lie down and cover your head.

When To Seek Medical Help

If you experience any of the symptoms of anaphylactic shock, you must go to the nearest emergency room or doctor immediately. This is also true if you experience severe symptoms due to multiple stings. You should also see a doctor immediately if you know you are allergic to stings, even if your reaction to a sting is mild.

Fortunately, there are effective short-term and long-term treatments for those who are highly allergic to bee stings. Once you are found to be allergic, your doctor can prescribe an emergency kit to deal with serious reactions to a sting. Long-term treatment involves going to an allergist for regular shots of a serum made from insect venom. This may gradually desensitize you until a sting poses little serious harm.

For More Information

• American Academy of Dermatology

▶ STINGS FROM MARINE ANIMALS

Stinging sea creatures include jellyfish, the Portuguese man-of-war, sea anemones, and some corals, all equipped with stinging cells called nematocysts. On contact with the skin they discharge a small barb and a dose of toxin.

You're more likely to encounter jellyfish and the Portuguese man-of-war while swimming; divers should watch out for coral and sea anemones. Sea urchins, which live on the sea bottom but may show up in shallow water, have poisonous spines that can puncture the skin even through thongs or sneakers.

Immediate Care for Different Stings

If you're stung or stuck by any of these animals, get out of the water as calmly as you can, and if possible identify the culprit so that you can choose appropriate first aid measures. If you weren't able to see what stung you, ask someone who knows the area. Then apply the remedies described here.

• **Jellyfish.** Only about 1 in 10 species of these translucent, bell-shaped blobs produces severe reactions in humans. But if you do come into contact with a toxic jellyfish's trailing tentacles, you'll feel mild burning and stinging; long red weals that look like the marks of a whip will develop.

If you have to pull the tentacles off, protect your hand with cloth or a glove to keep the stingers off your skin. To deactivate the stinging cells, wash with sea water, then apply rubbing alcohol, vinegar, or witch hazel. If possible, apply a papain-based meat tenderizer in paste form. This appears to break down the stinging cells (and the toxins in them) attached to your skin.

A paste made of talcum, baking soda, or flour mixed with sea water may also help. When the paste is scraped off, the cells come with it.

Don't rub the affected area or rinse with fresh water: this can discharge unactivated cells.

If pain persists, a nonprescription topical anesthetic (such as one containing a "-caine" ingredient) can be applied. (In some people, these medications can cause an allergic reaction.)

• **Portuguese man-of-war.** Bright blue or purple and red, this is actually a colony of many individual jellyfish at two stages of development. The floating colonies are easy to spot, but their transparent tentacles, which can trail invisibly for as far as 60 feet, are not.

Contact with the skin provokes red weals similar to jellyfish stings, but the burning and pain can be far more severe. Shortness of breath, nausea, stomach cramps, and shock may ensue. Treatment is similar to that for jellyfish stings (you can also try ammonia), but in some cases you may need to see a doctor.

• **Coral.** On contact, some corals release toxins; fragments may break off and become embedded in your skin.

Apply calamine lotion or rubbing alcohol, and if there is an abrasion, remove fragments with anything at hand: for instance, a towel, a handkerchief, tweezers, or a needle. Wash with soap and water.

• **Sea anemones.** These flowerlike creatures live fixed to the sea floor; their waving tentacles are equipped with stinging cells. If you step on one, follow the same measures as for jellyfish; do not rub the skin and do not rinse with fresh water.

• **Sea urchins.** Also floor dwellers, sea urchins are protected with toxic spines; broken-off spines can cause secondary infections if they are not removed. A scrub with soap and water will get rid of some. Extract others with a sterilized needle or tweezers; a doctor may have to pull out the remainder.

Hot compresses or immersion of the foot in hot water increases blood flow, which helps remove the toxins. Since the punctured foot may be numb, check the water temperature with your hand or uninjured foot.

Prevention Tips

Check ahead of time on the hazards that may be lurking off the beaches where you plan to spend your vacation. Pack a small first aid kit with the following items: needles and tweezers, rubbing alcohol or calamine lotion, and meat tenderizer.

133

When To Seek Medical Help

Sea stings are rarely fatal. However, when the reaction is severe, you should see a doctor as soon as possible.

For More Information

• American Academy of Dermatology

▶ STROKE

Strokes occur when an artery supplying blood to a part of the brain ruptures or becomes obstructed, restricting blood flow and oxygen to that portion of the brain. About 600,000 strokes occur each year in the United States, and about 160,000 of these are fatal—making stroke the third leading cause of death, behind cardiovascular disease and cancer. Stroke is also a leading cause of disability.

During the 1980s and early 1990s, the fatality rate from stroke declined dramatically, but in 1993 it increased for the first time in four decades. The fatality rate continues to be higher than it was a decade ago. According to research by the National Stroke Association, a major factor in this rising mortality rate is that many Americans are not aware of what a stroke is, what its warning signs are, and what to do when these signs occur.

Types of Stroke

With any stroke, the nerve cells in the affected area of the brain, deprived of oxygen and nutrients, can die within minutes. That's why a stroke can be so disabling: The parts of the body controlled by the injured area of the brain cease to function, permanently or temporarily.

Two types of stroke account for about 80% of all occurrences. *Ischemic stroke,* by far the most common type, result from a blocked blood vessel. The most common cause of ischemic stroke is cerebral thrombosis, in which a blood clot clogs an artery (usually one that has been partly blocked by deposits of fat and cholesterol). Another is cerebral embolism, which occurs when a clot is formed elsewhere and travels to blood vessels supplying the brain.

Hemorrhagic strokes, which account for 20 percent of all strokes, are caused by a rupture of a blood vessel either in the brain (cerebral hemorrhage) or on the brain's surface (subarachnoid hemorrhage). The rupture not only cuts off blood to those parts of the brain beyond the site of the rupture, but the escaped blood can form a mass that, because the skull is rigid, puts excessive pressure on the brain, causing damage. These hemorrhagic strokes are more likely to be fatal than those caused by a clot.

Warning Signs for Stroke

Knowing immediately when you or someone else has suffered a stroke is critical in order to get prompt treatment and thus minimize brain damage.

Here are the most common signs:

• Sudden numbness or weakness of the face, arm, or leg on one side of body.

• Sudden dimness of vision, particularly in one eye.

• Sudden difficulty speaking or understanding speech.

• Unexplained dizziness.

• Sudden severe headache with no known cause.

About one in ten major strokes is preceded by a "mini-stroke," or transient ischemic attack (TIA). Days, weeks, even months before a major stroke, temporary clogging of a cerebral artery can produce stroke symptoms—for anywhere from a few minutes to a few hours. However brief, a TIA is frequently a sign of worse to come. But prompt medical attention may prevent further attacks or a major stroke, depending on the underlying cause.

Immediate Care for Stroke

If you notice one or more of these warning signs, see a doctor or summon emergency medical help right away by calling 911.

- Until help arrives, make the person having the stroke as comfortable as possible. Do not let the person drink anything other than water, however.

- If there is no chance that an ambulance will arrive within a reasonable period of time, a family member or friend can drive the stroke patient to the hospital. But under no circumstances should the person experiencing the symptoms drive anywhere.

- Also be sure to notify the stroke patient's personal physician, since he or she can provide the hospital with the patient's history.

The best treatment for stroke is prevention. Fortunately, many risk factors for stroke are modifiable, as explained on page 66.

For More Information

- American Heart Association

▶ TICK AND CHIGGER BITES

Ticks and chiggers are biting parasitic creatures that can cause disease (in the case of ticks) or a strong allergic reaction (in the case of chigger mites).

Ticks probably exceed all other pests in the variety of diseases they transmit to man and domestic animals. Tiny, wingless, louselike creatures, they range in color from brown to gray and from one-sixteenth to one-quarter inch in length. Many species are known to carry diseases such as Rocky Mountain spotted fever, Colorado tick fever, tularemia, babesiosis, and Lyme disease, which they can spread by feeding off the blood of their hosts. They occur in every part of the United States, though large numbers are concentrated in certain areas.

Chigger mites hatch in April in the northern United States (year-round in warmer climes). They do not, as ticks do, feed off blood, nor do they spread disease. But the enzymes they secrete can cause an allergic reaction resulting in two weeks or more of intense itching—which leads to scratching that may result in serious bacterial infection.

Signs of Tick and Chigger Bites

A tick bite produces a slight stinging sensation, but is relatively painless. The tick is also visible in the skin, though because it is tiny (about the size of a pinhead), it is often overlooked.

If you become infected with a tickborne illness, various symptoms can develop, depending on the specific infection. Flulike symptoms (chills, fever, muscle pain) characterize some of these diseases, including Lyme disease (page 376). Fever, headache, and a tell-tale rash are characteristic of Rocky Mountain spotted fever (page 422). Tularemia produces a red bump at the site of the bite and swollen lymph nodes near the bite. Following a tick bite, therefore, you need to be on the alert for any developing symptoms.

Chigger bites can produce a red rash with intense itching; chiggers may be visible in the center of unscratched bumps as small red dots. Hives, blisters, and swelling may also occur.

Where Bites Occur

People usually pick up ticks and chiggers from woodsy underbrush, tall grass, and the fur of free-ranging pets.

The tick brushes against some part of the body and looks for a place to settle. It then bites the skin, embeds its head, and taps into a blood source, such as a small vein or capillary. As it feeds, the external part of its body swells to as much as three times its original size. The bite is relatively painless; the real danger is the viruses or bacteria that the tick may harbor and that may infect you.

Chigger mite larvae climb the nearest plant and wait for a bird, snake, small animal, or human to brush by. The mite drops off the plant and attaches itself with a pair of jawlike claws. It does not burrow, like a tick, but clings for about three days before dropping off. During that time it feeds by secreting enzymes that liquefy skin cells; these enzymes cause the initial symptoms of redness and itching.

Immediate Care for Tick and Chigger Bites

For ticks:

• **Remove the tick immediately.** The sooner a tick is removed, the smaller the likelihood any infectious organisms will be transferred. Don't try to detach a tick with your bare fingers; organisms from a crushed tick may be able to penetrate even unbroken skin. Instead, use a pair of fine-tipped tweezers (see box on page 137). If you cannot get the tick out, call a doctor.

• **Wash the bite area.** Use soap and water.

• **Relieve the discomfort.** An ice pack as well as calamine lotion will relieve any pain or itching.

• **Watch for symptoms.** In the days after a tick bite, be alert for symptoms of tickborne illness. Contact your doctor immediately if any develop.

For chiggers:

• **Remove the mite.** If a chigger mite attaches itself to you—it will look like a tiny red fleck—a needle, small knife, or even your fingernail will remove it.

• **Try starch baths and calamine lotion.** These two remedies can help relieve the persistent itch from chigger bites.

• **Don't scratch.** Chigger bites will cause an aggravating itch that can persist for weeks; constantly scratching the itch can lead to a bacterial infection.

Prevention Tips

The best treatment for chiggers and especially ticks is to ward them off. Take these precautions.

• **Dress protectively.** If you're hiking through grass or underbrush, fend off chigger mites and ticks by wearing a long-sleeved shirt secured at the wrist, waist, and throat; tuck your pants into your socks or boots. Cover your body as much as possible.

Wear light-colored, tightly woven fabrics: it's easier to spot ticks on white or tan slacks than on dark ones, and the ticks may not be able to grab onto the tight weave of slippery materials such as nylon. A hat may help, too, since ticks like to settle on the scalp.

• **Use insect repellent.** One of the best ways to ward off chiggers and ticks is to use an insect repellent containing DEET. Be sure to follow label directions. Also available are tick repellents that contain permethrin. Permethrin is applied to clothes before you put them on. The repellent must *not* be applied to your skin. Spray applications are effective for up to two weeks, even after laundering.

• **Check yourself.** Inspect your skin and clothing occasionally for ticks, especially when you're

How To Remove A Tick

Grip the tick with a pair of tweezers as close to your skin as possible and gently pull it straight out until it releases its hold. Don't twist it as you pull, and don't squeeze its bloated body—that may actually inject organisms into your skin. (If you spend much time hiking or gardening in overgrown areas, a pair of tick tweezers—available at many sporting goods stores—should be part of your first aid kit.) Afterward, thoroughly wash your hands and the bite area with soap and water and apply antiseptic (such as rubbing alcohol). If you must touch the tick, cover your fingers with tissue; then wash your hands thoroughly.

Home remedies for tick removal—gasoline, petroleum jelly, kerosene, nail polish remover, or a hot match—have not been shown to be effective and may actually increase your chance of becoming infected from the creature. These methods may cause the tick to respond by secreting more of the infecting toxins.

Save the tick in a tightly covered small container or jar (add a little alcohol). Label the jar with the date, the body location of the tick bite, and where you think the tick came from. You can show the tick to your doctor if necessary.

in underbrush or forests. Ticks often crawl around on clothing or even on the skin for a long time before they bite. Later do a thorough check of your entire body. Have someone look at your back and head, if possible, or use two mirrors.

- ***Try to stay near the center of trails.*** In overgrown countryside, walking in cleared areas reduces your risk.

- ***Shower and shampoo after your outing.*** This may help remove ticks and chiggers that haven't yet begun to feed. Check your clothes too; wash them immediately to remove any ticks that may be hidden in creases. Inspect any gear you were carrying.

- ***Check pets after they've been outdoors.*** Remove ticks from them as you would from yourself.

- ***Inspect your children.*** Check them over daily for ticks, perhaps before they go to bed. This is especially important during the summer, when they spend lots of time outdoors.

When To Seek Medical Attention

Call your doctor immediately if you notice symptoms that may be related to a tick bite. These can include fever, headache, muscle aches and pains, muscle weakness, rashes, and severe fatigue. Bring the tick with you in a container if you have it.

Also call a doctor if symptoms from a chigger bite become severe or if you develop a secondary infection from scratching.

Antibiotics are usually prescribed to treat the early stages of a tickborne disease. For severe reactions to chigger bites, lindane and crotamiton (a prescription drug) kill mites; crotamiton also alleviates itching. For more serious attacks your doctor may prescribe an oral antihistamine or topical steroid cream to control the itching. If you do develop a secondary infection, an antibiotic may be needed.

For More Information
- American Lyme Disease Foundation
- Centers for Disease Control and Prevention

Ailments & Disorders
A to Z Index

Ailments & Disorders
Problem Areas & Special Concerns

Acne

Symptoms

- The presence of blackheads, whiteheads, pustules, or cysts, with or without redness and inflammation around the eruptions.
- In adolescents the outbreak occurs mainly on the face, but also on the shoulders, back, neck, and buttocks. In adults it is usually confined to the chin and jawline. For women, symptoms may worsen before the start of each menstrual period.
- Groupings of red, inflamed cysts (cystic acne).
- Pockmarks and scarring (chronic acne).

What Is It?

Acne, a skin condition technically called acne vulgaris, is the bane of millions of teenagers, but it also strikes adults with its persistent and recurrent blemishes (red bumps, whiteheads, blackheads, nodules, or cysts) on the skin. It primarily affects adolescents, but one study indicates that even in their 50s, 6 percent of men and 8 percent of women continue to experience outbreaks. Except in severe cases, acne is generally harmless, although it can cause considerable psychological distress.

In both adults and adolescents, acne develops when oil glands in certain parts of the body—mostly glands associated with the pores from which face, chest, and back hairs emerge— secrete too much sebum, the thick waxy lubricant that acts to retain moisture. Excess sebum clogs the pores. If it remains beneath the skin, it results in whiteheads; blackheads occur if the plugs of sebum protrude above the skin. Angry red pimples appear if excess secretions invade and inflame surrounding tissue. The more extensive the inflammation, the more likely it will form abscesses and leave permanent scars and pits.

Prompt medical treatment of severe acne will help prevent scarring.

What Causes It?

Acne's causes at any age aren't completely understood. As in adolescents, acne flare-ups in adults are linked to various kinds of hormonal changes—for women, the hormonal fluctuations that accompany menstruation appear to be a factor. Contrary to conventional wisdom, acne is not a sign of poor health or a consequence of dietary indiscretions, nor is it caused by masturbation or constipation.

There may be a hereditary factor: if one of your parents had acne, there's a good chance you will have it as well. Other factors linked with acne include certain medications, such as oral contraceptives, corticosteroids, vitamin B_{12}, and lithium. Also, grease, cosmetics, tight clothing, or anything that can block your pores can cause acne. In some instances stress, exposure to dioxin (a contaminant found in herbicides), or climate changes may trigger an outbreak.

What If You Do Nothing?

Acne is not life-threatening, and a mild outbreak will clear up by itself. However, if acne causes emotional distress or if it worsens, a family physician or dermatologist should be consulted.

Home Remedies

Acne can't be cured, but you can take steps to keep mild symptoms under control until they go away.
• **Use a nonprescription drying lotion or cream.** The most effective over-the-counter preparations contain benzoyl peroxide, generally sold in either 5 percent or 10 percent solution. This active ingredient has a superficial irritant and drying action that helps loosen the plugs in the hair fol-

licles. It can take four to six weeks to experience the full therapeutic effect of the drug.

• **Wash daily, but not too roughly or too often.** Use ordinary soap and water. Don't waste money on medicated cleansers (the medication just rinses away) or granular facial scrubs (a washcloth does the same job). Facial saunas (actually facial steam baths) may aggravate acne.

• **Watch what you eat.** There is no scientific proof that nuts or colas can trigger flare-ups, but if they or other foods seem to act as a trigger for you, there's no harm in avoiding them. Numerous studies have failed to show that even large amounts of chocolate trigger outbreaks of acne. A few people are allergic to chocolate and may develop a rash when they eat it—but that's not acne.

• **Get your rest.** Flare-ups may also be related to emotional upset and too little rest, at least in some people.

• **Change your exercise gear.** Working up a sweat exercising while wearing tight-fitting, nonabsorbent clothes or sweatbands increases oil production and may contribute to acne.

• **Take care of your hair.** Style your hair away from your face to keep your complexion free of scalp oils, and avoid greasy hair dressings. Pull your hair away from your face when you sleep.

• **Use water-based makeup.** Oil-based cosmetics can block sebum from naturally reaching the skin's surface. Skip cosmetics entirely if acne is severe. When buying makeup, make sure it's "noncomedogenic" or "nonacnegenic." Be sure to remove all cosmetics with soap and water before going to bed. Don't overdo moisturizing.

• **Avoid prolonged exposure to the sun and ultraviolet lamps.** These light sources sometimes work to dry up acne, but they can cause long-term skin damage, which can result in skin atrophy and even cancer, and thus are ill-advised.

• **Don't pick at your face.** Squeezing and picking increase inflammation and the risks of pitting and scarring. Ask your doctor if you can use a black-head extractor (this device is available in most drugstores). Before you use the device, soften the affected area of skin with hot wet compresses for about 10 minutes. Make sure your hands and the extractor are very clean.

Prevention

Acne can't be prevented, but outbreaks can be lessened by following the measures outlined above.

When To Call Your Doctor

Acne can be emotionally upsetting and, in severe cases, disfiguring. Contact your physician if you have acne that is making you self-conscious, depressed, frustrated, or embarrassed, or if your acne is typified by cysts or nodules, or if unexplained symptoms develop after taking prescription acne medication.

What Your Doctor Will Do

After a close examination of your skin, your physician may open pimples or remove blackheads and whiteheads. The doctor may prescribe a wide variety of therapies, including lotions and ointments, antibiotics, and a drug called tretinoin.

Commonly called Retin-A, tretinoin—a derivative of vitamin A—is a topical prescription medication that has proved to be very effective for treating blackheads and has shown modest results for treating pimples. Tretinoin should be used in moderate to severe cases of acne after treatment with milder agents has failed. Anyone using it should be aware that the skin can become extremely irritated. The drug is available in cream-based preparations (the mildest form) as well as gels and liquids. Low concentrations are

143

tried first, then the strength may be increased, depending on the degree of peeling and irritation that occurs. There are also newer formulations of tretinoin (Avita and Retin A Micro) that claim to be milder than the original tretinoin.

Tretinoin cannot be used by pregnant women or those planning to become pregnant. Also, the drug may enhance the tendency to sunburn, so protective measures must be taken to limit sun exposure.

Topical antibiotics, such as clindamycin or erythromycin (administered as a cream, gel, lotion, or skin pad), can be useful in controlling the signs of acne. Your doctor may also recommend systemic oral antibiotics, such as erythromycin or tetracycline, which are effective in treating extensive acne pimples.

For severe acne that has proved resistant to other forms of treatment, a more powerful oral medication called isotretinoin (Accutane) may be prescribed. Accutane has a number of complications, including liver toxicity, so be sure to discuss these with your doctor. Also, the drug should never be taken if you are pregnant or trying to become pregnant.

Any acne therapy can take several months for improvement to occur. For teenagers prone to acne, the therapy may have to be continued throughout adolescence.

For More Information
- American Academy of Dermatology
- National Institute of Arthritis and Musculoskeletal and Skin Diseases Information Clearinghouse

Airplane Ears (Barotrauma)

Symptoms

- Muffled or partial hearing loss during and after a plane's descent.
- Mildly uncomfortable to extremely painful ears.

What Is It?

Even though today's aircraft are pressurized so that changes in air pressure are minimized, many air travelers are still afflicted with airplane ears (barotitis media), which causes partial hearing loss, ear pain, and a stuffed-up feeling in the ears. These symptoms typically begin while a plane is descending and can persist after it lands. Symptoms may range in intensity from mildly uncomfortable to extremely painful, but often clear within 20 or 30 minutes after landing.

What Causes It?

The cause of airplane ears is well understood. The eardrum retracts owing to rapid changes in pressure in the airplane cabin as the plane goes from a high altitude and low atmospheric pressure toward the ground, where the atmospheric pressure is much higher. The eustachian tube—which normally drains secretions from the middle ear into the throat—exchanges air between the ears and nose, but when there is a pressure differential, as there is in a descending plane, lower-pressure air may get trapped in the middle ear. The eustachian tube compensates by allowing a little more air to be pumped into or out of the middle ear, but this is sometimes difficult to do because the differences in air pressure in the ear and plane cabin create a vacuum that pulls the eardrum inward. In the process the eardrum is stretched (which is painful) and is unable to vibrate naturally (which impairs hearing).

Airplane ears can also be caused or made worse by a cold or allergy because the swollen nasal membranes can effectively block the opening of the eustachian tubes. When this swelling occurs, the eustachian tube, which is the size of a pencil lead, cannot open frequently and widely enough to equalize the pressure that starts to build on either side of the eardrum—and the result is pain. Airplane ears may also result from having narrowed eustachian tubes, typically the result of scarring from childhood ear infections.

What If You Do Nothing?

Most people recover quickly once air pressure has been equalized, and there are no long-lasting effects from airplane ears. However, if you travel frequently, you can take self-care measures rather than bear up to the pain and discomfort.

Home Remedies

Keeping your ears unblocked may require some experimentation with the methods described here.

- **Prepare for descent.** Once the "fasten seatbelt" sign is turned on and the plane begins its descent, swallow several times. This helps keep the eustachian tube open and equalizes ear pressure. If this doesn't work, blow your nose gently; this may also help open the eustachian tube.
- **Chew gum.** The act of chewing (like swallowing) activates the muscle that opens the eustachian tube. Once opened, a little droplet of air can pass from the nose and throat to the middle ear, thereby relieving pressure.
- **Yawn.** This is a more powerful way to activate the muscle that opens your eustachian tube.
- **Try a gentle blowing maneuver.** Another method to unblock your ears is to squeeze the nostrils shut with your thumb and forefinger, inhale

through your mouth, and then attempt to force the air back into the nose. Once you feel them "pop," you know your ears have unclogged. This popping sensation is often accompanied by mild pain, but it usually disappears quickly. You may have to repeat this several times during your descent.

• **Take a decongestant.** If you suffer pain from airplane ears on a regular basis, an hour before landing spray both nostrils with a decongestant nose spray or else take a decongestant pill (such as Sudafed or a generic containing pseudoephedrine). This will help shrink membranes, open your eustachian tube, and make your ears pop more easily.

• **Consider trying special ear plugs.** Small silicone rubber ear plugs marketed under the name EarPlanes have a filter that equalizes the effects of cabin air-pressure changes. These may be especially helpful if a cold or sinus congestion makes it hard to relieve ear discomfort by swallowing air. EarPlanes, which are safe for children, are available in drugstores and airport shops.

Prevention

• **Avoid alcoholic beverages in flight.** Alcohol causes the mucous membranes to become engorged and the eustachian tube to swell.

• **Try to avoid flying while suffering from a cold or allergy.** Any ear problems you normally have on descent will be magnified by these respiratory problems, so if it's possible to postpone your trip, do so.

When To Call Your Doctor

If your ears fail to open or if pain persists several hours after landing, contact your physician. If you fly frequently and often experience pain that lasts long after your flight, consult an ear specialist.

What Your Doctor Will Do

Your doctor will examine your ear. In extreme cases your eardrum may have to be lanced to equalize the pressure.

For More Information

• American Academy of Otolaryngology-Head and Neck Surgery

Altitude Sickness

Symptoms

■ Increased rate of breathing.
■ Headache.
■ Fatigue and insomnia.
■ Dizziness and nausea.
■ Shortness of breath and rapid heartbeat accompanying physical exertion.
■ Impaired thinking.

Symptoms usually begin 12 to 24 hours after arrival, are worse at night when respiration slows down, and typically decrease in severity by the third day.

What Is It?

Travelers going by plane from sea level to high elevations such as Denver, Aspen, or Mexico City may suddenly experience shortness of breath, fatigue, headaches, nausea, and other symptoms resembling flu. This condition, called acute mountain sickness (AMS), is the most common type of altitude sickness. It can occur at elevations as low as 5,000 feet, where it is likely to last only a day or so, but is more common above 8,000 feet. At elevations over 10,000 feet, three out of four people will have symptoms.

Not everyone feels sick at higher altitudes, and there is no way to predict a person's highest comfortable altitude. Being physically fit is not necessarily a protection. Indeed, athletes accustomed to working out daily at low altitudes may be the first to become ill if they continue intense workouts at high altitudes.

Susceptibility to AMS is greater in those under 40 years of age, perhaps because they are more likely to exert themselves at high altitudes. Skiers, hikers, and others who go above 8,000 feet risk getting more severe symptoms of AMS and at higher altitudes may even develop a serious med-

ical emergency known as high-altitude pulmonary edema (HAPE). This life-threatening condition is due to an accumulation of fluids in the lungs and can lead to death if not treated immediately. Those afflicted must immediately descend at least 2,000 to 3,000 feet and then be treated in a medical facility.

What Causes It?

As mountain climbers know, altitude sickness results from a lack of oxygen caused by going too high, too fast. Barometric pressure decreases as you go higher—that is, the air gets thinner—and you inhale less oxygen per usual breath. Trying to compensate for this, you breathe more deeply. The likelihood of symptoms increases the higher you go.

What If You Do Nothing?

Most people who develop acute mountain sickness will feel well within two to three days by taking it easy and avoiding strenuous activity. However, if you go up to 10,000 feet and higher and exert yourself without adequate acclimation, the more serious high-altitude pulmonary edema (HAPE) can develop.

Home Remedies

If you are going to the Rocky Mountains or another high-altitude region, you can probably alleviate symptoms of AMS quickly by taking the following measures.

• **Acclimatize and take it easy.** Spend your first day at high altitudes relaxing. Avoid even moderate exercise until you get accustomed to the new heights.

• **Drink extra water.** Drink as much as you can to remain properly hydrated, at least three to four quarts. Your urine should be clear and copious.

Avoid alcoholic beverages. The fast, deep breathing you must do at higher altitudes will tend to dehydrate you, an effect that alcohol intensifies.

• **Get headache relief.** Acetaminophen or an NSAID (such as ibuprofen) can be taken for headache.

• **Don't go up until symptoms go down.** If you start showing symptoms of moderate altitude sickness, don't go any higher until they decrease—or descend a few hundred feet to a lower altitude.

Prevention

The only established preventive strategy is to prepare for destinations above 8,000 feet. Spend a day acclimatizing at a lower level, or climb to a new level at a rate of 500 to 1,000 feet daily with an occasional day of rest. This allows the body to operate with decreased oxygen by increasing its depth of respiration, releasing more red blood cells to carry oxygen, and producing more of a particular enzyme that helps trigger the release of oxygen from hemoglobin to the body tissues.

When To Call Your Doctor

It's a good idea to seek medical advice in advance if you are planning to travel to extreme altitudes (8,000 feet or higher), particularly if you will be exerting yourself.

What Your Doctor Will Do

If you are affected by altitude sickness and/or if acclimatization takes too long or is not effective, your doctor may recommend acetazolamide (Diamox), a prescription medication that may reduce the incidence and severity of altitude sickness by as much as 75 percent. The drug improves pulmonary function and allows you to breathe faster and to obtain more oxygen without the adverse effects of breathing too strenuously.

For More Information

• Centers for Disease Control and Prevention
• Medlineplus (National Institutes of Health)

Anal Itching

Symptoms

■ Itching, often intense, that may be persistent or may occur only after a bowel movement.

■ Redness and irritation around anal skin.

What Is It?

Anal itching—known medically as *pruritus ani*—is generally regarded by physicians as a simple problem that home remedies can alleviate.

What Causes It?

The majority of cases are caused by skin irritation from fecal soilage. In older people, or in anybody with diarrhea, seepage of fecal matter may occur. Also, as people grow older, anal skin becomes more irregular and harder to clean. People with hemorrhoids (which may trap small fecal particles) are more prone to itching.

At any age, not taking the time to wipe thoroughly may contribute to poor hygiene, which causes itching and irritation. Then, too, being overzealously hygienic, such as rubbing energetically with dry toilet paper, can injure the skin. Another precipitating factor may be the hard stools of constipation, which can irritate the anal area.

Once the itch starts, many factors can exacerbate it. Hot weather and sweating, tight clothes that compress the buttocks, and nonabsorbent nylon panty hose and underpants may make matters worse, as can activities such as walking, sitting—particularly prolonged sitting on a plastic seat, which hampers the evaporation of any sweat—and bike riding. Some experts think stress may also be a factor in anal itching.

What If You Do Nothing?

Until the cause of anal itching is eliminated, the condition may persist indefinitely.

Home Remedies

• **Clean carefully.** Meticulous, gentle cleaning provides relief. One option is to regularly use premoistened wipes. You can also wash the anal area gently—in a shower or bath or over the toilet—with soap and water. Take care to rinse thoroughly, then gently pat the area dry with a towel or cotton ball.

• **Control the itch.** Corticoid lotions or creams can be effective if used for a short time. Avoid the "-caine" creams sold for topical relief, since they can further inflame sensitive skin.

• **Don't scratch.** It only causes additional irritation and invites infection.

• **Consider changing your toilet tissue.** Use

Anal Fissure
▼

An anal fissure is an elongated ulcer—or crack—in the skin lining the anal canal. Fissures usually result from constipation and the passage of hard stool, stool that is inadequately emptied, or in association with hemorrhoids. Subsequent bowel movements can irritate the fissure and cause spasms of the sphincter muscle—which can be extremely painful—and sometimes bleeding.

The best way to treat anal fissures is to avoid constipation by eating a diet high in fiber along with drinking plenty of fluids.

If you experience pain during bowel movements, or notice any bleeding, don't simply assume it's an anal fissure. Contact your physician to rule out potentially more serious problems. If your doctor diagnoses anal fissure, avoiding constipation can help make it less likely to cause pain. Warm baths can help ease the pain of spasms. Your doctor may prescribe stool softeners. Cleaning the anal area after each bowel movement is also important: use moistened cotton (and soap if necessary), then pat dry with dry cotton. A fissure will usually heal within two to three weeks.

149

plain, unscented, noncolored tissues.

• **Be prepared.** When away from home, carry a few premoistened, individually packaged wipes—the kind you use for a baby.

• **Manage leakage.** If you are bothered by leakage, wear a small cotton pad against the anal opening and change it frequently. Wear undergarments with cotton crotches and generally avoid tight clothing.

• **Don't schedule long bike rides—at least until the problem is resolved.** Also, avoid other activities that may cause excessive perspiration.

Prevention

• **Bathe regularly.** Wash your anal area with soap and water and dry thoroughly.

• **Make use of moistened tissue.** After a bowel movement, cleanse carefully with tissues moistened with vegetable or mineral oil. Several brands of premoistened varieties are now available in stores.

You can also use toilet tissue that you've moistened and lightly soaped, then rinse with plain wet tissue and dry the area.

• **Avoid tight underclothing.** Choose roomy, breathable underwear made of cotton rather than synthetics. This will keep the anal area ventilated and relatively dry.

When To Call Your Doctor

Contact your physician immediately if anal itching occurs along with bleeding or any unusual pain. Very rarely, persistent anal or rectal itching may be a sign of serious infection, so if it does not respond to simple treatments or the passage of time, contact your physician. Scabies and pinworms are possible causes that require a doctor's advice.

What Your Doctor Will Do

Your doctor will make a careful physical examination that may include a close inspection of the anal area using a plastic device known as an anoscope. You may also be examined for pinworm eggs or scabies.

For More Information

• American Gastroenterological Association
• International Foundation for Functional Gastrointestinal Disorders

Ankle Sprain

Symptoms

- Pain and tenderness, from mild aching to intense pain.
- Swelling of the ankle, usually occurring very quickly after the injury.
- Inability to move the ankle or to stand and put pressure on it.

What Is It?

In the architecture of your body, the ankles are among the most vulnerable elements. These complex hinges of bone, ligament, tendon, and muscle support your entire body weight and may absorb a force of impact equal to three to four times your weight when you run or jump. A sprained ankle is the most common of all joint injuries. It occurs when the bone is forced out of the ankle joint because of a tear of one or more of the multiple fascia and ligaments securing the bone in the joint.

Anyone is susceptible to ankle sprains—from the basketball pro to the average runner navigating an uneven surface to the woman in high heels stepping off a curb.

Ankle sprains are graded as mild (the ligament is strained or stretched), moderate (a partially torn ligament), and severe (a complete tear, meaning that the ligament can no longer control the ankle joint). If you hear a popping sound when your ankle turns, that probably means you have a severe sprain or a possible fracture.

Minor sprains, in which the ankle bone is tipped slightly out of place for an instant, often can be successfully treated at home. Moderate and especially severe sprains, however, need medical attention. Any sprain can put you at risk for another because, when the injury heals, it leaves the tendon weakened, less flexible, and more susceptible to injury.

What Causes It?

The great majority (about 85 percent) of sprains are inversion sprains. This happens when the sole of the foot turns inward, injuring the ligaments on the outside of the ankle. Basketball players who land on the edges of their feet and runners who step into potholes are among those who most commonly sustain inversion sprains. Eversion sprains occur when the foot turns outward, affecting ligaments on the inner side.

What If You Do Nothing?

Very minor sprains will improve on their own. However, in cases where there is swelling, discoloration, or intense pain, you should attend to the injury immediately.

Home Remedies

If you can put weight on the ankle and if the swelling and pain are slight, you may not need

---

Can High-Tops Help?

▼

For active sports where there is a tendency to roll over on the ankle, most (but not all) evidence shows that wearing snugly-laced high-top shoes is protective. These aren't floppy canvas high-tops but the padded, flexible shoes worn by basketball players. Such shoes stabilize the ankle and protect against injuries. According to the American Orthopaedic Foot and Ankle Society, a study of Israeli army recruits showed that high-top basketball shoes were as effective as army boots in protecting against ankle injuries. A study of basketball players at the University of Washington School of Medicine in Seattle also showed that ankle taping combined with high-tops offered good protection.

When shopping for high-top shoes, look for a pair with an ankle collar that is high enough to firmly support your ankles.

medical attention right away or at all. Icing the injury as soon as you can is essential; follow up the icing with the other steps of RICE (rest, ice, compression, elevation), as explained below. Maintain the treatment for up to 72 hours, if necessary.

Most sprains, even the most severe, do heal without complications. It takes about 10 days for a mild sprain to heal, though it takes longer for the full range of motion to return.

• **Rest.** Avoid any activity that causes pain. Keep weight off the ankle. Using crutches, even for mild sprains, is advisable for the first few days.

• **Ice.** Apply ice to the injury as soon as you can. Ice applied for 10 to 20 minutes about every 2 hours for 24 to 48 hours will reduce pain, inflammation, and any further bleeding into the ankle joint. You may apply ice at more frequent intervals if necessary. (See page 453 for more tips on icing.)

• **Compress.** Securely wrap the ankle in an elastic bandage and keep the bandage on during your waking hours. Be careful not to apply it so tightly that it causes pain or additional swelling or com-

promises blood flow to the area.

• **Elevate.** Whenever you are resting or sleeping, make sure your foot is elevated slightly higher than your heart. This helps draw fluids away from the injury, decreasing swelling.

• **Try over-the-counter pain relievers.** Nonsteroidal anti-inflammatory drugs (NSAIDs) such as aspirin, ibuprofen, or naproxen will help reduce pain and swelling, though they won't accelerate healing. Acetaminophen will help with pain but not inflammation.

Prevention

Preventive measures are unusually rewarding, since people who sustain an ankle injury once are nearly twice as likely to reinjure themselves.

• **Stretch.** Before and after exercising, stretch your calf muscles using the exercise illustrated below. Tight calf muscles pull on the Achilles tendon, attached to the heel bone, and can cut down on the range of motion in your foot, thus sometimes promoting twisted ankles.

Ankle Conditioners

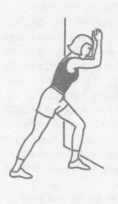

Calf stretch, for stretching muscles of the lower leg. Stand 2 to 3 feet from a wall, with feet perpendicular to wall, and lean against it for 10 to 30 seconds. Keep your feet parallel to each other; make sure the rear heel stays on floor. Switch legs and repeat. Variation: keep rear knee slightly bent during stretch. This will stretch the soleus, a flat muscle underneath the gastrocnemius, the major calf muscle.

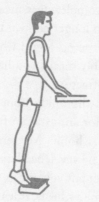

Heel raises and dips, for strengthening calf muscles. Standing with the balls of your feet on a thick book or step, slowly rise on your toes, then lower your heels as low as you can. Repeat. Use your hands for balance, not support. Gradually work up to 20 repetitions.

• **Wear supportive shoes.** When you're on your feet, especially if you're walking, wear stable shoes that offer some support. Replace or repair run-down heels and soles. Avoid platform soles and high heels, or any shoe that throws the foot off balance. Open shoes and sandals, which are less stable than other footgear, are a poor choice if you're trying to avoid ankle injury.

• **Exercise regularly.** Sedentary people are more likely to experience a sprain than those with strong muscles.

• **Strengthen your legs.** Start with heel raises: stand with your feet comfortably apart; rise on the balls of your feet as far as possible, hold for a few seconds, then lower. Gradually work up to 20 repetitions. Eventually try this exercise while standing with the balls of your feet on the edge of a step or a book, so that you carefully dip your heels lower than your toes.

Alternate these with toe raises: wearing flat shoes with smooth soles, stand on your heels and keep your toes as high off the ground as possible; walk like this, keeping your toes elevated, for three to five minutes. Also try walking on the insides of your feet, then the outsides.

When To Call Your Doctor

If you heard a pop, if the ankle looks abnormally bent, or if the swelling is severe and the skin discolored, you should suspect a severe sprain or fracture and contact your physician or go to an emergency room. Don't aggravate the sprain by flexing your ankle or putting weight on it.

Contact your physician if you initially suspected a mild sprain but find you can't put any weight on it after 36 hours of self-treatment. Also contact your doctor if you are having severe pain or swelling.

What Your Doctor Will Do

Your physician will review how the injury occurred and examine the ankle. X-rays may be taken to determine if a bone has been broken. Depending on the severity of the injury, your ankle may be taped or put in an air cast for several weeks. Anti-inflammatory medications may be prescribed.

For More Information

• American Academy of Orthopaedic Surgeons
• American Orthopaedic Foot and Ankle Society
• American Podiatric Medical Association

153

Asthma

Symptoms

Mild symptoms

■ Shortness of breath or breathing difficulty; coughing, wheezing, or rapid, shallow breathing that's eased by sitting up; coughing, especially at night, possibly with production of a thick, clear, or yellow sputum; a whistling sound when breathing; a sense of suffocation; painless tightness in the chest.

More severe symptoms

■ Inability to speak more than a few words without gasping for breath; clenched or constricted neck muscles; rapid pulse.

Emergency symptoms

■ Bluish tinge to the fingertips, lips, or face; extremely labored breathing; profound feeling of exhaustion.

What Is It?

Asthma is a chronic, yet reversible, lung disease that constricts the bronchial tubes (breathing passages). It affects an estimated 17 million Americans, including close to 5 million children. It's believed that many more have undetected asthma and go untreated.

Although asthma frequently begins in childhood, with half of all cases first occurring in children under the age of 10, it's no longer considered a disease that children "outgrow" when they become teens. Asthma can strike at any age and any time, causing even the most fit person to wheeze, cough, and gasp. These attacks can last for anywhere from a few minutes to more than a day.

During an asthma episode, the breathing passages are narrowed in three ways: the muscles surrounding the bronchial tubes constrict, the lining (mucosa) of the tubes becomes swollen, and there is increased mucus secretion. In all instances breathing becomes very difficult.

Experts now believe that asthma is an inflammatory disease that develops within the first few years of life. The air passages of people who have asthma, even those who suffer their first acute attack long after childhood, progressively become inflamed. This causes them to be swollen and to react strongly to inhaled irritants such as dust, pollen, tobacco smoke, air pollution, and cat dander. Even changes in weather can trigger an asthma episode. The main goal of asthma treatment is now to reduce this airway inflammation.

Patterns of asthma attacks differ from person to person, with symptoms ranging from mild and intermittent—shortness of breath and chest tightness, which require quick-relief medication—to severe and persistent, which require long-term control medications to keep the airways open.

It's critical that individuals understand the disease and their own symptoms and triggers. Asthma attacks may be predictable, occurring, for example, whenever a person comes into contact with a cat or performs strenuous exercise in cold weather. Conversely, the attacks may come on unexpectedly. Some people experience seasonal variations; some have nighttime episodes; some have continuous symptoms. Severe cases may warrant emergency hospitalization.

Asthma may stop on its own or with medication. Once an episode has subsided, breathing returns to normal. To date, there is no known cure for the disorder, but with new medications and techniques it can be managed to the point that most people with asthma can expect to have few or no symptoms or complications.

The number of Americans who have asthma has grown steadily in the past several years, but even more alarming has been the death rate,

Dealing with Dust Mites

▼

Dust mites—tiny members of the spider family—are not a problem for the great majority of nonasthmatics, but they may be the major indoor trigger of asthma attacks. It's estimated that 50 to 90 percent of asthmatics react adversely to dust. Actually, the main allergens in dust are certain proteins from dust mite droppings. The droppings are so small and light that they easily float in the air and are inhaled.

The mites live in carpeting, mattresses, clothing, and upholstered furniture. Bedrooms—particularly mattresses and pillows—are hot spots for them. They thrive in humid conditions, but even in cold winters dead mites and the droppings left behind can trigger allergic reactions.

Simply dusting or vacuuming can actually put more dust (and mite droppings) into the air. If you have asthma (or a dust allergy), take the following steps to combat dust mites.

- Vacuum your home regularly, especially the bedroom. Vacuuming is a necessary evil for those sensitive to dust, since even the best conventional machines spew out fine particles each time they are used. If possible, get someone else to vacuum while you're out of the house. Or wear a dust mask while vacuuming.
- Consider getting special microfiltration bags for your vacuum cleaner, or electrostatic filters that fit over the exhaust of some models. Make sure your vacuum cleaner doesn't leak a lot—for instance, through poorly fitting hoses. If your machine is old and leaky, consider replacing it (ask your allergist about specific models).
- Dust frequently with a damp or oiled cloth.
- Remove some or all carpets and upholstered furnishings, especially in the bedroom. To kill dust mites in area rugs, place them outdoors in direct sunlight. Vacuum the rugs afterwards to remove the dead mites.
- To reduce humidity (to below 50 percent), install an air conditioner and dehumidifier. Change or clean filters regularly. Don't use a humidifier in the winter.
- Wash all bedding weekly in hot water (at least 130°F). Use washable blankets and spreads. Dry cleaning is a little less effective in killing mites.
- Enclose your mattress, box springs, and pillows in zippered, nonallergenic casings. Some manufacturers now apply a special antimicrobial treatment to their bedding products, but this does not kill mites. It's unclear whether the treatment will help reduce dust-mite allergies.
- Wash curtains and draperies. Or replace them with blinds or shades.
- Get rid of stuffed toys, which collect dust mites, or wash them regularly. Don't allow pets into the bedroom.

which has risen sharply since 1979. The disease now kills more than 5,000 Americans each year. No one knows the reason for the increase, but some researchers suggest it's the greater amount of time people now spend in tightly sealed homes and workplaces where they are exposed to dust mites, pet dander, and other allergens. Most of these deaths are preventable if the asthma is properly diagnosed and treated.

What Causes It?

Asthma can be either extrinsic or intrinsic. Extrinsic asthma is caused by an overreaction or hypersensitivity to certain external triggers. These triggers aren't obvious with intrinsic asthma.

The triggers that cause extrinsic asthma episodes are many and varied. They include viral respiratory infections; exposure to pollen, mold, and dust mites; cockroach and animal dander (more than half the people with asthma have allergies);

exposure to chemicals or allergens; exposure to tobacco smoke, perfumes, hairsprays, air pollutants, vapors, gases and aerosols; emotional expressions such as fear, anger, frustration, crying, and laughing; medications such as aspirin, food additives, and preservatives; and changes in

---

Peak-Flow Meters

▼

You can measure your breathing capacity at home using a simple and inexpensive device called a peak-flow meter. This gadget measures how fast and how hard you are able to exhale air from your lungs. Flow rates may decrease several hours before an actual asthma episode occurs, so the meter can serve as an early warning long before you feel your first symptoms.

The peak-flow meter gives you a number indicating the velocity of air expelled in liters per second or liters per minute. You can compare the results with your predicted level and with your previous results. A drop of more than 10 percent below your normal readings may signal increased airflow resistance. A drop of 50 percent indicates you are in the danger zone. What you should do next will depend on the guidelines established by you and your physician.

The reason for the drop in the reading may be that your airways are constricted and swollen and mucus is accumulating; or that your particular medications may not be working as well as they usually do; or that you may be coming down with a cold.

Using a meter twice daily is especially helpful in teaching people with asthma, especially children, how to become attuned to reading their bodily sensations. The person with asthma soon learns, "So this is what it feels like when I'm beginning to have an asthma episode," and then he or she can better manage his or her condition.

Peak-flow meters are available through your physician, your local pharmacy, or by ordering directly from a manufacturer.

---

weather, humidity, and air temperature.

It's ironic that aerobic exercise, which helps strengthen the body and makes it more efficient in its use of oxygen, may also be a major trigger of asthma. This type of asthma, called exercise-induced asthma, or EIA, affects 1 in 10 people (60 to 80 percent of people with asthma). Because exertion soon triggers an uncomfortable attack, many people with asthma are afraid to exercise.

In cases of intrinsic asthma, no external allergen can be identified. However, a severe respiratory infection, such as bronchitis, generally precedes an intrinsic asthma episode. The asthma can then be aggravated by emotional stress, pollution, fatigue, and changes in temperature.

What If You Do Nothing?

Although there is no cure for asthma, trying to ignore asthma symptoms, however mild, is a mistake because the breathing difficulties it causes will prevent you from living a full and active life. While seldom fatal, asthma is a chronic disease that needs constant monitoring and medical attention.

Home Remedies

If you have asthma, you need to work with a physician to manage and control your condition. There is no known cure for asthma, but most asthma can be controlled by a two-pronged strategy aimed at preventing acute episodes and stopping those episodes that do occur. In addition to medications and other measures you will obtain from your doctor, take the following steps.

• **Remain calm.** Panic can worsen your condition during an asthma episode.

• **Breathe deeply.** When experiencing asthma, sit upright and lean forward, taking in deep, rhythmic breaths.

• **Avoid triggers.** The best treatment is to stay away

from substances that cause your asthma attacks.

• **Monitor your lung capacity.** A peak-flow meter is a hand-held device that measures how fast you can blow air out of your lungs; it should be an indispensable part of your treatment program. Since peak airflow often drops as much as a day or two before actual asthma symptoms become profound, regular peak-flow testing will help you assess the severity of your asthma (see page 156).

Prevention

• **Identify your asthma triggers.** Keep a diary and note when your episodes occur and what seems to trigger them. Include emotional and situational factors as well as environmental stimuli and foods. Check at home and at work. Common triggers include pollen, dust mites, aspirin, cat dander, chocolate, milk, nuts, and fish; avoid as many of these as possible.

• **Don't smoke.** If you do, quit. Avoid secondary smoke as well.

• **Vacuum regularly.** Reducing the amount of dust in your home will ease symptoms (see page 155). Get rid of (and avoid buying) carpets that are difficult to clean.

• **Drink plenty of water.** You will need at least eight glasses of liquid a day to help loosen airway secretions and maintain hydration.

• **Take precautions in cold weather.** Cold air can trigger an asthma attack. In cold weather, cover your nose and mouth with a scarf in order to filter, humidify, and warm the air that you breathe in.

• **Exercise regularly.** By staying physically fit, you will strengthen your body, especially your lungs. Water aerobics and swimming are two good choices since these exercises will allow you to be breathing humidified air. If a particular exercise triggers an asthma episode, talk with your physician about adjusting or changing your medication.

When To Call Your Doctor

Contact your doctor if you develop symptoms of asthma for the first time. If you have been diagnosed with asthma and you have an episode that does not respond to self-treatment, contact your physician immediately or go to a hospital emergency room.

Also contact your physician if your asthma medication isn't working as it's supposed to or if you develop new and unexplained symptoms.

What Your Doctor Will Do

A thorough medical history and physical exam focusing on the upper respiratory tract will be performed. Special tests may be taken to determine what triggers your acute attacks. Chest x-rays may be taken and a pulmonary function exam, a test to measure how much air you inhale and exhale, may be given.

Once a positive diagnosis has been made, the key is to work with your physician to find effective drugs and dosages that can prevent acute asthma episodes. Various asthma drugs may be prescribed to prevent attacks and halt symptoms when they occur. You should become thoroughly familiar with the medications prescribed for you and with how and when to take them. (Many of these drugs are available in oral inhalers; using an inhaler properly greatly increases the effectiveness of the medication.)

For More Information

• American Academy of Allergy, Asthma & Immunology
• American Lung Association
• Asthma and Allergy Foundation of America
• National Jewish Medical and Research Center

Athlete's Foot

Symptoms

- Scaling and peeling between the toes.
- Redness, itching, the appearance of tiny blisters, and scaling along the sides and soles of the feet.
- In severe cases cracks between the toes can develop, and the skin becomes soft and painful.
- If toenails are infected, they may become discolored and begin to thicken, scale, and crumble.

What Is It?

Athlete's foot is the most common infection of the skin. Despite its popular name, you don't have to be an athlete to contract this usually harmless fungal infection, which can develop in places other than locker rooms or gym showers. It occurs far more frequently among men than women and is more common in hot humid weather.

Once you have athlete's foot, it can be unusually persistent, so it's important to treat it. People with diabetes mellitus must be especially attentive to identifying athlete's foot, as it can be a major trigger for more serious bacterial infections.

What Causes It?

Trichophyton is the name of the most common group of fungi that causes athlete's foot. (The similarly itchy condition around the groin known as jock itch is also often due to *Trichophyton).* The fungus thrives best in warm, moist, enclosed environments. Snug, poorly ventilated shoes and damp, sweaty socks provide an ideal breeding ground. Your chances of catching athlete's foot from another person are slight, but the fungus can be spread to others by fragments of affected skin that have been shed.

What If You Do Nothing?

Athlete's foot should not be ignored. The condition can be easily treated, but if allowed to progress, it can be extremely bothersome and resistant to treatment, and can lead to cellulitis, a potentially serious bacterial infection.

Home Remedies

Once you have determined that athlete's foot is the problem, you should treat it immediately. The usual treatment is an over-the-counter antifungal cream, lotion, or powder containing antifungal agents such as clotrimazole.

Apply the cream on the soles of your feet. For between your toes, use the lotion or powder; it is more quickly absorbed than the cream and won't trap moisture, which could prolong the problem.

In most cases three consecutive days of treatment should clear up most of the symptoms of athlete's foot. It's common to assume that the infection has ended when the itching is gone and there is no sign of redness or cracking on the skin. This is not the case, however. In fact, six or more weeks of treatment are usually necessary to resolve the infection and prevent a relapse.

Prevention

Some people are more susceptible to the athlete's foot fungus than others. If you are susceptible, follow these commonsense rules, especially when you're very active and your feet tend to perspire.

- **Keep your feet clean.** Daily washing with soap and water is a good idea, but be sure you dry your feet thoroughly, especially between the toes (you can use a hair dryer on low heat).
- **After drying, apply antifungal lotion.** Follow this with an antifungal foot powder that does not contain cornstarch; cornstarch can encourage fungal growth.

• **Choose ventilated shoes.** This allows your feet to breathe. Also, don't wear the same pair of shoes every day, so that your shoes have a chance to air out.

• **When you can, go barefoot.** The next best thing to bare feet is sandals.

• **When you wear shoes, wear socks, too.** The best protection comes from socks made of synthetic materials (such as polypropylene) that wick away moisture. Change your socks daily.

When To Call Your Doctor

Contact your physician if the area turns red and swollen, or if nonprescription medication has provided no relief after two weeks.

What Your Doctor Will Do

Typically, your physician will examine your feet and, using a surgical blade, take a skin scraping that will be scrutinized under a microscope for fungal growth. If the problem is a minor case of athlete's foot, an antifungal lotion or powder will probably be prescribed. Severe or intractable cases can be treated with any of several newer oral antifungal agents.

For More Information

• American Academy of Dermatology
• American Podiatric Medical Association

Backache (Low-Back Pain)

Symptoms

- Persistent tenderness, stiffness, or pain in the lower back that can range from mild discomfort to excruciating pain that often limits motion.
- Gradual stiffening of the lower back, especially after sitting for extended periods.

What Is It?

About 80 percent of all Americans will have at least one backache during their lives. Every year articles and books about back pain appear, espousing new and old theories about its causes and how to treat it. However, there's room for controversy because the back is such a complicated, sophisticated structure, and while we can name all the bones, joints, nerves, muscles, and ligaments that constitute it, the sum total remains something of a mystery.

Pain and stiffness in the lower back can take several forms.

• Strain and sprain. The terms back strain and back sprain are often loosely applied to a broad spectrum of back disorders. Strain is generally used when a muscle is overstretched, and sprain when a ligament is partially torn. However, it is seldom clear whether it's a muscle or ligament that's been damaged, let alone whether it has been torn or not. Two other terms, muscle spasm and ruptured disk, are more clearly defined.

• Muscle spasm. The most common form of spasm is a sudden onset of sustained, painful, involuntary contractions of muscles in the back. This may serve to immobilize irritated back muscles, thereby protecting them and spinal nerves. A spasm usually results from a back injury but may also be caused or aggravated by poor posture, lots of sitting in the same position, tense back muscles, and weak abdominal muscles. Many researchers claim that psychological stress can also trigger muscle spasms.

• Disk problems. These are actually relatively uncommon. Only 2 to 4 percent of back ailments are due to what is commonly called a slipped disk. The term slipped is a misnomer, since the disk actually bulges (herniates) from between two vertebrae and may eventually rupture. If a displaced disk presses on a spinal nerve, the nerve can send shooting pains to the legs or arms, or create a sensation of tingling or numbness in them. If, as is common, the affected nerve is the sciatic, the condition is called sciatica (see page 432).

• Underlying diseases and structural problems. A small percentage of all backaches are related to identifiable medical problems such as kidney disease, cancer, arthritis, osteoporosis, or spinal infection. Sideways curvature (scoliosis), sway back (lordosis, or excessive curve in the lower back), or other structural defects may also be at the root of back pain.

What Causes It?

Low-back trouble is so common because the human spine hasn't evolved to the point where people can walk upright without some risk. Being erect puts extra pressure on the vertebrae of the lower back, or lumbar region, where the back curves most and where pain most often strikes. Backaches become more common between the ages of 30 and 50, as the disks—the fibrous pads that cushion the vertebrae—start to lose water and elasticity and thus some of their ability to absorb shock. In middle age, too, people tend to become less active, and their muscles grow lax, contributing to back instability.

A small portion of all backaches do have clear causes—for instance, a ruptured disk or some

Back-Care Products

One way people try to improve their posture and/or protect their backs is by using one of a variety of backrests, special pillows, and other devices now available in orthopedic-supply stores and catalogs. (Certain back products, especially those that immobilize the spine, should be prescribed by your doctor or other qualified practitioner and must be specially fitted.)

Choosing an off-the-shelf back-care product is largely a matter of personal preference and comfort. There is no scientific research showing, for instance, that a lumbar roll is better than a larger backrest, or vice versa. In fact, there is a great deal of disagreement among back experts (such as orthopedists, physical therapists, chiropractors, and product designers) about what's best for backs in general. Since backaches tend to be idiosyncratic, no single gadget will work for everyone, and for some backache sufferers no device will help.

Backrests
Sitting actually puts more pressure on your spinal disks than standing; slumping or hunching over in a chair is particularly straining. A chair that supports your lower back is essential. Backrests can also help encourage good sitting posture, especially when a chair is not adjustable. Backrests come in many sizes and shapes. Some contoured models are made for use in cars; others are inflatable and can be conveniently taken into planes, trains, or theaters.

Lumbar Rolls
These cylindrical foam pillows (four to five inches in diameter) are placed directly in the small of your back for support when seated. Many have straps for attaching to a chair.

Seat Wedges
When placed on a seat, one of these fabric-covered pieces of foam can tilt you forward and prevent you from sinking into an unsupportive chair. You can also place a seat wedge behind your back to adjust the angle of a chair's backrest.

Neck Supports
These pillows wrap around the neck and thus help keep your head upright and your cervical disks properly aligned. There are inflatable models.

Slant Boards
These angled boards, when placed on desks, make reading and writing more comfortable. Most boards are adjustable. They help prevent neck strain and slouching posture.

Pillows
Bad sleeping position is a common cause of aches and pains. If you have a stiff neck or shoulder most mornings, try a different pillow. New pillows can be expensive, and no one pillow is going to answer everybody's needs. Ideally, your neck should be straight most of the night. Some foam pillows are too high and firm, or too bouncy. Some down pillows are too soft and flat. If you generally sleep on your back or side, you might benefit from a cervical roll, a small round pillow for neck support. This can be used by itself or in addition to your regular pillow.

If your mattress is very firm and you sleep on your side, you may need a thicker pillow than you would on a mattress that allows your shoulder to sink into it. If you sleep on your stomach most of the night, try a soft, oversize pillow that goes under your chest but supports your head and neck. Try sleeping with different pillows or combinations of pillows. Or simply try a rolled-up towel as a cervical pillow. Some people prefer no pillow at all.

Bed Wedges
These help you stay comfortable while reading or watching TV in bed. You can also use them to elevate your knees to relieve pressure on your lower back if you sleep on your back.

Bed Boards
You can firm up a sagging mattress (a frequent contributor to low-back pain) by placing a board between it and the box spring. Lightweight folding models are available for travel.

161

Strengthening Your Back

Weak back muscles increase the risk of back problems, and exercise is essential for keeping these muscles strong and protecting the back from injury. The key to strengthening the back, according to a recent study, is to keep the pelvis from moving so that the back muscles do the work, not bigger muscles like the gluteals (in the buttocks) or hamstrings (in the thighs). Moreover, keeping the pelvis stable forces people to move their stiff spines, and movement alone may help promote healing.

Start any exercise program slowly, preferably under the guidance of a physical therapist. If your back hurts, talk to your doctor or therapist before starting to exercise. Stop if your back pain gets worse or you experience leg pain or numbness. Avoid exercises that increase the stress on the spine, such as straight-leg toe touches or backward bends. Before working out, always warm up and then gently stretch.

The exercises shown here—four strengtheners and two stretches—will get you started. They should be done at least twice a week. Start with low resistance and few repetitions.

If you belong to a gym or health club, you can use a "Roman chair" or a Nautilus-type machine that allows you to do back extensions by leaning backward against variable resistance, without arching your back, moving your pelvis, or using your leg muscles. If you want, you can do this exercise with an elastic band or tubing (see illustration); Thera-Band and Dyna-Band are some of the brands sold commercially.

For the trunk rotations, you can use a Nautilus-type machine that allows you to twist your torso against variable resistance while keeping your pelvis in place. You can also do this exercise with an elastic band (see illustration).

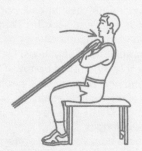

Back extension. Anchor elastic band to something stable below knee level. Sit upright, holding other end of band against your upper chest (band should be taut). Lean backward slowly 30 degrees, keeping your pelvis stable and back straight; don't arch. Hold for a few seconds, return slowly. Repeat 10 times.

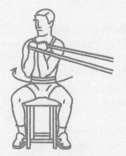

Trunk rotation. Anchor band to door knob. Sit at a 90-degree angle to closed door, holding other end of band against your upper chest; keep band taut. Keeping pelvis and knees in place and back straight, slowly rotate to one side against the tension. Hold for a few seconds, return slowly. Repeat 10 times, then switch sides.

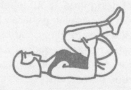

Lumbar stretch (for lower back). Lying on back, clasp one hand under each knee. Gently pull both knees toward chest, keeping lower back on floor. Hold for 10 to 30 seconds, relax, then repeat.

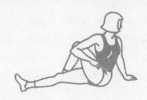

Spinal twist (for back and sides). Sit with right leg straight out, and left knee bent, with left foot placed on the outside of right knee. Bend right elbow and place it on outside of upper left thigh, just above knee, to keep that leg stationary. Place left hand behind you, slowly turn head to look over left shoulder, and twist upper body toward left arm. Hold for 10 to 30 seconds. Switch sides and repeat.

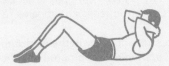

Crunches with feet on the floor. Lie on the floor with your knees bent and feet on the floor. Place your hands behind your head. Lift your shoulders slowly until they are completely off the floor. Pause and slowly lower yourself to the starting position. Repeat 10 to 15 times.

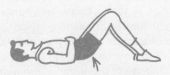

Pelvic tilt. Lie on your back with knees bent. Hold in your stomach and tighten your buttock muscles. Lift your buttocks slightly off the floor and hold for 10 seconds, keeping your lower back on the floor. Release. Repeat 20 times.

underlying disease. But in the great majority of cases the exact diagnosis isn't known. Is the cause of your backache that sudden movement yesterday when you bent down to pick up the newspaper, or is the problem that you get too little (or too much) exercise? Or could it be poor posture, or just everyday wear and tear? In fact, it's probably a combination of all these factors.

Usually x-rays show nothing wrong despite the pain—yet in some cases there is dramatic damage to disks but no pain whatsoever. Back injuries are often made worse by a number of contributing factors that include posture problems, tension and stress, a sedentary lifestyle, obesity, pregnancy, a sagging mattress, or poor body mechanics when lifting heavy objects.

What If You Do Nothing?

Fortunately, most backaches aren't serious and generally go away in a few weeks, with or without medical attention.

Home Remedies

The great majority of backaches (less serious strains, sprains, or spasms) usually don't require a doctor's attention. Depending on the severity of the pain, one or more of these measures should provide relief.

• **Avoid physically demanding tasks.** For soreness and minor pain in the back, avoiding physically demanding activity for a few days may be sufficient.

• **For mild to severe pain, lie down and rest.** Reclining may relieve the pain, and it takes mechanical pressure off the stressed back during the first day or two of injury. Some people find they are helped by putting a pillow under the knees when lying down. You may be able to take pressure off your back and get relief by lying on the floor, with your hips and knees bent, and your lower legs resting on the seat of a chair.

Allowing the inflamed tissue to repair itself can prevent a chronic cycle of back injury. Compared to standing, lying down reduces pressure on the lumbar disks by 70 percent, while unsupported sitting increases it by 40 percent.

• **Don't overstay your time in bed.** The current trend in treating common backaches is to get people out of bed as soon as they can get up comfortably. While doctors traditionally recommended a week or two of bed rest, research has found that two days in bed are usually sufficient for run-of-the-mill backaches, while longer bed rest should be reserved only for disk problems. Moreover, shorter periods of bed rest tend to reduce the likelihood of the adverse effects associated with prolonged bed rest, such as weakening of muscles from inactivity, that can lead to further back injury. (As patients bedridden for other reasons often discover, a couple weeks of bed rest can actually produce a painful back.) It's also a good idea to begin walking as soon as possible.

• **Try over-the-counter anti-inflammatory pain relievers.** Nonprescription NSAIDs—aspirin, ibuprofen, and naproxen—will help reduce the intensity of pain and inhibit inflammation.

• **Apply ice and heat.** If you feel soreness in one specific area of the lower back, put an ice pack on the area to temporarily block the transmission of pain messages to the brain. Wrap the ice in a towel to avoid damaging the skin. Keep the ice on for no longer than 20 minutes at a time to avoid chilling the back muscles, which can lead to a muscle spasm.

You may find that heat provides better pain relief than ice. Hot compresses applied with a hot water bottle, a heating pad (on a low or medium setting), or a towel heated in water can help

relieve spasm symptoms after the first 24 hours. Keep the heat on the lower back for no longer than 30 minutes. Reapply it up to four times a day. A hot bath or shower or sitting in a hot tub will also increase blood flow to the lower back

Alternative Therapies for Back Pain

▼

In an effort to cope with recurring back pain, many people turn to alternative modes of treatment, in particular seeking relief from chiropractors and acupuncturists. Do these therapies work?

Chiropractic may be worth trying, but the problem is that spinal manipulation does not appear to be any more effective than medical treatments at the other end of the spectrum. A study from the North Carolina Back Pain Project found that the benefits from treatment provided by primary-care physicians, chiropractors, or orthopedic surgeons were about equal.

A more recent study in the *New England Journal of Medicine* compared patients receiving physical therapy (the McKenzie method, which consists of certain exercises), chiropractic manipulation, or simply a good informational booklet about back pain. All three groups fared about the same. X-rays done by a chiropractor are no more likely to be useful than those done by an MD. (See page 99 for more information on chiropractors.)

Some people find that acupuncture provides relief. In 1997, a Consensus Panel at the National Institutes of Health concluded that acupuncture might be useful as an adjunct treatment for low back pain in a "comprehensive management program." (Such a program would include preventive measures.) A study in *Archives of Internal Medicine* found acupuncture more effective than conventional treatments (including surgery), but possibly no better than sham acupuncture (placebo). However, acupuncture is hard to study scientifically. (See page 98 for information on acupuncture.)

and contribute to pain relief.

• **Take it easy.** Remember, any resumption of activity must be gradual, since your back needs time to heal completely. Once the pain is gone, avoid heavy chores and sports for at least two weeks. If you wish, continue taking aspirin or other anti-inflammatories to reduce pain. However, do not use a corset or back brace unless your doctor prescribes it.

Prevention

Because most backaches are due at least in part to excessive strain or to weak or tense muscles, there is much you can do to prevent them. In more than half of all cases, back pain eventually recurs, so it's a good idea to consider the following preventive measures, especially if you have a history of back problems.

• **Maintain a good weight for your height.** A paunch can strain back muscles, distort posture, and overly compress the disks in the lower back. Not surprisingly, then, most obese people have chronic back problems. Excess weight, particularly if it has been recently gained, puts increased strain on back muscles and ligaments. Being pregnant can have a similar adverse effect because it alters an expectant mother's center of gravity.

• **Improve your posture.** Sitting and standing put considerable pressure on the lower back. Correct posture keeps the head and chest high, neck straight, pelvis forward, and stomach and buttocks tucked in.

• **Change your sleeping position.** Don't lie on your stomach, since that makes the stomach muscles sag and increases sway back. Instead, lie on your side with your knees bent to relieve pressure on the disks. For the same reason, if you lie on your back, keep your knees slightly bent by putting a pillow under them. For most people the

ideal mattress has firm inner support but adequate surface cushioning. If your mattress is too soft, insert a board under it.

• **Exercise.** Regular exercise is vital to the health of your back. Calisthenics and stretching routines can help strengthen the back (see pages 162-163). In addition, low-impact activities like walking, swimming (but not the butterfly or breast stroke, which can put excessive strain on the lower back), and cycling (with an upright posture or recumbent position) are good for the back. You should concentrate not only on exercises that stretch and strengthen back muscles, but also on those that strengthen the abdominal muscles (such as pelvic tilts), which help support the back .

However, sports that involve lifting, twisting, excessive arching of the spine, jumping, sudden starts and stops, and/or collisions with other players (including racket sports, golf, bowling, football, and basketball) are usually not recommended for people with chronic back problems.

• **Think before lifting and carrying.** Bending to pick up an object puts maximum strain on your back and is probably the primary cause of backaches. When you lift, bend at the knees, not at the waist, making your leg muscles do most of the work. To pick up something heavy, squat with your legs apart, tighten your stomach muscles, keep your back straight, and hold the object close to your body. Better yet, push a heavy object instead of lifting it. Pulling is more likely to injure your back.

When carrying a heavy load, don't arch your back or twist your body—try to let your arms and abdominal muscles bear the weight. Because a heavy purse or briefcase can pull your back out of alignment, alternate the load from side to side.

• **Dress for ease of movement.** Prolonged use of tight pants and girdles may induce weak abdom-

165

inal muscles and result in back trouble. Avoid high heels since they tend to increase the curvature of the back and increase the risk of a fall.

• **Sit in a straight-backed chair.** Whenever you sit, hold your spine against the back of the chair. Try to keep your knees a little higher than your hips.

• **Check your shoes.** Wear flat shoes or shoes with low heels (one inch or lower.)

• **Stop any activity that hurts.** Any twisting, bending, turning, and stretching that contributes to pain can create back problems that could take weeks to cure.

When To Call Your Doctor

Contact your physician if the pain from backache or sciatica is severe, or if it doesn't improve after two days. In addition, call your doctor if you have any of the following symptoms: pain, numbness, or tingling that radiates down an arm or leg; back pain that continues unabated when you're lying down; back pain after a fall or car accident; vomiting or fever associated with back pain; or backache in an elderly person or child. Any of these may indicate a more serious problem.

Many people have found relief from acute (not chronic) back pain with chiropractors. If you have acute low-back pain and wish to consult a chiropractor or seek some other alternative treatment such as acupuncture, see pages 97-103 for more information and guidelines.

What Your Doctor Will Do

On your first visit your doctor will probably just examine you and take a history. Bed rest and anti-inflammatory painkillers are often the first choice for treatment of low-back pain. Your doctor may prescribe a stronger painkiller or may refer you to a physical therapist for a course of exercises and treatment, or to a specialist in back problems for further examination.

If you don't get better, your doctor may need to determine whether your problem comes from a herniated disk, an inflamed piriformis muscle (which can trigger sciatica), or other causes. X-rays may be called for, along with magnetic resonance imaging (MRI), a diagnostic technique that uses magnetic fields and radio waves. An MRI reveals spinal architecture accurately and in much more detail than an x-ray.

Back experts urge physicians not to rush to use MRIs to diagnose patients with sciatica or uncomplicated acute low-back pain (that is, pain not due to an underlying illness or injury and not involving nerve damage or paralysis). These problems are usually self-limited, and an MRI reveals little information that helps with a prognosis.

Whatever the diagnosis, opt for the most conservative treatments—rest, exercise, painkillers, and physical therapy. Surgery may be an option in some persistent cases, but it is expensive and requires a long period of recuperation. It is also frequently unsuccessful. Before considering surgery, you should exhaust all other forms of treatment. If your doctor suggests surgery, consider a second opinion. Don't consent to traction, which has not been shown to be beneficial for low-back pain.

For More Information

• American Academy of Orthopaedic Surgeons
• American Osteopathic Association
• Back Pain Hotline
• American Pain Foundation

Bad Breath

Symptoms

- Exhaled breath has an unpleasant odor.
- Bad taste in the mouth.
- Bleeding gums.

What Is It?

Millions of Americans—perhaps as many as 85 million—have chronically bad breath, or halitosis. Concern about halitosis has given rise to a billion-dollar-a-year industry of products that are intended to eliminate or conceal mouth odor. You can even take advantage of one of hundreds of "breath clinics" being offered all over the country. But the most effective steps involve simple oral hygiene.

What Causes It?

Bad breath has many causes, but often the underlying cause is the activity of bacteria in the mouth. Most cases of bad breath are due to the breakdown of food particles in and around your teeth, which can create foul-smelling gases. If you have healthy teeth and gums but still experience bad breath, it usually comes from the back region of the tongue, possibly because of postnasal drip to the tongue surface.

Periodontal disease (inflammation of the gums) can also cause bad breath (see Gingivitis, page 287), as can a dry mouth, which contributes to halitosis because saliva helps keep bacteria in check. This helps explain "morning breath," since the mouth dries out during sleep. Mouthwashes with a high alcohol content can also dry the mouth, allowing bacteria to thrive. And certain medical conditions and medications can cause chronic dry mouth, or xerostomia.

Halitosis can also be caused by certain respiratory or gastrointestinal disorders as well as diabetes mellitus, chronic sinusitis or bronchitis, a liver or kidney ailment, and emphysema.

Other contributing factors include smoking, alcoholic drinks, and such foods as garlic and onions, which contain volatile oils that are absorbed into your bloodstream, carried to your lungs, and released in your breath.

What If You Do Nothing?

Most cases of bad breath are temporary, and if a particular food contributed to it, then the problem will clear up when you stop eating that food. But if you often have bad breath, you'll need to take stronger measures like the self-care remedies that follow.

Home Remedies

Mints and mouthwashes will only temporarily quell bad breath; they cannot cure the underlying problem. Instead, take these measures.

Mouthwash Tips

▼

Mouthwashes, also called mouth rinses, have been around for centuries; the oldest of all is plain water. The great majority of nonprescription mouth rinses are simply breath fresheners—they have little effect against plaque (the thin film on teeth where decay-causing bacteria live), and they don't prevent gingivitis (the early stage of periodontal disease).

- If you simply want temporary breath freshening, nearly any mouthwash will do. The effect lasts up to half an hour.
- Don't overuse rinses. A tablespoon or two should do. Swish it around in your mouth for about 30 seconds. Never swallow rinses. Don't eat or drink for half an hour after use.
- No mouthwash or other breath freshener can take the place of thorough flossing and brushing, as well as semiannual visits to the dentist.

• **Brush more frequently.** Brushing your teeth after each meal will improve most cases of mild bad breath. When you're finished with your teeth, gently scrub the roof of your mouth and your gums.

• **Clean your tongue.** This can be one of the most effective steps for eliminating bad breath. The tongue's microscopic hairs harbor plaque and food particles that can give rise to breath-fouling bacteria. In fact, the tongue can become coated with bacteria that ferment proteins and give off unpleasant odors. Therefore, brush the surface of the tongue when you finish with your teeth in order to dislodge the culprits, or else use a special plastic tongue scraper, sold in most pharmacies.

Choose a brush with soft bristles; stroke from the rear of the throat (as far back as you can go without gagging) and gently brush outward. For better results, wet your brush with an effective mouthwash.

• **Floss.** Clean the spaces between your teeth at least once a day.

• **Get regular dental checkups.** Have your teeth examined and cleaned periodically by your dentist and/or a dental hygienist.

• **Take care of dentures.** Soak your dentures overnight in an antiseptic solution.

• **If you smoke, quit.** In addition to being linked with lung and other cancers, tobacco is a major cause of bad breath.

• **Drink more water.** Keeping your mouth moist will help disperse the bacteria living there. Drink at least eight glasses of water daily.

• **Avoid foods that trigger bad breath.** There are many common spices and foods that can cause bad breath. Obvious culprits include anchovies, garlic, onions, and anything containing alcohol.

Prevention
Follow the measures listed above.

When To Call Your Doctor
If your bad breath does not respond to the measures suggested above, contact your dentist to see if gum or tooth disease is the culprit. Also contact your dentist if your bad breath is accompanied by tooth pain. This may signal a cavity, a lost filling, or an abscess. If you have bad breath and your gums bleed often after brushing, this can be a sign of gum disease.

What Your Doctor Will Do
After taking a careful history to determine the possible causes of the odor, your dentist may recommend a mouthwash that has been shown to be effective in fighting bad breath. If the problem can't be traced to a tooth or gum condition, particularly if you are maintaining good oral hygiene, then you should see a physician to check on the possibility of lung or gastric disorders or some other underlying medical condition.

For More Information
• American Dental Association

Bed-Wetting

Symptoms

■ Involuntary loss of nighttime bladder control that persists beyond the age of five or six years.

What Is It?

As they grow and mature, young children gradually gain mastery over bodily processes, including bladder control. Many children stay dry at night by age three or four, about six months after they have mastered daytime bladder control. But in about 15 percent of children, bed-wetting persists past the age of five (and acquires a medical name, enuresis). It may occur occasionally, or almost every night, and is more common in boys than girls. Many such children continue to have the problem for several years, though virtually all cases resolve by adolescence. It's also not uncommon for children who previously had no trouble to have periodic lapses, particularly during times of stress.

What Causes It?

Less than 10 percent of the time, underlying medical problems are the cause. These can be easily identified by a physician and include an unusually small bladder, diabetes mellitus, kidney problems, epilepsy, sickle cell anemia, urinary tract infections, or developmental disorders like autism or mental retardation. If a child who is toilet trained is also having trouble staying dry during the day, it's a good indication that the bed-wetting has a physical cause.

A genetic component appears to be included as well: the disorder often runs in families. Some studies suggest that bed-wetting may be linked to a deficiency in a naturally occurring substance called antidiuretic hormone, or vasopressin, which helps regulate the amount of urine produced.

Emotional factors (for example, acting out by the child) were once thought to be an important contributing factor. Although the stress of a move or a new sibling can cause periodic lapses in nighttime bladder control, persistent bed-wetting is rarely psychological in origin.

What If You Do Nothing?

Most children outgrow the problem without any adverse consequences. The best thing to do is to be patient and supportive. Anger or disgust from parents or taunting by siblings can lead to shame and anxiety in a child, leading to more serious psychological problems.

Home Remedies

• **Maintain a supportive environment.** A child will be frustrated and embarrassed by bed-wetting. Parents, too, will have their patience tried. Stay calm, and reassure your child (and yourself) that bed-wetting is a condition that can, and will, be overcome. Let the child know that others (particularly if they are family members) have had the problem but outgrew it.

Praise your child for dry nights; a calendar with gold stars or other rewards may help. Don't become angry or blame your child for wetting the bed, and explain the importance of a sympathetic and encouraging home environment to other family members.

• **Watch your child's fluid intake at night.** Get him or her to drink plenty of fluids in the morning or the afternoon to stretch the bladder and increase its capacity. Your child can drink fluids at night as well, but not in excess, and should avoid beverages that contain caffeine.

• **Encourage bladder control practice.** Have your child hold his or her urine for increasingly longer periods during the day—up to 10 to 15 extra minutes. This may help improve bladder control.

• **Encourage urination before bedtime.** Get your child in the habit of emptying the bladder as much as possible before going to bed. Once in bed, try positive imaging: have the child imagine waking up in the morning with clean, dry sheets.

• **Consider wake-up breaks.** Some experts suggest setting the alarm for several hours after bedtime and encouraging the child to get up and urinate at that time—though others say this needlessly disrupts the child's natural sleep cycles. Special bed-wetting alarms that attach to the underwear and that are set off by the first hint of moisture are also available. You can discuss these options with your doctor. With time, your child will learn to recognize a full bladder and get up on his or her own.

• **Protect your child's bedding.** To help minimize stress, make cleanup as easy as possible. Use two sets of sheets, with a rubber pad between them, and a plastic cover over the mattress. Children may wear an extra thick pair, or two pairs, of underwear, to help absorb urine. Don't use diapers on children older than four; it will only humiliate them.

• **Work in partnership with your child.** Have your child assist with tasks: laundering the sheets, making up the bed, putting out a fresh pair of pajamas and a towel before retiring. The job should be fun and not punitive. Involving your child may increase his or her sense of control and help to resolve the problem.

Prevention

No specific measures can prevent persistent bed-wetting. Some experts believe that toilet training at too early an age and at too rapid a pace can be stressful for a child and may cause psychological conflicts that contribute to the problem. Recognize bed-wetting as a normal stage of child development—one that, like walking and talking, comes at different times for different children.

When To Call Your Doctor

If bed-wetting is accompanied by fever, abdominal pain, or blood in the urine, or by urinary pain, burning, or dribbling, it may be a sign of a urinary tract infection or some other physical problem; contact your doctor immediately. Also seek medical guidance if bed-wetting persists past age five or six and your child is unduly upset about it, or if bed-wetting newly develops in an otherwise healthy older child and persists for more than a month.

What Your Doctor Will Do

Your pediatrician will ask for a detailed history of the child's medical condition, take a urine sample, and do a thorough physical examination, including careful inspection of the genital area to look for any physical causes for the problem. X-rays are sometimes also needed. Very small doses of the antidepressant medications imipramine or amitriptyline, which may help curb bed-wetting through an unknown mechanism, are sometimes prescribed. Another medication your doctor may recommend is desmopressin (DDAVP), a vasopressin-like hormone drug that reduces urine output during the night. If underlying psychological issues are suspected, counseling may be recommended.

For More Information

• American Academy of Pediatrics

Belching

Symptoms

- An eruptive noise from the mouth and throat.
- Possible nausea.
- Possible burning sensation in the throat or mouth.

What Is It?
Belching (or burping) is an escape of air from the stomach and is usually a way to relieve abdominal distress caused by excessive air buildup, particularly after eating a large meal or drinking a carbonated beverage.

What Causes It?
One cause of belching is swallowing air, which can occur if you eat too quickly, chew with your mouth open, talk while you are chewing, chew gum, or drink through a straw. Drinking carbonated beverages can also increase the amount of air that reaches your stomach.

Belching can also be brought on by certain ailments such as heartburn, hiatal hernia, and peptic ulcer, but in these instances it is typically accompanied by other symptoms.

What If You Do Nothing?
Although belching is a social faux pas and can be embarrassing, for the vast majority of people belching is not a problem that requires treatment.

Home Remedies
Once you are aware that the cause of your excessive belching may be linked with the unconscious swallowing of too much air, you should be able to eliminate it by making the conscious effort to swallow much less. Take these measures.
- **Avoid rapid eating.** Eat four to six mini-meals throughout the day, which can stave off hunger pangs and curb your desire to eat too rapidly.
- **Take small bites when you eat.**
- **Chew food with your mouth closed.** This will keep you from taking in extra air when you swallow. Also avoid talking with food in your mouth.
- **Cut back or eliminate gum chewing.**
- **Cut back or eliminate carbonated beverages.** The carbon dioxide gas in the beverages can cause excessive belching.
- **Don't take calcium carbonate.** Calcium supplements made from calcium carbonate can release carbon dioxide in some people, creating excess gas in the stomach. If you take calcium supplements regularly, choose another form of calcium, such as calcium citrate.

Prevention
The measures under Home Remedies will help prevent belching.

When To Call Your Doctor
Belching is often an insignificant problem. However, excessive belching often results from aerophagia, an unconscious nervous habit of swallowing too much air. Professional help is required if this becomes a chronic problem.

What Your Doctor Will Do
If excessive belching becomes a problem, your physician will review your diet and check for specific foods or drinks that are causing the distress. Your doctor will also point out personal habits, such as sucking on candy, eating too quickly, smoking, and gum chewing, that can cause excessive swallowing and may be the source of your belching.

For More Information
- American Gastroenterological Association

171

Blepharitis

Symptoms

- Scaly, red eyelids that are inflamed around the margins.
- Itching and burning, with a sensation that there is something in the eyes.
- Awakening to a sticky crust sealing the eyelids.
- Dandruff-like flakes of skin on the eyelids.

What Is It?

Your eyelids protect and clean your eyes but are also sources of bacterial infection. Blepharitis, or "granulated lids," is an inflammation of the edges of the eyelids. This results in a persistent red-rimmed, scaly appearance that usually affects both eyes at once. The ailment is generally not serious and is rarely a threat to vision. But blepharitis tends to be a chronic condition and may require long-term treatment.

What Causes It?

Blepharitis is often associated with seborrhea (seborrheic dermatitis)—red, scaly, itchy patches of skin that affect the scalp and parts of the face. A bacterial infection also often causes or complicates the problem: eyelashes each grow out of separate follicles, and bacteria can enter readily, resulting in infection. Pus oozes out along the eyelash, where it dries, crusts, and falls into the eye, causing chronic red eyes.

In rare cases blepharitis may be caused by an infestation of lice in the eyelashes.

What If You Do Nothing?

Sometimes blepharitis clears up on its own, but it can easily recur and become chronic. Early treatment is essential to prevent recurrence or complications.

Home Remedies

- **Keep your eyelids clean.** Wash your eyelids three times daily with warm saltwater or baby shampoo diluted with water. Use a cotton-tip applicator to gently scrub the eyelid margins, upper and lower, removing all traces of the dry crust. Use a new tip for each margin. Do this procedure when you awaken, at midday when oils and pus accumulate, and at bedtime.
- **Don't wear eye makeup until the inflammation subsides.** Mascara or eye shadow may result in contact dermatitis of the eyelids.
- **Don't wear contact lenses until the condition is resolved.** If your case is chronic, discuss with your ophthalmologist when you can continue wearing the lenses.

Prevention

Controlling blepharitis with the remedies outlined above will also prevent it from recurring or worsening. Also, use a medicated shampoo to control any seborrhea of the scalp.

When To Call Your Doctor

If your case doesn't clear up after two weeks of self-care measures, contact your ophthalmologist. If you notice lice on yourself (or on a child who is infected), call a doctor right away.

What Your Doctor Will Do

After a careful examination your physician may prescribe an antibiotic ointment to rub onto the eyelids to counteract the bacteria. If lice are the cause, the doctor will recommend an ophthalmic ointment and/or will remove the nits by hand.

For More Information

- American Academy of Ophthalmology

Blisters

Symptoms

■ Fluid-filled, raised areas on the skin that are often tender to the touch.

What Is It?

Blisters are raised or loose areas of skin in which fluid accumulates under the outer layer. A blister may not be painful at first, but if the outer layer of skin—the epidermis—is opened, the sensitive skin underneath can become quite painful and may also get infected.

What Causes It?

Blisters have many causes, including burns, cold sores, and allergic reactions to plants or insects. But the most common nonmedical cause is friction or pressure from ill-fitting shoes, socks, or stockings (either too big or small) that rub against skin. Going without socks or stockings in normally well-fitting shoes can also blister heels and toes, particularly in hot weather, when feet are likely to swell and sweat. Sandals and other shoes with straps are particularly likely to blister bare skin.

What If You Do Nothing?

If it's a small blister, it will heal by itself if you eliminate the pressure that is causing it. Just make sure it stays clean.

Home Remedies

If the blister is less than an inch across, don't break it open or try to drain it. Not only is the skin underneath extremely sensitive, but it can also become infected. If necessary, take the following steps.

• **Relieve pressure.** If the blister is in a weight-bearing spot, cover it with a moleskin pad with a hole cut in the middle.

• **Relieve pain.** If you have a large blister that hurts when you walk on it, you may want to puncture it. First wash it, then make a small hole near its edge with a sterile needle (hold it in a flame for a few seconds). Don't remove the "roof" of skin. Gently squeeze out the liquid and cover it with a tight sterile bandage; try to keep it dry.

• **Cleanse and protect.** If the blister breaks, wash it with soap and water, and protect it with a light bandage.

Avoiding Blisters: The Fitted Shoe

▼

Shoes that don't fit well are a major cause of blisters. However, this all-too-common problem can be avoided by following these simple steps. Start with proper measurement: the shoe store's metal Brannock device is more accurate than a wooden ruler. Always put your full weight on the foot being measured. Try the size that fits the larger foot.

Sizes indicate very little: size 8½ C in one brand may be a 9B in another. Imported shoes are likely to run small.

Follow these other tips:

• Try to shop in the middle or towards the end of a normal day, not early in the morning, since your feet swell as the day progresses owing to friction, heat, and use.

• Wear the kind of socks or stockings that you intend to wear with the shoes. Avoid socks and stockings that constrict your feet or bunch up.

• When testing new shoes, stand on one foot at a time. Wiggle your toes. Stand on tiptoe. The shoe should bend where your foot bends.

• Never buy a shoe with the idea of breaking it in over a period of time. Your foot may alter in an uncomfortable shoe, but the shoe won't.

• Check to see that you have one-half inch of space between the end of your big toe and the tip of the shoe.

• Make sure the widest part of your foot—the metatarsal arch—fits comfortably in the widest part of the shoe.

Prevention

- **Buy shoes that fit.** This is your first line of defense.
- **Keep your feet dry.** Cotton or woolen socks, though able to absorb moisture better than nylon, still hold moisture against your skin, thus increasing the risk of blisters. Athletic socks made from a variety of polyesters, such as polypropylene, acrylic, or Capilene, draw moisture away from your feet so that it can evaporate. Foot powders also help absorb excess moisture.
- **For hiking, an antiperspirant may help.** If your feet tend to sweat heavily and you are prone to blisters, you can try an aluminum-containing antiperspirant to keep feet super dry. In a study of West Point cadets, the cadets found that applying such an antiperspirant daily for three days before a long hike significantly reduced the risk of blisters. However, half the cadets experienced skin irritation from the antiperspirants they used, so if antiperspirants irritate your underarms, this approach isn't for you. Otherwise, try it using a roll-on or stick product.

- **Protect blister-prone areas.** Use foot powder, breathable adhesive tape (sometimes labeled "first aid"), moleskin, "Second Skin" (a slippery pad that absorbs friction), or petroleum jelly to reduce pressure and friction. If you typically develop blisters on your hands after using tools or sports equipment, don't forget to put on gloves before beginning your activity.

When To Call Your Doctor

Contact your physician if a blister shows reddening, swelling, or pus—each is a sign of infection. Also contact your physician if you have a history of diabetes or circulatory disease and have developed a blister.

What Your Doctor Will Do

If infection is suspected after a close examination, your physician may prescribe an antibiotic medication.

For More Information

- American Academy of Dermatology

Bloodshot Eyes

Symptoms

■ Red spidery veins on the white of the eyeball.

What Is It?

Bloodshot means that the small vessels on the surface of the eyeball are dilated and visible.

What Causes It?

Many people notice that their eyes are red on awakening. Lack of sleep, alcohol consumption the night before, overuse of contact lenses, or an allergy are among the possible causes. Bloodshot eyes during the day can be caused by an irritant, eyestrain, rubbing your eyes excessively, or anything that tends to dry your eyes (high heat and low humidity, or insufficient tear production).

Colds, flu, and hay fever can produce bloodshot eyes as well, but occasionally the condition can be a sign of underlying disease or injury. Conjunctivitis, or pinkeye, which is usually more alarming in appearance than bloodshot eyes, is an infection that produces very red, irritated eyes, as well as itching and a discharge. Blepharitis is another eye infection (of the eyelid) that produces redness, typically accompanied by a crust forming over the eyelashes (see page 172).

What If You Do Nothing?

Most commonly, if the cause is external and temporary, bloodshot eyes improve by themselves.

Home Remedies

• **Wash your face and eyelids.** Using cold water can help and so can cold compresses.
• **Try over-the-counter eyedrops and eyewashes.** Drops usually contain a decongestant to constrict blood vessels; eyewashes usually contain boric acid or a saline solution. Both may help. But be sure to follow instructions carefully with any eye product. Overuse of some eyedrops can actually increase redness. And eyecups can be a source of infection, so use only the disposable kind.

When To Call Your Doctor

If you think you have an eye infection, or if your eyes don't clear up right away, or if you have eye pain or changes in vision, you should seek medical advice.

What Your Doctor Will Do

Your doctor will check your vision, your eyes, and eyelids. If there is an infection, antibiotic eyedrops or ointments may be prescribed.

For More Information

• American Academy of Ophthalmology

Over-the-Counter Eyedrops
▼

Most eyedrops are rarely necessary. Normal eyes do not need "cleansing," "soothing," or "refreshing" solutions. Your tears, which contain antibacterial agents, are the most effective eye cleansers. Though they may be soothing, over-the-counter drops can mask symptoms of eye infection and disease. If there is irritation or redness for more than a day or two, seek professional advice. And if you wear contact lenses, use only eyedrops recommended by your eye-care specialist. (For more information on eyedrops, see pages 581-585.)

Any liquid you put in your eyes should be sterile and should therefore be bought in a drugstore. There's one exception: emergencies. If you get dirt or a toxic chemical in your eye, there won't be time to find a sterile solution—just wash your eye with plenty of tap water.

Boils

Symptoms

- A lump, often pea-size, that forms under the skin on the face, neck, armpits, or buttocks. Red and tender to the touch, the lump fills with white or yellowish pus, forming a head or tip.
- Fever (occasionally).

What Is It?

A boil, or furuncle, is an inflamed, painful, pus-filled skin sore. It first forms as a nodule under the skin, then after several days it develops into a raised reddish sore with a white or yellow pus-filled center. Because of pus accumulating under the skin, the boil may become more painful. Eventually the pocket of pus rises towards the skin surface and finally bursts and drains. Once this occurs, pain diminishes and healing begins.

What Causes It?

Boils are typically caused by bacteria, usually *Staphylococcus*, that infect the oil gland of hair follicles, typically on the back of the neck, buttocks, groin, and armpits. Once germs proliferate in the gland, infection and inflammation of the skin begins rapidly. The staph germs may enter the body through cuts, scratches, or other skin breaks (and for this reason the bacteria can be spread to family members).

Anyone can get a boil, but some circumstances can predispose people to them. These include diabetes, a suppressed immune system, exposure to certain industrial chemicals, treatment of skin problems with corticosteroids, and poor hygiene.

What If You Do Nothing?

Boils are usually minor skin ailments. Most boils will rupture and drain on their own within two weeks. However, if left untreated, a boil can reach enormous size and become quite painful in a matter of days.

Home Remedies

- **Don't squeeze.** Using your fingers to squeeze a boil may force infected matter deeper into the skin.
- **Relieve pain and inflammation.** Take aspirin, ibuprofen, or naproxen according to label directions to relieve pain and inflammation.
- **Use a hot compress.** A boil on any body part except the face can often be treated effectively at home using hot, wet compresses. To make a compress, take a cotton cloth—a washcloth or a folded cotton handkerchief—dip it into hot water, and wring it out. Gently apply it to the infected area on and off for 10 minutes, remoistening the cloth when necessary. Repeat this process three times a day. The compress will help both to relieve pain and swelling and to bring the infection to a head, causing the boil to rupture and the pus to drain.
- **Keep the area clean.** To prevent reinfection, wash the area thoroughly with soap and water, then apply antibacterial ointment and cover the boil with a sterile gauze bandage. Change the bandage once a day, first washing the site and reapplying the ointment.

Prevention

- **Practice good hygiene.** Keep the site of the boil as clean as possible by washing it regularly with soap and water. If you are prone to boils, bathe regularly with a solution containing chlorhexidine, an antibacterial agent that is available in over-the-counter formulations (such as Hibiclens).
- **Don't share.** To avoid spreading bacteria, don't let anyone else use your towels, bedding, athletic equipment, or clothing. And change clothes and bedsheets regularly.

How to Treat Carbuncles

▼

A carbuncle is an oversized boil or cluster of boils that grows sideways in the tissue beneath the skin, usually in areas where the skin is thick and inelastic—for example, the back of the neck. It is less common than a boil.

Carbuncles can be very painful and usually require medical attention—especially if they are on your face, if you notice red streaking around it, or if you have a fever. As with boils, carbuncles on your face are of great concern because the infection can spread, even to your brain.

Carbuncles may require a doctor or nurse to incise and drain them. You should never squeeze a carbuncle or try to drain it yourself. You'll be instructed to keep the area clean and to apply an antibacterial ointment and sterile gauze. You may also need to take antibiotics.

When To Call Your Doctor

If the self-care measures for boils don't work after three or four days, contact your physician for treatment. However, contact your physician immediately if you develop a boil on the face above the lips, on the nose, or in the ear. These boils are especially dangerous because of their tendency to seep and drain directly into the brain, which may cause a life-threatening infection.

Also contact your physician if a fever accompanies your boil or if you have recurring boils. Medical attention is also required if you develop a carbuncle (see box at left).

What Your Doctor Will Do

Your physician will examine the infected area. For boils on the face, your doctor may lance the boil to drain the pus; he or she may also prescribe antibiotics.

If boils are recurring, blood or urine tests may be taken to diagnose the cause of the condition, which can include diabetes mellitus or other systemic diseases. Oral antibiotics may be prescribed to treat boils that aren't localized.

For More Information

• American Academy of Dermatology

177

BPH (Benign Prostatic Hyperplasia)

Symptoms

In some cases, there are no symptoms.

- More urgent and frequent need to urinate.
- Awakening at night with the need to urinate.
- A stop-and-start flow of urine, or urinary dribbling after completing urination.
- A sensation that the bladder is not completely emptied.
- Urinary hesitancy (difficulty with starting to urinate).
- Decreased volume and force of stream.

What Is It?

BPH (benign prostatic hyperplasia) is an enlargement of the prostate that is common in men over 40—not just in this country but throughout the world. The prostate is a walnut-size gland in men located just below the bladder. It wraps around the urethra, the tube that carries urine from the bladder out through the penis. Normally, the prostate produces the seminal fluid that carries sperm outward during an ejaculation. If the gland enlarges, however, it can interfere with urination.

Many people fear that an enlarged prostate is a prelude to cancer, or is cancer, but this is not the case. Hyperplasia simply means an overgrowth of cells. Although BPH can cause unpleasant symptoms, such as the need to urinate frequently, it is not harmful in itself—hence the term "benign." After age 60 more than half of all men have some degree of BPH.

BPH does not affect sexual function.

What Causes It?

No one knows what causes BPH. Diet has no known connection with this condition, but heredity may be a factor in its development. Another theory is that BPH is caused by normal changes in hormone levels, especially a drop in testosterone. (Testosterone therapy, however, is not a safe or recognized treatment for BPH.) Still another theory is that a substance called dihydrotestosterone (DHT), produced by aging men, promotes cell growth.

What If You Do Nothing?

Because urinary discomfort is largely subjective, how aggressively to deal with BPH is largely up to the patient. For men with mild symptoms, "watchful waiting" is usually the best course, since mild symptoms sometimes clear up or remain stable without treatment. Studies show that about 40 percent of men with mild symptoms improve without treatment, 45 percent continue with no change, and only 15 percent deteriorate. You should nonetheless get regular checkups to monitor the condition.

BPH requires treatment only if the symptoms are truly bothersome and begin to limit a man's activities, or if the urinary tract is threatened. Sometimes urinary flow stops altogether, which is a life-threatening medical emergency.

Home Remedies

The following lifestyle changes can help manage mild BPH. Keep in mind that you should have regular checkups if you have BPH.

- **Avoid certain medications.** Avoid tranquilizers, as well as over-the-counter cold remedies containing decongestants and antihistamines. These can worsen urinary symptoms.
- **Cut down on fluids—especially alcoholic beverages—in the evening.** This will decrease the need to urinate during the night.
- **Go easy on caffeinated drinks.** These are diuretics, which don't help and can be harmful.

Prevention

As of now, there are no measures known to prevent BPH.

When To Call Your Doctor

If you have any urinary difficulties, it's wise to discuss them with your doctor. They may be caused by something more serious that needs immediate treatment.

Herbs and the Prostate

▼

Plant-derived substances used as drugs are in wide use for treating BPH in Europe, and indeed are preferred by German urologists. Not classified as drugs in this country or regulated as such, these are sold over the counter in health-food stores.

Probably the best-known such therapy is saw palmetto, derived from berries of the saw palm tree (*Serenoa repens, Serenoa serrulata,* and other species). Saw palmetto appears to have a similar action to that of finasteride—that is, it may shrink the prostate. Some studies tend to support its effectiveness, though the evidence is fairly sparse.

Unfortunately, there is still a lack of real scientific information based on well-designed clinical trials of saw palmetto and other herbal remedies. Meanwhile, supplement manufacturers can market saw palmetto without any further proof of efficacy. And since their products are not regulated, you may or may not be getting what the label says.

If you want to try saw palmetto, do so only after seeing a doctor; don't dose yourself if you have prostate symptoms, since your condition could be cancer. Get a diagnosis. Also, if you are having a PSA test, tell your doctor if you are taking any over-the-counter remedies, since they may alter the results and thus make prostate cancer hard to diagnose.

For more information about saw palmetto, see page 634.

What Your Doctor Will Do

If you have BPH, your doctor should be able to diagnose it. The digital rectal exam is one method, plus tests to measure the rate of urine flow and lab tests of urine and blood. You may also be referred to a urologist for diagnosis and treatment. Most urologists also have a device in their offices that can measure the size of your prostate gland using ultrasound.

If your symptoms worsen, the first line of treatment is usually drugs. Finasteride (Proscar) can shrink the prostate. Studies have shown that finasteride works best if the prostate is greatly enlarged, but not in cases of mild enlargement. It may take six months to produce any improvement and may cause side effects, including reduced sexual function and desire.

Certain alpha blocker medications (Cardura, Flomax, Hytrin), which are also used to treat hypertension, act to relax the sphincter at the bladder outlet, facilitating urination. While the alpha blockers may reduce symptoms, they can produce such side effects as reduced sexual function, low blood pressure, and dizziness.

In cases of severe BPH, surgery may be the best option. One of two forms of surgery is usually undertaken, one involving removal of some prostate tissue (TURP, or transurethral resection of the prostate), and the other an incision in the tissue to relieve pressure (TUIP, transurethral incision of the prostate). Several other approaches are now available, including laser, radiowave, and microwave reduction of the prostate. But surgery is not necessary in most cases.

For More Information

• American Foundation for Urologic Disease
• National Kidney and Urologic Diseases Information Clearinghouse

179

Bronchitis (Acute)

Symptoms

- Persistent coughing that may be initially dry and hacking, but usually becomes productive, bringing up sputum that is green, yellow, or gray.
- Shortness of breath and wheezing.
- Fever (occasionally), usually below 101°F.
- Chest pain and discomfort behind the breastbone.

What Is It?

Many people suffer an attack of acute bronchitis as part of a severe cold. Bronchitis occurs when an irritant or infection causes inflammation and swelling of the lining of the bronchial tubes. These tubes, the bronchi, are the major air passages that lead from the trachea (the windpipe) into the lungs. The bronchi are lined with cilia, or tiny hairs, that sweep foreign matter out of the respiratory tract. When the bronchi are inflamed, the cilia don't function properly, and coughing—the chief symptom of bronchitis—becomes the body's way of coping with the irritants and mucus that build up and threaten to clog the bronchi.

About 5 percent of Americans suffer from chronic bronchitis, which is characterized by a deep mucus-producing cough that over time becomes constant and lasts for months. Most people who get chronic bronchitis are smokers.

What Causes It?

Most cases of acute bronchitis are caused by viruses, including some of the viruses that cause the common cold. Occasionally, however, bacteria cause the condition. Chemical fumes, dust, smoke, or other irritating air pollutants may also cause or aggravate bronchitis. In addition, smoking, asthma, cold weather, and congestive heart failure may increase the risk of an attack.

What If You Do Nothing?

Attacks of acute bronchitis are common but usually not a major health threat. Symptoms generally clear in about a week, but if you are a smoker or have a chronic lung disease such as asthma or emphysema, you must take care of the bronchitis to prevent possible complications.

Home Remedies

- **Relieve the discomfort.** Take nonprescription NSAIDs—aspirin, ibuprofen, or naproxen—or acetaminophen to reduce fever and pain.
- **Don't stop a wet cough.** If you have a wet productive cough (coughing up phlegm), do not suppress it with nonprescription cough suppressants unless the cough keeps you from sleeping. It's not recommended to stop a cough entirely because mucus can become trapped in the bronchial tubes, leading to breathing difficulties or triggering pneumonia.
- **Suppress a dry cough.** If you have a persistent dry cough that interferes with sleep and everyday activities, take an over-the-counter cough suppressant containing dextromethorphan, a medicine that relieves a cough by acting directly on the brain's cough center. Cough medicines with a name that ends in "DM" contain dextromethorphan.
- **Drink plenty of fluids.** This will liquefy the mucus and loosen phlegm, making it easier to expel them when coughing. Drink at least eight glasses of water or other nonalcoholic fluids a day, until your urine is virtually colorless.
- **Humidify the air.** Take hot steamy showers or use a humidifier or vaporizer in your bedroom to keep your bronchial tubes moist. However, home humidifiers can harbor fungi and other potential allergens, so be sure to keep the system scrupulously clean and in good working order. Change the water daily, and replace filters as often as directed.

Prevention

• **Don't smoke.** Avoid secondhand smoke as well.

• **Take it easy.** If you are at risk for bronchitis, avoid strenuous outdoor work and outdoor exercise on poor air-quality days.

• **Steer clear of all respiratory irritants.** Try to avoid paints, dust, smoke, chemical vapors, or other irritants. If these are unavoidable at your workplace, be sure to use a mask or other protective gear.

• **Filter the air.** If you live in an area with high pollution levels and your bronchitis has become chronic, consider installing a home air-conditioning unit to filter the air. Like humidifiers, home air conditioners can provide an ideal environment for fungi that have the potential to worsen your symptoms, so it's important to keep the system clean and to replace filters as often as directed.

When To Call Your Doctor

Contact your doctor if symptoms don't begin to ease up within 72 hours or if episodes of acute bronchitis recur. Also contact your physician if you develop bronchitis and you suffer from a lung ailment or congestive heart failure. If you cough up blood during an attack of bronchitis, or if you have a fever above 102°F, contact your physician right away.

What Your Doctor Will Do

Your doctor will take a complete medical history and then examine you. Blood tests and chest x-rays may also be taken. An expectorant may be prescribed to treat a dry, hacking cough. In most cases the underlying infection is caused by a virus, but after a positive diagnosis of a bacterial infection (about 10 percent of the cases), a course of antibiotics may be prescribed.

For More Information

• American Lung Association
• National Jewish Medical and Research Center
• National Heart, Lung, and Blood Institute Information Center

181

Bunions

Symptoms

- Pain and swelling of the joint where the big toe joins the foot.
- Inward leaning of the big toe toward the second toe.

What Is It?

A bunion occurs when the large metatarsal bone angles outward at the big-toe joint, thus forcing the toe inward; pressure over this distended joint can cause swelling and eventually a bony outgrowth. In the formation of a bunion, the bursa—a small, fluid-filled sac—around the base of the big toe becomes inflamed, forcing the toe out of proper alignment. (Bursae, which are found around most joints, help minimize friction between tendons and muscles as they pass over bone.)

Smaller bunions—bunionettes—may occasionally appear on the fifth metatarsal bone and the little-toe joint.

What Causes It?

Developing a bunion may be the result of an inherited tendency, and flat-footed people are more likely to get bunions than others. Poorly-fitted shoes—especially those with high heels and narrow toes—are undoubtedly the worst bunion makers, which is why women are far more prone to bunions than men.

What If You Do Nothing?

Not only is a bunion painful, it can also become disfiguring. Neglecting bunions over a period of years can eventually interfere with standing and walking.

Home Remedies

- **Change shoes.** If you think you are developing a bunion, switch to shoes with a low heel, ample toe room, and a proper last, so that the big toe is not forced against the second toe. Avoid any shoes or stockings that put pressure on the big toe joint. If practical, consider wearing sandals or other types of open shoes.
- **Pamper your feet.** Soaking them in warm water may offer relief. Gentle massage can also help.

Prevention

Wearing well-fitting shoes is the best way to prevent bunions. Corrective pads can help as well.

When To Call Your Doctor

If persistent bunions become painful or hinder walking, seek professional advice.

What Your Doctor Will Do

Medical measures include attaching a splint along the inner side of the foot to align the big toe into proper position. Various surgical procedures have been devised for treating severe cases. If you decide to undergo surgery for bunions, get a second opinion. Also find out if patients treated by the physician performing the surgery are satisfied with the results.

For More Information

- American Orthopaedic Foot and Ankle Society
- American Podiatric Medical Association

Bursitis

Symptoms

- Nagging ache and swelling in or around a joint.
- Painful and restricted movement in the affected joint.
- Pain radiating into the neck or arms when bursitis strikes the shoulder (the most common site).
- Fever, when associated with an infection.

What Is It?

That dull misery in the shoulder, knee, or elbow known as bursitis can and does strike anybody, from the couch potato to the highly trained athlete. Though bursitis may hurt as much as arthritis, it isn't a joint disease. Rather, it's an acute or chronic painful inflammation of a bursa. Bursae (from the Greek word for wine-skin and related to the English word purse) are small, closed, fluid-filled sacs that protect muscles and tendons from irritation produced by contact with bones. If friction becomes too great—from overexercising, hard work, or injury, for instance—the bursae themselves may get inflamed.

Though the shoulder is a common locale for bursitis, any of the bursae in the human body—there are approximately 150—can become irritated. Occupational bursitis is not uncommon and is known by old, familiar names such as "housemaid's knee," and "policeman's heel." One of the most common foot ailments, the bunion, is a form of bursitis.

What Causes It?

Repetitive, vigorous movement, strenuous and unaccustomed activities that put pressure on a joint, or a blow or other injury can bring on bursitis. The cause can vary depending on where the bursitis occurs. In the shoulder, for example, it can be brought on by excessive strain, such as from serving in tennis. Kneeling on a hard floor can cause bursitis of the knee, and similarly, repeatedly resting the elbow on a hard surface (such as a desk) can cause bursitis in that joint. Arthritis, gout, and certain infections can also contribute to the problem. Bursitis, in fact, may signal the onset of arthritis.

While getting older isn't a cause of bursitis, older people, especially older athletes, are more likely to develop the condition.

What If You Do Nothing?

Bursitis is not in itself a serious ailment. It often clears up on its own in a week or so, especially if you are careful to protect the injured area from further aggravation. However, bursitis sometimes recurs and becomes chronic, in which case you should seek medical attention.

Home Remedies

If you follow these steps, most attacks of bursitis should subside in four or five days and all symptoms should be gone within two weeks.

• **Rest the body part that hurts.** If you suspect that one activity has caused the pain, stop it until the pain is entirely gone. A sling, splint, or padding may be needed to protect the area from possible bumps or irritation.

• **Try over-the-counter pain relievers.** Nonprescription NSAIDs (aspirin, ibuprofen, and naproxen) will help reduce pain and swelling, though they won't accelerate healing. Acetaminophen will help with pain but it doesn't reduce inflammation.

• **Ice it, then heat it.** Apply ice packs during the first two days to bring down swelling (see page 453 for tips on icing). Then use heat—warm baths or a heating pad (on a medium or low setting)—to ease pain and stimulate blood flow.

• **Don't push it.** Resume exercising only after you feel better. Start with gentle activity.

• **Skip the liniments.** Liniments and balms are no help for bursitis. Liniments don't penetrate deeply enough to treat bursitis; they mainly warm the skin and make it tingle, thus distracting attention from the pain beneath. Massage is likely to make matters worse.

Prevention

It isn't always possible to avoid the sudden blow, bump, or fall that may produce bursitis. But you can protect your body with measures similar to those that protect you from other kinds of overuse injuries, such as tendinitis.

• **Keep yourself in good shape.** Strengthening and flexibility exercises tone muscles that support joints and help increase joint mobility.

• **Don't push yourself too hard (or too long).** If you're engaged in physical labor, pace yourself and take frequent breaks. If you're beginning a new exercise program or a new sport, work up gradually to higher levels of fitness. And anytime you're in pain, stop.

• **Work on technique.** Make sure your technique is correct if you play tennis, golf, or any sport that may strain your shoulder.

• **Watch out for "elbow-itis."** If you habitually lean on your elbow at your work desk, this may be a sign that your chair is uncomfortable or the wrong height. Try to arrange your work space so that you don't have to lean on your elbow to read, write, or view your computer screen.

• **Take knee precautions.** If you have a task that calls for lots of kneeling (for example, refinishing or waxing a floor), cushion your knees, change position frequently, and take breaks.

• **Wear the right shoes.** High-heeled or ill-fitting shoes cause bunions, and tight shoes can also cause bursitis in the heel. Problems in the feet can also affect the hips. In particular, the tendons and bursae in the hips can be put under excessive strain by worn-down heels. Buy shoes that fit and keep them in good repair. Never wear a shoe that's too short or narrow. Women should save their high heels for special occasions only.

When To Call Your Doctor

Contact your physician if bursitis pain is disabling (when movement of the joint is largely or entirely restricted), if the pain doesn't subside after a week of self-care, or if the joint is red and swollen. Also call your doctor if you develop a fever, which could signal infectious bursitis—a condition that especially can afflict the elbow. Except for the fever, symptoms resemble other forms of bursitis, but infectious bursitis requires immediate medical attention.

What Your Doctor Will Do

After taking a history and performing a physical examination, your physician may order x-rays to rule out other disorders. Your doctor may administer injections of corticosteroids and a local anesthetic to reduce swelling and ease pain. Also, to reduce swelling, your physician may draw excess fluid from the bursa with a syringe and then tightly wrap and compress the joint with an elastic bandage. In severe, persistent cases surgery to remove the bursa may be necessary. For infectious bursitis, antibiotics will be prescribed.

For More Information

• American College of Rheumatology

184

Canker Sores and Cold Sores

Symptoms

Canker sores

- Small white or yellow sores ringed by a red area on the tongue or inside the lips or cheek.
- Pain or tingling preceding the appearance of the sore.
- Local pain when eating and talking, especially during the first two or three days.

Cold sores (also called fever blisters)

- Painful, itchy, fluid-filled blisters that commonly occur on the lips.
- Burning, itching, and/or tingling sensation often preceding the blister by a few days.
- Rupture of the blisters within hours, followed by crusting.

What Is It?

These very common sores are often confused because they both usually occur in or around the mouth. But there are crucial differences—in appearance, causes, and specific locations.

Canker sores have bothered humanity since ancient times. Hippocrates coined the medical term for them—*aphthous stomatitis*—in the fourth century B.C. These craterlike lesions can occur on or under the tongue or inside the cheek. They have not been proved to have a viral origin, nor are they known to be contagious or a sign of an underlying disease.

Cold sores are tiny, unsightly, and often painful blisters that occur most frequently on the lips and adjacent skin, though occasionally on gums or the nose. Any reactivation of cold sores is usually, but not always, signaled 24 to 48 hours prior to an outbreak by an itching or tingling sensation in the lips. A small red area develops, followed by a blister or group of tiny blisters that fill with liquid.

What Causes It?

No one is sure what causes canker sores, and there are no known remedies. Canker sores seem to be brought on by stress in some people; stress can also be a side effect. Heredity may play a role, and some women find that the sores recur with menstrual periods. Some people believe that irritation from such foods as chocolate, salted nuts, or potato chips can cause an outbreak or that food allergies can cause the problem. There's no proof, but it certainly won't hurt to follow your hunches.

Another suspect is trauma—the kind that comes from biting your tongue or the inside of your cheek, or from using a hard-bristled toothbrush, having a jagged tooth, rough dentures, or being burned from hot food or liquids.

Cold sores, on the other hand, are caused by the herpes simplex virus (HSV)—usually by HSV Type 1, which is different from the Type 2 virus more commonly associated with genital herpes. The infection is contagious, but most people have already contracted the virus by early adulthood (though often with no symptoms). The virus lies dormant in the body until it is triggered by factors such as a cold, fever, fatigue, sunlight, or emotional stress—though in many cases the cause of the virus being activated isn't known.

What If You Do Nothing?

Painful and irritating as they are, canker sores usually go away in 5 to 15 days, with or without treatment.

Similarly, cold sores, although unsightly, pose no health threat and will clear up on their own within 7 to 10 days.

Home Remedies

Canker sores

The Food and Drug Administration (FDA) has

approved the first drug for canker sores, called amlexanox (Aphthasol). This prescription oral paste, intended only for canker sores, has been shown to ease pain and accelerate healing by a day or two. The following remedies may also help ease discomfort.

• **Ice it.** Apply crushed ice to the sore. This will numb the pain and provide some relief.

• **Avoid spicy foods.** Abrasive, acidic, and spicy food can irritate the sores.

• **Brush carefully.** Using a soft brush will minimize irritation.

• **Try over-the-counter pain relief.** If canker sores become very painful, ask your pharmacist to recommend an anesthetic drug or protective gel to reduce pain and inflammation.

Cold sores

The first over-the-counter medication for healing cold sores, called Abreva, was recently approved by the FDA. By applying this topical cream as soon as the tell-tale tingling of a cold sore occurs, you may be able to prevent the blister from developing or, if it does appear, speed up the time it takes to heal (though the drug won't help everyone). For severe outbreaks, prescription medications are likely to offer the most benefit (see What Your Doctor Will Do).

Other products (such as the amino acid lysine) have been suggested for treating cold sores, but there is no evidence that they work.

The following remedies may help relieve the discomfort of a cold sore.

• **Rinse with salt water.** Rinse your mouth several times a day with a cup of warm water to which you've added a half teaspoon of salt.

• **Try ice.** Applying an ice cube to the infected area may help relieve pain. Wrap an ice cube in a damp washcloth and keep it on the area for five minutes. Reapply it every hour.

• **Apply an ointment.** An over-the-counter anesthetic ointment can help relieve pain.

• **Don't pick.** Do not squeeze, pick, or pinch a blister or scab. A light coating of petroleum jelly on the scab will prevent cracking and bleeding.

• **Wash carefully.** This will help prevent infection. Avoid touching your eyes, genital area, or another person.

Prevention

Canker sores

It's not clear how to prevent canker sores, but the following steps can help.

• **Keep the mouth clean and healthy.** Brush at least twice daily and floss regularly. And consider switching tooth cleansers: a study conducted in Norway suggested that a detergent found in most toothpastes, sodium laurel sulfate, can aggravate canker sores. If you have recurrent sores, try switching to a tooth powder, baking soda, or other dentrifice without this ingredient.

• **Stop biting.** Any mouth injury can get infected, so if you unconsciously bite the inside of your cheek, try to break the habit.

• **Stay away from anything that can hurt the lining of the mouth.** This includes hard-bristled toothbrushes, toothpicks, and bones in meats.

• **Determine if specific foods trigger attacks.** Avoid those foods that seem to cause problems.

Cold sores

• **Use sunblock.** Outbreaks due to sun exposure can be prevented by applying sunscreen with a sun protection factor (SPF) of 15 on the lips before going outside and reapplying it frequently during the day.

• **Avoid touching the blisters.** Touching the blisters and then other people is a possible way of spreading the virus. Kissing is one of the most common ways this transmission occurs.

• **Don't share.** During an outbreak, don't lend personal items such as towels, razors, cups, or toothbrushes.

• **Consider medication.** If you get frequent outbreaks, speak with your physician about taking an antiviral drug for prevention.

When To Call Your Doctor

Canker sores

Contact your physician if the pain becomes severe, you're unable to drink adequate fluids, the mouth ulcers increase to four or more in number or last longer than two weeks, or if a fever develops. If a canker sore is caused by your dentures or braces, consult your dentist to eliminate the problem. Also contact your physician if you develop canker sores more than two or three times a year.

Cold sores

Contact your physician if you develop a fever, if your cold sores last longer than two weeks despite treatment, or if cold sores recur frequently during the course of a year.

What Your Doctor Will Do

Canker sores

After a careful examination, your physician may apply a topical anesthetic to relieve pain or may prescribe medications to reduce inflammation and prevent pain. A prescription for amlexanox (Aphthasol), a canker sore medication, can be worthwhile if your lesions are very painful and if they tend to recur.

Cold sores

After a careful examination, your physician may prescribe penciclovir (Denavir), an antiviral cream, to help speed the healing of existing sores. If you get frequent cold sores, ask your doctor about oral acyclovir (Zovirax), a prescription antiviral medication that can help reduce the severity and duration of cold sores if taken as soon as you notice the early warning signs of itching and tingling. Two related drugs, famciclovir (Famvir) and valacyclovir (Valtrex), are also used as preventive agents.

For More Information

• American Academy of Dermatology
• American Dental Association

Carpal Tunnel Syndrome

Symptoms

- Burning, tingling, and numbness in your hands, especially in the thumb and first three fingers. Usually symptoms first occur early in the morning or at night, and may also awaken you at night. Nocturnal awakening occurs in up to 95 percent of all patients. Flexing your hand in your sleep or sleeping on it may aggravate the discomfort.
- Weakness in the hands and fingers that may make it difficult to pick up or hold onto objects. Carpal tunnel syndrome usually affects the dominant hand and begins with pain and tingling or numbness.
- A sensation of swelling in the fingers without any visible swelling.

What Is It?

If you put in long hours at a repetitive hand-intensive task—working on an assembly line or in the garment industry, typing or computer keyboarding, or knitting or playing piano—you could develop carpal tunnel syndrome, or CTS. Deriving its name from the Greek *karpos,* or wrist, CTS is a painful disorder of the wrist and hand that results from compression of the median nerve at the wrist by surrounding tissue or excess fluid.

The carpal tunnel is the passageway, composed of bone and ligament, through which a major nerve system of the forearm passes into the hand. These nerves control the muscles in this area, as well as the nine tendons that allow your fingers to flex. The wear and tear of repeated movement thickens the lubricating membrane of the tendons and presses the nerves against the hard bone. This process, called nerve entrapment, can be caused not only by repetitive strain, but by bone dislocation or fracture, arthritis, and fluid reten-tion (as may occur in pregnancy)—anything that narrows the tunnel and compresses the nerve.

Thousands of cases of CTS are diagnosed each year, and women are far more susceptible to it than men because women tend to do the kinds of industrial, office, and domestic jobs that promote CTS. In addition, their carpal tunnel space is smaller by nature.

What Causes It?

CTS is brought on by repetitive work or movement. In addition to the examples mentioned above, carpenters and dentists, people working with electric drills or other vibrating instruments, and indeed anyone who works with his or her hands for long hours can get CTS. Tennis and squash players are also candidates, as are people who frequently work out with handweights, rowing machines, or other exercise equipment involving repetitive hand movements.

CTS is also associated with pregnancy and with certain medical conditions, including arthritis, diabetes mellitus, and hypothyroidism (underactive thyroid).

What If You Do Nothing?

In some instances the symptoms of carpal tunnel syndrome disappear without any treatment. Usually, however, if you do nothing to alleviate the problem, the tingling and numbness can progress to a weakened grip and severe pain in the forearm or shoulder. By all means get medical advice before this happens.

Home Remedies

Symptoms of mild CTS may improve with the following measures.

- **Elevate.** When you lie down, elevate your arm with pillows.

• **Try ice.** Icing the wrist for 20 minutes at a time can offer temporary pain relief.

• **Take over-the-counter anti-inflammatory pain relievers.** Nonprescription NSAIDs (aspirin, ibuprofen, and naproxen) will help reduce pain and swelling.

• **Avoid smoking.** This may help prevent the constriction of the small blood vessels of the hand, which can aggravate the condition.

• **A wrist splint may help.** For mild CTS symptoms, a splint that keeps your wrist and fingers in a neutral position can help ward off pain that occurs at night from bending your wrist in your sleep. Your doctor or a physical therapist can advise you about obtaining a splint and how often to wear it.

• **Be wary of other CTS devices.** The marketplace is full of devices—braces, wristrests, wrist trolleys, fingerless gloves—that supposedly head off CTS or help correct it. But there's little, if any, evidence that any of them are worth much.

Prevention

A few simple precautions can help minimize the risk of CTS.

• **Don't flex.** When working with your hands, keep your wrists straight. Flexing and twisting them stresses the carpal tunnel.

• **Think before lifting.** Lift objects with your whole hand—or better yet, with both hands—to reduce stress on the wrist.

• **Adjust your keyboard.** If you work at a computer keyboard, make sure your fingers are lower than your wrists; don't rest the heels of your hands on the keyboard.

• **Give your hands a rest.** Take breaks frequently when working with your hands. Working too rapidly may contribute to the problem.

• **Type with a soft touch.** Don't pound the keys, which aggravates pressure on the wrist.

• **Stop when it hurts.** If your hands hurt while you're exercising or playing a racket sport, stop. If you carry handweights while running or exercising, make sure they aren't too heavy.

• **Don't grip the steering wheel.** Hold it gently to reduce pressure on your wrists.

• **Share work tasks.** If the work you do is stressing your hands, see if you can rotate tasks or share work with someone else.

When To Call Your Doctor

Contact your physician if carpal tunnel syndrome symptoms become bothersome, begin to interfere with normal daily activity, of if you find yourself having to take aspirin or other painkillers to keep working. The syndrome is much easier to treat and much less likely to cause long-term problems when it's diagnosed early.

What Your Doctor Will Do

After taking a thorough history, your doctor will perform a physical exam that will include one or more tests to assess the extent of pain in your wrist. Your hand and wrist may also be x-rayed. Although CTS is usually not difficult to diagnose, you may be referred to a neurologist for testing the nerves' ability to transmit impulses. If your condition is mild, wearing a splint at night may be all you need. If that doesn't work, your doctor may suggest anti-inflammatory drugs, such as aspirin or ibuprofen, or injections of cortisone.

If nerve injury or muscle damage progresses, surgery may prove advisable. Surgery is usually successful in restoring full hand function unless the condition has been present for several years.

For More Information

• American Academy of Orthopaedic Surgeons

189

Cataracts

Symptoms

- Gradual, painless blurring and/or dimming of vision.
- Increased sensitivity to light; poor vision in sunlight or glaring light (such as car headlights).
- Halos encircling lights; sometimes the impression of a film over the eyes.
- Diminishing color perception (as cataracts progress).
- In advanced cases, cloudy appearance of the lens, so that the normally black pupil turns milky white.

What Is It?

The lens of your eye, which focuses light on the retina at the back of the eyeball, is normally colorless and clear. With age, however, the lens may grow cloudy and opaque, impairing your vision—a condition called a cataract. Although cataract surgery, in which the lens is removed, is almost always successful, cataracts are still a major cause of treatable blindness worldwide. In the United States, over a million cataract operations are performed each year, accounting for about 12 percent of the entire Medicare budget.

Until recently, cataracts were thought to be an inevitable part of growing older: as you age, the lens of your eye deteriorates. Now, however, there's hope that with good health habits you may be able to postpone or in some cases prevent cataracts.

What Causes It?

Though aging is the single greatest risk factor, lifelong exposure to ultraviolet light appears to be a primary cause in promoting cataracts, which are most common in regions where the duration and intensity of sunlight are greatest.

In addition, it's long been suspected that smoking increases your risk of cataracts, and that the risk rises with the number of cigarettes smoked. The *Journal of the American Medical Association* has published two studies (one involving 17,000 male physicians, the other 69,000 female nurses), both of which showed a strong association between cigarette smoking and cataracts, with the heaviest smokers running the greatest risk. An accompanying editorial estimated that at least 20 percent of all cataracts could be attributed to smoking.

Finally, there is some evidence suggesting that dietary factors may affect your risk of cataracts. Carotenoids—a family of nutrients not classified as vitamins but similar to them—appear to be especially important. Some carotenoids can be detected in high concentrations in eye tissues. They function as antioxidants—that is, they neutralize damage to cells caused by free radicals (highly reactive oxygen molecules), which are created by such factors as sunlight and exposure to cigarette smoke. People who regularly eat lots of carotenoid-rich foods (which include leafy greens, corn, kiwis, and other green, red, or yellow fruits and vegetables) seem to have the healthiest eyes. Vitamins C and E, other antioxidants, may also help prevent cataracts.

In younger people, diabetes can cause cataracts. And taking certain medications (such as corticosteroids for inflammation) for long periods is linked to the formation of cataracts in some people.

What If You Do Nothing?

Cataracts will usually worsen gradually, and eventually you may need surgery to correct the problem. But in most cases cataracts develop very slowly, and you may be able to postpone surgery or avoid it altogether. In recent years increasing knowledge about the risk factors for cataracts makes it likely that their rate of progression can be slowed even further.

Home Remedies

Surgery is the only true cure for cataracts, but if cataracts aren't interfering with normal activities, surgery can be postponed, sometimes indefinitely. In the meantime you can take steps to slow or minimize the impact of cataracts on your vision.

Prevention

The following steps may help forestall or prevent cataracts as you grow older. Because the causes of cataracts are not completely understood, there is no guarantee that these measures will help. But they may, and some have obvious auxiliary benefits, including a lower risk of some cancers and heart disease.

• **Wear ultraviolet-protective sunglasses.** This is the most important step you can take to prevent additional damage to your eyes. Sunglasses with lenses tinted yellow, brown, or amber will absorb blue light, which is the light most readily scattered—and so transformed into glare—by incipient cataracts.

• **Outdoors, wear a hat with a brim or visor.** The right hat can reduce glare. Sitting under an umbrella also helps minimize glare. Try to stay in the shade as much as possible rather than in direct sunlight.

• **If you smoke, quit.** No one knows exactly how smoking damages the lens, but smokers are about twice as likely to develop cataracts as nonsmokers.

• **Eat a diet high in carotenoids.** Two large studies of health-care professionals suggest that foods rich in two carotenoids, lutein and zeaxanthin, are associated with a lower risk of cataracts. The best sources for lutein are corn, kale, spinach, and other dark leafy greens, pumpkin, zucchini, yellow squash, red grapes, and green peas; for zeaxanthin, orange bell peppers, oranges, corn, honeydew melon, and mango. (Of course, these are not the only beneficial carotenoids you should eat, but they scored high in this study.)

When To Call Your Doctor

If you notice any symptoms of cataracts, consult your ophthalmologist.

191

What Your Doctor Will Do

The ophthalmologist will perform an eye exam to determine the presence and stage of any cataract formation. If recommended, surgery for cataracts involves removal of the lens and replacement with an intraocular lens implanted in the eye, or with a contact lens, or with eyeglasses. Surgery is usually performed on an outpatient basis. Treatment is safe and 90 percent effective at improving vision.

For More Information

• American Academy of Ophthalmology

Celiac Disease

Symptoms

- Diarrhea that may be chronic or intermittent, pale and foul-smelling.
- Loss of appetite; weight loss.
- Fatigue.
- Flatulence.
- In infants: Gastrointestinal distress after starting to eat cereal.
- In infants and children: Failure to gain weight or grow taller.

What Is It?

Celiac (pronounced SEE-lee-yak) disease, also called celiac sprue, is a chronic toxic reaction in the small intestine that's triggered by gliadin, a component in gluten found in wheat and wheat products, rye, oats, and barley. The intestine can't break down the gliadin, and undigested gliadin damages the lining of the small intestine, which causes malabsorption: water and nutrients aren't properly absorbed by the intestine.

The ailment usually surfaces during infancy or early childhood, shortly after the child begins eating food containing gluten. Symptoms typically diminish or disappear in late childhood, but then reappear in the third to sixth decade.

The prevalence of celiac disease isn't known. It's estimated to affect about 1 in 3,000 people, but many cases may not be diagnosed because symptoms are mild or absent. The disease primarily affects whites of northwestern European heritage; it rarely affects African-Americans, Asians, or Jews. Twice as many females develop it as men.

What Causes It?

The exact cause of celiac disease is unknown, but it appears to be a type of autoimmune disease.

The disease appears to run in families, so it probably has a genetic component, but how it is passed on hasn't been determined.

What If You Do Nothing?

Celiac disease is difficult to diagnose but relatively easy to treat, and so should not be ignored. Untreated celiac disease can lead to malabsorption of necessary nutrients, weight loss, fatigue, and retarded growth.

Home Remedies

Treatment for children and adults is the same. After a diagnosis from a gastroenterologist, the following measures will restore normal absorption and bowel function within a few months.

• **Go gluten-free.** This means absolutely avoiding any foods made with wheat, barley, rye, or oats. You will feel better in two to four weeks, and be symptom-free within a year.

• **Be careful of hidden gluten.** Even small amounts of gluten can cause an adverse reaction, so you need to be aware of products that contain hidden sources of gluten. These range from some soy sauces and vinegars to the backing on postage stamps and even the flour used on chewing gum (which keeps it from sticking to the wrapper). Wheat flour is also used in hundreds of prepared foods, but its presence may not always be indicated on a food label. Information on these foods can be obtained from celiac sprue organizations and books on gluten-free diets. A good dietician can also be helpful.

• **Buy gluten-free products.** This may add time to your shopping at first, but you will quickly learn what you can and cannot eat. Specialty mail-order companies have a wide variety of gluten-free products, including those made with safe substitutes such as rice, corn, and soybean flours.

• **Speak up.** When eating out or traveling by plane, tell your waiter or flight attendant about your special dietary needs.

• **Avoid foods you aren't sure about.** If you can't be sure a food is gluten-free, don't eat it.

Prevention

There is no way to prevent celiac disease. However, you can avoid celiac flare-ups by maintaining a gluten-free diet.

When To Call Your Doctor

Contact your physician if you suddenly lose your appetite and develop persistent, runny, foul-smelling diarrhea. If you already have celiac disease and are following a gluten-free diet for at least three weeks, contact your physician if new abdominal pain, diarrhea, or weight loss begins. Also contact your physician if your child does not improve within a few days after gluten has been removed from the daily diet.

What Your Doctor Will Do

Celiac disease is extremely difficult to diagnose and often goes undiagnosed for years. For testing, you should go to a gastroenterologist or—for a child—a pediatric gastroenterologist. After taking a thorough history, the doctor will test your blood for antibodies and their response to gluten. In order to make a positive diagnosis, a biopsy of the small intestine will be performed. If it is positive, over the next few months the physician will then monitor your response to a gluten-free diet.

For More Information

• Celiac Disease Foundation
• Celiac Sprue Association/USA
• National Digestive Diseases Information Clearinghouse

Chicken Pox

Symptoms

The chief symptom of chicken pox is a rash. However, one or two days before the rash appears, some children develop a fever, which may be accompanied by headache, malaise, and/or a lack of appetite. It is important that you never give aspirin to children for fever. The combination of aspirin or aspirin-like drugs (salicylates) and the chicken pox virus is associated with an increased risk of Reye's syndrome, a rare but potentially fatal liver and brain illness.

When the rash appears, it typically goes through several stages:

- Splotchy, red spots (pox) or pimples appear and, over the first few days, progress to small, fragile, fluid-filled blisters on top of an itchy, red rash.
- Over a period of about seven days, the blisters erupt and form a scab or crust; at this stage there may be intense itching.
- The rash often begins on the face or trunk and then spreads over the extremities in successive waves. Spots may also spread to the mouth, vagina, anus, or ears. There may be only a few sores or hundreds. Rashes at varying stages of eruption and healing may be present at the same time. When all the blisters have scabbed, the scabs may last for another week.
- Any fever generally subsides once the rash has reached the scab stage.

What Is It?

Chicken pox is a very common, highly contagious disease that is usually mild in its course, which is marked by fever and a characteristic itchy rash. More than 90 percent of cases occur in children

younger than nine years of age. Outbreaks are common among children in a household and in schools and day-care centers, often during the winter and spring.

Most adults have been exposed to chicken pox as children and, with rare exceptions, possess life-long immunity to the disease. But unexposed adults are susceptible, and those who do get chicken pox generally have more severe symptoms and are at greater risk of complications than children.

What Causes It?

Chicken pox is caused by a form of herpes virus called *Varicella zoster*. The virus is easily and rapidly spread from person to person through exposure either to cells from the skin lesions that are suspended in air or droplets from the mouth or nose.

A child who first shows symptoms is infectious for a week or so, beginning about a day before a rash appears and continuing until all the pox have dried up. Once the virus has been transmitted to a susceptible child, it will incubate in the body for 10 to 23 days before symptoms appear.

After lesions heal, the *Varicella zoster* virus remains inside the body in a latent (inactive) form. Many years later the virus may become reactivated, causing the painful ailment shingles *(Herpes zoster)*, which occurs in about 20 percent of people who have had chicken pox.

What If You Do Nothing?

The rash may be uncomfortable, but most cases of chicken pox clear up without complications in 10 to 14 days—though some scabs may take up to 20 days to heal. The scabs may leave behind light scars, but these will fade.

One possible complication is a secondary bacterial infection of the skin. Infection with Group A *Streptococci*, for example, can spread through cracks in the skin and invade the body, causing potentially life-threatening disease. Those with cancer or compromised immune systems may take a longer time to heal and are at greater risk of serious complications, including pneumonia or brain infections.

Pregnant women who have never had chicken pox should avoid anyone with the disease: in rare cases chicken pox in pregnant women damages the fetus. Newborns should also be kept away from those with the disease. Chicken pox in newborns can be quite severe and is sometimes fatal—although most infants possess protective maternal antibodies against the illness.

Home Remedies

There is no cure for chicken pox, but you can relieve the symptoms. Remember to never give children aspirin for lowering fever. Also be aware that many over-the-counter remedies, including herbal preparations, contain aspirin. To reduce fever and relieve aches in children, use acetaminophen instead.

• **Plenty of rest is helpful.** Children need not be kept in bed constantly, but their activity should be limited.

• **Relieve itching.** Dab calamine lotion on affected areas twice a day with sterile gauze. Over-the-counter antihistamine creams may also help, as can cool baths. Add a handful of ground instant or colloidal oatmeal (available in pharmacies), or a half a cup of baking soda or cornstarch, to the bath water. Pat, don't rub, the skin dry.

• **Keep skin clean.** Sponge baths a few times a day will also help to keep scabs and blisters clean and free of infection. Have infected children wash their hands frequently with antibacterial soap.

• **Don't scratch.** Scratching can cause blisters to become infected, leading to permanent scarring. Cut a child's fingernails short. Gloves or mittens may be worn to prevent scratching during sleep.

• **Gargle with salt water.** If blisters have formed in the mouth, a salt water gargle (a half teaspoon of salt per cup of water) may bring relief.

Prevention

• **Get vaccinated.** A safe and effective chicken pox vaccine is available. It is recommended for children a year old or older who are in good health, and for adults who have never had the disease. A single dose is given to children 1 to 12 years of age. Adolescents and adults get two doses four to eight weeks apart.

• **Avoid infecting others.** A child with chicken pox should stay home at least until all scabs have dried completely—at which point the infection won't be spread. (This applies to infected adults as well.) Friends, playmates, or schoolmates—indeed, anyone who has come in contact with the infected person in the preceding few days—should be informed about the situation. Susceptible adults, especially pregnant women, should take care to avoid contact with anyone infected—and newborns should be kept away. Children can return to school once the last blisters have crusted over.

When To Call Your Doctor

Call your doctor to confirm the diagnosis. A description of the rash is usually sufficient to determine that the illness is chicken pox. Avoid visiting the doctor's office, where others could catch the infection, unless your doctor tells you to come in. Routine chicken pox in otherwise healthy children is best treated at home.

Call the doctor at once if there are convulsions, a stiff neck, severe headaches, listlessness, confusion, or rapid breathing. These may be signs of a brain infection or pneumonia, which require immediate medical attention. Call your physician if blisters have become infected (red and oozing pus) or have spread to the eye area; also call if fever exceeds 102°F, persists for more than four days, or is accompanied by a sore throat.

Pregnant women and newborns who develop symptoms should be seen by a doctor at once.

What Your Doctor Will Do

If itching is severe, your doctor may prescribe an oral or topical antihistamine. Antibiotics will be prescribed if a secondary infection develops. Some patients may also be treated with an antiviral drug (acyclovir), which helps to reduce the severity and shorten the course of illness.

Pregnant women and newborns who become infected may be treated with immune-boosting agents as well as acyclovir. Drugs may also be needed for lesions that are affecting the eye area to prevent damage to vision.

For More Information

• American Academy of Pediatrics

Chlamydia

Symptoms

- Most of those infected have only mild symptoms or no symptoms at all.
- If a woman has any symptom of chlamydia, it is likely to be a vaginal discharge. If the infection gets into the urinary tract, there is likely to be pain, burning, and/or a frequent urge to urinate.
- The symptoms most likely to occur in men are painful urination or a discharge from the penis.

What Is It?

Chlamydia is the most common bacterial sexually transmitted disease (STD), affecting three to four million Americans annually. While it is most common among teenagers and young adults, anybody can get it: half of all sexually active people between 18 and 30 may be infected. The bad news about it is threefold: it's usually symptomless until very advanced; it's the leading cause of pelvic inflammatory disease and infertility in women, while in men, the ailment can lead to disease of the urinary tract; and it is easily transmitted sexually, through contact with infected membranes.

Chlamydia can infect the eye, throat, and rectum, as well as the reproductive tract. Since symptoms seldom occur, testing is the only way to diagnose it with certainty. The good news is that chlamydia is also easy to detect and treat. Unlike herpes or AIDS (both viral in origin), chlamydia can be cured with antibiotics.

What Causes It?

The *Chlamydia* bacterium comes in three recognized species. One version, *Chlamydia trachomatis,* has strains that cause the STD as well as eye and lung infections in newborns. Other strains can cause psittacosis (a respiratory disease transmitted by birds), and pneumonia. Recent research suggests that one strain of *Chlamydia* can infect the interior of the arteries, possibly becoming a factor in hardening of the arteries and, thus, heart disease.

But the type of *Chlamydia* that infects the reproductive tract is most common among teenagers and young adults, though anybody who is sexually active can get it. Like other sexually transmitted diseases, it is spread by contact with infected mucous membranes, typically through vaginal or anal sex. The infection is similar to gonorrhea and sometimes hard to distinguish from it—and it often occurs simultaneously with gonorrhea. (The presence of one STD is always a risk factor for another, including HIV infection.)

Infection can also be passed from a mother to her newborn during birth, leading to eye infection or pneumonia in the child.

What If You Do Nothing?

Chlamydia should be treated immediately, otherwise it may become chronic and lead to extensive inflammation and scarring of the genital tract in both men and women. In women, untreated infections can lead to pelvic inflammatory disease (PID), which may result in ectopic pregnancy and infertility, even in women who never develop clinical PID.

Home Remedies

As with other bacterial STDs, such as syphilis and gonorrhea, there are no home remedies for chlamydia. It requires diagnosis by a physician and treatment with antibiotic medications. Abstain from sexual activity until tests show no more infection.

197

Prevention

• **If you have sex, make it safer.** Abstinence, obviously, prevents chlamydia. So does remaining monogamous with a healthy monogamous partner. But the true key to prevention is knowledge. Any sexually active person not in a long-term, monogamous relationship, or any young person about to become sexually active, should understand the importance of a male sex partner using latex condoms consistently and correctly (see page 58). Oral contraceptives do not protect against STDs and may even increase the risk for chlamydia.

• **Test regularly.** Now there are quick and reliable tests for chlamydia. Contrary to what many women believe, however, a Pap test does not detect any kind of STD. If your health-care provider does not mention the subject, ask to be tested. Early diagnosis and treatment with antibiotics can cure the disease and prevent complications like infertility or the birth of infected infants.

The U.S. Preventive Services Task Force recommends routine screening for all sexually active female adolescents, women with new or multiple sex partners (and particularly those who don't use condoms consistently), and women with a history of STDs. Pregnant women who fall into one of these high-risk categories should also be tested. If you are in a risk group, ask your health-care provider to test you.

Anybody diagnosed with chlamydia should inform his or her sexual partners, who can then be treated as well.

• **Talk to your kids.** If you are the parent of adolescents or young adults, talk to them. Unwillingness of parents to discuss sex, and especially STDs such as chlamydia, is one reason for the current epidemic. Ignorance is never protective.

When To Call Your Doctor

Contact your physician if you develop any symptoms or if symptoms persist for more than a week after undergoing treatment. Even if you have no symptoms but fall into one of the high-risk categories mentioned above, you should arrange to be tested.

Also contact your doctor if your sexual partner has developed the infection, whether or not you have symptoms.

What Your Doctor Will Do

After a careful physical examination, your doctor will take a specimen from the cervix or urethra. For women, a culture from the cervical cells has been the most reliable test, but new testing methods that deliver results more rapidly are becoming increasingly popular alternatives. If the results are positive, a course of antibiotic medication will be prescribed.

For More Information

• American Social Health Association
• American Urological Association
• CDC National Prevention Information Network

198

Cholesterol (Elevated)

Symptoms

There are no obvious symptoms for high levels of blood cholesterol, but the problem is linked to other conditions that have recognizable symptoms, including heart disease, stroke, and high blood pressure.

What Is It?

Cholesterol is a white, waxy, fatlike substance. Although we usually think of it as found only in the bloodstream, it is actually present in all tissues in humans and other animals. It is thus present in all foods from animal sources. It it not present in any plants.

Cholesterol is essential to life: among other things, it is used in the outer membranes of cells; as a fatty insulation sheath around nerve fibers; and as a building block for certain hormones.

Despite its importance to life, cholesterol isn't an essential nutrient—you don't have to consume any to stay healthy. Most of the cholesterol in your bloodstream is manufactured in your body—primarily by the liver—from the fats, proteins, and carbohydrates you eat.

Just how cholesterol is distributed throughout the body is not entirely clear, but researchers now hypothesize that the mechanism works in this way: the liver puts together packages called lipoproteins, made of proteins, cholesterol, and triglycerides (fats either made by the body or derived directly from foods). Low-density

Who's At Risk?

▼

The chart at right shows guidelines for total cholesterol as well as HDL ("good") and LDL ("bad") cholesterol for people free of coronary artery disease, or CAD. (The recommended total and LDL levels for people with CAD are lower.) The chart also indicates desirable levels of triglycerides—fats similar to cholesterol that, at elevated levels and especially in combination with low levels of HDL, may increase the risk of a heart attack. Triglyceride counts are also used in calculating LDL levels.

In the United States, cholesterol is measured in milligrams per deciliter (mg/dl) of blood. In Canada and many other countries, it's measured in millimoles per liter (mmol/L). The latter is known as the International System. (To convert from milligrams to that system, multiply the number by 0.0259. To convert from millimoles to milligrams, multiply by 38.67.)

Total Cholesterol	
DESIRABLE	Less than 200 mg/dl (5.2 mmol/L)
BORDERLINE-HIGH	200–239 mg/dl (5.2–6.19 mmol/L)
HIGH	240 mg/dl or higher (6.2 mmol/L or higher)

HDL Cholesterol	
LOW	Below 35 mg/dl (1.6 mmol/L)

LDL Cholesterol	
DESIRABLE	Below 130 mg/dl (3.4 mmol/L)
BORDERLINE-HIGH	130-159 mg/dl (3.4-4.1 mmol/L)
HIGH	160 mg/dl or higher (4.1 mmol/L or higher)

Triglycerides	
DESIRABLE	50-200 mg/dl (1.3-5.2 mmol/L)
BORDERLINE-HIGH	200-400 mg/dl (5.2-10.36 mmol/L)
HIGH	Above 400 (10.36 mmol/L)

199

lipoprotein, or LDL, carries cholesterol throughout the system, dropping it off where it can be used for cell metabolism. Cholesterol carried by LDL that is not used, broken down by the liver, or excreted is left to circulate in the bloodstream, where it accumulates in the arterial walls. Nodules, called plaques, are eventually formed, decreasing the flow of blood over time—a condition known as atherosclerosis—and favoring the formation of blood clots. This may ultimately cut off the flow of blood; in the coronary arteries, this leads to a heart attack, and in the cerebral arteries, a stroke.

The liver makes another molecular package known as high-density lipoprotein, or HDL. Like the other lipoproteins, HDL is composed of triglycerides, protein, and cholesterol, but HDL carries less cholesterol than LDL. As it circulates through the bloodstream, HDL seems to have the beneficial capacity to pick up cholesterol and bring it back to the liver for reprocessing or excretion.

In simple terms, then, LDL brings cholesterol into the system, so it's often called "bad" cholesterol, and because HDL clears cholesterol out of the system, it has been dubbed "good" cholesterol. HDL (as well as LDL) is formed only in the body. You can't eat "good" cholesterol; no type of cholesterol you eat is good for you.

• **Cholesterol and heart disease.** Generally speaking, a high total cholesterol level, along with a high LDL level, is associated with an increased risk of heart disease. Low HDL, defined as less than 35 milligrams per deciliter (mg/dl), is also considered a risk factor for heart disease. One study by researchers in Israel and at Case Western Reserve University in Cleveland showed that the risk of dying from heart disease was 38 percent higher in men with HDL under 35, even if their total cholesterol was below 200. Stroke risk in such men was higher, too.

The higher your HDL, the better. A high HDL level, defined as 60 mg/dl or more, is considered protective against heart disease. (Female sex hormones tend to raise HDL; this may help explain why women are usually protected against atherosclerosis during their childbearing years, when estrogen production is high.)

Experts now believe that to be at low risk for heart disease, adults should reduce their total blood cholesterol levels to less than 200 mg/dl (see box on page 199). While there is no magic number—a point at which your blood cholesterol level automatically passes from safe to dangerous—the risk of heart disease rises continually with increasing levels of blood cholesterol, though it doesn't rise markedly until levels exceed 200 mg/dl. And the rate of coronary heart disease begins to accelerate rapidly above the 220 mg/dl level. Thus, many researchers believe that cholesterol levels should be as low as possible; well below 200 mg/dl is excellent.

Some experts question whether high blood cholesterol levels cause heart disease in everybody, and certainly your cholesterol level needs to be put in perspective within your total risk scenario for heart disease, based on such factors as age, sex, and health habits like exercise levels and whether you smoke. But there is substantial evidence that, in most cases, the connection between high blood cholesterol levels and heart disease is as incontrovertible as the link between smoking and lung cancer. This connection is strongest in men under 50 years of age. For young women and for everybody over 50, the link is weaker but still significant.

What Causes It?

A diet rich in cholesterol and—even more significantly—in saturated fat can increase your

Cholesterol Testing Guidelines

▼

According to guidelines from the National Cholesterol Education Program (NCEP), all adults over the age of 20 should be tested for HDL and total cholesterol at least once every five years. Some people should be retested more frequently.

- If your total cholesterol is in the desirable range (see page 199) and your HDL is above 35 mg/dl, you can wait up to five years to have them rechecked. If your total cholesterol is borderline-high and your HDL is above 35 mg/dl, you should be rechecked in a year or two.
- If your total cholesterol is borderline-high or high and/or your HDL is below 35 mg/dl, especially if you have two or more risk factors for coronary artery disease (CAD), you should have a complete lipid profile (which requires fasting overnight) to determine LDL. Then, if your LDL is in the desirable range, you can wait up to five years to be retested. But if your LDL is borderline-high or high, and depending on your other risk factors, you'll need to be retested annually as well as modifying your diet and take other steps to reduce your risk of CAD.

Note: Calculating LDL isn't simply a matter of subtracting your HDL from your total cholesterol. The blood fats known as triglycerides figure into the equation for arriving at total cholesterol and are used in deriving LDL.

Risk Factors

The recommendations for testing are more stringent if you have other risk factors for CAD besides high cholesterol and/or low HDL. These risk factors are age, family history of premature CAD (a heart attack in your father before age 55, in your mother before age 65), smoking, high blood pressure, and diabetes. The guidelines are even stricter for those who already have CAD: for instance, your LDL should be below 100, rather than 130.

Men and Women

Women need to be monitored as carefully as men. But women tend to develop CAD about a decade later than men do, so while age is considered a risk factor for men starting at age 45, for women it's at age 55. Women over 55 who have high cholesterol should make as great an effort as men to reduce it.

The Elderly

People in their 70s or even older should be treated just like people in their 50s or 60s, according to the NCEP guidelines. It is true that blood cholesterol levels naturally start to decline after age 75. But a recent report from the National Cholesterol Education Program found that nearly three-fourths of older people have substantial cholesterol build-up in their arteries. To reduce heart attack risk, therefore, it is important to have your blood cholesterol checked every five years even if you're over 70. If your cholesterol is high, you and your physician should discuss your other risk factors, lifestyle changes to lower cholesterol levels, and whether to consider taking cholesterol-lowering medication.

Children

According to the NCEP, only children who have a family history of very high cholesterol levels and/or heart disease—particularly those with a parent who suffered a heart attack before age 50—should be tested. That includes as many as one-quarter of the nation's children. Many authorities have concluded that screening all youngsters is unnecessary, since high blood cholesterol levels in childhood do not necessarily predict high levels later in life. But all children, whatever their family history, can benefit from a low-fat, heart-healthy diet after age two.

blood cholesterol level. (Sources of saturated fat include beef, butter, whole-milk dairy products, dark meat poultry, poultry skin, and coconut, palm, and kernel oils.) Many other factors affect your blood cholesterol level, and some people, no matter how small their fat and cholesterol intake, may continue to have high blood cholesterol levels because of genetic disorders, diabetes, or other metabolic diseases. For most people, though, diet remains the first defense against elevated blood cholesterol.

Other factors that can raise cholesterol levels are excess weight (each pound gained adds to total blood cholesterol) and smoking (which increases total cholesterol and decreases HDL cholesterol).

Before menopause, women tend to have higher HDL levels than men of the same age, and some researchers think that the higher HDL levels (as well as lower LDL) may be linked to estrogen. At menopause, estrogen production declines, and so does HDL.

What If You Do Nothing?

A high total cholesterol level isn't likely to decrease significantly unless you make some or all of the lifestyle changes described below, particularly those regarding weight control and diet. Some individuals may also require cholesterol-lowering medication to control their cholesterol levels.

Home Remedies

The following measures tend to lower total cholesterol and LDL levels, and also tend to raise HDL levels—or may at least stabilize HDL while bringing down LDL. (Not everyone responds to these changes, and if your total cholesterol level remains high after several months of adopting these changes, you should consult your doctor

about taking cholesterol-lowering drugs, as explained on page 203.

• **Lose weight.** Not only does excess body fat raise LDL levels and reduce HDL, but it also appears to be an independent risk factor for heart disease. Where the fat accumulates is also important: excess weight around the waist (the so-called apple-shape body) seems to reduce HDL more than weight in the hips and thighs (pear shape).

• **Cut down on saturated fats.** This is the most important dietary step you can take. First, keep your total fat intake at or below 30 percent of your daily calories. Secondly, substitute unsaturated fats for saturated fats. Studies have shown that polyunsaturated fats (such as safflower and corn oil) and monounsaturated fats (such as olive oil) help to lower blood cholesterol levels. Monounsaturated fats may help maintain or increase the level of HDL cholesterol as well.

• **Cut down on dietary cholesterol.** It's estimated that reducing cholesterol intake from food from 500 to 250 milligrams a day will lower total blood cholesterol by an average of 10 milligrams. This response is variable, however; some people have little or no response, and others a far greater one.

• **Watch out for "trans fats."** Manufacturers hydrogenate—that is, add hydrogen to—corn, soybean, and other liquid vegetable oils to make them more stable. This prolongs the shelf life of margarines, crackers, cookies, potato chips, and other foods that contain the semisolid oils. Hydrogenated oils are also often used for deep-frying in fast-food restaurants. But hydrogenation alters many of the oils' unsaturated fatty acids, making them more saturated and changing their structure in other ways that transforms them into trans fatty acids, or simply trans fats. Studies have shown that trans fats act like saturated fats—raising total and LDL cholesterol lev-

Should You Take A Cholesterol-Lowering Drug?

▼

Unfortunately, because of genetics, not everyone with high cholesterol responds to a low-fat diet—though the vast majority do, and the higher the cholesterol level to begin with, usually the greater the response. But many other people simply can't stick to a low-fat diet. (Likewise, not everyone with a low level of HDL is able to raise HDL through lifestyle changes.) If your cholesterol level remains unchanged after several months of effort at lifestyle changes, your doctor may prescribe a cholesterol-lowering drug, particularly if you have other risk factors and/or symptoms of CAD.

Not long ago, such medications were recommended only for people who could not reduce their cholesterol by any other means and who have significant risk factors for, or symptoms of, heart disease. Recently, however, some new studies have suggested that even healthy people with desirable, but not optimal, cholesterol levels can reduce their risk of a heart attack by taking "statin" drugs, the most effective and widely-used medications for lowering cholesterol. These drugs—which include lovastatin (Mevacor), pravastatin (Pravachol), and atorvastatin (Lipitor)—not only improve cholesterol levels (primarily by lowering LDL), but may also have a beneficial effect directly on artery walls

themselves. (Some recent studies have suggested that statins may have other health benefits, such as lowering the the risk of stroke in people with heart disease—but more research is needed to confirm this.)

Not A Clear-Cut Decision

No one should elect to take any type of drug to lower cholesterol without first consulting his or her doctor. Some people experience side effects such as muscle pain and/or weakness and liver damage. And no one knows how safe these drugs are over a lifetime, though they appear to be quite safe. Therefore, the decision to take a drug should be made in light of an overall evaluation of a person's risk for heart disease.

You will need advice from your doctor, and you will also need a fasting test to obtain a cholesterol profile of your HDL and LDL. Your doctor will also need to check for adverse reactions to any drug you start taking, regulate dosages, and judge the effects of medication on your cholesterol levels.

Some Guidelines

- **You probably don't need a statin drug** if your LDL cholesterol is 130 or lower, your HDL is at least 40, and you have good health habits and few, if any, coronary risk factors.
- **You may want to discuss statin drugs with your doctor** if your LDL is above 130, your

HDL is below 40, and you have any other risk factors for heart disease: you smoke, have high blood pressure, are sedentary, overweight, have diabetes, eat a lot of foods high in saturated fat, or are a man over 45 or a woman over 55. Also be sure to ask your doctor about possible interactions between statins and any other medication you are taking.

- **You may want to discuss taking low-dose aspirin.** Depending on your risk factor profile, a daily low-dose aspirin may be a more appropriate, and much less expensive, measure to reduce your risk of a heart attack. But don't start taking aspirin without talking to your doctor (see page 600).
- **If you're a woman at or past menopause,** you might consider starting hormone replacement therapy. The hormone estrogen tends to raise HDL. But there are a number of factors to weigh in deciding whether to take hormones, and you'll need to discuss these with your doctor (see page 382).

Remember that there is no substitute for a healthy lifestyle if you want to reduce your risk of heart disease. The heart-healthy habits outlined under "Home Remedies" and on pages 64-65 are always something to try before taking drugs—and while taking drugs.

els—and there is some evidence that they lower HDL cholesterol as well.

Nutrition labels have not specified how much trans fat is in the foods, and it's not counted as saturated fat. Hence, trans fats have remained invisible on food labels. The Food and Drug Administration (FDA) has recommended that the amount of trans fatty acids in foods be included in nutrition labels (a final ruling on the proposal is expected in 2001). In the meantime, if you eat lots of margarine and also many processed foods, cut back, or switch to a tub or liquid "squeeze" margarine, which has fewer trans fatty acids. "Diet" margarines are even better—they contain more water and only half the fat of other margarines.

• **Exercise more.** Results of studies have been inconsistent concerning the effect of aerobic exercise or strength-training exercise on total cholesterol and LDL. But the evidence is stronger that an exercise program can help raise HDL, and its effect on lowering the risk of coronary artery disease (CAD) is overwhelming. The exercise doesn't have to be strenuous—walking a mile or two or even gardening several times a week can help.

• **Combine diet and exercise for better results.** In a study at the Stanford School of Medicine, a group of subjects who followed both a low-fat diet and a moderate exercise program (equivalent to briskly walking for three hours a week) had an average drop of about 18 points in total cholesterol, while subjects who followed only a dietary or exercise regimen experienced just a small improvement not considered significant.

• **Consume more soluble fiber.** Eat more legumes, oats, fruits, and vegetables such as carrots, split peas, and corn. Sweet potatoes, zucchini, and broccoli have some soluble fiber, as do bananas, apples, pears, and oranges. If you regularly eat a high-fiber, low-fat diet that includes a variety of the these vegetables and fruits and some oatmeal or oat bran daily, you may see results the

What About "Natural" Remedies?

▼

Several products marketed as dietary supplements claim to help lower blood cholesterol. Some may do just that—but read on before you try them.

There are varying degrees of evidence that three such supplements—guggulipid, niacin, and red yeast rice (sold under the brand name "Cholestin")—can effectively (and inexpensively) reduce cholesterol levels.

However, if your cholesterol is high, you first need to talk to your doctor, who will consider all of your risk factors for heart disease in arriving at a treatment plan, which may include a prescription drug. Actually, though niacin and Cholestin can be obtained without a prescription, both act as drugs and should not be taken without medical advice and supervision, since dosages must be individually designed.

The dosage for guggulipid is difficult to determine, since there is no guarantee that what you are buying standardized. If you decide to try it, be sure to tell your doctor.

Garlic is also widely advertised as having cholesterol-lowering properties. Here the claims are doubtful. Two recent well-designed studies—one appearing in the *Archives of Internal Medicine*, the other in the *Journal of the American Medical Association*—found that garlic had no effect on cholesterol levels. Both studies, which lasted 12 weeks, involved people with elevated cholesterol levels and compared results of garlic against a placebo, or dummy pill.

Interestingly, the studies used two entirely different types of garlic supplement—a garlic oil preparation and a popular garlic powder tablet—yet neither had any cholesterol-lowering benefit.

next time you have a cholesterol test—particularly if the level was previously elevated.

• **Eat fish instead of meat.** According to some studies, the oil in fish—polyunsaturated fatty acids called omega-3s—can lower elevated cholesterol. Evidence from other studies disputes this, but substituting some fish for meat (or other sources of saturated fat) should help lower blood cholesterol. Eating fish is preferable to taking fish oil supplements. Not only is fish one of the best nutrient-rich foods around, but it is unclear whether omega-3s, by themselves in supplements, provide the same health benefits as eating the fish itself.

• **Consider a drink or two a day.** A number of studies have shown that moderate alcohol consumption—defined as no more than two drinks a day for a man, one drink a day for a woman—may boost HDL. The health risks of heavier drinking, however, outweigh the potential benefit for the heart. (See page 47 for more information on alcohol consumption and health.)

• **Don't smoke.** Smoking increases total cholesterol and reduces HDL. In addition, it is an independent risk factor for heart disease.

Prevention

The same measures that help lower high cholesterol levels can also help prevent cholesterol levels from rising in the first place, so follow the recommendations described above. You should also have your blood cholesterol level tested periodically by your doctor (see page 201).

When To Call Your Doctor

If you are over the age of 20, consult your doctor about having your cholesterol levels measured. Children who have a family history of heart disease or of high cholesterol levels should also be tested. You can also call your local hospital, health department, or American Heart Association chapter for advice.

Don't rely on home cholesterol tests. When your doctor does the test, it should be part of an overall evaluation of your risk of heart disease. Also, home tests cannot measure HDL levels.

What Your Doctor Will Do

Blood will be drawn for the test, and beforehand your doctor should give you instructions that will help to ensure the best possible result. These may include not eating anything for 12 hours before the test (if you are having your LDL and triglyceride levels measured); not exercising before your test (which can cause a temporary rise in cholesterol levels for up to an hour after the activity); and sitting down for at least five minutes before your blood is taken. At least two weeks should have elapsed since any surgery, trauma, illness, or physical strain, since these factors can also affect the test results.

Your doctor may want you to have at least two tests performed, separated by a month or two, since cholesterol levels fluctuate.

Your doctor will discuss the results of your test with you. If your cholesterol is high or your HDL is low, the two of you will discuss measures to take—including the possibility of using cholesterol-lowering drugs—to try and bring your cholesterol levels into a desirable range.

For More Information

• American Heart Association
• National Heart, Lung, and Blood Institute Information Center

Chronic Fatigue Syndrome

Symptoms

- Recurrent flulike symptoms, including fever, sore throat, headache, muscle pain, and joint pain.
- Severe, debilitating fatigue that is not relieved by rest or sleep and is made worse by exercise.
- Depression and irritability.

What Is It?

A person who has chronic fatigue syndrome (CFS) feels weak and enervated much or all of the time and may have difficulty performing daily tasks, even those that are routine and undemanding. Having difficulty sleeping and finding it hard to concentrate are also common symptoms.

No specific cause has been linked to CFS, and because the symptoms associated with CFS are connected to many other disorders, it is difficult to establish a diagnosis. Generally, according to guidelines established by the Centers for Disease Control and Prevention, the problem isn't considered to be CFS unless severe fatigue and other symptoms have interfered with the ability to work and function for at least six months.

Those who are most likely to develop the problem are 25 to 45 years old, but CFS can occur at any age. In the United States about 80 percent of those diagnosed with CFS are women, for reasons that aren't understood. (It may be that women have simply reported the problem more often than men.) A majority of those who report having the problem are allergy sufferers.

While there are anecdotal reports of increased rates of other illnesses (such as cancer and multiple sclerosis) among those with CFS, there is no evidence to support these claims.

What Causes It?

Researchers have tried to pin down a cause, but the goal has proved elusive. In the early 1980s the disorder was called Epstein-Barr syndrome because most chronic sufferers were found to be infected with the Epstein-Barr virus, which causes mononucleosis. However, since then many people complaining of CFS symptoms show no sign of the virus, and many healthy people have been exposed to the virus with no ill effects. There is no evidence, in fact, that CFS is caused by any virus or that it is contagious.

According to another theory, people with this syndrome have an autoimmune disorder in which the immune system reacts (or overreacts) to a perceived threat (such as a virus) by attacking otherwise healthy tissues. This has led to CFS also being referred to as chronic fatigue and immune

Chronic Fatigue and Alternative Remedies

▼

Claims have been made for a number of treatments for CFS, including herbal preparations, liver extract, antiviral drugs, vitamins, and infusions of immunoglobulin. Many of these therapies are either untested or haven't been confirmed when subjected to scientific study, so that positive responses may be due to a placebo effect rather than to an effective therapy.

It's important to discuss with your doctor any alternative remedies you pursue. Many may be harmless, but some unproven treatments can have adverse effects. More important, there is a danger that someone who has never been formally diagnosed as having CFS may actually have a much more serious underlying disorder. In that case alternative therapies are a poor, and possibly dangerous, substitute for getting a thorough physical examination and a proven course of treatment.

dysfunction syndrome, or CFIDS.

Some researchers also think that emotional and psychological factors play a role in causing or exacerbating CFS.

What If You Do Nothing?

Most people who have CFS recover, with or without treatment; symptoms disappear and normal levels of activity can eventually be resumed. But recovery can take months or even years. The course of the illness varies greatly among individuals, and often the presence of symptoms follows a cyclical pattern, with periods of illness alternating with periods of relatively good health.

Home Remedies

There is no cure for CFS, but a few measures may provide relief.

• **Take it easy—but not too easy.** Get plenty of rest and try not to overexert yourself, since doing so can aggravate symptoms. But do try to stay physically active and perform some light exercise.

• **Try over-the-counter pain relievers.** Aspirin, ibuprofen, and naproxen can relieve joint pain and headaches and reduce fever.

• **Contact support groups and hotlines.** There are growing numbers of groups that offer psychological support and information about CFS. Some publish newsletters that describe recent research efforts, offer advice about how to cope with the illness, and list doctors who are experienced in diagnosing and treating CFS.

Prevention

There is no established way to prevent chronic fatigue syndrome.

When To Call Your Doctor

If you experience symptoms of CFS, consult your doctor. You may have CFS, but the problem may turn out to be another disorder.

What Your Doctor Will Do

No specific diagnostic tests are available to identify CFS. Your doctor will obtain a detailed medical history and order blood and urine tests to rule out other causes for your fatigue. If no other cause for chronic fatigue can be established, then your physician will probably want to monitor your symptoms for three to six months to arrive at a diagnosis of CFS.

Certain prescription medications may help. A drug called cyclobenzaprine (Flexeril), which can relieve pain, tenderness, and muscle spasm, is sometimes prescribed for CFS. Low doses of certain antidepressants may help improve sleep and decrease fatigue and mood swings.

For More Information

• American Association for Chronic Fatigue Syndrome
• Centers for Disease Control and Prevention
• Chronic Fatigue and Immune Dysfunction Syndrome (CFIDS)

Cold, Common

Symptoms

- Runny nose (discharge is usually clear, but may be yellow, or greenish).
- Sneezing.
- Sore or scratchy throat, with hoarseness.
- Coughing.
- Inflamed membranes in the nose and throat, which may cause discomfort day and night.
- Fatigue and general malaise.
- Occasional low-grade fever (more often found in children than adults).
- Muscle aches and pains.

What Is It?

Just about everyone gets colds—a general term referring to a group of minor but highly contagious upper respiratory viral infections that cause inflammation of the mucous linings of the nose and throat. Symptoms generally develop one to two days after exposure to the virus, and anyone with a common cold is contagious for about two to three days, starting the day before symptoms appear. There is no cure, but there are measures that alleviate symptoms during recovery, which generally takes about a week.

Scientists estimate that there are as many as 200 different cold viruses, the most common being the rhinoviruses (nose viruses), which are estimated to cause 30 percent of all colds. No one knows what makes a person susceptible to colds in general or to any particular cold. Although newborns are thought to be immune to 20 percent of rhinoviruses (they get the antibodies from their mothers), they quickly lose their immunity. Small children are the most susceptible to colds, and can have six or eight a year. People who spend a lot of time with children, such as teachers, also tend to have numerous colds.

There is also evidence that smokers are more likely to catch colds and to have longer-lasting symptoms than nonsmokers. Tobacco smoke paralyzes the hairlike projections that line the nose and throat. Thus, these cilia are less efficient at moving mucus out.

In one sense every cold is your last—from that particular virus for a period of time. One compensation for growing older is that you develop immunity to a progressively larger number of viruses and thus catch fewer colds. By age 60, most people have an average of one cold per year, if any.

Colds and the Weather Factor

▼

Colds do occur seasonally—peak periods in the United States are September, October, and early spring—and it is hard to keep from blaming them on the weather. Puzzlingly enough, researchers have never been able to connect cold viruses with the weather. (One theory says that people catch colds in September because the schools open then, and the most susceptible population—that is, children—begins transmitting viruses.)

Getting chilled or undergoing rapid weather changes cannot cause you to catch cold. At least in the laboratory, low temperatures do not seem to increase susceptibility. In one study reported in the *New England Journal of Medicine,* one group of volunteers in a 40°F environment was exposed to cold viruses, while another group received its viruses in an environment warmed to 86°F. Both groups caught colds at about the same rate.

Some people believe winter is a prime time for colds because indoor heat removes humidity from the air, which dries out your nasal passages and makes you more susceptible. But while dry air may make you feel more uncomfortable, there is no evidence that it increases your susceptibility.

What Causes It?

Researchers know more than they used to about how colds are transmitted and about the viruses that cause them. Rhinoviruses tend to infect people in late summer and early autumn. Other types of viruses, not so well understood, are more likely to cause winter and early spring colds.

A sure way to "catch" a cold virus to which you are not already immune is to get a dose of it directly in the upper nose, where the temperature and humidity are ideal for its growth. In laboratory experiments, putting rhinovirus in the noses of volunteers almost always gives them a cold, no matter what their state of physical or emotional resistance or whether they are cold and wet or warm and dry.

Three possibilities exist for the way cold viruses get into your nasal passages: they may travel through the air (from the sneezing or coughing of others); they may be transmitted through direct contact (shaking hands with a cold sufferer, for example, and then touching your eyes or nose); or they may spread via a telephone, toy, or cup used by a cold sufferer. One study has found that airborne transmission is common in adults, whereas children tend to transmit secretions directly.

But, in fact, unless the virus gains access to the upper nose, the body has many lines of defense against it. Simply putting a cold virus near the nose usually has no effect, because it cannot penetrate the skin. The mucous membranes of the mouth are usually an effective barrier, so that kissing is not an efficient way to spread a cold. Simply being in the same room with a cold sufferer won't do it. Workers in the same office usually don't share colds. They may have colds at the same time, but they are usually due to different viruses.

Family members, though, do tend to share their colds. The three factors that primarily influence transmission are the amount of time spent around the cold sufferer, the volume of his secretions, and the amount of virus in them.

Cold Products: Are They Helpful?

▼

There are more than 800 over-the-counter cold remedies that promise to alleviate your symptoms. Some of the ingredients in these products can provide a degree of temporary relief. But many products contain multiple ingredients, which may actually work against one another and also increase the risk of side effects. Moreover, none of them may prove to be helpful.

If you do want to try a remedy, chose a product to match the symptoms that are really bothering you.

• **Decongestants** open nasal passages temporarily and may dry up mucus. If overused, however, they can have a rebound effect—an increase in swelling and congestion. In some people they can elevate blood pressure and induce insomnia.

• **Cough syrups** come in two types, suppressants and expectorants. The latter can help to loosen mucus if you're congested. For a dry, nonproductive cough, suppressants may help you get a good night's sleep. But don't use them during the day—the coughing serves a useful purpose by clearing secretions from your throat.

• **Over-the-counter NSAIDs**, such as aspirin and ibuprofen, as well as acetaminophen, can relieve fever and muscle aches. Children age 19 and younger should not take aspirin for fever because of the risk of Reye's syndrome. Pregnant women, especially in the last trimester, should avoid NSAIDs.

• **Antihistamines** are actually intended for hay fever, but are included in cold products. They may make mucus too thick, and thus difficult to expel by coughing. They can also induce drowsiness. It's best to avoid them for cold relief.

(See "Cold and Cough Medications" on page 575 for more information.)

209

What If You Do Nothing?

People seldom develop serious complications from colds. The discomfort can be debilitating, but a cold is by definition temporary and self-limiting. Most colds last a week or less, but two-week colds are not unheard of.

Home Remedies

Colds cannot be cured by antibiotics, including penicillin, or any other drug. Nor is it wise to take antibiotics in an attempt to prevent later bacterial infection. Take antibiotics only when your doctor prescribes them—and certainly don't take them on your own for a cold or flu.

Your symptoms, however uncomfortable, are a sign that your body's defenses are working against the virus. Keep the following pointers in mind for your general well-being.

• **Don't automatically "take something" for a cold.** Over-the-counter cold remedies won't necessarily make you feel better. If you do use them, do so sparingly (see page 575). Also, don't insist on giving medicine or vitamins to a child. Many cold medications made for adults contain ingredients that are harmful when taken by children.

• **Gargle to ease a sore throat.** A salt or sugar-water gargle (one-quarter teaspoon of salt or one tablespoon of Karo syrup added to eight ounces of water) can be helpful in relieving sore throat symptoms.

• **Saline nose drops may clear nasal passages.** Like the gargle, these can also be made with one-quarter teaspoon of salt to eight ounces of water.

• **Choose your fluids.** "Drink plenty of fluids" is time-honored advice, but there is no evidence that increasing fluid intake will do anything but increase the need to urinate. Drink as many fluids as you want—they ease a dry throat—but you don't need to force yourself or anyone else to consume liquids.

Hot drinks, on the other hand, are definitely comforting. In one study chicken soup (as compared with cold water and hot water) was shown to increase the flow of nasal secretions. The taste and aroma was thought to be part of the therapy, as well as inhalation of the vapor. Some other hot soup might do as well, if you prefer it. Tea with honey isn't bad, either.

• **Skip the hot toddies.** Hot alcoholic beverages or a shot of brandy may sound tempting, but alcohol dilates blood vessels and may produce more

---

Can Supplements Help?

▼

Several dietary supplements are promoted as cold remedies:

Vitamin C. Though megadoses of vitamin C have been highly touted as a means of preventing a cold, no clinical trial has ever shown vitamin C to be more than marginally useful. At most it may shorten the duration of a cold by an insignificant amount. Megadoses of vitamin C—defined as more than 10 times the recommended dietary allowance (RDA) of 90 milligrams—may cause side effects, including nausea, abdominal cramps, and diarrhea.

Echinacea. This herb is prescribed in Germany for colds and flu, but studies have yielded conflicting results. The plant is a complicated mix of chemicals; some might actually stimulate the immune system or promote healing. But you don't know what you're getting in the bottle, and little is known about the plant's toxicity.

Zinc. The evidence on zinc is mixed. A few studies have indicated that taking zinc lozenges soon after the onset of symptoms can help shorten the duration of a cold. Yet in other studies, cold sufferers taking the lozenges were just as likely as those taking placebo pills to still have the cold after seven days. There is no evidence zinc will actually prevent a cold.

nasal congestion. Overindulgence, obviously, may bring on stomach upset and headache. Pregnant women are advised never to drink.

• **Rest if you feel like it.** Bed rest will not cure a cold or even alleviate symptoms, but if you feel exhausted or your symptoms are distractingly painful, rest at home—either in bed or just around the house.

Increased humidity in the air you breathe can sometimes make you feel better, at least temporarily. Hot-water vaporizers offer some advantages, but can cause burns and scalding. For safety's sake, use a cool-mist vaporizer or humidifier. There is no value in adding medications to the water.

Remember that humidifiers can harbor molds, which may cause allergic reactions. Clean the tank daily, rinsing with a mild solution of chlorine bleach and refilling with fresh water.

• **Ease up on exercise.** There's no harm in exercising if you feel up to it, but you should never force yourself if you feel too tired or unfit, or if you have a fever. A break of two or three days in your exercise program won't be a significant setback.

• **Soothe your red, sore nose and lips.** The irritation, which is caused by mucous secretions and aggravated by nose blowing, can often be relieved with petroleum jelly or skin lotion.

• **Consider keeping kids at home for a day.** If a child has a cold, going to school will do him no harm. But for the protection of other children, a child in the first stages who has a severe runny nose should probably stay at home. The most infectious period generally begins about a day before symptoms appear and lasts only another day or two.

Prevention

• **Wash your hands—often.** The most effective way to keep a cold from spreading is hand washing. If you have a cold, remember that it spreads

---

Antibiotics: Too Many, Too Often

Antibiotics are truly "miracle drugs." Many terrifying infectious diseases of the past, such as strep infections and bacterial pneumonia, are usually easily curable with a course of these agents. But, tragically, these miracle drugs are losing their power, as many bacteria are becoming resistant to them. In large part, this resistance is due to the enormous amount of antibiotics used by humans, for ourselves as well as in animals and agriculture. The more often antibiotics are used, the more often bacteria have the opportunity to mutate into new, resistant strains.

Each year in the United States, doctors write about 100 million prescriptions for antibiotics—the equivalent of nearly one pound of antibiotic drugs for every person. Yet probably half of all of the prescriptions are unnecessary. Most of this unnecessary prescribing is for upper respiratory infections including colds, which are caused by viruses, as are the vast majority of sore throats and coughs. No antibiotic ever killed a virus.

Why are doctors writing so many inappropriate prescriptions? They may be motivated by pressure to deal with patients quickly (it takes much more time to explain why an antibiotic is not needed than to write a prescription for one). And patients often demand the drugs ("whenever I get this cough, the antibiotic seems to clear it right up").

What you can do. Most important, do not ask for antibiotics for a cold, a sore throat, or a cough. Also, don't stockpile antibiotics for use in an "emergency." ("I've got a meeting tomorrow—this should help.") If you think you may have a bacterial infection, ask your physician for an examination. If antibiotics are prescribed for a bacterial infection, always complete the entire course.

You can find more information about the safe use of antibiotics online at the Web site for the Alliance for the Prudent Use of Antibiotics (www.apua.org).

via your fingers, so wash them often in soap and warm water. If you are around people with colds, wash your hands often and try to avoid putting your fingers to your nose and eyes.

• **Try not to share objects with cold sufferers.** This means not touching their telephones, pencils, typewriters and other tools, drinking glasses, or towels. Paper towels and paper cups are worthwhile investments during cold season. See that used tissues are disposed of promptly and properly. They should be discarded in a plastic-lined receptacle or paper bag, or in any manner that makes rehandling them unnecessary.

When To Call Your Doctor

There is virtually nothing a doctor can do for a cold. But contact your doctor if you have any of the following symptoms, which may seem cold-like but can indicate something more serious.

* High fever.
* Severe pain in the stomach, chest, head, or ears.
* Enlarged neck glands.
* Fever, sore throat, or severe runny nose that persists for more than a week.

For children: Shortness of breath or wheezing (particularly difficult breathing), marked irritability or lethargy.

Don't assume that a nasal discharge that thickens and looks greenish indicates a bacterial infection. By itself, a greenish secretion is nothing to worry about. It is not caused by invading bacteria, but is part of your immune system's response to the cold virus, and does not call for antibiotics.

What Your Doctor Will Do

The ears, nose, throat, and chest will be examined, and a chest x-ray may be taken. If a bacterial infection is diagnosed, your doctor may prescribe an antibiotic. But if a cold is found to be uncomplicated, home treatment is the most likely recommendation.

For More Information

* National Institute of Allergy and Infectious Diseases

Colic

Symptoms

- Persistent, inconsolable crying spells in otherwise healthy infants. The spells typically begin after two weeks of age, then quickly subside around three months of age.
- Crying typically starts suddenly, often in the late afternoon or early evening, and may persist for several hours or occur fitfully through the night. The passage of gas or a bowel movement may temporarily halt the crying.
- Crying or screaming may be accompanied by a red or flushed face, clenched fists, drawn-in legs, a tense abdomen, and rumbling in the stomach.
- During an episode, a colicky child may initially suck hungrily at a bottle, breast, or pacifier but then suddenly refuse it and resume crying.

What Is It?

Colic is a common childhood condition marked by prolonged episodes of intense crying, usually during the evening hours. The crying arises suddenly for no apparent reason, and little can be done to stop it: holding, cajoling, burping, changing the diaper, or engaging the infant has no apparent effect. Crying may stop only after the baby (and caregiver) appears exhausted.

Typically, a contented and restful newborn will be brought home from the hospital, only to start the pained screaming fits after a week or two. Crying continues for several months, often at the same time each evening. The condition is sometimes referred to as three-month colic, because at that age the fits quickly dissipate. Needless to say, colic is a major source of distress for new parents and a major reason for frantic calls to the pediatrician.

What Causes It?

The cause of colic is unknown. The word *colic* means "of the abdomen," and the condition may be a response to abdominal spasm and pain, perhaps caused in part by air that is swallowed during crying. Some experts think it may be triggered by an infant's frustration at being unable to interact with the environment. Fatigue may also be a contributing factor.

It is important to distinguish colic from specific disorders that can produce abdominal pain or cramping and prolonged crying, including infection, food allergies, or intestinal obstruction. If no physical causes can be found, colic is usually the diagnosis.

What If You Do Nothing?

Colic is not a serious illness. All infants outgrow it, usually soon after their third month. Excessive crying is not harmful. Infants with colic are otherwise healthy, and they grow and gain weight at a normal rate.

Home Remedies

Effective treatments are difficult for a condition in which the cause is so uncertain. Supportive reassurance is the best approach. Holding, snuggling, gentle rocking or swaying, walking with your infant, and other hands-on measures that reinforce the child's sense of security are always a good idea. In addition, you can try the following measures.

• **Divert the child.** Take the baby for a ride in the car. Play soft music, or use the gentle hum of an air conditioner or radio static in the child's room. Give the baby a pacifier, but don't automatically feed the child every time he or she cries; this can contribute to bloating. Also, try not to overstimulate the child with too much distraction.

213

• **Use proper feeding techniques.** Feed the baby in a semi-upright position, and continue holding the baby upright for about 15 minutes after feeding. Whether you are bottle- or breast-feeding, it's important to burp the baby. If you are bottle-feeding, also be sure to use the appropriate bottle and nipple size for the child's age.

• **Use gentle stroking.** Massage the stomach using smooth, gentle strokes. Or, drape the child, stomach down, along your forearm with the head in the crook of your elbow and arms and legs dangling over either side of your arm; then gently massage the back.

• **Try gentle warmth.** Place the child's stomach down on a warm heating pad or washcloth or on a hot water bottle placed on your lap. You can also try warm baths or swaddling the baby in a soft blanket.

• **Stay calm and rested.** If you are anxious and upset, your child may become more irritable. Take turns caring for the baby with other caregivers. Periodic breaks will increase your coping skills.

Prevention

Nothing can be done to prevent colic, since so little is known about its cause. Other causes of crying should be ruled out. A supportive, attentive home environment may be the best safeguard.

When To Call Your Doctor

Call your pediatrician if a crying episode lasts longer than four hours. Also consult your doctor if your baby seems sick between bouts of crying or has constipation, fever, diarrhea, or loss of appetite; these may be symptoms of infection or another underlying disorder. Episodes of colic should decrease quickly after the child reaches three months of age; call your doctor if fits persist past the fourth month.

What Your Doctor Will Do

Your doctor will do a thorough physical examination to look for signs of infection or illness that may be causing the crying. A urine sample may be taken to check for possible urinary tract infection. Your doctor may ask you to try a different baby formula or, if you are breast-feeding, to eliminate certain foods from your diet; this will test for possible food allergies that can cause intestinal discomfort in the child.

In the past, colic was treated with various medications, but these are generally no longer recommended for infants younger than six months.

For More Information

• American Academy of Pediatrics

Conjunctivitis

Symptoms

- Pink or reddish tinge to the white(s) of the eye(s).
- Oozing, pus-like discharge (bacterial conjunctivitis) or profuse tearing with slight discharge (viral conjunctivitis). Upon awakening, eyelids may be crusted over.
- Swollen eyelids.
- Sandy or gritty sensation upon blinking.
- Itching and tearing (allergic conjunctivitis).

What Is It?

Conjunctivitis, or pinkeye as it is popularly called (because of the dilation and reddening of the blood vessels in the whites of the eyes), is an infection or inflammation that affects the conjunctiva, the thin transparent lubricating membrane that lines the eyeballs and inner eyelids. It can be triggered by an infection, an allergic reaction, or exposure to an irritant. The conjunctiva becomes red and inflamed, and this redness may be combined with a discharge from the eye. If the infection is bacterial, a yellow or white discharge typically occurs. If the whites of both eyes are red, and there is tearing but little or no discharge, this is more symptomatic of a viral infection. One or both eyes may be affected.

What Causes It?

Conjunctivitis usually results from either a bacterial or viral infection, and either type of infection is highly contagious. Children who have conjunctivitis in one eye frequently spread it to the other eye with their fingers. The infection also can be easily passed from one person to another by direct contact (for example, shaking hands with an infected person and then touching your face) or by sharing towels or washcloths that have been used to wipe infected eyes. Improperly cleaned contact lenses, or lenses cleaned with expired solutions, can also be the cause of infections.

Allergies to cosmetics or contact lens solutions, or exposure to pollen, chemical fumes, or other irritants, may also cause conjunctivitis. In these cases the condition is not contagious.

What If You Do Nothing?

Viral conjunctivitis is usually not a serious eye ailment and typically clears up in a week, though symptoms can be bothersome for adults and children alike. Bacterial conjunctivitis is more serious than the viral form and may require treatment by a doctor. Allergic conjunctivitis can persist until the source of the reaction has been identified and dealt with.

Some childhood diseases—measles, German measles (rubella), and chicken pox—can also cause conjunctivitis.

Home Remedies

The following measures are usually effective for soothing conjunctivitis.

• **Apply a compress.** For bacterial or viral conjunctivitis, dip a clean washcloth in warm water, wring it out, and place it over the eyes for five minutes. Once it cools, apply another warm one. Repeat two or three times throughout the day.

If the cause is allergic, applying cool compresses on the eyes can bring relief. Over-the-counter antihistamines may also help reduce redness and itching.

• **Keep the infection from spreading.** When the cause is viral or bacterial, wash and wipe away any discharge with tissue and avoid touching or rubbing the infected eye(s). If only one eye is infected, these steps will keep the infection from spreading to the other eye and also help prevent other people from becoming infected. Also, don't use contact lenses or eye makeup, which can spread the infection to the other eye.

Prevention

• **Practice good hygiene.** Make it a habit to wash your hands frequently with soap and water. This is especially important if you are in contact with a child who has conjunctivitis.

• **Try to avoid touching or rubbing your eyes.** This can easily transmit an infection. Most of us touch our eyes without thinking, so not touching them requires a deliberate effort.

• **Don't share.** Don't share towels, washcloths, or eye makeup with others. If you have an infection, be sure to keep your washcloths and towels separate from those used by anyone living with you—and launder your towels separately as well.

When To Call Your Doctor

Consult your doctor if any discharge is severe, if redness becomes noticeably worse, if your eye is very painful, or if your vision is persistently blurred. These indicate a bacterial infection or some other complication that should be medically treated. Also call your doctor if a chemical irritant has caused a severe reaction that is not relieved by washing the eye with water.

What Your Doctor Will Do

A thorough examination is often sufficient to determine the cause of the conjunctivitis, though swab samples may also be taken and cultured to pinpoint the type of bacterial infection that is present. Antibiotic ointment or eyedrops will clear up most bacterial infections.

For persistent or severe cases of allergic conjunctivitis, a trial course of oral antihistamines and/or appropriate eyedrops may be prescribed.

For More Information

• American Academy of Ophthalmology

Constipation

Symptoms

- Infrequent bowel movements.
- Hard stools that can cause strain and pain when passing.
- Abdominal swelling.
- Continued sensation of fullness after a bowel movement.
- No bowel movement in at least three days (four days for children).

What Is It?

Constipation is really more a complaint than a disorder—in fact, it is the most common gastrointestinal complaint in the United States. It is usually defined as the failure to have a bowel movement after three days or more and is often accompanied by a hardening of the stool and by straining during defecation. Though constipation can be a sign of an underlying health problem, in most cases it's nothing you need to worry about and can be remedied with self-care measures.

One of the biggest myths about constipation is that you're constipated if you don't have a daily bowel movement. Although a daily bowel movement is often thought of as "regular," there is no norm for regularity. It is perfectly normal for a person to have a bowel movement once a day, twice a day, every other day, or perhaps only two or three times a week.

What Causes It?

A lack of fiber in the diet is probably the most common cause; fiber adds bulk to stool, it absorbs water to help soften stool, and it stimulates peristalsis, the colonic contractions that produce the urge to defecate. A lack of fiber and fluids can result in hardened stools that are slow to pass.

Other common causes of constipation include not drinking enough fluids on a daily basis; a sedentary lifestyle; emotional stress, obsessive-compulsive disorder, or depression, which can bring about a change in bowel habits; ignoring the urge to defecate; travel or any other shift in your daily routine that changes your regular toilet habits; laxative abuse; and a lack of access to toilet facilities.

Constipation can be caused by various medications, including pain medications, calcium sup-

217

Constipation in Children

▼

Constipation is frequently encountered in infants and children, particularly when the diet is composed largely of highly refined foods. As with adults, bowel movement frequency for children varies tremendously, from several times a day to as little as once a week.

A decrease in normal bowel habits can be triggered by several causes, including
- a sudden change in diet,
- a resistance to toilet training due to parental pressure,
- stress or emotional turmoil, such as the birth of a sibling, divorce, or the death or departure of a loved one, and
- the memory of a painful bowel movement.

The child's pediatrician or your family physician should be contacted if
- the child suffers discomfort or severe pain while defecating,
- blood is in the stool,
- the child has not had a bowel movement within four days,
- the child has an urge to defecate but can't pass anything, or
- you have concerns you want answered.

Dietary changes usually relieve childhood constipation, so be sure to increase the child's daily intake of fiber-rich food (whole grain products, fruits, and vegetables) and liquids. If the constipation stems from toilet training, stop the training and use diapers until the child actually has the urge to use a toilet.

plements, antacids containing aluminum, iron supplements, antidepressants, and diuretics. There are also medical conditions associated with constipation, including diabetes, kidney failure, backache, bowel disease, and irritable bowel syndrome. Pregnancy can also cause constipation because of hormonal changes.

What If You Do Nothing?

If you have no other symptoms, constipation may clear up on its own in a matter of days; however, at the very least you may need to make some changes in your diet or other lifestyle habits to alleviate it.

Home Remedies

Treatment depends on the specific cause, severity, and duration of the problem, but in most cases these straightforward measures will quickly bring relief.

• **Drink plenty of nonalcoholic fluids.** These will soften the stool, and soft stools are easier to pass than hard ones. Be sure to drink at least eight glasses of water or fruit juice a day.

• **Eat a diet high in fiber.** Examples of high-fiber foods are grains (including unprocessed wheat bran), fruits, vegetables, and legumes. As your grandmother may have told you, prunes are particularly effective in preventing constipation, as are raisins and figs. Try to eat five to six servings of fiber-rich foods daily (which should provide 20 to 30 grams of dietary fiber). But be careful to increase your fiber intake gradually: consuming excessive amounts of fiber can lead to bloating and gas.

• **Get regular exercise.** Physical activity helps stimulate bowel movements by strengthening your abdominal and pelvic floor muscles.

• **Set aside regular bathroom time.** Try not to ignore the urge to defecate, even when it may not be convenient.

• **Use laxatives or enemas sparingly, if at all.** Chronic use of either interferes with the colon's ability to contract.

Prevention

The steps for alleviating constipation should also prevent its recurrence. In short, keep your fiber intake high; drink a minimum of eight glasses of water or other nonalcoholic fluid daily; exercise on a regular basis; try to keep regular toilet hours; and don't ignore the urge to defecate.

Don't Rely on Laxatives

Worry about "irregularity" leads many people to rely routinely, chronically, and unnecessarily on laxatives or enemas. Americans spend more than $400 million annually on laxatives—a mostly useless expenditure that fails to promote normal bowel movements or accomplish any health objective. In fact, excessive laxative use often causes diarrhea and vomiting.

While a mild laxative may occasionally be appropriate if your eating or exercise habits have been altered by travel or some other circumstance, relying on laxatives can actually weaken bowel function and cause irritable bowel syndrome or other problems that will intensify constipation. A laxative is a drug and should not have a permanent place in your medicine cabinet. The most habit-forming laxatives are the so-called stimulants, which work by irritating the walls of the intestine. Laxatives that increase stool bulk (such as psyllium-containing products) are less of a problem, but any laxative can cause dependency.

If you feel in need of one, consult your physician about the type of laxative, the dosage, and frequency. (For more information on laxatives, see page 589.)

Constipation *continued*

When To Call Your Doctor

Constipation that lasts longer than a week without apparent cause and continues despite self-care measures is a signal to consult a doctor, for it can occasionally be a symptom of some underlying disorder. You also should contact your physician if any of the following occurs.

- Constipation accompanied by fever, severe lower abdominal cramping, bloating, or pain. This may indicate a diverticular disorder.
- Bright red bloody streaks on your bowel movement. This can be a sign of hemorrhoids, caused when the hardened stool stretches and tears the anal opening. Bloody streaks can also signal anal fissures (see page 149) or even rectal carcinoma.
- Constipation after beginning a new prescription medication, vitamin, or mineral. You may need to discontinue the medication, change it, or reduce the dosage.
- Impacted bowel movement. The fecal mass becomes hardened, cannot be excreted, and must be removed by a physician.
- Any other significant changes in your bowel habits.

What Your Doctor Will Do

After taking a thorough history, the doctor may perform a physical examination, including a digital rectal exam (DRE) with a gloved finger to evaluate the anal sphincter (the muscle that closes off the anus) and to detect any signs of impaction, tenderness, or blood. Diagnostic tests may also be prescribed, including one or more of the following: special blood tests, stool study, upper GI (gastrointestinal) series, barium enema x-ray, proctosigmoidoscopy.

For More Information

- American Gastroenterological Association
- Intestinal Disease Foundation
- National Digestive Diseases Information Clearinghouse

219

Corns and Calluses

Symptoms

- **Corns:** patches of hardened, thick, tough skin that appear on the tops of toes or between the toes, and may or may not be tender or painful.
- **Calluses:** hardened, tough, thickened areas of skin that typically appear on the soles of the feet, palms, and fingertips.

What Is It?

Corns and calluses are thick, hard growths of skin formed in response to excessive pressure and chafing. Corns, which usually appear on the toes, are thickenings of skin around a core, whose apex points inward. Most hard corns appear on the little toe; soft corns appear on the web between toes.

Calluses are thickened pads of skin, usually on weight-bearing portions of the sole. They also can develop on the hands if excessive pressure and friction occur.

What Causes It?

A hard corn, which often develops on the toe joint, is generally caused by pressure from ill-fitting shoes. Soft corns are generally caused by excessive moisture between toes or from pressure of toes rubbing against each other.

With calluses, rubbing against the skin, typically from ill-fitting shoes, will first cause blisters. If these aren't treated, continued rubbing will cause the skin to thicken into a callus as a layer of dead skin builds up. On the hand, calluses develop from the pressure of repetitive motion.

What If You Do Nothing?

Corns and calluses are minor inconveniences and need no special care. (However, if you have diabetes mellitus, special care must be taken because of the possibility of infection.) Once the cause is eliminated, corns and calluses generally go away within four weeks.

Home Remedies

- **Soak.** The best way to treat corns and calluses at home is to soak the foot in warm (never hot) water until the hardened skin softens, then gently apply a pumice stone or callus file; don't rub the area raw. It may take several treatments.
- **Protect the area.** Use a light pad or bandage. Moleskin comes with adhesive and can be trimmed to fit the spot and relieve pressure.
- **Remove the corn.** Many over-the-counter corn remedies are available, most containing salicylic acid. Though the Food and Drug Administration (FDA) has approved these products, most doctors advise using them only with caution; they can burn the surrounding healthy skin.

Prevention

- **Make sure shoes fit properly.** Have your feet accurately measured by an experienced shoe salesperson. Shoes should be wide enough and sufficiently cushioned to protect the feet.
- **Avoid extended high-heel use.** These shoes put pressure on the toes and can lead to corns.
- **Wear appropriate gloves.** Gloves will protect your hands during gardening or other activities.

When To Call Your Doctor

Contact your physician if a corn or callus becomes infected or inflamed.

What Your Doctor Will Do

After a close examination your physician may remove the callus or corn with a scalpel. In some cases an orthotic—a special shoe insert—may be recommended to correct abnormal foot mechanics that are causing the problem.

Coughs

Symptoms

A cough is a symptom itself rather than an ailment, and coughs can have a number of different patterns and causes, as described below. The production of mucus, phlegm, or blood can indicate an infection. The mucus may be thin or thick in consistency, clear, green, yellow, white, or blood-stained.

What Is It?

A cough is one of the most common reasons that people see a doctor. It is an important reflex that keeps lungs and airways free of secretions or foreign objects that might interfere with breathing. Coughing can be a response to an irritation or obstruction in the throat, larynx, bronchial tubes, or lungs, but in most cases a cough doesn't require medical attention.

Your lungs, sinuses, and throat contain a network of cough receptors—nerve endings that transmit cough messages to the brain. Basically, a cough begins with a deep inhalation of air and closing of the epiglottis and vocal cords, which keeps the air in the lungs. Your diaphragm and chest muscles contract, creating pressure. The epiglottis and vocal cords open abruptly, so that the trapped air bursts out of the lungs, loosening and expelling foreign objects and mucus.

You may not notice it, but people normally cough once or twice an hour—an action that clears the throat. That's all well and good, until you get the dry hacking type of cough that keeps you awake at night and turns into a social liability by day.

There are two distinct types of coughs, productive and nonproductive. A productive cough brings up sputum from the respiratory tract; this process helps speed recovery from inflammation of the airways and lungs. A nonproductive cough is dry and scratchy, raises no sputum, and is typically a response to allergies or medication.

When you have a cold, a cough is usually dry during the first stages; later you may have a productive cough, which usually means that your cold is on the way out.

What Causes It?

Along with colds, flu is a common cause of coughing that can last for several days. Other respiratory tract conditions associated with coughing include asthma, which produces mucus and triggers a productive cough, and bronchitis. One of the leading causes of chronic coughing is cigarette smoking because it increases the production of mucus in the bronchial tubes, which then has to be moved out by coughing.

Coughing can also be triggered by dust, an object or piece of food trapped in the airways, and pollution or other environmental irritants (including second-hand smoke from cigars and cigarettes).

Gastroesophageal reflux (heartburn) can also cause paroxysms of coughing. And certain medications can produce coughing bouts. For example, many people who take ACE inhibitors—a type of drug for treating high blood pressure—develop a dry cough.

In children, croup typically causes a loud harsh cough that sounds like a seal's bark. A loud gasping cough can be triggered by pertussis, or whooping cough.

Coughing, especially when accompanied by chest pain or breathing difficulty, can indicate a more serious medical condition, such as pneumonia, lung cancer, cancer of the larynx, congestive heart failure, or some other severe problem.

What If You Do Nothing?

A cough will generally subside on its own. However, a persistent cough is a telling symptom for a number of serious diseases. If a cough continues for more than five days without any obvious reason or if it interferes with your everyday activities, contact your physician.

Home Remedies

The following remedies should help make a common cough more bearable and shorten its duration.

• **Drink plenty of water.** Water is the best expectorant because it helps thin secretions and makes them easier to bring up. For most coughs, water is often more effective than medications.

• **Loosen up with an expectorant.** If you're congested but your cough is not productive, you may wish you had something to loosen up the mucus. Plenty of products, known as expectorants, claim to do just that. All contain guaifenesin, the only expectorant approved by the Food and Drug Administration (FDA), which has classified it as "safe and effective." You should know, however, that guaifenesin has never been proved effective in clinical trials, nor has the necessary dosage been established. There is also no standard amount of this ingredient in cough medicines.

• **Suppress a dry, hacking cough.** The most common kind of single-ingredient cough medicine is a suppressant, which acts on the cough center in the brain. Some suppressants contain the narcotic drug codeine or a codeine derivative, which are approved for over-the-counter sales in several states. Codeine is effective, but can cause stomach upset and constipation.

A better choice is a suppressant with dextromethorphan, a synthetic relative of codeine that works on the same nerve center to suppress coughing but with much milder side effects. A third type is one containing diphenhydramine (such as Benadryl), the only antihistamine rec-

ommended for treating coughs. Like codeine, it may make you drowsy.

If you decide to use a cough medicine, remember that generics are as effective as the comparable brand-name product and usually a lot less expensive.

• **Steer clear of combinations.** Be cautious about combinations of ingredients. If your cough is allergic in origin, an antihistamine can help, but you probably won't also need an expectorant. Antihistamines dry up secretions, and expectorants are supposed to loosen them, so if you combine these two ingredients, you are working against yourself. And combinations of ingredients may not have sufficient doses of any one of them.

• **Read and follow warning labels on all cough medicines.** Some cause drowsiness and should not be taken if you're driving; some can interact with other medications. If you're pregnant or giving cough medicines to children, it's a good idea to get professional advice.

• **Try cough drops—or hard candy.** Despite the medicinal taste and smell of some of the more serious-looking cough drops and throat lozenges, there's no clinical evidence that they're better than hard candy. Eucalyptus and menthol oils, topical anesthetics, and other ingredients may not help you any more than a plain old lemon drop. Sucking on a hard candy (or cough drop) probably works by promoting saliva flow, which is soothing; the sugar can also soothe the throat.

Cough drops are generally harmless, but aromatic oils can irritate mucous membranes or upset your stomach. Like hard candies, cough drops that contain sugar can contribute to tooth decay.

• **Try a vaporizer.** If your home is dry and overheated, use a vaporizer in your room to add moisture to the dry air. This is especially important at night when you sleep. The humidified air helps liquefy the mucus and make your cough more productive. Since vaporizers can harbor bacteria and fungi that can aggravate and even cause a cough, be sure to clean your machine regularly.

• **Don't forget ointments and salves.** Camphor ointments (such as Vapo Rub) also help ease coughing and are the only topical treatment approved by the FDA. In addition, rubbing your chest with menthol salves or pure peppermint oil and breathing the vapors may also help quell coughing.

• **If you smoke, quit.** Smoking poisons the breathing tubes, and the chronic cough that results from smoking—the so-called smoker's cough—is often a precursor of fatal diseases, such as lung cancer.

• **If your cough is due to heartburn, treat the heartburn.** If you have persistent heartburn along with a cough, stopping the heartburn may clear up your cough (see page 315).

Prevention

• **Avoid tobacco smoke.** Coughing may result from exposure to cigarette smoke. Encourage your spouse, family members, or co-workers to quit smoking.

• **Reduce exposure to irritants.** If you are regularly exposed to dust, chemicals, or smoke at work, be sure that you wear a mask and that your work area is properly ventilated.

• **Avoid air pollution.** If you exercise outdoors, be sure to exercise early in the day. In most major cities, air pollution levels are lowest during the early morning hours, until about 10 A.M.

• **Consider air filters.** An air conditioner or special air filter can be useful, especially if you have seasonal allergies or asthma.

When To Call Your Doctor

If coughing brings up mucus that is yellow, brown, or green, it may indicate infection that needs to be treated by your physician. If the mucus is blood-tinged or bright red in color, contact your physician immediately. Excessive coughing can cause blood vessels in the throat to rupture and bleed, which is not a serious problem. However, you may have an acute respiratory ailment that causes bleeding, and this needs to be treated immediately.

Also contact your doctor if you are coughing frequently for more than five days or for no obvious reason, or you have a cough attributable to a cold, flu, or some other known cause that fails to get better within three weeks.

You should also call your doctor if coughing is accompanied by a fever, skin rash, thick sputum, an earache, chest pain, shortness of breath, lethargy, or pain in the teeth or sinuses.

What Your Doctor Will Do

After taking a medical history, the doctor may x-ray your chest and sinuses, take a culture of your sputum, and prescribe medication. If it's warranted, you may be sent to a medical specialist to treat the underlying illness causing your cough.

For More Information

• American Academy of Otolaryngology-Head and Neck Surgery

Cradle Cap

Symptoms

- Thick, oily, yellow scales or patches on the scalp, usually in infants three to nine months of age.
- Scales may also be present behind the ears, around the eyebrows, or, infrequently, in the skin creases of the groin.
- Skin in affected areas may be slightly red; only rarely does the skin itch.

What Is It?

Cradle cap is a common skin condition in infants marked by oily, yellow patches of scales on the scalp. It is very similar to dandruff in older children and adults. When it spreads to other areas of the skin, such as the eyebrows or behind the ears, it is known by the medical name seborrhea (seborrheic dermatitis). Cradle cap is most common in infants between three and nine months of age, but it can occur in children up to three years of age. It is not contagious. Typically, flare-ups will last for several weeks and then subside, but the condition often reappears.

What Causes It?

No one knows the exact cause of cradle cap. A likely cause is the excessive release of sebum, an oily substance produced by glands in the scalp and other areas. Sebum accumulates in these glands, and then skin cells die and slough off, producing the oily, sticky scales.

What If You Do Nothing?

Cradle cap is usually harmless, although it may be unsightly and does tend to recur. It should not, however, be left unattended, because the buildup of scales may weaken the underlying skin, predisposing it to infection. In fact, if the scales are left to accumulate, an infection or inflammation may develop under the dead skin. Cradle cap does not leave any scars or other lasting effects.

Home Remedies

Most cases of cradle cap are easily treated at home. You will probably need to apply these measures for at least several consecutive days to clear up the condition. Cradle cap often recurs, so take preventive steps as well.

- **Loosen the scales.** Massage warm mineral oil or baby oil into the scalp to loosen and soften scales. Leave it on overnight, or apply warm, moist towels over the oiled scalp for an hour or so. Make sure the towels stay warm so that the baby's body temperature does not drop.
- **Then shampoo.** In the morning, or after warm towels have been applied, wash the hair with a mild baby shampoo. Use special care when washing around the fontanelle, or soft spot, but don't overlook this area of the scalp. (New mothers may hesitate to wash the area thoroughly because of concern about the soft spot—but the skin there is as resilient as the rest of the baby's skin.) Rinse thoroughly.

  Avoid using over-the-counter dandruff shampoos on infants and young children unless your doctor instructs otherwise. These shampoos contain chemicals that could be harmful to an infant or young child.
- **Brush.** To help minimize scale buildup, brush the baby's hair daily using a soft-bristle brush, which will loosen any remaining scales. Scales can then be removed with a fine-tooth comb.
- **Use an OTC cream.** Applying an over-the-counter corticoid cream or ointment two to three times a day, especially if the skin is inflamed, can help bring relief.

Prevention

No specific measures will prevent the first episode of cradle cap. Regular applications of oil as well as daily hair brushing may help prevent recurrences. Gentle shampooing at least twice a week may also help.

When To Call Your Doctor

Call your physician if the condition seems to be getting worse despite several weeks of home treatment, or if it spreads to other areas of the body. Also call your doctor if affected areas appear to be infected or inflamed, with excessive redness, pain, crusting, itching, or oozing.

What Your Doctor Will Do

Your doctor will examine the skin to make sure your child has cradle cap and not some other condition, such as dermatitis, a fungal infection, or an allergic reaction. Some sample flakes from the scalp may be taken for laboratory examination. The doctor may prescribe a mild topical corticosteroid cream, such as 1 percent hydrocortisone, to reduce inflammation. If any areas have become infected, antibiotics or antifungal creams may also be prescribed.

For More Information

• American Academy of Pediatrics

225

Croup

Symptoms

- Shrill, wheezing inhalations.
- A harsh, barking cough (sometimes described as "seal-like") that often occurs in sudden and spasmodic bouts.
- Fever (usually less than 102°F, though some children will not have any fever.
- Hoarseness.
- Symptoms typically appear or worsen late at night and may continue for several consecutive nights.

What Is It?

Because its symptoms involve breathing, croup is one of the most upsetting illnesses of childhood—but most cases are relatively mild and do not cause any lasting damage. It's an inflammation of the area just below the voice box that causes swelling of the air passages and difficulty breathing. Croup most commonly affects children younger than three or four years of age, waking them in the middle of the night with rasping breaths and a barking cough. It can affect children as young as three months or as old as six years. Most cases can be safely and effectively managed at home, and symptoms usually subside within three to seven days. Some children are prone to recurring bouts of croup and seem to get it with any respiratory illness.

What Causes It?

Croup is usually caused by one of several viruses, which are spread from child to child, usually during the fall or winter months. Typically, a child will be sick for a day or two with a cold or a flu-like illness before excessive secretions and swelling in the child's small airways lead to labored breathing and the characteristic barking cough. In other cases, symptoms come on very suddenly, perhaps in response to an allergy. In general, the younger the child, the more severe the symptoms. By age seven, children's respiratory tracts are usually large enough so that croup is uncommon.

What If You Do Nothing?

Symptoms of croup should be monitored closely; although croup rarely is serious, it can become severe and lead to potentially life-threatening airway obstruction.

Home Remedies

Even though the harsh and troubled breathing may be upsetting to both parents and child, croup is almost always easily treated at home.

- **Comfort your child.** It's important that you and your child stay calm. Agitation and crying can make symptoms worse. Your child may prefer to sit up or lie down—whichever position makes it easier for the child to breathe and relax should be encouraged.

- **Soothe the throat with warm mist.** Run the bathroom faucets and shower with hot water to create a steam room effect. Keep the child in the bathroom for 20 minutes or so, perhaps by reading to him or her, until breathing becomes easier. Don't place the child over a steaming teapot or hot-steam vaporizer because of the risk of accidental burns.

- **If heat does not provide relief, try cool air.** Use a cool-mist vaporizer or open the bedroom windows and let the child breathe cool air. This sometimes provides relief if heat does not work. Many parents have found their child's breathing was improved after a nighttime car ride to the emergency room. The moist night air streaming through the open windows seems to break the cycle of labored breathing.

• **Keep the bedroom moist.** Run a cool-mist vaporizer in the bedroom for several days, until the cough and other symptoms subside. If you don't have a vaporizer, try hanging damp sheets or towels in the room to help keep it moist.

• **Reduce fever.** Acetaminophen is effective for reducing fever.

• **Drink plenty of clear fluids.** Encourage your child to drink plenty of water, tea, ginger ale, apple juice, or other clear liquids to prevent dehydration and to help moisten the throat and loosen mucus. Avoid milk, since it can thicken the mucus, so coughing it up becomes harder.

Prevention

Little can be done to prevent croup. The viral infections that cause it are easily transmitted from one person to the next. Avoiding contact with infected children will help to minimize your child's chances of contracting croup, although most children who get viral respiratory infections don't get croup.

Children who are prone to recurrent bouts of croup may benefit from the use of a cool-mist vaporizer whenever they have a respiratory infection. These children will eventually outgrow it, usually by age seven.

When To Call Your Doctor

Call your doctor if:

• your child continues to have trouble breathing for more than an hour, despite use of home treatments.

• breathing is rapid (more than 60 breaths a minute) or heart rate fast (more than 160 beats a minute).

• fever exceeds 102°F.

You should take your child to the emergency room if any of the following are present:

• your child is gasping for breath and seems exhausted.

• your child has pale skin, blue or gray lips, or blueness around the fingernails.

• your child maintains a position with the head tilted forward and the jaw jutting out and appears to be working hard to breathe.

• your child has great difficulty swallowing or is drooling because it is too difficult to swallow saliva.

These may be signs of airway obstruction, perhaps brought on by a serious disorder called epiglottitis. Immediate medical attention is required. However, epiglottitis, which is caused by infection with a bacterium *(Hemophilus influenzae* type B), is becoming increasingly uncommon since the introduction of an HiB vaccine.

What Your Doctor Will Do

In severe cases of croup, a child will be admitted to the hospital and placed in a mist tent, which makes breathing easier. The child may also receive inhaled drugs, such as epinephrine and corticosteroids, to reduce inflammation and spasm. A tube may be placed down the mouth or nose to aid breathing. If croup is complicated by a bacterial infection, the doctor will prescribe antibiotics. X-rays of the neck may be taken if the doctor suspects the child may have epiglottitis.

For More Information

• American Academy of Pediatrics

Dandruff

Symptoms

■ Dry, flaking, white skin scales on the scalp that collect in the hair and fall onto the shoulders. Scaling may also occur in the eyebrows, causing redness and flaking. Scales may be accompanied by mild itching.

What Is It?

Your whole body continually sheds outer layers of dead skin. Usually the process isn't noticeable, but when the scalp sheds skin in large clumps, flakes (dandruff) can collect in the hair with dirt and oil. The condition may be a form of seborrhea (see page 434). Mild dandruff isn't so much a medical problem as it is a cosmetic concern.

What Causes It?

Dead skin cells are typically shed almost invisibly, but in some people, skin-cell turnover may increase rapidly, and the visible flakes called dandruff appear. People with oily scalps tend to be more susceptible to dandruff, probably because oil helps the growth of yeast that is thought to be instrumental in scaling.

What If You Do Nothing?

Dandruff may be an unsightly nuisance, but it's generally not a cause for alarm; dandruff does not signal hair loss, for instance.

Home Remedies

• **Start with regular shampooing.** An ordinary shampoo may work if used often enough—usually every two to four days—but consider daily shampooing for more serious cases.
• **Try a dandruff shampoo.** Dandruff shampoos may control the problem for a few days longer, usually by helping to slough off the scales. Look for these effective antidandruff ingredients: zinc pyrithione, sulfosalicylic compounds, selenium sulfide, or coal tar. While there is some concern that hair dyes containing coal tar may be carcinogenic, dandruff shampoos have much smaller concentrations of the substance and are considered safe and effective by the Food and Drug Administration (FDA). Also, tar shampoos can give hair a brownish tinge—a consideration for people with blond or silver hair. Use special care with products that contain any of these ingredients—they can hurt your eyes. And since continually using any shampoo may leave a residue buildup, alternate your chosen brand with another dandruff shampoo or regular shampoo.

Prevention

There's no way to prevent dandruff from forming, but frequent shampooing can remove excessive scalp buildup and keep it under control.

When To Call Your Doctor

Contact your physician if dandruff doesn't improve within two weeks after following self-help measures, or if more extreme symptoms develop. Severe flaking, crusting, itching, and redness may be signs of medically treatable problems.

What Your Doctor Will Do

After taking a careful history and performing an examination, your physician will determine whether or not you have dandruff, a fungus infection of the scalp, or seborrhea, a skin condition that triggers dandruff-like scales. Prescription medications may be recommended to treat the problem.

For More Information

• American Academy of Dermatology

Dermatitis (Eczema)

Symptoms

- Itching, initially, followed by redness, swelling, and dryness that occurs in specific areas, typically the hands, face, scalp, wrists, behind the knees, and in front of the elbows.
- Oozing blisters and crusting of the affected areas.
- Peeling and chafing.
- Thick and scaling patches of skin (chronic cases) due to scratching.

What Is It?

Dermatitis and eczema are general terms for many recurring noncontagious skin rashes. Sometimes eczema is used to refer to rashes that occur chronically and often without an identifiable external cause, while dermatitis includes symptoms caused by specific triggers that affect many people in much the same way. Often the two terms are used interchangeably. (Technically, dermatitis means inflammation of the skin and refers to the symptoms, not the cause of the irritation.)

There are various types of dermatitis, some grouped by causes, others by specific symptoms and locations on the body. All of them have symptoms of itching and redness, and they often worsen if scratched. The following are among the most common types.

• **Atopic dermatitis.** A chronic skin irritation, this condition is characterized by a hypersensitivity, or allergy, to common substances that don't bother most people. (Atopic is derived from a Greek word meaning "away from the place.") The condition is primarily inherited and usually affects people with a family history of the disorder, or of asthma or hay fever. Symptoms typically first appear in infancy, then flare up at intervals during adulthood.

• **Contact dermatitis.** This form of eczema, also known as allergic contact dermatitis, is an acute rash or irritation caused by substances—such as soaps, detergents, cosmetics, and other types of chemicals—that come in direct contact with the skin. Because the irritation is usually localized, you can often discover what the cause is—though sometimes the reaction won't occur until several hours after you've come in contact with the allergen. Also, it may take more than one contact with a substance before dermatitis first occurs. But then the skin becomes sensitized so that any repeated contact produces a reaction.

• **Seborrheic dermatitis.** Flaking and scaling are typical of seborrheic dermatitis, which tends to occur around the scalp, eyebrows, and face (see page 434 for more information). Dandruff may also be a form of seborrhea.

• **Stasis dermatitis.** A chronic ailment of middle-aged adults, this is caused by pooling of blood in the lower legs. Symptoms, which include red, scaly patches, usually first appear on the inside of the lower leg around the ankles.

What Causes It?

Dermatitis may be caused by allergies, as well as by irritants, sweating, and infections—though it may occur for no apparent reason. Sensitivity to irritants and/or allergens sometimes takes years to develop, and symptoms in some cases may appear only after prolonged exposure.

Common triggers can include clothing (wool and silk, especially), skin lotions, detergents and soaps, stressful situations, antiperspirants, plants (poison ivy, oak, sumac), and medications.

Next to poison ivy, the most common cause of allergic skin rashes is nickel, which is used in costume jewelry, coins, keys, tools, zippers, and other fasteners. An estimated 6 percent of Americans

229

are allergic to nickel. The incidence of an allergic reaction to nickel is higher among women than men because the needles used for ear piercing often contain nickel.

Other common allergens linked to contact dermatitis are cosmetics (especially nail polish), dyes, and leather. Some people are allergic to latex, which is used in a wide range of medical and consumer products; however, the allergy is relatively uncommon except among health-care workers who are frequently exposed to the material.

In some people, foods (especially wheat, milk, seafood, eggs) can trigger an outbreak. And occasionally, a previously tolerated medication turns into an allergen and causes itching.

Stasis dermatitis is often linked to varicose veins.

What If You Do Nothing?

Some cases of dermatitis will clear up on their own. But if your skin is very itchy, it's hard to avoid scratching, which can aggravate the eczema and cause it to appear in other areas where you scratch. When you can't avoid the urge to scratch, make use of the self-care remedies or contact your physician for more potent treatments.

Home Remedies

Self-care for most forms of dermatitis entails stopping the itch-scratch cycle and avoiding known triggers. Therefore, in addition to easing your discomfort, try to identify the substance that's causing your symptoms. If you can discontinue using it or coming in contact with it, you may not need medical help.

• **Don't scratch.** Scratching worsens dermatitis, so try to resist the urge. Keep your fingernails clean and as short as possible to prevent possible infection.

• **Suppress the itch.** Over-the-counter cortisone ointments and creams may help if the allergy or irritation is mild. As a rule, you should use creams or ointments only on dry rashes. If a lesion is oozing, use lotion or liquids. Oral antihistamines may also help relieve the itching. Be wary of "-caine" preparations, such as benzocaine. These deaden the itching, which may feel good momentarily, but they can cause secondary allergic reactions.

• **Compress the itch.** Try a cold compress and that old standby, calamine lotion. Some people have also found temporary relief with milk compresses: pour very cold milk onto a washcloth and leave it on the affected area for three minutes or so; apply another wet cloth for three minutes; repeat several times throughout the day as needed.

• **Bathe less frequently.** Limiting yourself to as few as two baths or showers per week can help keep your skin from drying out. It's also helpful to bathe in lukewarm water rather than hot water.

• **Wear loose cotton clothing.** Cotton clothing allows perspiration—a potential irritant—to evaporate easily. Avoid woolen and silk garments; their fibers may irritate your skin.

• **Try support stockings for stasis dermatitis.** These special stockings can improve circulation in the legs.

Prevention

• **Pinpoint the source of irritation.** If your face is itchy and irritated, suspect a cosmetic. If your hands are cracked and itchy, suspect some chemical you handle (dish detergent, for example). Some people become allergic to nickel after having their ears pierced, and any form of nickel that touches the body produces intense itching and sometimes a rash that looks like poison ivy. The rash may appear anywhere on the body, not necessarily on the ear lobes.

Cosmetics and Sensitive Skin

▼

While true allergic reactions to cosmetics may be few, many people may be irritated by products like deodorant soaps, bath salts, hair removers, hair straighteners, permanent-wave solutions, and hair dyes containing ammonia. Even if you don't think of yourself as having sensitive skin, be cautious about products that promise to kill bacteria or dissolve, curl, or straighten hair. They may leave you itching and burning, so be sure to follow instructions carefully if you do decide to use them.

If you do tend to have allergic reactions to cosmetics, follow these tips.

- Use only one new product at a time when you get cosmetics as gifts or you decide to try a new brand. If you have a bad reaction, you'll be able to nail the perpetrator at once.
- Be wary of labels. Products that are labeled "hypoallergenic" are less likely to cause dermatitis, since the term means less allergic—but there's no guarantee. The Food and Drug Administration (FDA) has no list of allergens nor any rules governing the use of this term on a label. "Allergy-tested" and "dermatology-tested" presumably indicate that the manufacturer has tested the product on animals or people. But again, there is no FDA regulation about using this term.
- Don't skip the patch test whenever it's part of the instructions. If you're wary of any product, try your own patch test: put a dab of the new product on your forearm and cover it with a small bandage; repeat daily for three or four days, and then wait another day or two. If you have no reaction, it's probably safe to use.
- If you do get a reaction and don't know what caused it, stop using all cosmetics. An over-the-counter hydrocortisone cream can help relieve itching or rash. Resume cosmetic use only after doing a series of patch tests, trying one product at a time until you find the culprit (if you're so lucky). If the irritation lasts more than 10 days or is severe, you should see a physician.

231

- **Avoid irritants.** Stay away from substances to which you are hypersensitive. If soap or detergent or other chemicals cause problems, wear rubber gloves. Make sure any jewelry is nickel-free. If you have your ears pierced, make sure it's done with a stainless-steel needle, and be sure that your first pair of earrings are stainless steel or high-quality 18-carat gold studs. Let your doctor or dentist know if you're allergic to latex, since gloves, surgical tubing, elastic bandages, and many other medical supplies contain latex.
- **Moisturize.** After bathing, apply unscented moisturizer on damp skin immediately to seal in the moisture. If you develop dermatitis on your hands in cold weather, apply moisturizer regularly to keep your hands soft. If you live in a dry climate, or are experiencing dry weather, moisten indoor air with a cool-mist humidifier.
- **When washing or bathing, avoid harsh soaps or detergents.** Use your automatic dishwasher and clothes washer as much as possible to avoid contact with detergents.
- **Relax.** Some dermatitis is triggered by stress. If that appears to be true for you, try to maintain emotional stability. Stress reduction techniques such as yoga or meditation can help.
- **Avoid swimming in chlorinated pools.** Chlorine is an irritant. However, you may find that swimming in saltwater bays and the ocean isn't a problem.

When To Call Your Doctor

Contact your physician immediately if a bacterial infection develops (typically signaled by crusting or weeping sores). Also call your physician if a rash or other irritation doesn't respond to self-treatment after a week, or if it keeps recurring.

An allergic reaction to latex is typically an itchy rash that develops at the site of exposure. But in some people, latex allergy can produce hives, breathing difficulties, and even anaphylactic shock—the same kind of potentially fatal reaction bee stings can cause (see page 130). If you've ever had a serious reaction to latex, be sure to discuss it with your doctor. You should also carry some identification stating that you are latex-sensitive, in case you have to be treated in an emergency.

What Your Doctor Will Do

After a thorough examination, stronger prescription medications—including corticosteroid creams, antihistamines, and steroid pills—may be prescribed for symptom relief. Recently, the Food and Drug Administration (FDA) approved the first new type of drug in many years for treating eczema. Called Protopic, it is an ointment that can ease the itching of moderate to severe eczema in both adults and children. It is intended for use when other treatments either don't work or can't be tolerated because of side effects.

For More Information

- American Academy of Dermatology
- National Eczema Association for Science and Education

Diabetes Mellitus

Symptoms

The onset of symptoms in type 1 diabetes is usually sudden. Symptoms due to type 2 diabetes often develop gradually over years.

- Increased frequency of urination.
- Excessive thirst and fluid intake.
- Increased hunger.
- Weight loss that is not deliberate.
- Weakness and fatigue.
- Blurred vision.
- Numbness and/or tingling in the hands and feet.
- Recurring infections, such as urinary tract and vaginal yeast infections.
- Slow healing of cuts and wounds.

Complicating symptoms requiring immediate care:

- Diabetic ketoacidosis. This is a potentially life-threatening complication caused by insufficient insulin. It is most common in people with type 1 diabetes, but can also occur in those with type 2 diabetes. *Symptoms:* dry mouth, flushed skin, fruity-smelling breath, difficulty breathing, vomiting, and abdominal pain.
- Hyperosmolar nonketotic states. This is another potentially fatal complication, usually associated with extremely high blood glucose levels in type 2 diabetes patients. *Symptoms:* Extreme thirst, lethargy, weakness and confusion. In about one third of people with type 2 diabetes, these symptoms are the first sign of their disease.

People experiencing symptoms indicating either of these conditions should contact their doctors at once. If unconsciousness occurs, an ambulance should be called immediately.

What Is It?

Perhaps the most important fact to recognize about diabetes—a disorder that affects about 16 million Americans—is that a great many people who have the disorder, as many as one half, don't know they have it. Like high blood pressure or high cholesterol, diabetes doesn't produce symptoms right away in the vast majority of people affected by it. But in common with those two chronic disorders, diabetes can be detected before symptoms appear—and it also can be controlled and in some cases prevented with straightforward lifestyle measures.

Diabetes is a metabolic disorder characterized by a breakdown in the body's ability to utilize glucose efficiently. Glucose is the main type of sugar produced when foods are digested, and all cells in the body need glucose for energy. But most cells can absorb adequate glucose only in the presence of the hormone insulin, which is produced by the pancreas. A person who has diabetes either isn't producing enough insulin or isn't able to utilize it efficiently—two underlying problems that have led medical experts to make a distinction between the two types of diabetes. In both types, initial symptoms are usually related to hyperglycemia, the medical term for high blood glucose. And in both types, high levels of excess sugar pass into the urine, a characteristic that gives the disorder its proper name, diabetes (Greek for "siphon") mellitus (Latin for "honey-sweet").

In type 1 diabetes, previously known as juvenile diabetes or insulin-dependent diabetes mellitus (IDDM), the body produces little or no insulin. This type of diabetes develops suddenly, usually in people under age 30 (the average age of onset is 12 to 14 years).

In type 2 diabetes, insulin production is normal or close to normal, but cells respond to insulin inefficiently—a condition called insulin resistance. Previously known as adult-onset diabetes and non-insulin dependent diabetes mellitus, or

NIDDM, type 2 diabetes is far more common than type 1, accounting for at least 90 percent of cases. It develops gradually and primarily affects people over age 40, particularly individuals who are overweight. Only about 50 percent of people diagnosed with type 2 diabetes present with classic symptoms; the rest are diagnosed through routine screenings or during exams for unrelated medical problems.

In recent years, the rise in type 2 diabetes in the United States has been dramatic. It is three times as common today as it was in 1960. This increase is due in large part to the fact that Americans are living longer, are becoming fatter, and are less physically active. Also, more people are being screened for the disease. About 800,000 cases are now diagnosed each year.

Diabetes also develops in some women during pregnancy. Although gestational diabetes, as it is called, usually disappears after childbirth, it does increase a woman's risk of developing type 2 diabetes later in life.

Treating type 1 diabetes entails taking daily insulin injections, usually for life. Type 2 diabetes can be controlled with lifestyle measures if it is detected early enough. And in recent years there has been growing evidence that diet and exercise in particular may actually help prevent or delay the onset of the disease (see Prevention). With more advanced stages of type 2 diabetes, treatment with medications is usually necessary to control symptoms.

What Causes It?

The exact cause of diabetes is unknown. Type 1 diabetes is thought to be an autoimmune disorder, in which the body's immune system mistakenly attacks and damages the cells in the pancreas that produce insulin. Type 2 diabetes is clearly linked to obesity—most people with type 2 diabetes are significantly overweight. Heredity appears to play a role in both types, but figures more prominently in type 2 diabetes than in type 1. Certain racial and cultural groups are at increased risk of type 2 diabetes, including

---

Exercise: Prescription for Prevention

Doctors have long recommended exercise as a way to help control diabetes (including Type 1 diabetes, which is usually diagnosed in young people). But in recent years studies have offered strong evidence that physical activity may actually help prevent Type 2 diabetes.

Exercise can help you maintain a healthy weight and reduce body fat, which in turn reduces the risk of diabetes. But the protective effect of exercise against diabetes is due only in part to its effect on weight control. Exercise makes the body more sensitive to insulin's action, so blood sugar is controlled better. Physical activity also tends to reduce abdominal fat, which is associated with early metabolic changes that can lead to diabetes. It's well known that a loss of abdominal fat boosts insulin sensitivity and glucose tolerance, both of which reduce the risk of diabetes. In addition, physical activity enhances the entire series of metabolic events by which your body uses glucose.

The exercise does not have to be strenuous; the point is to not be sedentary. But you do have to exercise regularly to reduce your risk of diabetes, since the effects on glucose and insulin last only a few days at most.

It's best to do activities that work a variety of muscle groups. But any increase in activity improves your odds against diabetes—as well as against other related "diseases of civilization," namely hypertension and heart disease. You can't change some things that put you at risk, such as family history of diabetes or advancing age, but staying active is up to you.

African-Americans, Hispanics, Native Americans, and Pacific Islanders.

Less commonly, diabetes can develop because of certain medical disorders that affect the pancreas or that increase the production of hormones that interfere with insulin action. Certain medications, such as corticosteroids, can increase the risk of type 2 diabetes.

What If You Do Nothing?

If untreated, either type of diabetes will lead to abnormally high levels of glucose in the blood (hyperglycemia). In the case of type 1 diabetes, this can quickly become an emergency. Letting type 2 diabetes go uncontrolled will eventually precipitate a number of serious long-term complications, including cardiac and other vascular diseases, hypertension, stroke, and diseases of the eyes, nerves, and kidneys.

Home Remedies

There are no home remedies, *per se*, for diabetes. Lifestyle measures, especially exercise and dietary modifications, play a crucial role in controlling diabetes, but anyone diagnosed with the disorder should be under the care of a physician. Your doctor needs to monitor the progress of your symptoms, be alert to possible complications from diabetes, prescribe appropriate medications, and instruct you in the use of those medications (see When To Call Your Doctor).

At the same time, the most intelligent step a person with diabetes can take is to become well educated about the condition. The American Diabetic Association and the National Institute of Diabetes and Digestive and Kidney Diseases are excellent starting points for information. In addition, your doctor or health plan may refer you to a diabetes educator—a specialist who is skilled in teaching you about healthful eating, exercise, medications, insulin administration, and overall psychological adjustment.

Prevention

There is no way known to prevent type 1 diabetes, though a large-scale study has been underway to determine if medication can be used for prevention. However, there is growing evidence that lifestyle measures, especially exercise, may be effective tools for preventing type 2 diabetes. If you are at risk for type 2 diabetes, the following steps may prevent symptoms from develop-

---

The Evidence for Exercise

▼

• Studies have found that physical activity has an independent beneficial effect against diabetes in obese and non-obese people, and older and middle-aged ones, as well as among those with a family history of diabetes and those without. Still, those people at highest risk for developing diabetes are likely to benefit most from exercise.

• A 1999 study of 8,600 men who visited the Cooper Clinic in Dallas found that those who were least fit were three times more likely to develop diabetes than fit men over a six-year period.

• While most studies have focused on men, the well-known Nurses' Health Study has shown that women also enjoy the protection afforded by being physically active. Moderate-intensity activity such as daily brisk walking was found to cut the risk of diabetes in these middle-aged women by 60%—as much as more vigorous kinds of exercise.

• Aging itself may play a smaller role than the inactivity that usually accompanies it. When older people stay fit (and don't gain weight), studies have found that the increased risk of diabetes is small. For instance, older athletes have blood glucose and insulin levels similar to those of young people.

ing and may also help prevent or reduce any later complications of the disease.

• **Maintain a healthy weight.** Losing weight through diet and exercise if you are overweight is the key to reducing your risk for type 2 diabetes. For more information on losing weight, see page 33.

• **Improve your diet.** Try to maintain a semivegetarian diet that is low in fat and emphasizes complex carbohydrates over simple sugars. Such a diet is also known to lower the risk of heart disease and some cancers.

• **Get daily exercise.** Studies have shown that exercise may be especially helpful—and that even small amounts of exercise can significantly reduce the risk of developing the disease (see the boxes on pages 234 and 235).

• **Consider vitamin E supplements.** Studies suggest that this vitamin may improve control of blood sugar, notably by enhancing the action of insulin and by affecting cell membranes. Vitamin E also helps combat free radicals, which cause oxidative stress that contributes to an increased risk for cardiovascular disease as well as diabetic complications. A daily recommended dose is 200-400 IU of vitamin E, and people who are at risk for diabetes (or those who have the disorder) should probably be taking this supplement.

• **Get screened for diabetes.** Early detection of type 2 diabetes can identify cases that are mild or borderline, when it is possible to prevent diabetes or control it without medication. For this reason, it's important that all adults age 45 or older undergo regular blood and urine testing for diabetes as part of their regular checkups (see page 82).

• **Keep your heart healthy.** To prevent the cardiovascular complications of diabetes, you should follow the recommendations for preventing heart disease outlined on pages 63-65. Also be sure to take any prescribed medications for cholesterol or hypertension faithfully.

When To Call Your Doctor

You need to call your doctor if you experience any of the symptoms of diabetes, especially a sudden or gradual increase in hunger, thirst, or urine output.

If you have diabetes, you should contact your doctor if you contract an illness with fever and chills, such as flu, urinary infections, dental infections, or wintertime bronchial infections, which can cause your blood glucose levels to go out of control. You should also see your doctor if you develop any skin sores, rashes, or other skin changes that don't heal.

In particular, diabetes reduces sensation in the feet, so that small sores or other foot problems may go unnoticed and can subsequently turn into major infections. Therefore, it's important to inspect your feet every day for irritation and sores and to see your doctor if you develop a foot problem. And because diabetes can cause serious eye complications, everyone with diabetes should get an annual eye examination.

Also call your doctor right away if you experience signs or symptoms of diabetic ketoacidosis or hyperosmolar nonketotic states (described under Symptoms). If you are with someone who experiences these symptoms and unconsciousness occurs, call an ambulance.

What Your Doctor Will Do

Diabetes is diagnosed by measuring blood glucose levels. Your doctor may also order additional tests to evaluate possible kidney damage and risk factors for heart disease.

If you are diagnosed with diabetes, your doctor will work with you to set up a diabetes care plan aimed at keeping your blood sugar levels as close to normal as possible. For type 2 diabetes, if your symptoms are mild, your doctor may initially recommend dietary changes, weight control, and exercise. Later, your doctor may add any of a number of oral medications that reduce the level of blood sugar. If an oral drug or combination of drugs fails to bring your blood sugar under control, your doctor may recommend that you also start using insulin. No matter what medications are used, however, it's important that you continue lifestyle measures.

In addition, people with either type of diabetes should, under the guidance of their doctors, perform blood tests at home to measure glucose levels. Your doctor, a nutritionist, and/or a diabetes educator who specializes in instruction on day-to-day care will advise you about dietary guidelines and exercise. Your doctor will also provide a daily timetable to coordinate eating, exercising, monitoring your blood glucose, and taking any medications, including insulin. It's important to follow the timetable.

As part of your diabetes care plan, your doctor may refer you to other specialists, including a dietitian, a podiatrist (for routine foot care), and an endocrinologist (who specializes in the treatment of diabetes and other disorders of the hormonal system).

For More Information

- American Diabetes Association
- National Diabetes Information Clearinghouse

Diaper Rash

Symptoms

■ Rough, red patches of skin on the buttocks, upper thighs, genitals, or other areas over which a diaper is worn.
■ The rash may be accompanied by the smell of ammonia.

What Is It?

Diaper rash is irritation of the skin from a moist diaper. Most babies get it occasionally, even very well cared-for babies with normal, healthy skin. (Diapering is a way to make infants manageable and socially acceptable, but in fact it inevitably causes diaper rash. In societies that don't diaper, diaper rash is unknown.)

Most diaper rashes can be classified as simple contact dermatitis, though others can become complicated by fungal infections. Diaper rash is not contagious, but it can recur. As babies age, their skin grows less sensitive, and diaper rash is apt to be less of a problem.

What Causes It?

A wet or soiled diaper keeps the skin moist and traps urine, which can react with the bacteria in a baby's feces to produce strong skin irritants, including ammonia. Diaper rash can also occur as a reaction to new foods or to chemicals, such as fragrances found in some lotions, creams, detergents, disposable diapers, or other products. Breast-feeding may offer some protection against diaper rash, perhaps because breast-fed babies have fewer irritants in their urine and feces, though breast-fed babies also get diaper rash.

What If You Do Nothing?

Diaper rash may be irritating and unpleasant for the child. Without proper care, it is unlikely to get better, and it can also lead to more serious complications, such as bacterial or fungal (yeast) infections.

Home Remedies

Most diaper rashes go away after several days with proper home care. Improvement should be noted in a day or two, with complete clearing of the rash by the third or fourth day. Home-care measures are simple and effective.

• **Change diapers frequently, even more frequently than usual.** This will discourage any moisture buildup. To avoid further irritating a rash, rinse the baby's bottom instead of wiping. That is, pour water from your hand or a small container. Then, pat the area gently with cotton or tissue to dry it; don't use a hair dryer for this purpose, since it can easily lead to accidental burns. Also, you should not wash a baby under running water, since the water temperature might suddenly change.

• **Allow the affected area to air.** Although it may be messy, allow the baby to go diaperless for an hour or more each day. If you're using cloth diapers, leave the plastic pants off as much as possible. Avoid plastic-coated disposable diapers or plastic pants. These measures will encourage air circulation to the affected areas.

• **Apply ointment.** When diapering, apply zinc oxide paste to protect the skin from irritants in urine and feces. Petroleum jelly can also be used, but it allows more moisture to be trapped under the ointment. (Products such as A and D Ointment or Desitin, though popular, do not appear to perform any better than plain zinc oxide or petroleum jelly.) Avoid any ointment, however, if the skin is severely inflamed or cracked.

Prevention

Along with other advantages they enjoy, among them reduced illness and infection, breast-fed babies have less trouble with diaper rash—possibly because they have fewer irritants in their urine and feces. So breast-feeding mothers are already a step ahead. But even a breast-fed baby can get a rash. Here are ways to head it off.

• **Keep the bottom dry.** Diapers should be changed as soon as possible when they are wet or soiled to keep the baby's bottom dry. Newborns, however, urinate about 20 times a day (dropping to an average of 6.5 times at 12 months). And most newborns have a bowel movement after each feeding. Obviously, you cannot change diapers every hour around the clock, but you should aim to keep the baby as dry and clean as you can.

• **Gently wash the diaper area.** Use plain water, and pat dry. It's not necessary to use soap—which may be irritating—for diaper changes. Also, no ointments or creams are needed on healthy skin.

• **If you use disposable diapers, use super-absorbent ones.** Disposable diapers constructed with a highly absorbent middle layer keep skin drier and retain more urine at the center, away from the skin, than conventional disposable or cloth diapers. This should not discourage parents from using cloth diapers. What's important is changing diapers often, rather than relying on a diaper to keep the baby dry. A super-absorbent disposable might be best for naps or at night. When washing cloth diapers, rinse them thoroughly. Detergent residue can be irritating.

• **Fit diapers loosely.** Diapers should probably be more loosely fitted than the ads show. Tight-fitting diapers block the circulation of air and may contribute to skin irritation.

• **Powders help keep skin drier.** If you wish to use a powder, choose one that is pure cornstarch.

Don't use talc, which has been linked to a small risk of cancer. To keep the infant from inhaling any powder, apply the powder to your hand first and spread it onto the baby.

• **Be careful with wipes.** In some babies the baby wipes now widely used for cleansing may promote skin irritation. These products contain cleansers, fragrances, alcohol, and preservatives that may be irritating, although some are alcohol-free. If your baby's skin isn't irritated by them, it's fine to use them. If a rash develops, switch to plain water.

• **Introduce solid foods slowly.** To prevent a rash brought on by a reaction to new foods, avoid introducing solid foods until your baby is four to six months old. If you think a particular food may be causing a rash, wait a while before reintroducing it.

When To Call Your Doctor

Call your doctor if diaper rash doesn't improve with home treatments after two or three days. Also let the doctor know if the rash has spread to other areas of the skin, if there is redness within the skin creases, if blisters have developed, or if the child also has fever or loss of appetite; these may be signs of a complicating infection or an allergic reaction.

What Your Doctor Will Do

If a fungal or bacterial infection is present, your doctor will prescribe antifungal drugs or antibiotics. Your doctor may also suggest a corticosteroid cream to reduce inflammation if an allergic reaction is present.

For More Information

• American Academy of Dermatology
• American Academy of Pediatrics

239

Diarrhea

Symptoms

- A change in bowel habits with unformed, watery and/or frequent bowel movements.
- Abdominal pain and cramping.
- Excessive gas.
- Nausea.

What Is It?

Diarrhea occurs when too much fluid is passed along with the stool during a bowel movement. Normally, fluids in the digestive tract are mostly reabsorbed through the intestinal walls, so that fecal matter solidifies as it travels through the digestive tract. If something interferes with the effectiveness of this process, you'll pass excess fluid as you defecate.

It's important to distinguish between two basic types of diarrhea. Non-inflammatory diarrhea is characterized by unformed, watery, and frequent bowel movements, often accompanied by abdominal cramps, gas, and nausea. This type of diarrhea is common, and an acute bout that is mild to moderate is often simply unpleasant and inconvenient (though it can be serious, particularly for children and the elderly, because of the risk of dehydration).

Inflammatory diarrhea is another matter. This is signaled by small stools, blood and/or pus in the stool, fever, and abdominal pain. These symptoms are indicative of a more serious bowel disease and should not be self-treated with an anti-diarrheal remedy or any other over-the-counter product. Anyone with these symptoms needs to be diagnosed by a physician before beginning treatment (see When to Call Your Doctor).

What Causes It?

Simple non-inflammatory diarrhea has many causes. The leading cause is bacterial or viral infection from eating contaminated food or drinking water. (Examples of diarrhea-causing agents are also discussed in Food Poisoning on page 267 and Traveler's Diarrhea on page 476.)

In addition, specific types of diarrhea can occur after taking antibiotics as well as from excessive use of certain over-the-counter antacids that contain magnesium. People with lactose intolerance (who have trouble digesting milk products) may also suffer from recurrent diarrhea if they eat dairy products. Diarrhea may also be triggered by emotional stress.

Chronic diarrhea that persists for days or weeks can result from an excessive use of laxatives. Another cause of persistent diarrhea, often alternating with bouts of constipation, is irritable bowel syndrome. (In these cases, or whenever diarrhea lasts for more than 48 hours, medical evaluation is recommended for pinpointing the cause and determining the appropriate measures.)

What If You Do Nothing?

Fortunately, simple diarrhea is usually self-limiting—it gets better without treatment in a day or two as long as you drink plenty of fluids. However, diarrhea can have serious consequences when it causes dehydration.

Home Remedies

You can obtain symptomatic relief with the following steps.

• **First and foremost, drink fluids.** You need to replace the water you've lost and—in more severe cases—restore the proper balance of electrolytes (sodium, potassium, and chloride salts) that your body requires for the proper functioning of many organs, including the heart. Glucose or some other carbohydrate should also be consumed, to aid the absorption of electrolytes.

Diarrhea in Children

▼

Only illnesses such as colds occur more frequently during childhood than diarrhea. Often a child will develop diarrhea at the same time as, or immediately following, the start of an infection of the upper respiratory tract. Most diarrheas are short-term and usually run their course and improve without medication. Home treatment of children with short-term diarrhea is usually successful in a few days; severe cases may require a week or more until all signs and symptoms disappear.

For many mild cases of diarrhea, effective home treatment is usually sufficient to comfort your child. However, children require or can benefit from certain measures that aren't necessary for adults.

Drinking Guidelines
Make sure the child drinks plenty of fluids. Fluids are most important, even if no solid food is eaten during the several days of an episode. As the frequency of stools increases, so does the need for fluids to keep up with losses. When a child is having frequent stools, a liquids-only diet is recommended. Once diarrhea begins to diminish, soft solid foods may be introduced, followed eventually by a normal diet.

Simple, clear liquids are most helpful. However, liquids like apple juice, cola drinks, and sports drinks contain too much sugar, which can exacerbate a child's diarrhea. Plain water doesn't replace lost minerals. Therefore, in infants and children up to 12, replace lost fluid with specially made oral rehydration drinks such as Infalyte, Naturalyte, Pedialyte, and Rehydrate. These products contain the right amount of fluid, salts, and carbohydrates to prevent dehydration.

Children older than 12 can also consume sports drinks or the home rehydration mix described on page 242. Decaffeinated tea with sugar, flat (defizzed) soda such as ginger ale, or diluted fruit-flavored gelatin are other acceptable choices.

Infant Feeding
For babies who are breast-feeding, continue regular feedings. Although breast milk contains lactose, it doesn't appear to worsen diarrhea; some substance in the milk may actually enhance the digestion of lactose. For infants on formula, diluted versions of the formulas they are taking is satisfactory.

Sipping Guidelines
Here is a suggested drinking schedule indicating the minimum amounts of fluid a child should consume. (If a child balks at drinking, encourage the child to take small sips. Sucking on ice chips or licking ice that has been frozen in a paper cup may be a welcome variation.)
- Infants: 2 ounces every hour (12 ounces, or one and a half cups, every 6 hours).
- Preschool children: 4 ounces every hour (24 ounces—3 cups—every 6 hours).
- School-age children: 5 ounces every hour (30 ounces—almost 4 cups—every 6 hours).

Follow the Regular Diet
If diarrhea occurs no more than twice in 24 hours, continue the same eating patterns. Contact your physician if stools are still loose after 36 hours.

Start the BRAT Diet
If diarrhea occurs as often as once every four hours, clear liquids and the BRAT diet (bananas, rice, applesauce, toast) can be started. These bland, easily digested foods will help speed recovery. If no change in diarrhea occurs within 24 hours, consult your physician.

Avoid fats, at least for several days. Fats won't remain long enough in the intestines to be digested. While not harmful, this undigested food leads to foul-smelling bowel movements.

Protect the Sensitive Areas
Once an infant develops diarrhea, protect the diaper area with zinc oxide paste or petroleum jelly to prevent painful skin irritation. Change diapers more often, and with each change wash the child's bottom with plain water and then rinse and pat dry with a clean towel.

For adults with little or no dehydration, drinking several types of clear liquids—fruit juices, clear broths, flat (de-fizzed) soft drinks—provides adequate rehydration. Sip small amounts for the first few hours, increasing your intake to as much as your stomach can handle. Try to drink at least one pint of fluid (16 ounces) every hour.

• **For a severe attack of diarrhea, or when a child has diarrhea, it is more effective to consume an oral rehydration solution.** You can buy a solution or make it yourself. These solutions don't taste very good, however, and some people will balk at drinking them. An acceptable second choice is a sports drink like Gatorade. Sports drinks typically don't contain enough sodium or potassium, and their high sugar content can sometimes aggravate the diarrhea. But they are better than plain water, caffeine-free soda, or apple juice.

To make up your own oral rehydration solution, dissolve a half teaspoon of salt and four teaspoons of sugar in one quart of water. (Be accurate—too much salt or sugar can cause further dehydration.) Younger children should drink a commercial solution (see page 241).

• **Avoid alcohol, caffeine, milk and dairy products, and any products containing the sweeteners sorbitol, xylitol, and mannitol.** The latter are most commonly found in sugarless gums, vitamins, and diet foods.

• **If you suspect food poisoning, you are probably better off letting the diarrhea run its course.** This allows you to get the harmful bacteria and/or toxins out of your system. But also consult your doctor just to be sure that your diarrhea isn't serious. (Traveler's diarrhea may require different treatment strategies—see page 476).

• **If you suspect diarrhea is caused by a drug you are taking, call your doctor.** This is especially true if you are taking an antibiotic (see When To Call Your Doctor). Also, stop using any over-the-counter antacids or laxatives until you've spoken to your doctor.

• **Be careful with antidiarrheal medications.** Wait a few hours after the onset of diarrhea before using one of these medications: you want to give your system a chance to get rid of whatever irritant is causing the problem. Once that occurs, some of the medications designed to alleviate diarrhea can be useful in certain cases. However, don't use these medications if you have a fever or if there is blood or pus present in your stool.

Over-the-counter products helpful for simple diarrhea include those containing loperamide (Imodium AD) and bismuth subsalicylate (Pepto-Bismol). Both are available in generic formulations that are just as effective as the name brands. Diphenoxylate hydrochloride (Lomotil) is an effective prescription medication. None of these products should be used, however, for diarrhea caused by taking an antibiotic.

Alert: Signs of Dehydration

▼

Contact your physician for any child who cannot retain fluids because of diarrhea. Dehydration, the severe loss of essential body fluids and salts, can occur rapidly and be life-threatening, especially for infants under six months of age. Signs of dehydration include

- fewer wet diapers,
- cool, dry, pale skin,
- dry tongue and no drooling,
- thirst,
- listlessness,
- rapid pulse,
- sunken eyes,
- no tears when crying, and
- sunken fontanelle, the soft spot on the top of an infant's head.

Products containing attapulgite (for example, Donnagel or Kaopectate) or kaolin and pectin (for example, Kaolin Pectin or Kao-Spen) are generally not effective.

• **Don't stop eating.** Cutting back on food aggravates dehydration and limits the nourishment necessary for the body to overcome dehydration. Follow the BRAT diet (bananas, rice, applesauce, toast). If you can't hold down any food, continue to drink rehydration solutions, de-fizzed soda, or an eight-ounce glass of fruit juice to which a pinch of table salt and a half teaspoon of table sugar have been added.

Prevention

The most easily prevented cause of diarrhea is food poisoning. You simply need to take precautions when preparing, cooking, and storing food (see pages 269-273). Above all, don't consume any unpasteurized foods or beverages.

Also, avoid foods you know your body can't tolerate well. People who are lactose-intolerant should avoid the dairy products that seem to trigger symptoms or should drink milk treated with lactase. Avoid taking large doses of vitamin C; too much vitamin C can cause diarrhea.

When To Call Your Doctor

If you started taking—or have recently taken—a prescription drug, contact your physician. Antibiotics in particular can sometimes cause diarrhea by allowing a resistant organism normally present in your gastrointestinal tract (called *Clostridium difficile*) to grow excessively and produce enough toxin to cause a serious bout of diarrhea. Be sure to tell your doctor if you have been on a course of antibiotics.

At any age, diarrhea requires prompt medical attention if it lasts more than 48 hours or is accompanied by any of these symptoms.
• Severe abdominal cramping.
• Blood or pus in your stool.
• Lightheadedness or dizziness (indicating dehydration).
• Fever.
You should also consult a physician if you get frequent bouts of diarrhea or if you have alternate bouts of diarrhea and constipation, since this may be a sign of an underlying disorder.

For children: Call your doctor right away if diarrhea is accompanied by other symptoms such as severe abdominal pain or vomiting or if diarrhea lasts for more than one day in a child under the age of two, or two days in an older child. Call sooner if diarrhea worsens or if the child has a fever or bloody stools, or the number of bowel movements has not decreased in two days.

What Your Doctor Will Do

For acute diarrhea your doctor will examine your abdomen and often will have the stools examined in a laboratory. If a bacterial infection is present, antibiotics may need to be prescribed. Although the course of the diarrhea may not be shortened, the number of bowel movements will be reduced sharply and promptly in many cases. Chronic diarrhea will require more extensive evaluation of the stools, as well as blood tests and other examinations of the intestinal tract.

For More Information

• American Gastroenterological Association
• National Digestive Diseases Information Clearinghouse

Diverticular Disorders

Symptoms

Diverticulosis

- In most cases there are no symptoms.
- Some people develop mild cramping or tenderness, usually in the left side of the abdomen, which disappears after a bowel movement or passing gas. Nausea, gas, and constipation are also occasional symptoms.

Diverticulitis

- The most prominent symptom is intermittent lower left abdominal cramping (or tenderness or acute pain) that usually appears suddenly and may be mild to severe. The discomfort may stop and then recur, or it can become continuous.
- During attacks, fever may occur, accompanied by chills and nausea.
- Constipation is common, diarrhea is less common.
- In some instances rectal bleeding occurs.
- Rarely, breaks and leaks in the bowel wall lead to a fistula, or channel, that typically connects the colon and the bladder (though it can also occur between the colon and other organs). This is signaled by bladder irritation and the passing of fecal matter and gas in the urine.

What Is It?

Diverticulosis is a condition, not a disease. It occurs when tiny grape-size pouches (diverticula) form in the stomach or intestine, typically along the lower wall of the colon (large bowel). These are small, self-contained pouches that often produce no symptoms, and typically are discovered by an x-ray or other types of intestinal examination for an unrelated problem.

According to the National Institutes of Health, 1 in 10 people over 40 and half those over 60 have diverticulosis. Though the condition is common, most people who have it never know, since they experience no symptoms. However, the condition is associated with irritable bowel syndrome, which may cause such symptoms as gas, bloating, and diarrhea. And if your diverticulosis turns into diverticulitis, as happens with some people, you will definitely have symptoms.

Diverticulitis occurs when one or more of the pouches becomes infected from bacteria in the digestive tract. A mild infection can produce bloating, gas, and nausea, and most people don't immediately see a doctor for these symptoms, especially if they improve. Pain is usually on the left side of the abdomen, unlike appendicitis, which affects the right side.

However, some symptoms—abdominal pain and/or rectal bleeding—are severe and shouldn't be ignored. They can be signs of complications or other serious problems. The intestinal wall may become perforated, causing surrounding tissues in the abdominal cavity to become infected. These cases, fortunately rare, can be life-threatening and call for immediate hospitalization, and possibly surgery.

What Causes It?

Exactly why diverticulosis occurs isn't known, but it appears to be caused by excess pressure (and possible weakening) within the colon that pushes an area outward, creating a pouch (diverticulum). This pressure buildup often gets worse with age.

Research done on different populations suggests that a lack of fiber in the diet is associated with diverticulosis. The condition occurs most frequently in industrialized societies, where fiber intake tends to be low. It is rare in regions (such as rural Asia and Africa) where the diet is high in fiber. Fiber helps soften stools so they move more easily through the colon; hard stools require the colon to exert more pressure, which may lead to the formation of diverticula.

What If You Do Nothing?

For most people, diverticulosis poses no problems, and mild flare-ups of diverticulitis, with symptoms of abdominal distress, often clear up with no special measures taken. More serious cases of diverticulitis cannot be ignored because an inflamed diverticulum may rupture and cause a life-threatening infection.

Home Remedies

Diverticulosis is rarely a problem for most people, but you can take measures to prevent the condition or to prevent existing diverticula from becoming inflamed (see Prevention).

Treatment for diverticulitis generally consists of bed rest, a liquid diet, and antibiotics to combat the infection. An attack without complications may respond to antibiotics within a few days. Some patients—about 15 to 30 percent—who experience severe or multiple attacks may require hospitalization and possibly surgery.

Prevention

The best way to reduce your odds of developing diverticular problems is to avoid constipation and straining during bowel movements. Perhaps because fiber used to be called roughage, it was once commonly thought that a high-fiber diet—fruits, grains, and vegetables—was somehow rough on the bowels and that a person with symptoms of diverticulitis should immediately go on a low-fiber or even a liquid diet. It's now thought that this is about the worst thing you can do. Indeed such a diet can even cause the large intestine to go into spasm.

Fiber, on the other hand, provides bulk in the intestine when the fiber is consumed with an adequate amount of fluid, and this enables food and waste to pass more easily and efficiently.

Of course, if you have an acute case of diverticulitis, you may have to follow a liquid diet and take antibiotics until your colon has begun to heal. Soon after, though, you will be advised to increase your fiber intake.

Here are steps you can take to keep diverticulosis "silent."

• **Eat a lot of fruits, whole grains, and vegetables to boost your fiber intake.** (If you aren't used to a high-fiber diet, start gradually.) Choose whole-wheat bread over white, brown rice over white. Add a little bran to baked goods. Eat whole-grain cereals for breakfast. Eat fruits and vegetables unpeeled when you can. Raw produce is good, but cooking does not destroy fiber.

• **Drink plenty of fluids.** At the very least, try to

245

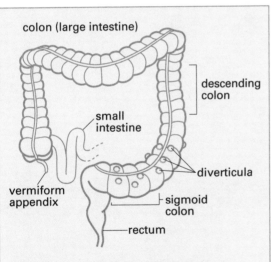

In diverticulosis, small pouches, called diverticula, form in the large intestine, usually in the sigmoid colon (which descends to the rectum). If one or more of the diverticula become inflamed, the condition is called diverticulitis.

consume the equivalent of eight eight-ounce glasses daily, including juices and soups. Fruits and vegetables also contain a high percentage of water, which is another benefit of adding them to your diet.

• **Get regular exercise.** There is some evidence that physically active people are less prone to diverticulitis and that exercise may help prevent constipation.

• **Eat a few prunes for occasional constipation.** They are not only a good source of fiber but also contain a natural laxative. You can also ease constipation and increase dietary fiber with over-the-counter "bulk" laxative products such as psyllium (see page 590). Do not rely on stimulant laxatives, however.

When To Call Your Doctor

For most people, diverticulosis is not a serious problem and rarely requires medical assistance.

Diverticulitis, by contrast, often requires medical diagnosis and intervention, so consult a physician right away when symptoms develop.

What Your Doctor Will Do

After taking a thorough history, your doctor will perform a physical examination, checking the tender areas on the abdomen. Diagnostic tests may also be prescribed, including one or more of the following: blood cell count, urinalysis, x-ray, barium enema, sigmoidoscopy and/or colonoscopy. (The latter three tests should not be performed during or for a few weeks after an episode of diverticulitis.)

For More Information

• American Gastroenterological Association
• Intestinal Disease Foundation
• National Digestive Diseases Information Clearinghouse

Dry Eyes

Symptoms

- Excessive tearing, persistent scratchy and/or stinging sensation in the eye.
- Redness, swelling, or irritation (as if some gritty foreign body is under the eyelid).
- Blurred vision.

What Is It?

Your eyes are regularly bathed by tears, which help lubricate the blinking action of the eyelids and wash away any debris that lodges on the cornea—the clear protective coating on the eye. One of the most common external eye complaints among people over age 40 is dry eye syndrome, or keratoconjunctivitis sicca (KCS), which produces an itchy, gritty feeling in your eyes. Surprisingly, overflowing tears are often a symptom of the condition, produced in response to underlying dryness.

Dry eyes are more likely to occur with age because the tear glands tend to shrink. This condition is also more common in women, especially after menopause.

What Causes It?

The discomfort of dry eyes is usually due to insufficient tear production by the lachrymal glands. Certain eyelid abnormalities or surface infections may also be responsible. The problem can also occur as a side effect of certain medications (diuretics and antidepressants), and it can be associated with rheumatoid arthritis. It also occurs in Sjögren's syndrome, a type of autoimmune disorder in which the glands that produce lubricating solutions—including those for the mouth and vagina as well as the eyes—are attacked.

The environment can also contribute to the problem. Too much exposure to direct sunlight or extremes of wind and low humidity may quickly dry out the eyes, and in arid parts of the country many people develop dry-eye problems because tears evaporate quickly in the heat. When this happens, tears quickly flood the eyes as a protective measure, blurring vision in the process and leading people to mistakenly think the excessive tearing is a condition called wet eye, or epiphora. In reality, the excessive tears are masking the problem.

High altitudes, air conditioning, and air pollution can also contribute to dry eyes by increasing the rate of tear evaporation. Soft contact lenses can also have the same effect.

What If You Do Nothing?

Dry eyes may clear on their own if you are able to avoid or remove the source of the problem. But if you have persistent dryness, you should obtain a professional diagnosis.

247

Home Remedies

• **Use "artificial tears" eyedrops on a regular basis.** In some cases this may mean two drops, three to four times daily, of a nonprescription tear preparation. These nonprescription drops are often completely effective. Some solutions are thicker than others, but all can help protect the delicate front surface of the eye. Try several solutions and see which one works best for you. Be aware that most products will lose their effectiveness within an hour after application.

You may find that while the thicker gel lubrication solutions relieve symptoms for a longer time, they may cause slightly blurred vision for a short period after they've been applied. (A good time to use the thicker products is at night, just before going to bed.)

Some people have allergic reactions to the

preservatives in these products; if you do, look for preservative-free artificial tears. As noted on the package, these products must be kept refrigerated after opening.

• **Try a cooling soak.** With a cool, wet facecloth, soak your closed eyes for three to five minutes. This helps constrict the blood vessels and ease the gritty sensation.

• **Splash water in your eyes.** This will help to quickly relubricate your eyes.

(In addition, see the prevention tips below.)

Prevention

• **Protect your eyes from the wind.** If you find that your eyes dry out because of high winds, be sure to wear goggles or glasses with protective side shields. These are available in many pharmacies as well as outdoor-equipment stores.

• **Avoid smoky environments.** Smoking dries the eyes, as does secondhand cigarette smoke.

• **Keep alcohol and caffeine intake to a minimum.** Both types of beverages have a diuretic effect that can exacerbate dryness.

• **Alternate contact lenses with eyeglasses.** If you work or live in a low-humidity environment, this will help ease the strain of dry eyes brought on by daily-wear or extended-wear lenses. When you wear your lenses, be sure to use rewetting drops at the first sign of dryness.

• **Humidify your home.** Cold winter air coupled with indoor heat can produce an extremely dry environment, particularly if rooms are overheated.

A home humidifier can help reduce dryness, as can turning down the heat.

• **Break up your computer time.** As you work in front of a computer screen, you tend to blink less, which can cause eyes to become drier. Taking a break every hour or so can help prevent excessive dryness.

• **Speak to your physician about your medications.** Certain antihistamines, oral contraceptives, and antidepressants can contribute to dry eye. If it's possible, try an alternative drug that doesn't produce this particular side effect.

When To Call Your Doctor

Contact your ophthalmologist if you don't find relief for dry eyes in a day or two, or if you find that you need artificial tears on a daily basis.

What Your Doctor Will Do

The ophthalmologist will test your rate of tear production and check your eyes' blinking mechanism and possibly the chemical composition of your tears. If you have a dry mouth, joint pain, or other symptoms indicative of Sjögren's syndrome or another autoimmune disorder, blood tests may also be ordered for indicators of autoimmune activity. Along with artificial tear solutions, your doctor may prescribe antibiotics to treat any associated bacterial eye infection.

For More Information

• American Academy of Ophthalmology

Dry Skin

Symptoms

- Skin that appears dry, scaly, brittle, rough.
- Itching (moderate to severe cases).

What Is It?

Itching, scaling, cracking, flaking, and chapping are the chief signs—and consequences—of dry skin. Dry skin is an annoying problem for elderly people, who have lost much of the natural moisture and oil from their skin. For people of all ages, dryness is aggravated by winter weather, when outdoor chill and particularly indoor heat become the enemies of the epidermis. Common sites of dry skin include the lower legs, thighs, and upper arms. Cold weather can also cause nails to break and cuticles to roughen.

What Causes It?

Throughout much of life, secretions from oil and sweat glands help to moisten the skin and prevent dryness. As you age, however, natural secretions decrease and the skin gradually dries out. Also contributing to the problem is the fact that skin sags more (because the fat just under the skin diminishes) and it loses elasticity because of changes in connective tissue. In addition, cold weather, dry air, harsh skin-care products, and too-frequent bathing contribute to the overall drying effect.

What If You Do Nothing?

In most cases dry skin will eventually clear on its own once the humidity increases. However, the unsightly appearance and accompanying itching may be too much to bear until that time finally arrives.

Home Remedies

There are effective and inexpensive ways to take care of dry skin.

- **Take short baths or showers and use lukewarm water.** Cut bathing back to two or three times a week during the cold winter months. Sponge bathe the rest of the time. Overbathing in a tub may cause damage to skin cell membranes, possibly by removing essential body oils.
- **If you take tub baths, add bath oil.** This will help soothe the skin. Cornstarch, instant oatmeal, or colloidal (finely ground) oatmeal are good alternatives.
- **Don't use deodorant soaps.** Choose a milder soap and use as little of it as you can.
- **Pat yourself dry instead of rubbing.** Gentle patting is less irritating than vigorous rubbing.
- **Moisturize.** Apply a moisturizing oil or lotion, especially after a bath or shower. Avoid products that contain rubbing alcohol.
- **Make sure all clothing that touches your skin is well rinsed when washed.** Try switching to a detergent that contains no perfume. Discontinue fabric softeners, bleaches, and other wash ingredients. (You may be able to return to your regular washing routine later.)
- **Wear cotton.** It's easier on your skin compared with wool or synthetics, whose rough texture tends to catch and move the skin scales, leading to a vicious cycle of itching and scratching. Permanent press and wrinkle-resistant fabrics may have formaldehyde or other irritating chemicals in their finish. Wash new clothing and towels before using them.
- **Try not to scratch.** You may irritate the skin further. If symptoms persist, apply a hydrocortisone cream to your skin. Don't use alcohol-based products, which are drying, to combat itching.

Prevention

• **Keep the indoor temperature at 68°F in the winter.** This saves fuel as well as skin by increasing the relative humidity. If this isn't possible, use a humidifier to raise humidity and slow dehydration.

• **Avoid toasting yourself in front of a fire or woodstove.** Wood heat—because it is so hot if you're near enough to get really warm—is extremely drying.

• **Stay out of direct sunlight as much as possible.** Too much sun causes dryness, and it is the leading cause of skin cancer. Use facial moisturizers that contain sunblocking agents.

• **Use a moisturizer after bathing.** Moisturizing ingredients trap moisture and change the surface of the skin (see box at left).

• **Avoid air conditioning whenever possible.** Going from a humid environment into an air-conditioned room where the relative humidity is low causes water to be lost from your skin.

• **Use liquid soap whenever possible.** Liquid soaps are milder than most soap bars.

How Moisturizers Can Help

▼

Moisturizers work just on the skin's surface to relieve the flaking, itching, and tightness that characterize dry skin. Despite the claims in advertisements, these creams and lotions—even if they contain vitamin E, hormones, and other "skin foods"—can't penetrate and "nourish" the deeper layers of the skin, slow the aging process, or reduce wrinkling. Still, moisturizers can help relieve the symptoms of dry skin.

There are two types of moisturizers:

Emollients, also called occlusives (such as petroleum jelly, lanolin, and mineral oil). These work very much like your skin's natural oils; they form an oily barrier on the skin's surface that seals in moisture to some extent and thus blocks its evaporation.

Humectants (such as glycerin, sorbitol, lactic acid, and urea). These attract and hold water on your skin's surface.

Which moisturizer will work best for you? This depends on the moisturizer's ingredients and how chapped, dry, or sensitive your skin is. The simpler the moisturizer, the better. The more ingredients in a moisturizer—perfumes, colors, thickeners, emulsifiers—the greater the chance of a sensitivity reaction, especially if you have delicate skin. If you are prone to acne, overuse of any moisturizer may cause your skin to break out.

The best advice: buy by price. In a comparison of more than 30 moisturizers, *Consumer Reports* found that the least expensive (Vaseline Intensive Care Dry Skin formula) worked best. When you find a product you like, you'll find that it works on your face, hands, and body. You don't need different products for various body parts.

When To Call Your Doctor

Contact your physician if you develop a severe rash accompanied by itching or if you are bothered by persistent itching.

What Your Doctor Will Do

After a careful examination to rule out other disorders, your physician may prescribe a powerful corticosteroid cream to diminish the itching and lubricate the skin.

For More Information

• American Academy of Dermatology

Ear Infection (Middle Ear)

Symptoms

- Congested feeling in the affected ear(s).
- A sharp or sudden pain, or a dull, continuous pain in the ear.
- Muffled hearing or temporary hearing loss.
- Pain when pulling on the earlobe.
- Fever (when bacterial infection is present).
- Discharge from the ear, headache, dizziness, and profound hearing loss are serious symptoms.
- In children: Young children may act extremely irritated and/or cry persistently as well as tug at their ears.

What Is It?

Middle ear infections—technically called otitis media—are the most common cause of earache. They can occur at any age, though they are especially common among children up to age eight. Some children will experience these infections only occasionally, but in other children the infections can be chronic, occurring frequently and/or not clearing up readily.

Symptoms develop when the eustachian tube, which helps drain fluid from the middle ear into the nasal passages, becomes swollen and then blocked. This is often preceded by a cold or other upper respiratory infection. Fluid and pressure build up in the cavity between the eardrum and the inner ear, and the discomfort this causes can range in severity from a mild, dull ache that won't let up to an intense searing pain felt in front of, above, or behind the ear. Typically, the fluid that accumulates in the middle ear allows bacteria and viruses drawn in from the back of the throat to breed and cause infection. Sufferers often experience some temporary hearing loss.

Middle ear infections can afflict one or both ears, and they typically occur in the winter and early spring months, when respiratory tract infections are common.

(For information on the most common infection of the external ear, see Swimmer's Ear on page 458.)

What Causes It?

Viral or bacterial infections of the upper respiratory tract, especially a cold or sore throat, are often the cause of middle ear infections. Some allergies can also cause middle ear infections, as can the abrupt change in altitude when flying.

The fact that the eustachian tube is smaller and more horizontal during early childhood, which helps spread infection from the upper respiratory tract to the middle ear, may be why children are more vulnerable to the infection.

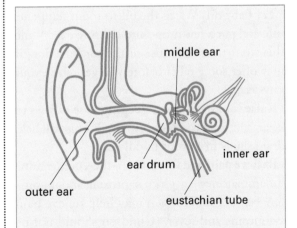

middle ear

inner ear

ear drum

outer ear

eustachian tube

Middle ear infections affect the cavity between the ear drum and the inner ear (where sound waves are converted into nerve impulses). Infections occur when the eustachian tube, which connects the middle ear to the nasal passages, becomes blocked, allowing fluid and pressure to build up.

What If You Do Nothing?

Otitis media can clear up spontaneously within 10 days. Some infections can persist for weeks. Because the pain and discomfort are often too much to bear, treatment by a physician, supplemented by home treatment, is advisable. Also, in some cases an untreated ear infection can worsen to the point where the eardrum becomes inflamed or pressure causes the eardrum to rupture. Hearing loss is another possible complication, though it is usually reversible.

Home Remedies

Whenever you (or a child) develop middle-ear symptoms, these measures can alleviate some of the discomfort. Nonetheless, you should also contact your doctor, since most middle ear infections can be cleared up quickly with medication.

• **Warm the ear.** Hold a heating pad or warm compress to the ear.

• **Try baby oil.** Warm the oil to room temperature and put a few drops into the sore ear. While this won't treat the cause of the ear infection, it may offer some relief before you get to see your physician.

• **Raise your head when sleeping.** Use pillows to keep your head comfortably raised. This will help drain fluids from your middle ear.

• **Relieve pain and fever.** Over-the-counter anti-inflammatories—aspirin, naproxen, and ibuprofen—or acetaminophen may help relieve pain symptoms and fever. (Children should not be given aspirin for fever because of its association with Reye's syndrome.) Nonprescription ear drops may also bring some pain relief.

• **Take an over-the-counter decongestant.** Decongestants can help shrink mucous membranes to open the eustachian tube and relieve middle ear pressure and discomfort. It's impor-

tant to follow warnings and instructions carefully when taking these medications. Some are made for adults and contain ingredients that are harmful when taken by children.

• **Sugarless gum may help.** In a Finnish study, children chewing gum containing xylitol, a sugar substitute, had 40 percent fewer ear infections than those chewing regular gum. But kids in the study had to chew two pieces of gum five times daily—quite a mouthful, even if the child loves gum.

Prevention

It is usually not possible to prevent otitis media. But children who have recurrent infections may be able to take medications to prevent bacterial infections. You can also take steps to prevent ear pain when flying (see page 142.)

When To Call Your Doctor

Contact your doctor if you or your child has symptoms of middle ear infection. Also call your doctor if symptoms have not cleared up after a week.

What Your Doctor Will Do

Your physician will examine the ears, checking for redness and fluid. Once an ear infection has been diagnosed, medications, including prescription nose drops, may be prescribed to help open up the eustachian tubes. Antibiotics may be prescribed to fight infection and reduce the chance of complications. Your physician may also recommend that drainage tubes be inserted into one or both ears to keep the passage open at all times.

For More Information

• American Academy of Otolaryngology-Head and Neck Surgery

Earwax

Symptoms

- Diminution of hearing, with or without pain.
- Pain of varying intensity (sometimes).
- Balance problems (rare).

What Is It?

Cerumen, or earwax, is the yellow-orange substance normally secreted by glands in the outer portion of the ear canal (the tube leading to the eardrum). The main function of wax is to lubricate the canal, protecting the skin from infection and other conditions. The wax can cause serious problems when it's oversecreted and builds up excessively in the ear, or when it's pushed deep into the ear canal. This often "plugs" the ear, leading to discomfort and a feeling of fullness.

What Causes It?

Ordinarily, earwax gradually dries up in small particles and migrates to the outer ear, where it falls out or is washed off. Buildup occurs when the wax inexplicably moves inward instead. Many times, earwax problems are self-induced. Some people use cotton swabs or even bobby pins to clean wax from their ear canal . Such objects can push wax up against the eardrum and temporarily impair hearing. They can also irritate the skin or, far worse, perforate the drum.

What If You Do Nothing?

Serious buildups of wax need to be initially treated by a physician, otherwise pain, hearing, and balance problems may develop.

Home Remedies

• **Clean your ears methodically.** If wax does accumulate, use an eyedropper to put a drop or two of warm (not hot) mineral or vegetable oil in each ear twice a day. (Over-the-counter earwax softeners are generally safe, but are no more effective than mineral oil and occasionally can cause allergic reactions.) Then, using a bulb syringe, flush the ear with warm water, holding your head upright and then turning it sideways to allow the water to drain. (However, if you have a perforated eardrum, never put any liquid in your ear.)

Don't use hydrogen peroxide or any other product that causes fizzing in your ear, since pressure can build up that might injure your eardrum.

Prevention

If you don't have a tendency to produce excess earwax, simply avoid using cotton-tip applicators for cleaning your ears. Instead, clean and dry your outer ears with cotton balls after bathing.

When To Call Your Doctor

If your ear remains blocked because of impacted wax, consult your doctor. Contact your physician if you develop pain, swelling, tenderness, and have persistent hearing loss and milky discharge. These may be signs of an ear infection.

What Your Doctor Will Do

After a careful examination, if an infection has been ruled out, your physician may irrigate your ear and soften the wax for removal. If you regularly develop painful earwax buildups, you may need to schedule regular appointments for wax removal every 6 or 12 months.

For More Information

• American Academy of Otolaryngology-Head and Neck Surgery

Fibromyalgia

Symptoms

- Chronic and widespread musculoskeletal pain and stiffness (often worst in the morning).
- Extreme sensitivity to pressure at multiple specific sites (tender points) on the body.
- Chronic or occasional deep fatigue.
- Unrefreshing, fragmented, non-dreaming sleep.
- Common associated symptoms include tension-type headaches, sensitivity to cold, low-grade depression and anxiety, and abdominal pain.

What Is It?

Fibromyalgia is a poorly understood but increasingly recognized condition characterized by muscle pain and stiffness, troubled sleeping patterns, and fatigue. Most often people with fibromyalgia complain of widespread pain and achiness, similar to symptoms associated with a bad case of flu or with certain forms of arthritis. However, the pain *(algia)* is not in the joints (as it is in arthritis), but in the body's fibrous *(fibro)* ligaments and tendons as well as in the muscles *(my)*.

Most people with fibromyalgia report that some level of pain is present much or all of the time. The severity of pain may vary from day to day, however, and may flare up under certain circumstances, such as sudden physical exertion. Often there is aching and fatigue upon waking up. Depression may also accompany fibromyalgia, but it isn't clear whether depression causes the disorder or is a consequence of it.

According to the American College of Rheumatology, three to six million Americans are affected; other estimates put the figure as high as 10 percent of the general population. Most patients (70 to 90 percent) are women of child-bearing age, but men, children, and the elderly can also be affected.

Fibromyalgia is considered a syndrome rather than a discrete disease, with symptoms that exist on a continuum—much like chronic fatigue syndrome, which has some of the same symptoms. Diagnosing fibromyalgia is further complicated by the fact that its symptoms mimic or overlap those associated with a number of other more established diseases, most especially rheumatoid arthritis, but also osteoarthritis, Lyme disease, sleep apnea, restless leg syndrome, Sjögren's syndrome, and irritable bowel syndrome. Moreover, fibromyalgia does not produce physiological changes that can be detected through conventional diagnostic tools. Blood tests, x-rays, and biopsy tissue samples will all be normal (unless another condition is also present).

In 1990 the American College of Rheumatology developed criteria for diagnosing fibromyalgia that include checking for tenderness that occurs in precise, localized areas, particularly in the neck, spine, shoulders, and hips. The existence of these "tender points" is considered a distinguishing feature.

Nevertheless, because symptoms of the syndrome mimic those of other disorders, and because fibromyalgia often occurs in association with other disorders, arriving at the diagnosis is difficult. Many people who eventually are found to have fibromyalgia have been misdiagnosed by physicians not familiar with the syndrome. And although more and more doctors are informed about fibromyalgia, there continues to be much controversy about how to classify, diagnose, and treat the condition.

What Causes It?

Doctors still don't know what causes fibromyalgia. It was once thought to be an inflammatory condition, but no good evidence of inflammation has been discovered. Because anxiety and depression often accompany it, some experts suggested it was a psychiatric disorder. However, studies have shown that people with fibromyalgia are not any more likely to be depressed than people with arthritis or other chronic painful disorders.

Some cases, researchers think, may be caused by an injury or trauma, possibly affecting the central nervous system. Another theory links fibromyalgia to abnormal patterns of deep sleep, which may affect levels of growth hormone that in turn affect muscle health. The frequency of depression has led some researchers to propose that the mechanisms that trigger depression may be similar to those causing fibromyalgia. Still others suggest that fibromyalgia causes changes in the immune system as if the body is fighting a virus (though no virus or other infectious agent has been identified).

Many experts have come to believe that a number of such factors, rather than a single cause, may contribute to fibromyalgia. As with other chronic disorders such as diabetes or heart disease, a genetic predisposition may also play a role.

What If You Do Nothing?

Fibromyalgia does not appear to progressively worsen over time, it does not damage or deform joints or muscles, nor is it life-threatening. But without treatment, symptoms may become more irritating or new symptoms may develop. In addition, most patients find it increasingly hard psychologically to deal with a frustrating condition that health-care providers and others may regard with skepticism. Once they are accurately diagnosed and treated, most fibromyalgia sufferers have a positive response to self-care measures and

proper medical intervention, though improvement can take months.

Home Remedies

If you have symptoms of fibromyalgia, it's important that you see a doctor to rule out other disorders. Never assume that chronic pain is due to fibromyalgia. If fibromyalgia is diagnosed, you may benefit from medication (see What Your Doctor Will Do), but active self-care plays a critical role in managing the condition.

• **For immediate relief, try heat.** To relieve pain and stiffness, soak in a hot bath or apply a heating pad on low heat. On days you awaken with a lot of discomfort, take a hot shower right away.

• **Use over-the-counter pain relievers sparingly.** Nonprescription NSAIDs such as aspirin and ibuprofen, as well as acetaminophen, may provide limited relief from pain and stiffness (though since there is little or no inflammation, NSAIDs seldom help much). Don't take any OTC drug on a long-term basis without consulting your doctor. Generally, prescription medications are more effective for easing fibromyalgia pain.

• **Get enough sleep.** Interrupted sleep is often a consequence of—and may contribute to—the pain of fibromyalgia. Though medication may be needed to restore normal sleeping patterns, before considering that step, try lifestyle measures. These include maintaining a regular wake/sleep schedule and avoiding heavy meals, alcohol, or caffeine before bedtime. (See page 353 for more detailed recommendations.)

• **Exercise provides real benefits.** Lack of physical activity appears to make symptoms get worse, perhaps because unconditioned muscle are more pain sensitive. Exercise may increase your pain at first, but studies have shown that symptoms improve after six to eight weeks of moderate aerobic exercise such as brisk walking, swimming, or cycling. Stretching and strengthening exercises can also help reduce pain and stiffness, but it's a good idea to develop this kind of exercise program with your doctor or a physical therapist.

• **Be careful not to overdo it.** Start with 5-to-10-minute sessions of low-intensity aerobic exercise and gradually increase your exercise time to 30 or 40 minutes per session. Try to exercise at least three times a week. (See page 31 for more information on aerobic exercise.)

• **Pace yourself each day.** Fatigue and emotional stress can aggravate physical discomfort, so it's important to balance daily activities with periods of rest. Prolonged or repetitive tasks, such as sitting and typing for hours, can also make symptoms worse. You can avoid this by frequently rotating the types of tasks you perform.

• **Get support and information.** Fibromyalgia has received a great deal of attention in recent years, and there are now many books, newsletters, Web sites, and organizations that can help you educate yourself about the condition and also provide psychological support. It can also be helpful to provide family, friends, and co-workers with information in asking for their support.

• **Be skeptical of alternative remedies.** Like other conditions whose chief symptom is chronic pain, fibromyalgia has attracted its share of unproven treatments. Claims are made for vitamin and herbal supplements, dietary regimens, antiviral drugs, and body therapies that have not been scientifically tested. Some of these remedies may be helpful, but many will not. Some can also have adverse effects. If you do try alternative remedies, be sure to tell your physician. And don't substitute unproven treatments for medical care from a knowledgeable practitioner.

• **Be patient.** Dealing with fibromyalgia can have many frustrations—from trying to find a sympathetic physician to day-to-day coping with pain and fatigue. But many people with fibromyalgia can improve how they feel given enough time, effort, and understanding.

Prevention

There is no known way to prevent fibromyalgia.

When To Call Your Doctor

You should see a physician if you experience any symptoms related to fibromyalgia for three months. Call your doctor sooner if pain, sleeping difficulty, depression, or other symptoms interfere with daily activities.

What Your Doctor Will Do

Your doctor should review your symptoms and take a careful history of any other medical problems you've had. Some basic diagnostic tests, including x-rays and blood tests, may be ordered to see if your symptoms are due to another ail-

---

Finding The Right Doctor

▼

If you suspect you have fibromyalgia, it's important to consult a doctor who is experienced at diagnosing and managing the syndrome. If your primary-care doctor isn't knowledgeable, look for a fibromyalgia specialist. This may be a rheumatologist (a physician who specializes in joint diseases) or a physiatrist (a practitioner who specializes in physical medicine and rehabilitation). Some internists and neurologists are also skilled at treating fibromyalgia.

One way to locate a specialist, or to confirm one who's been recommended, is to check with the organizations listed on page 257. You can also check with a local support group and ask for recommendations.

ment with similar symptoms such as rheumatoid arthritis or Lyme disease.

Once other medical conditions have been ruled out, your doctor will evaluate you using a number of diagnostic guidelines. These include applying consistent pressure at specific sites on your body to see whether you have pain at sensitive tender points. Your doctor will also ask you about secondary symptoms, such as headaches, depression, anxiety, and diarrhea or constipation, to see if any are related to fibromyalgia or might signal a coexisting condition.

Your doctor will develop a treatment plan with you. Typically, this will include guidelines for an exercise program and for getting enough sleep, along with therapies (such as heat) to help reduce pain. Depending on the severity of your symptoms, medications may be prescribed to help control pain and improve sleep. If depression is a component of your fibromyalgia, your doctor may prescribe an antidepressant medication and/or recommend that you see a psychologist or other licensed counselor for therapy.

In addition, your doctor may recommend that you see a physical therapist, who can design stretching and strengthening exercises and also treat acute flare-ups of muscle pain. A physical therapist can also advise you about how to best manage work or recreational activities that aggravate symptoms.

Treating fibromyalgia often entails trying a number of strategies to see which one—or which combination—offers the most help. You can also discuss alternative therapies with your doctor. Massage therapy and acupuncture may be effective at helping control pain associated with fibromyalgia. In particular, pinching and lifting the skin and subcutaneous tissue at tender points is often helpful. But any alternative therapy should complement, not replace, the treatment plan your doctor has recommended.

For More Information

- American College of Rheumatology
- American Pain Foundation
- Arthritis Foundation
- Fibromyalgia Network

257

Fifth Disease

Symptoms

In children, fifth disease produces a characteristic rash that progresses through three stages.

■ Initially, a bright red rash develops on both cheeks (as if the cheeks have been slapped). The area around the mouth will look relatively pale.

■ One to four days later, a slightly raised pink rash appears on the upper part of the arms and legs and spreads to the lower limbs and sometimes the trunk. The rash has a lacelike pattern, with some areas of clearing.

■ In the third stage, the rash comes and goes over one to three weeks. The rash may be reactivated by sunlight, trauma, exercise, or exposure to heat (such as a warm bath) or cold.

■ Children may also experience a slight fever, sore throat, and headache.

■ Arthritis and achy joints are common in adults and sometimes in older children, particularly in females. The joint pain may occur without a rash and linger for weeks. Affected joints may include hands, wrists, knees, or ankles. Both sides of the body are usually affected equally.

■ Most adults who get fifth disease develop only a mild rash or have no rash at all.

What Is It?

Fifth disease, so named by turn-of-the-century physicians because it was the fifth most common contagious rash in children, is a mild infection that commonly affects children 5 to 15 years of age, though adults can also get it. Its medical name is erythema infectiosum, and its main feature is a characteristic red rash that begins on the cheeks and spreads to the limbs and trunk. In some instances, however, the rash is so mild it goes unnoticed. In fact, children usually do not feel sick after being infected. Other symptoms, including fever, are unusual, though in some cases the rash is accompanied by headache, sore throat, itching, and mild fever.

For otherwise healthy people, fifth disease doesn't pose a problem. However, children or adults with certain blood disorders—such as leukemia or sickle cell disease—can become quite ill, since the virus causing fifth disease can temporarily suppress the body's production of red blood cells. Individuals with compromised immune systems can also develop complications from fifth disease. In addition, pregnant women who get fifth disease are at risk for miscarriage or fetal damage, usually four to six weeks after becoming infected.

What Causes It?

Fifth disease is caused by a virus called parvovirus B19. The disease is easily spread from one person to another through contact with respiratory droplets, often through coughing, sneezing, or breathing. A child may also rub a runny nose and then infect another person by touching. Outbreaks of the disease are common during the late winter and spring.

The virus typically incubates in the blood for four to 14 days. During this time, the infected person may spread the virus to others, but the virus causes no symptoms until the appearance of the characteristic slapped-cheek rash. Once the rash appears, a person is no longer contagious.

After a bout of fifth disease, a person produces antibodies against the virus that persist for years. Those who have had the disease are generally immune to it for the rest of their lives. Only about 5 to 10 percent of preschool-age children have antibodies against the fifth disease virus. But well over half of adults older than 35 have the antibodies.

What If You Do Nothing?

There is little you can do for a child with fifth disease, except watch and wait for symptoms to subside. The vast majority of cases resolve uneventfully on their own after a week or so. In pregnant women who contract the disease, fewer than 10 percent have any fetal complications. In rare cases, there may be some blood or nervous system complications, particularly in those with blood or immune system disorders.

Home Remedies

Since most children and adults with fifth disease usually feel well, home treatment typically isn't necessary. It's important to watch for fever or any other symptoms in addition to the rash, since these may indicate the presence of another infection (see When to Call Your Doctor).

• **Pain relievers can help.** Adults or older children with joint pains can use over-the-counter pain relievers—either acetaminophen or one of the NSAIDs (aspirin, ibuprofen, naproxen)—for several weeks until the aches subside. Children age 19 and younger should not take aspirin because of the risk of Reye's syndrome, a potentially life-threatening condition.

Prevention

There is little you can do to prevent fifth disease. The illness is highly contagious, and infected persons may harbor and spread the virus for a week or more before the identifying rash appears. Good hygiene, including frequent handwashing, can help decrease the risk of infection.

Once a child is known to have fifth disease, there is generally no reason to restrict the child's activities, since he or she is no longer contagious. However, if possible, try to keep an infected child from coming in close contact with pregnant women or anyone with impaired immunity or blood disorders. Likewise, these people should avoid known outbreaks of fifth disease in schools, hospitals, or other settings.

When To Call Your Doctor

Because the rash from fifth disease can mimic certain rashes caused by drugs, you should consult with your pediatrician about any medications your child is taking.

Also call your doctor if the rash is accompanied by fever, or it spreads to areas such as the palms or soles of the feet, or if you or a child develops other symptoms; it may be an illness other than fifth disease.

If you are pregnant, or if you have a blood or immune system disorder (such as sickle cell disease, thalassemia, anemia, HIV infection), you should call your doctor if you suspect you have contracted fifth disease.

What Your Doctor Will Do

The doctor may test pregnant women to see if they have previously had fifth disease and are therefore immune. Persons at risk for complications from fifth disease may receive an injection of immune-boosting agents, which may confer some protection against the disease. In the rare instance when a fetus is in danger, the fetus may receive an intrauterine blood transfusion.

For More Information

• American Academy of Pediatrics

259

Flatulence

Symptoms

- Passage of intestinal gas from the rectum.
- Abdominal bloating and discomfort.

What Is It?

Flatulence, or intestinal gas expelled through the rectum, is one of the oldest human complaints. The typical adult passes gas 15 to 20 times a day, an amount deemed normal by gastroenterologists. Despite the occasional embarrassment it may cause, flatulence is rarely a symptom of bowel cancer or any other serious disease.

What Causes It?

The offending gases, including carbon dioxide, hydrogen, methane, nitrogen, and sulfur dioxide, are produced when bacteria normally present in the large intestine ferment incompletely digested carbohydrates—which are notoriously present in legumes like beans and lentils, and in cruciferous vegetables like broccoli or brussels sprouts. People who have trouble digesting certain foods, such as those with celiac disease or lactose intolerance, are also potential flatulence sufferers. Gas can also be caused by stress and the nervous habit of frequent swallowing. Carbonation in soft drinks and other beverages is also a trigger.

What If You Do Nothing?

Unless the flatulence is excessive, there is no reason to do anything about it. If it does become excessive, it can usually be reduced with basic changes in daily diet.

Home Remedies

Although it is usually not a serious symptom, flatulence can cause embarrassment and discomfort. Here's how to reduce intestinal gas production.

- **Be aware of foods that cause flatulence.** Foods with the fewest complex carbohydrates cause the fewest flatulent consequences. These include fish, meat, grapes, berries, nuts, and eggs. Foods that are highest in complex carbohydrates and produce excess intestinal gas include certain pink beans, soybeans, cabbage, cauliflower, and Brussels sprouts. In some people, prune juice, milk, and milk products can also produce gas.
- **Gradually increase your fiber intake.** Eating food rich in fiber is one of the best ways to prevent constipation and ensure soft, bulky stools. If you're eating less than the recommended 20 to 30 grams of fiber daily, you need to increase your fiber intake. Be prudent, because introducing too much fiber at once may quickly lead to increased flatulence. Eat moderate amounts of fiber-rich foods at first, gradually increasing your intake over a period of time. If specific fiber-rich foods continue to disturb your system, reduce or eliminate them from your diet.
- **Soak beans before cooking.** Soaking uncooked beans four to five hours or overnight will remove some of the water-soluble carbohydrates that cause gas. You must discard the soaking water and then cook and simmer the beans slowly, then discard the water once again.
- **Chew food thoroughly.** If you gulp it, you swallow harder-to-digest lumps that remain longer in the intestine, where their residue may ferment.
- **Avoid constipation.** When you're constipated, the passage of food through the gastrointestinal tract is slowed, thereby stepping up fermentation. Eat high-fiber foods and drink plenty of fluids.
- **Avoid diet candies containing sorbitol.** Read labels carefully. This artificial sweetener is often used in sugarless gums and candies and can cause or contribute to flatulence and diarrhea.
- **Beano may help.** Beano is a dietary supplement

containing an enzyme that is said to help break down the complex sugars found in high-fiber foods into simple sugars that can be comfortably digested. A few small controlled studies found that it reduces flatulence, but the evidence for its effectiveness is not conclusive and it won't help everyone.

• **Don't expect relief from other over-the-counter remedies.** Antifoaming agents (such as simethicone), found in some "antacid-antigas" preparations, merely change large gas bubbles into smaller ones—hardly a remedy for flatulence. Bulk-forming laxatives can actually promote the kind of fermented residues that cause the problem in the first place. As for products containing "activated charcoal," there's little or no evidence that—contrary to what they claim—they can actually absorb gas in humans; they can, however, interfere with the absorption of birth-control pills and other drugs.

Prevention

Use the home remedies described above to avoid excessive flatulence.

When To Call Your Doctor

Although sometimes embarrassing, flatulence is generally not a medical problem. Contact your physician if you suddenly develop intestinal gas accompanied by abdominal bloating or diarrhea that lasts for a few days. This could be a sign of irritable bowel syndrome. Persistent and severe flatulence may also be a symptom of gallbladder problems, inflammation of the intestines such as ileitis or colitis, or cancer that affects the colon and intestinal tract. Also contact your physician if the self-care remedies suggested on the previous pages don't work and you have questions or concerns.

What Your Doctor Will Do

After a physical examination and detailed history to rule out any serious ailment, your physician may recommend diagnostic tests if some digestive disorder is suspected. No treatment is necessary if there is not a gastrointestinal disorder. Your doctor will probably recommend a low-flatulence diet. There are measures you should adopt if lactose intolerance is discovered (see page 369).

261

For More Information

• American Gastroenterological Association
• Intestinal Disease Foundation

Floaters and Flashes

Symptoms

- **Floaters:** jagged specks, little lines, spider webs, or circles floating in your field of vision.
- **Flashes:** Flashing, flickering, brilliant streaks of light in your line of vision.

A dramatic onset of floaters and flashes, a sudden wavy, watery quality in vision, or a sudden, partial loss of vision are symptoms of a detached retina, an emergency that requires immediate treatment (see box at right).

What Is It?

Floaters are spots or lines that drift across your eyeball from time to time—and they are generally nothing to worry about. Called entoptic phenomena, they are sloughed-off retinal cells floating in the vitreous—the jellylike substance that fills much of your eyeball. From time to time floaters may be bothersome when you're reading or if they happen to appear directly in your line of vision. In rare instances floaters can be a warning sign of a detached retina—a condition that requires immediate medical attention.

Between the ages of 40 and 60, flashes of light will randomly appear in the line of vision for no apparent reason. People who get hit in the eye may also notice streaks of light, claiming that they have seen stars.

What Causes It?

Floaters tend to appear when you tilt your head or suddenly glance up or down, causing cellular debris to cross the center of the retina.

The causes of flashes are spontaneous and linked directly to the aging process. The gel inside the eye starts to liquefy and peel off from the retina. The tugging and pulling that goes on causes the retina to be stimulated, and the ensu-ing flashing lightning streaks and stars may continue on and off for several weeks until a layer of gel is stripped away.

The brilliant streaks of light people notice after getting hit in the eye have nothing to do with stars but are caused by the mechanical stimulation of the retina, the light-sensing inner layer of the eye.

What If You Do Nothing?

Most floaters are quite benign, not a cause for alarm, and will move away very quickly.

Over 90 percent of the time flashes of light in the field of vision are a benign event related to aging and not associated with anything that produces long-term problems. However, if you are struck in the eye and see stars, do not casually

---

Detached Retina: An Emergency

▼

Flashing lights, a sudden onset of floaters, or a rapid increase in them (especially if they are confined to one eye or appear in large clumps), blurry vision, or the disappearance of part of your visual field may indicate that your retina has, or is about to become, detached from your eye.

A detached retina is a tear or dislocation of the eye's back layer of light-sensitive cells and nerve endings. This can be caused by a severe blow, but it is more commonly the result of a shrinking of the vitreous inside the eyeball, which may occur with aging. Severe shortsightedness is a risk factor, as is diabetes. Retinal detachment also occurs in about 3 percent of people who have undergone cataract surgery.

It is essential to seek treatment immediately, since a detached retina can cause complete loss of vision. Go to the nearest emergency room or ophthalmologist. Many treatments are now available, including laser or surgical repair, that can successfully correct early retinal detachments in 90 percent of cases.

dismiss the incident but go immediately to an ophthalmologist for an eye exam to make sure your retina was not damaged in the accident.

Home Remedies

For floaters, try looking up and down several times. This movement within the eye will often cause the floaters to disappear.

There is no home treatment for flashes.

Prevention

Nothing can be done to stop the progressive liquefaction of the vitreous gel inside the eye and the resulting floaters. There is no way to prevent flashes.

When To Call Your Doctor

If you experience a sudden shower of floaters or flashes, including floaters that accompany a blow to the eye, you may have a detached retina and should seek immediate medical help (see box on page 262).

What Your Doctor Will Do

An ophthalmologist will perform an eye exam and use special diagnostic tools—including fluorescein angiography (which allows photographic images to be taken of the eye's blood vessels)—to assess the condition and determine which surgical procedure may be necessary.

For More Information

• American Academy of Ophthalmology

Flu

Symptoms

Within 72 hours of exposure to a flu virus, the following symptoms develop.

- Rapid onset of moderate to high fever, between 101°F and 103°F, that lasts for three to five days.
- Dry cough.
- Sore throat.
- Runny nose.
- Headache.
- Joint pain.
- Chills.
- Stuffy nose.
- Burning sensation in the eyes.
- Loss of appetite.

What Is It?

Influenza, more commonly known as flu, is a viral infection of the nose, throat, and lungs that infects many Americans each winter. It's virtually impossible to tell the difference between a mild flu and a cold. But although flu is considered a respiratory ailment, it generally affects the whole body, with symptoms ranging from sore throat and dry cough to fever, body aches, and burning eyes. The accompanying fever rises quickly, often to 103°F or higher, and stays there for several days. Even after the fever has subsided, physical exhaustion may last for days afterward.

Flu viruses are highly contagious and they also mutate frequently, so that new variations, or strains, can emerge or spread to a new location every year. Epidemics occur about every four years, and about every decade a flu virus strain appears that is so different from others that a pandemic—a worldwide epidemic—soon follows. Flu viruses are often given names based on their place of assumed origin, for example, the Beijing flu.

Having the flu once does not confer lasting immunity as it does with some childhood viral diseases. The antibodies produced in response to one flu virus don't provide immunity to a different flu virus that may occur the next year.

Most outbreaks of flu in the United States occur between October and May, with the peak months falling between late December and early March. (In the Southern Hemisphere, flu season occurs from April to September—though in some tropical areas it lasts all year.)

Most of the millions of Americans who contract flu each year may feel extremely uncomfortable while they have it, but they recover within 10 days or so without further problems. However, the virus can lead to further, sometimes serious, complications, including bronchitis. If the flu spreads from the upper respiratory tract and bronchi to the lungs, secondary bacterial pneumonia can develop. Those at greatest risk for these problems—which can sometimes cause a bout of the flu to be fatal—are the elderly, pregnant women, cancer patients, people with heart disease or respiratory illness, those with diabetes, and those with compromised immune systems.

What Causes It?

You usually catch the flu by being in close proximity to an infected person, who expels droplets containing flu viruses during coughing or sneezing bouts. The droplets travel through the air and can be inhaled by others. You can also catch flu from direct contact—touching hands or kissing—with someone who is infectious, and the viruses can even live for hours in dried mucus that may have been left on objects touched by a flu-infected person's unwashed hands.

What If You Do Nothing?

Flu is a self-limiting ailment, generally not dangerous, and will normally clear by itself within 10 days or less—though weakness and fatigue can persist for several weeks or longer. However, if you are in a high-risk group and develop flu, you should be aware of possible complications and consider contacting your physician.

Home Remedies

Flu is a viral infection and antibiotics are ineffective against it. You can help lessen its symptoms at home with the following measures.

• **Stay in bed.** Bed rest is important to help your body battle the flu, so stay there until your temperature returns to normal and you no longer have body aches and pains.

• **Drink plenty of fluids.** Fluids prevent dehydration and keep the protective mucous lining of the respiratory system moist so it can fight off the virus. It doesn't matter if the fluid is hot or cold as long as you drink at least eight glasses a day.

• **Be judicious in lowering your temperature.** A fever of up to 102°F acts as an antiviral agent, so don't take acetaminophen or ibuprofen to lower your fever if it's in this range. However, if your fever is 103°F or higher, take two acetaminophen or ibuprofen every four hours. (Aspirin should not be taken by anyone age 19 or younger because of its association with Reye's syndrome, a rare but fast-progressing and often fatal disorder that can be triggered by aspirin.)

• **Use a cough suppressant.** A flu infection generally causes a dry, hacking cough, which is unproductive and does not speed recovery. In

---

Everyone Should Get a Flu Shot

The most effective tool for fighting a flu virus is immunization with a special vaccine made of inactivated or fragmented flu virus. Because the viruses are inactivated, you cannot get influenza from the vaccine. Instead, a vaccinated person's immune system responds by forming antibodies that can fight the active virus.

Since it takes one to two months after being vaccinated to build up sufficient antibodies, mid-October to mid-November is the best time to get your flu inoculation—well before the start of the annual late-December flu season. Flu vaccine contains the flu viruses expected to cause illness that year, so new batches must be created at the start of each flu season.

The U. S. Public Health Service now recommends annual flu shots for everyone age 50 or older, instead of age 65.

People in the following groups are considered at high risk for serious complications from flu, and so should be vaccinated, no matter what their age: those with lung disease (asthma, emphysema, chronic bronchitis, tuberculosis, or cystic fibrosis), heart disease, chronic kidney disease, diabetes, severe anemia, HIV infection, or certain other chronic disorders.

People who are likely to be exposed to influenza infections, such as health-care workers, hospital workers, and police officers, should also consider annual vaccinations.

Even younger, healthy people can benefit from the flu shot and should consider getting it. If you are pregnant, however, consult your doctor before getting inoculated.

People allergic to eggs should consult their doctors about flu shots. The inactivated viruses used in flu vaccine are grown on egg embryos, and though these undergo a purification process, some egg protein may be carried over—enough that it may trigger reactions such as hives, allergic asthma, difficulty breathing, and other symptoms.

addition to causing a sore throat, coughing can spread the virus into the lungs. Choose an over-the-counter cough suppressant product that contains dextromethorphan. This medication inhibits coughing by affecting the cough reflex in the brain.

Copious amounts of green, yellow, or blood-tinged mucus indicate a possible bacterial infection. Stop all cough suppressants and contact your physician.

• **Wash your hands frequently.** This will help prevent spreading germs to others.

Prevention

• **Get a flu vaccination in the fall.** An annual vaccination is the number-one method of flu prevention, and it is now recommended for all adults 50 or older, as well as for certain other people considered at high risk (see page 265).

• **Avoid unnecessary contact with people who have the flu.** The flu virus is highly communicable and can be transmitted by a kiss, grasping a doorknob, or inhaling the virus from a sneeze or cough.

When To Call Your Doctor

You should call your doctor if you don't feel better after the fifth day of your flu, or if you begin to feel better but then suffer a relapse.

What Your Doctor Will Do

Once your doctor diagnoses your condition as the flu, you may be able to benefit from antiviral medications. There are four medications that can be used to treat as well as prevent flu. Two of them, amantadine and rimantadine, work only against the influenza A strains, not the B strains, so they are not meant to be a substitute for a shot of flu vaccine. But they can be used preventively for people who have not been vaccinated or who don't respond to flu vaccine. When given as a treatment within the first 48 hours of the onset of flu symptoms, these drugs can reduce the severity and duration of influenza A.

Two newer, more expensive drugs, zanamivir (Relenza), which is a nasal spray, and oseltamivir (Tamiflu), are effective against both influenza A and B viruses. These drugs are approved only for treatment of flu, not as a preventive measure. Like amantadine and rimantadine, they must be used within two days of the onset of symptoms and can provide relief and shorten the duration of flu, but are not an immediate cure.

For More Information

• Centers for Disease Control and Prevention
• National Institute of Allergy and Infectious Diseases

Food Poisoning

Symptoms

The onset of symptoms can occur anywhere from one hour to seven days after eating contaminated food, depending on the infectious agent.

■ Diarrhea (the most common symptom).

■ Abdominal pain and cramps).

■ Nausea and vomiting (sometimes severe).

■ Fever (may not be present).

■ Headaches (may not be present).

■ Bloody stool (may not be present).

Another sign of food poisoning is that people who have eaten the same food(s) all become ill.

What Is It?

Food poisoning is any illness caused by foodborne bacteria, parasites, viruses, or chemicals. Every home, and every person, is host to a variety of bacteria that can cause serious illness if they get into food and multiply. You can get mild food poisoning without realizing it. When people come down with a "bug" accompanied by symptoms such as headache and stomach distress, it's often dismissed as "stomach flu" or "24-hour virus"—but it may be food poisoning. And some types of microbes can cause severe illness that can be fatal in the elderly, in children, in people with certain disorders (such as diabetes), and in people whose immune systems are depressed, such as cancer patients. The Centers for Disease Control and Prevention (CDC) estimates that 76 million cases of food poisoning occur each year. Most go unreported since they are mild and last for only a day or two. But more than 300,000 cases are serious enough to require hospitalization, and an estimated 5,000 deaths each year are related to foodborne infections.

What Causes It?

Food poisoning is primarily caused by a number of different bacteria and some viruses, with bacteria being responsible for the majority of cases. Just about every type of food—unless it has been sterilized—has bacteria in or on it, but most of them are harmless. In addition, bacteria can be introduced into foods from external sources. For example, fresh fruits and vegetables can become contaminated if they are washed or irrigated with water that contains animal manure or sewage. Contaminants can also be introduced during food processing by food handlers who are infected.

The mere presence of bacteria or viruses in food isn't enough to make you sick. They cause problems only when the food is improperly handled and prepared. Bacteria begin to multiply quickly in food left at room temperature and thrive on food that is kept warm on a stove. Moist foods, such as stuffing or cooked rice, are especially susceptible to bacterial growth. Refrigeration retards the growth of bacteria, and cooking at high temperature kills most of them. But if food has been left out long enough, some types of bacteria can form a toxin that will survive heat or freezing.

The bacterium *Salmonella* is by far the most frequent cause of foodborne illness, and it is rapidly becoming more prevalent. The CDC estimates that poisoning by *Salmonella*, called salmonellosis, accounts for several million cases annually—though only about 35,000 cases are actually reported. That's because many individuals and even doctors mistake salmonellosis for "intestinal flu." The increase in salmonellosis has been attributed principally to high-speed mechanical methods of slaughtering and eviscerating animals, especially poultry. According to a variety of estimates, at least half of all raw chicken marketed is contaminated by *Salmonella* and/or *Campylobacter jejuni*, another bacterium that causes diarrhea, fever, and abdominal cramps,

Cutting Boards: Plastic vs. Wood

Common sense might tell you that plastic cutting boards would be less subject to bacterial contamination than wooden ones. The fact is that both types of boards are likely to spread bacteria that can cause food poisoning if they're not kept clean.

Whether you use wood or plastic for cutting raw meat and poultry, scrub the board well afterward with hot soapy water (and don't forget to wash the knife and your hands thoroughly as well). If the surface has fat on it, or if the plastic is deeply scarred, it's especially important to get it very clean. Plastic cutting boards can also be cleaned in the dishwasher.

There is no advantage to using a board impregnated with disinfectant, because you must still wash it thoroughly.

and which may cause blood in the stool. *Campylobacter* has been implicated in millions of cases of food poisoning.

Any animal may harbor *Salmonella*. Raw eggs, too, can be a source. But in these cases poor handling may not be the only cause. Researchers suggest that the bacteria can come from inside the hen and are in the raw egg itself, rather than getting there by the usual route of cracked or dirty eggshells. While raw or soft-cooked eggs—or foods made with them, such as eggnog or Caesar salad—are potentially risky, commercial products made with eggs, such as mayonnaise, are safe because the eggs have been pasteurized.

Each year an estimated 25,000 cases of food poisoning are attributed to *E. coli* 0157:H7, a particularly dangerous strain of *E. coli*—a bacteria widely present in fecal matter—that can spread to humans when they consume food or water contaminated with microscopic amounts of cow feces. Most cases are associated with undercooked, contaminated ground beef, but cases have

also occurred from many other sources, including people eating unpasteurized apple juice and apple cider made from fallen apples contaminated with manure.

Fish and shellfish are another common source of food poisoning, particularly when they are eaten raw. Any fish or shellfish, no matter how fresh, may carry some bacteria and viruses—and animals from sewage-polluted waters may carry large doses of them. Certain shellfish—clams, oysters, mussels—live by filtering water, and if the water they inhabit is polluted, they will retain bacteria and viruses along with the microscopic foodstuff they absorb. Raw shellfish can thus be a source of hepatitis, gastroenteritis, and other diseases. Raw fish, as used in sushi and sashimi, may be a source of parasites such as tapeworms and roundworms, as well as bacteria and viruses.

Other causes of food poisoning are shown in the chart on pages 270-271.

What If You Do Nothing?

Most cases of food poisoning are not serious and recovery usually occurs within three days without any medical care. However, the disease can be fatal if the treatment of a serious food poisoning case is delayed. Symptoms to be concerned about include the following.

• bloody diarrhea or pus in the stool (possible *Campylobacter* or *Shigella* infection).

• headache, stiff neck, and fever (possible *Listeria monocytogenes* infection).

• rapid heart rate or dizziness after standing up suddenly, when accompanied by vomiting, nausea, or diarrhea (possible dehydration).

• tingling in the arms and legs, sometimes around the mouth, blurred vision, weakness, or numbness (possible botulism poisoning).

Home Remedies

• **Get in bed and keep warm.** Resting enhances recovery. Make sure you have easy access to a bedpan or bathroom.

• **Drink plenty of fluids.** Diarrhea and vomiting function to clear the toxins out of your system, but they can result in a substantial loss of body fluids. To prevent dehydration from developing, drink six to eight ounces of clear fluids per hour throughout the day. These can include water, tea with sugar, bouillon, or any of the commercially prepared sports drinks. If vomiting continues and you can't keep anything down, try to take small sips or suck on ice chips. (See page 241 for managing dehydration in children.)

For children: Have a child with food poisoning drink five ounces of clear liquids per hour; infants should drink at least one ounce per hour.

• **Apply heat.** If you have stomach pain or cramps you may get some relief by placing a heating pad (on the low setting) or a hot water bottle on your abdomen.

• **Reintroduce foods gradually.** After your symptoms diminish, gradually reintroduce soft and easily digested foods such as cooked cereal, bananas, rice, applesauce, toast, potatoes, eggs, and noodles. Once the diarrhea has stopped and your appetite increases, you can return to your normal diet.

• **Avoid milk and milk-based products for several days after diarrhea has subsided.** This will allow the enzymes in the small intestine—needed to handle the lactose contained in milk and milk-based products—to be replenished.

Prevention

You can take a number of simple measures to prevent food contamination and reduce your risk of getting sick from tainted food.

• **Keep your refrigerator below 40°F and the freezer below zero.** Check them periodically with a thermometer, especially in the summer months. If needed, adjust the temperature-control dial.

• **Always refrigerate raw meat or poultry immediately.** Once it's in the refrigerator, however, don't keep it for more than two or three days.

• **Don't leave food sitting in a hot car.**

• **Wash your hands thoroughly before and after you handle food.** The proper way is to use soap and warm water for at least 20 seconds, working

Botulism: Rare but Dangerous

Botulism is caused by potent toxins produced by the spore-forming bacterium *Clostridium botulinum,* which is common in soil. Any food that is contaminated by soil and is subsequently carelessly washed or mishandled may be a source of botulism. However, this microbe produces poisons only at temperatures above 38°F and under certain conditions—notably an almost complete lack of oxygen—and so is quite rare.

Canned goods are a potential source of botulism. Modern commercial canning methods have gone far toward eliminating botulism from canned foods, but outbreaks still occur as a result of home canning. Though contamination usually causes cans to swell, the absence of swelling does not guarantee safety. Other warning signs in a can's contents are gas bubbles, discoloration, and milky liquids that normally should be clear.

Even if the spores are present, toxins won't be produced unless food is left at room temperature for at least 12 to 24 hours and under relatively airless conditions—for example, a tight wrap or a coating of fat. The spores can be destroyed only by moist heat at 248°F under pressure (in a pressure cooker, for instance) for 30 minutes, but the toxin will be inactivated if the food is brought to the boiling point (212°F) for 10 minutes.

269

Types of Food Poisoning

DISEASE/ORGANISM	SOURCES OF INFECTION	SYMPTOMS	WHEN SYMPTOMS BEGIN
Campylobacteriosis (*Campylobacter jejuni*)	Food can become contaminated during processing of meat and poultry. Sources of infection include raw or undercooked beef and poultry and raw milk. Can also be present in untreated water and in shellfish.	Fever, diarrhea, abdominal cramps, and bloody stool.	2 to 5 days
Botulism (*Clostridium botulinum*)	Improperly processed, low-acid canned goods (usually home-canned products), such as green beans; foods contaminated by soil and then left in an oxygen-free environment, such as potatoes coated with oil or butter, at room temperature.	Nervous system affected: double vision, problems swallowing, trouble breathing. Can be fatal.	8 to 36 hours
Perfringens food poisoning (*Clostridium perfringens*)	Grows rapidly in large portions of food that are cooling slowly or at room temperature. Can grow in any dish made with meat or poultry as well.	Abdominal pain and diarrhea. Sometimes nausea and vomiting. Symptoms are usually mild, but can be more severe in the ill and the elderly.	8 to 24 hours
Salmonellosis (*Salmonella*)	Raw or undercooked beef and poultry or foods contaminated by coming into contact with them. Raw or undercooked eggs or products made with them. Food handlers with poor hygiene.	Nausea, vomiting, abdominal cramps, fever. Can be fatal in infants, the elderly, and individuals with depressed immune systems.	12 to 48 hours
Shigellosis (*Shigella*)	Food can become infected by a food handler with poor hygiene and can cause illness if the food is not cooked properly. Multiplies when food is kept at room temperature for long periods.	Abdominal cramps and pain, nausea, vomiting, diarrhea, bloody stool, fever. Can be serious in infants, the elderly, and those with depressed immune systems.	1 to 7 days

DISEASE/ORGANISM	SOURCES OF INFECTION	SYMPTOMS	WHEN SYMPTOMS BEGIN
Staphylococcal food poisoning *(Staphylococcus aureus)*	Food that has been coughed or sneezed on or otherwise handled in an unsanitary manner. Staph is present on the skin, around pimples and boils, and thus can be introduced into foods by a food handler with a skin infection. It is particularly common in foods that require a lot of handling, such as tuna or potato salad. Multiplies rapidly at room temperature.	Nausea, vomiting, abdominal cramps, diarrhea.	1 to 8 hours
Cholera *(Vibrio cholera)*	Fish and shellfish from waters infected with sewage.	Diarrhea and abdominal pain. Can be mild or severe. Cholera can be fatal.	1 to 3 days
Parahaemolyticus food poisoning *(Vibrio para-haemolyticus)*	Fish and shellfish. Proliferates in warm weather.	Abdominal pain, diarrhea, nausea, fever, headaches, chills, bloody stool.	15 to 24 hours
Gastroenteritis *(E. coli,* some enteroviruses, rotaviruses, and Norwalk virus)	Viruses present in human intestine. Can be passed on by food handlers with poor hygiene. Also in shellfish from waters contaminated with sewage.	Vomiting, nausea, diarrhea.	12 to 48 hours
Infectious Hepatitis (Hepatitis A)	Can be passed on by a food handler who has the disease. Also in shellfish from contaminated waters.	Fatigue, jaundice, nausea. Can cause liver damage. Can be fatal.	15 to 50 days

the soap into the hands, including the fingernail area and between the fingers.

• **Use a fresh dish towel every time you cook.**

• **Defrost frozen foods in the refrigerator, in the microwave, or under cold running water.** You can defrost at room temperature, but only if you monitor the food carefully and cook it as soon as it has thawed. Use a microwave only if you plan to cook the food right away or re-refrigerate it until cooking time.

• **Wash thoroughly.** After preparing raw meat or poultry, wash the utensils, counter, cutting board, and your hands—anything that touched the food—thoroughly in hot soapy water before making a salad or handling vegetables.

• **Marinate meats and poultry only under refrigeration.** And don't put cooked meat back into an uncooked marinade or serve the used marinade as a sauce unless you heat it to a rolling boil for several minutes.

• **Be aware of cooking temperatures for meats.** An internal temperature of 160° should kill all bacteria in red meat. Rare roast beef or steak (140°) carries some risk, though healthy people may wish to take the risk occasionally. Ground beef should never be eaten rare. Because trichinosis in hogs is now extremely rare, the USDA recommends that pork can be cooked to 160° (instead of 170°, or "well-done"). This leaves the meat juicy and with traces of pink. Chicken should be thoroughly cooked—not pink at all. Whole chicken should be cooked to 180°.

• **Be careful at barbecues.** Don't serve barbecued meat on the same plate you used for the raw meat and don't use the cooking utensils for serving.

• **Avoid uncooked meats.** Whether at home or eating out, pass up the steak tartare and any other uncooked meat.

• **Take special care if you eat sushi.** Eating any

272

Microwaving Microbes

▼

While microwave ovens cook foods quickly and tend to destroy fewer vitamins than conventional cooking methods, they also may heat foods unevenly and leave some parts undercooked. This leaves open the possibility that bacteria may survive cooking. To be sure that your microwaved food doesn't cause food poisoning, follow these guidelines:

• To be sure that foods cook evenly, rotate all foods at various intervals during cooking.

• Check the internal temperature of meat and poultry to be sure that they are cooked all the way through.

• Wrap plastic made to be used in microwave ovens around the dish, or cover it with glass or ceramic. The trapped steam will help decrease evaporation and will heat the surface. Prick a hole in the plastic wrap to vent steam. The plastic wrap shouldn't touch the food.

• Allow microwaved food to stand covered after cooking. Heat concentrated on the inside will radiate outward through the food, cooking the exterior and equalizing the temperature throughout. Food will taste better this way, too, since it will be consistently hot.

• Thaw meats before cooking in a microwave oven; most models have defrost settings for this purpose. Ice crystals in frozen foods are not heated well by microwaves and can leave cold spots.

• If you're used to conventional cooking, remember that the more food you're microwaving, the longer it will take. For example, four baked potatoes will take much longer than two.

---

kind of raw seafood is risky. However, well-trained sushi chefs know how to purchase, examine, and prepare fish so as to minimize the risk of illness and parasitic infection. There is also little risk of parasites with most tuna species, including yellowtail, sold in the United States. Avoid raw freshwater fish (such as brook trout), which carry a high risk of parasites. Don't prepare sushi at home—home-prepared raw fish is the most common source of parasitic infection from fish—and don't risk eating sushi or other raw fish if you are in frail health or are pregnant. Foodborne illness could be dangerous to you.

• **Avoid raw shellfish.** The risk of illness from raw clams or oysters is simply too high. If you can't resist, at least make sure that the shellfish is fresh and has been prepared by an experienced chef.

• **Don't leave normally refrigerated foods sitting out.** Hold foods at room temperature no longer than an hour before or after cooking. Given the right conditions, the bacterial content in some foods can double in 20 minutes.

• **Promptly refrigerate leftovers**—particularly anything with a coating (bread or fat) or a tight wrapping. Divide large amounts of leftovers—such as sauces, soups, stews, and casseroles—into smaller containers so that they cool faster. Throw away any questionable leftovers.

• **Store all starchy stuffing (rice, bread) separately from the poultry in which it was cooked.**

• **Be careful canning.** If you can fruits and vegetables at home, ask your county health depart-ment for guidelines about safe procedures to protect against botulism.

• **Be prudent.** Pass up all food that smells or looks spoiled. Don't buy or use any food in bulging, rusty, or leaky cans.

• **Inspect the salad bar.** Make sure food is protected by a sneeze guard. Cold foods should be kept well chilled, and hot items should be steaming hot.

• **Use only pasteurized milk and products made from pasteurized milk.**

• **Keep pets away from food preparation areas.**

When To Call Your Doctor

Contact your physician immediately if you develop any of the following: sudden and severe diarrhea, bloody diarrhea, severe abdominal pain, or a fever of 100°F or higher.

Certain people need medical attention if they develop mild symptoms of food poisoning. These include the elderly, young children, heavy antacid users, pregnant women, people with diabetes, alcoholics, or anyone with a weakened immune system. These people are at greater risk of life-threatening complications.

Also contact your physician if symptoms of mild food poisoning don't subside in a week.

What Your Doctor Will Do

After taking a personal history, your physician will try to identify the source of the food poisoning. Laboratory cultures of vomit, feces, and blood may be taken. Suspected foods will also be examined for contaminants. If you have botulism, you will be given a prescription medication. If you have severe vomiting and diarrhea, you may be given medication to stop them.

For More Information

• Centers for Disease Control and Prevention

Frozen Shoulder

Symptoms

- A slow onset of shoulder pain and stiffness. The pain is generally dull but becomes sharp with movement. It may become so severe that it limits your ability to use your shoulder and interferes with sleep.
- Over time, as shoulder motion becomes limited and the shoulder becomes stiffer, pain diminishes, creating a vicious cycle: shoulder stiffness prevents normal movement, while reduced movement increases stiffness.

What Is It?

The shoulder, which is the most flexible joint in the body, is akin to an engine—don't use it for awhile and chances are it won't start up as quickly and function as smoothly as the last time. Similarly, if you avoid using the shoulder (because of tendinitis or bursitis pain, an injury to your arm, or a general feeling of stiffness and discomfort), you risk developing adhesions—constricting bands of tissue—in the shoulder joint capsule that will severely limit your shoulder's natural range of motion. As a result, even brushing your hair or putting on a shirt can become a painful, if not impossible, task. This condition is known as adhesive capsulitis, or more familiarly as frozen shoulder.

Since it doesn't get as much use, the shoulder that is opposite the favored hand—usually the left shoulder in right-handed people—is the one most often affected.

What Causes It?

Although underuse of the shoulder is the most evident reason for frozen shoulder, researchers are still uncertain about the exact cause. Sometimes trauma to the shoulder may bring about the condition, but many cases occur for no apparent reason.

A minor injury such as bursitis can initially cause frozen shoulder, with the subsequent lack of use causing adhesions to form within 7 to 10 days, making movement increasingly difficult. After three to four weeks of disuse, the adhesions can become so severe that movement is seriously restricted in the shoulder joint, making a simple motion, such as raising your arm, extremely painful.

What If You Do Nothing?

The longer you continue to neglect a frozen shoulder, the greater the possibility of developing a permanent shoulder disability. Prompt action is recommended to restore a normal range of motion to the shoulder.

Home Remedies

If you develop shoulder pain, start the following measures right away to prevent adhesions from forming. For any persistent pain, however, you should get medical advice.

- **Try heat or cold.** Depending on which works best for you for pain relief, try a hot compress or heating pad for 15 minutes several times daily, or else apply an ice pack to the shoulder for 15 minutes, several times daily.
- **Take anti-inflammatory medication.** For minor pain, take aspirin, ibuprofen, or naproxen according to label directions.
- **Support the shoulder.** Using a sling may help ease your discomfort.

Prevention

- **Stretch and strengthen.** Performing an exercise routine that helps maintain overall shoulder strength and flexibility will help prevent frozen shoulder. The exercises on page 426 for rotator cuff tendinitis can help get you started (though you should discuss them with your doctor first).

When To Call Your Doctor

Contact your physician if you have symptoms of a frozen shoulder or if you have persistent shoulder pain or stiffness that won't clear up.

What Your Doctor Will Do

After taking a medical history, your doctor will examine your shoulder for range of motion, stiffness, and pain. You may also be asked to undergo magnetic resonance imaging (MRI), a diagnostic test that provides a far more detailed picture of the shoulder than a conventional x-ray.

Depending on the severity of the case, your physician may prescribe anti-inflammatory medications or inject cortisone into the joint to reduce inflammation and pain. He or she may also recommend therapy and exercises. In more advanced cases your physician may recommend a procedure to manipulate the shoulder under general anesthesia and break up the adhesions.

For More Information

- American Academy of Orthopaedic Surgeons
- National Institute of Arthritis and Musculoskeletal and Skin Diseases Information Clearinghouse

275

Ganglion Cyst

Symptoms

- A round lump—which can be soft or hard—
  under the skin, often on the back of the wrist.
- Usually painless, but sometimes pain and tenderness are present.

What Is It?

Though it may look peculiar and even worrisome,
a ganglion is a benign cyst that forms under the
skin and attaches to a tendon sheath or a joint,
usually on the back of the wrist but also on the
top of the foot.

Each of your movable joints is enclosed within
a fibrous capsule that has an inner lining known
as the synovium, which also forms a sheath for
certain tendons. Ganglia (plural) are formed when
a thick, jellylike fluid secreted by the synovium—
a fluid that normally lubricates a joint or tendon—accumulates around the joint or tendon
instead of being reabsorbed by the body. As the
fluid accumulates, the area balloons out.

The cysts are typically pea-size but can grow
as large as a golf ball.

What Causes It?

Although the cysts can form after trauma to a
tendon or joint, the cause is unknown.

What If You Do Nothing?

A ganglion cyst is harmless and often disappears
without treatment. If your cyst does not go away
and its appearance disturbs you, or if it becomes
painful or limits your range of motion, you may
want to consider removal.

Home Remedies

There are no home remedies for ganglia. Removing a ganglion should be left to a doctor.

Prevention

There are no known ways to prevent ganglia.

When To Call Your Doctor

To rule out a tumor, contact your physician when
you notice a lump anywhere on your body. Also
contact your doctor if the cyst becomes unsightly
or painful.

What Your Doctor Will Do

After a careful examination, your physician may
remove the built-up fluid with a needle or recommend surgery to remove the cyst. Ganglia frequently recur, however.

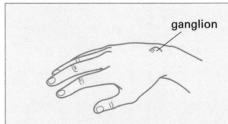

ganglion

A ganglion is a lump just under the skin that
usually appears on the back of the wrist.

Gastritis

Symptoms

- Abdominal discomfort or pain under the rib cage.
- Nausea, occasionally with vomiting, that may last 24 to 48 hours.
- Loss of appetite.
- Swollen abdomen.
- Vomiting blood (infrequent, but requires immediate attention).

What Is It?

Gastritis is a general medical term for any mild irritation, inflammation, or infection of the stomach lining. Acute gastritis occurs as a sudden attack that can last from a few hours to a few days. Chronic gastritis, which is fairly common among the elderly, can occur over a long period and may produce similar symptoms or only mild discomfort, along with loss of appetite and nausea.

What Causes It?

Gastritis has many causes. Infection with *Helicobacter pylori,* the bacterium that causes most ulcers, is the most common cause of acute gastritis. The condition can also be triggered by any substances that irritate the stomach lining. These include anti-inflammatory drugs, such as ibuprofen, aspirin, and arthritis medications, particularly when these drugs are used over the long term. Many other prescription and over-the-counter medications may also irritate the stomach lining, as can tobacco smoke, alcohol, and foods that you have trouble digesting.

Gastritis may also be caused by stress and anxiety, which trigger stomach acid production.

Chronic gastritis can be caused by prolonged irritation of the stomach by alcohol, smoking tobacco, and medications; by bile and other acids that back up into the stomach; by pernicious anemia, an autoimmune disorder that can damage the stomach lining; and by degeneration of the stomach lining with age.

What If You Do Nothing?

Mild cases of acute gastritis are often self-limiting and will clear up within two days. However, any instances of severe acute gastritis or chronic gastritis should receive medical attention.

Home Remedies

Most cases of mild gastritis respond well to the following self-care measures within 48 hours.

- **Don't eat.** Fast for 24 hours after the gastritis attack begins; you should drink water and nonalcoholic beverages. The next day, begin to eat small meals consisting of bland foods like rice, toast, cooked vegetables, and applesauce, which shouldn't irritate your stomach.
- **Avoid all products that contain anti-inflammatory drugs.** Pain relief medications or other products (such as some cold remedies) that contain aspirin, ibuprofen, naproxen, or other so-called NSAIDs can be harsh on your stomach.
- **Take nonprescription antacids or acetaminophen for stomach pain.** Follow your doctor's orders or the label directions.
- **Stop smoking and abstain from alcohol and caffeine for as long as you have symptoms.**

Prevention

- **Know your medications.** If you must take a medication that ends up irritating your stomach, ask your physician about taking an enteric form. Enteric pills have a special coating that allows them to pass undissolved directly from your stomach to your small intestine. In some instances this may help prevent gastritis symptoms.

277

• **Keep a food diary.** Certain spicy, fatty, or fried foods may trigger your gastritis. Cut back or eliminate them from your diet.

• **Eat frequent, small meals.** This may help reduce any excessive acid buildup in the stomach.

• **Quit smoking; reduce or eliminate alcohol intake.** These are two common causes of both acute and chronic gastritis.

• **Try to minimize stress.** If stress is a cause of your gastritis, try to figure out what is causing the stress in your life and what changes you can make to reduce it.

When To Call Your Doctor

Most cases of gastritis are mild and require no attention. However, contact your physician if abdominal pains accompanied by fever or nausea persist and do not respond to self-care measures within 24 hours, or if there is any blood in your vomit.

Contact your physician immediately if stomach pain becomes severe.

What Your Doctor Will Do

Your physician may order tests to confirm the gastritis diagnosis. Prescription antacids may be recommended. If smoking or alcohol consumption is the cause, you will be urged to quit. Your doctor may also check for *Helicobacter pylori* infection and, if it is present, prescribe a course of antibiotics. For persistent cases, an endoscopy may be performed for confirmation.

For More Information

• American Gastroenterological Association
• Intestinal Disease Foundation
• National Digestive Diseases Information Clearinghouse

Gastroenteritis

Symptoms

Gastroenteritis symptoms will vary according to the cause and the gastrointestinal area that's affected and may include one or more of the following.

- Nausea, vomiting.
- Loss of appetite.
- Diarrhea.
- Abdominal pain or cramps.
- Fever.

What Is It?

Gastroenteritis is a generic medical term for a self-limiting irritation or infection of the stomach, small intestine and/or colon that typically leads to sudden and often violent gastrointestinal upset. It may be identified as traveler's diarrhea, stomach flu, food poisoning, or intestinal flu. After the common cold, gastroenteritis is the second most common cause of work absenteeism among adults and a major cause of sickness and mortality among young children.

What Causes It?

Gastroenteritis has a number of causes, but specific causes are often unknown or uncertain at best. Bacterial infections are a major cause of traveler's diarrhea. Food poisoning, caused by food-borne bacteria and viruses, can cause serious illness.

The disorder may also be caused by a sudden change in the normal bacterial state of your gastrointestinal tract owing to an illness, the use of antibiotics, or a trip to a foreign country.

What If You Do Nothing?

Gastroenteritis is typically self-limiting, and the associated diarrhea, nausea, vomiting, and abdominal cramping will generally clear within 48 hours. More severe cases must be treated by a physician.

Home Remedies

You can treat mild gastroenteritis with the following self-care measures. (However, if you are taking an antibiotic, call your doctor. The medication may be causing your symptoms.)

Children and Gastroenteritis

▼

Infants and very young children are at special risk if they contract gastroenteritis because of the speed with which dehydration often develops. Once the water, salts, and nutrients used by the cells drop below optimal levels, the condition may rapidly become life-threatening, especially for infants under six months of age.

Contact your physician immediately if your child complains of abdominal pain that persists for a half hour or longer or if the child's stool is flecked or streaked with blood.

Also contact your physician immediately if dehydration is suspected. Signs of dehydration include one or more of the following: skin that is dry, cool, and pale; abnormal thirst; dry tongue; listlessness; rapid pulse; and, in infants, a sunken and soft fontanelle, the space between the bones on the top of the infant's skull.

Your physician might suggest that, for a bottle-fed infant, you substitute an electrolyte replacement drink (available at supermarkets and pharmacies) for 24 hours to boost fluid levels. On the second day, dilute the baby's formula to half the normal strength; two-thirds strength on day three; and three-quarters strength on day four. Give the baby the normal volume, but in small amounts every hour or so. You can resume normal feedings on the fifth day.

For breast-fed infants, resume normal feeding within 12 to 24 hours after using the electrolyte solution.

• **Rest.** Get plenty of bed rest until your major symptoms have cleared.

• **Drink to replace lost fluids.** To prevent dehydration from diarrhea or vomiting, drink clear fluids—tea, de-fizzed ginger ale, or lemon-lime soda—throughout the day. For fluid replacement, drink sports beverages (for adults) or commercially prepared electrolyte-sugar solutions (for infants and children) throughout the day as well. If you are unable to keep any fluids down, take very small sips or try sucking on ice chips.

• **Eat a BRAT diet.** A mild bland diet consisting of bananas, rice, applesauce and toast is recommended on the second day of the illness and for the following two days after all symptoms have disappeared.

Prevention

Gastroenteritis may be communicable, so you should take the following preventive measures to avoid it or keep it from spreading.

• **Practice good hygiene.** To avoid germs that cause gastroenteritis, wash your hands frequently throughout the day, especially after going to the bathroom.

• **Don't share.** Use your own eating utensils and dishes and store them separately.

• **Use travel sense.** To avoid traveler's diarrhea when traveling in underdeveloped countries, don't eat fresh fruits and vegetables and uncooked foods. Don't drink unbottled water or beverages.

• **Be careful with food preparation and storage.** You can take a number of simple steps to prevent food contamination and reduce your risk of getting sick from tainted food (see page 269).

When To Call Your Doctor

Most people recover from a mild attack of gastroenteritis within 48 hours without any special medical treatment. However, contact your physician if the symptoms are severe, persist longer than two days, fever is 100°F or higher, or there are signs of dehydration, including excessive thirst, dry mouth, or confusion.

What Your Doctor Will Do

Your physician will take a complete medical history and then examine you. If gastroenteritis is severe, with repeated vomiting, diarrhea, and cramps, medication to stop these symptoms may be prescribed.

If a child or an elderly or debilitated person shows severe symptoms, or if anyone is severely dehydrated, hospitalization may be recommended in order to replace the lost fluids intravenously. For patients who have recently traveled to underdeveloped countries or the tropics, a stool sample may be examined for the presence of organisms causing dysentery.

For More Information

• American Gastroenterological Association
• Center for Disease Control and Prevention
• Intestinal Disease Foundation
• National Digestive Diseases Information Clearinghouse

Genital Herpes

Symptoms

- Within 7-21 days after exposure, flulike symptoms—muscle aches, swollen glands, fever, and sometimes shooting pains in the legs or abdomen.
- Painful blisters and sores on genitals, occasionally accompanied by blisters and sores around the mouth.
- In women, painful urination.

Symptoms subside without treatment, but sores recur at unpredictable intervals in about two-thirds of the cases.

What Is It?

Genital herpes is a contagious viral infection of the genitals that's transmitted through vaginal intercourse as well as through oral or anal sex. An estimated 45 million people in the United States are infected with the virus, and experts estimate that a many as 500,000 new cases may occur each year. Once a person is infected, the virus establishes itself permanently in the nerve cells, staying dormant for months or years.

Many people who become infected are asymptomatic. In about one-third of those who develop clinical symptoms, permanent remission occurs after the initial attack, most likely due to the ability of the body's immune system to contain the virus. The remaining two-thirds of people with symptoms will suffer additional outbreaks at unpredictable intervals. The first outbreak, which can last from one to three weeks, is usually the most severe. The subsequent outbreaks become less severe over time, though the frequency and severity of recurrent episodes vary greatly from person to person.

Genital herpes is highly contagious, and transmission can occur with or without the presence of visible sores. In most cases the virus is more easily transmitted from male to female partners. Pregnant mothers must be especially careful since herpes is readily transmitted during childbirth and can result in severe health problems for the baby.

What Causes It?

The most common cause of genital herpes is the herpes simplex virus, or HSV. There are two types of virus, and genital herpes is usually caused by HSV Type 2, though Type 1—the same virus that causes cold sores—can also produce sores in the genital area. In fact, both viruses can infect either area, causing roughly the same symptoms. Both viruses are transmitted through direct contact, including kissing, sexual contact (vaginal, oral, or anal sex), or skin-to-skin contact.

After remission, herpes may recur again and again. The triggers for subsequent outbreaks are not clearly understood, but may include sexual intercourse, sunlight, stress, fatigue, and extremes of heat and cold. People with a weakened immune system (including those with AIDS) are at risk for severe outbreaks of genital herpes.

What If You Do Nothing?

Genital herpes is incurable; once you are infected, the virus remains dormant in your body and symptoms may reappear. The level of discomfort will vary from person to person, but symptoms can be lessened with treatment. If you have recurrent herpes, refrain from sexual contact when you have sores, since you are certainly contagious during this period.

Home Remedies

Although genital herpes cannot be cured, the following measures can be taken to help lessen the discomfort. (However, when symptoms occur, be sure to contact your doctor for evaluation and diagnosis.)

• **Relieve the pain.** Take over-the-counter pain relievers—either NSAIDs (aspirin, ibuprofen, or naproxen) or acetaminophen, according to label directions. Also, frequent warm baths and warm compresses may bring temporary relief.

• **Avoid discomfort during urination.** To prevent urine from irritating any vaginal sores, women can urinate in the shower or through a tube, such as a toilet-paper roll.

• **Avoid tight-fitting garments.** Snug underwear and pants may irritate the genitals.

Prevention

• **Be careful about sexual contact.** If either partner has a blister or sore, avoid sexual intercourse. Abstain from oral sex if you or your partner has a cold sore on the mouth.

• **Use a condom.** If either sex partner has inactive genital herpes, use a latex condom during intercourse. Remember, though, that a condom may not cover all infected areas.

• **If you are infected and pregnant, tell your physician, so precautions can be taken to prevent passing the virus to the baby.** You can be monitored for a herpes outbreak during your pregnancy and at the time of delivery, if necessary, undergo a cesarian section to prevent the baby from being infected during delivery through an infected birth canal.

When To Call Your Doctor

Contact your physician if you have any symptoms of genital herpes. Also contact your doctor if you've started treatment but your symptoms don't improve within seven days, or if a fever returns during treatment.

What Your Doctor Will Do

Because the symptoms associated with herpes can vary, your doctor will carefully examine you and may also order a lab culture taken from an active sore to confirm the presence of the herpes virus. (A negative result from these tests does not mean that the virus isn't present, however; the virus is notoriously hard to pinpoint.)

The disease does not respond to usual antibiotics. Acyclovir (Zovirax), a prescription antiviral medication available in ointment or capsule form, is not a cure but can ease symptoms and may reduce the length of an attack. The capsules are more effective than the topical preparation. If taken continually, this drug usually prevents or decreases the incidence of recurrences. Two other drugs, famciclovir (Famvir) and valacyclovir (Valtrex), have been approved specifically for treating recurrences.

For More Information

Herpes support groups may be helpful in combating depression and other emotional problems that sometimes result from the disease. For links to support groups and other information, contact the following:

• American Social Health Association
• CDC National Prevention Information Network
• CDC National STD and AIDS Hotline

Genital Warts

Symptoms

- Local irritation and itching, followed by soft, flat, irregularly surfaced growths that appear around the anus, on the cervix, inside the vagina, on the shaft and tip of the penis, or in the urethra, as well as in the mouth and throat. The warts may increase in size and number.
- Warts may also be barely visible, small, flat elevations of skin that otherwise cause no symptoms.
- Some warts are so small they cannot be seen by the naked eye.

What Is It?

The virus that causes genital warts is the most common sexually transmitted infection in the United States. As many as 24 million Americans may be infected, and the frequency of infection appears to be increasing. One study suggests that nearly 40 percent of college-age women have these warts on the cervix. The growths appear on, in, and around the genitals anywhere from one to eight months after a person has been infected by the human papilloma virus (HPV).

The virus is highly contagious, spreading by sexual or other intimate bodily contact, and a person can be infected with the virus and spread it even though no warts are visible. HPV occurs among all ages and all classes, though it is most prevalent among young people and the poor.

The warts, which may have no obvious symptoms, are benign, but some strains of HPV are believed to be precursors of genital cancers, notably of the cervix and possibly the penis. Most women with cervical cancer are infected with HPV, but only a relatively small proportion of HPV-infected women eventually develop a related cancer. Of the more than 70 types of HPV that have been identified, only two or three are known to be commonly linked to cancer.

What Causes It?

HPV is the same virus that causes warts on the hands, feet, and face. Genital warts, however, are passed from person to person through sexual activity, and they spread more easily than other types of warts. Scientists attribute the increase in genital wart cases in part to changes in sexual behavior (namely, sexual activity starting at an earlier age and/or with multiple partners) in recent decades.

What If You Do Nothing?

The warts themselves are benign, and if left untreated, they may disappear on their own. They are more likely to grow larger and more numerous, however, and treatment is necessary to prevent further growth and reinfection.

Home Remedies

Drugstore remedies for most warts are useless and may be harmful. Such remedies should never be used with genital warts. It's generally recommended that genital warts be removed surgically or chemically as soon as possible (see When To Call Your Doctor). However, the virus may remain dormant for years, so the warts can be hard to eradicate. Even after warts have been removed, an infected person may still be able to transmit the virus, and the warts often recur.

Prevention

Apart from abstinence, the most reliable preventive is long-term monogamy with a monogamous partner. If you're healthy and have a long-term monogamous relationship with a healthy partner, you're at no risk. But if you have not had a long-standing monogamous relationship, always take the following measures.

• **Check your partner.** If you notice any wartlike bumps on or around the genitals of a sexual partner, ask that he or she seek medical attention.

• **Always use a latex condom.** It will not offer complete protection against genital warts, but it will significantly reduce the degree of contagion.

• **Women should get Pap tests.** Early identification of HPV is important in identifying women at high risk for cervical cancer. Once diagnosed with HPV infection, a woman must have annual Pap smears (for the early detection of cervical cancer) as recommended for the rest of her life.

• **Make sure your partner is examined and treated.** It's important that both partners in a sexual relationship receive care if one of them has genital warts. If both partners are infected but only one is treated, then reinfection may occur.

When To Call Your Doctor

Contact your physician immediately if you suspect you have genital warts.

What Your Doctor Will Do

A close examination will be undertaken. Small warts often cannot be seen by the naked eye, so your doctor will use a special magnifying instrument called a colposcope to closely examine the cervix. Men may be checked for warts in the bladder or urethra.

No standard treatment for genital warts exists; you must be evaluated and treated individually based on the extent of the infected area. A number of treatments have been used with varying success, including surgically removing the warts, removing them by freezing, using a laser to vaporize the warts, or using chemicals to burn them off. Two prescription creams for treating genital warts, imiquimod (Aldara) and podofilox (Condylox), are also available, and your doctor may prescribe one of these.

For More Information

• American Social Health Association
• CDC National Prevention Information Network
• CDC National STD and AIDS Hotline

Giardiasis

Symptoms

The following symptoms may occur (though about two-thirds of infected people have no symptoms):

- Mild to severe diarrhea that is foul-smelling (rotten-egg odor) and frequent (2 to 10 stools a day). Diarrhea may last one or more weeks, accompanied by one or more of the following: fatigue, abdominal pain, cramps, gas, bloating, or swelling. (Diarrhea from giardiasis is not associated with fever or blood in the stool.)
- Loss of appetite and possible weight loss.

What Is It?

Giardiasis, an intestinal infection of the small bowel caused by the microscopic parasite *Giardia lamblia*, is the most common parasitic infection in the United States. Most commonly, the parasite passes from the feces of an infected person or animal into a food or water supply and is then ingested. The parasite can also pass from one person to another through oral-genital sexual contact and, more rarely, by hand contact. The parasites then colonize in the small intestine. Symptoms usually appear within one to two weeks after exposure, but may take as long as 25 days—so you may have trouble pinpointing exactly when you became infected.

What Causes It?

Most infections stem from ingesting fecally contaminated water or the fecal-oral transfer of the *Giardia lamblia* from an infected person. Giardia infection occurs worldwide and is most common in developing countries or areas where sanitation and hygiene are substandard.

In the United States it also turns up among campers and hikers who have drunk unpurified water from streams contaminated by animal and human feces. Up to 80 percent of all water in the wild contains this protozoan, according to the Environmental Protection Agency (EPA). But the most common sites of infection are daycare centers and preschools, which now account for about half of the giardiasis cases. In many centers children's soiled diapers harbor millions of the parasites, and both staff and children risk becoming infected after diaper changes if they don't carefully wash their hands.

You can also get giardiasis from food poisoning (caused by someone who is infected handling food without washing his hands). And pets can become infected and then spread the parasite to humans.

What If You Do Nothing?

Giardiasis with mild diarrhea typically clears up by itself without any treatment—usually within one to four weeks. However, in some cases, if left untreated, symptoms become chronic and recur intermittently. With proper medical treatment, recovery is complete.

Home Remedies

There are no effective home remedies to treat giardiasis. It is usually treated with prescription medication—typically metronidazole (Flagyl) for adults and furazolidone (Furoxone) for children. No alcohol can be consumed while taking metronidazole and it shouldn't be taken pregnancy.

Prevention

• **Wash your hands carefully after toilet visits.** Wash thoroughly and often, throughout the day, to avoid catching the infection from other people. Pay special attention to the fingernails, which can harbor the parasite. If you have young children who attend preschool or daycare centers, giardia

285

infection is one more reason to wash your hands well after handling soiled diapers or underwear.

• **Boil water gathered outdoors.** When you are camping or hiking, no matter how crystal clear and safe water from a stream, pond, river, or lake may seem, boil any water for three minutes before drinking it. If in doubt, carry your own bottled water or use an appropriate water filter.

• **In developing countries, don't drink from the tap.** If you are traveling in developing areas of Latin America, Asia, or Africa, or if you are in any location where conditions seem unsanitary, drink only bottled water, carbonated drinks, or drinks you open yourself. Don't brush your teeth or wash dishes with any water that hasn't been bottled or boiled. Also, don't add ice cubes to drinks.

• **Wash your food.** When traveling in developing countries, be sure to peel all raw fruits and vegetables before eating them in case the foods have been rinsed in contaminated water or handled by an infected person.

When To Call Your Doctor

Contact your physician if you have symptoms of giardiasis. Be aware that many physicians are unfamiliar with this condition. The infection may be misdiagnosed as gallbladder inflammation, irritable bowel syndrome, or a peptic ulcer.

What Your Doctor Will Do

A doctor familiar with the disorder will ascertain if you have traveled or have been camping within the past few weeks, or if you work or have children in a daycare center. A laboratory stool test will be ordered to detect the presence of *Giardia lamblia*. The skill of the lab technician is important, and the test may need to be repeated as many as three times over a two-week period if early studies are negative, since many of the tests are false-negative (negative even though you may have the infection).

A newer test, an antigen detection test, also produces many false negatives, but yields false-positives only rarely. It is also cheaper than previous tests and consequently has become the diagnostic tool of choice.

Because the likelihood of false-negatives is high with any test, your physician may still prescribe antiparasitic medications even if your test results are negative, basing the decision on your history and symptoms. The drugs are extremely effective, though they have a wide range of side effects.

For More Information

• Centers for Disease Control and Prevention

Gingivitis (Gum Disease)

Symptoms

- Gum swelling, tenderness, and redness. Gums may bleed easily during brushing.
- Chronic bad breath; a bad taste in the mouth.

What Is It?

Gingivitis is the medical name for gum (gingiva) inflammation. The ailment is usually caused by an acid generated by bacteria in the mouth. These bacteria live in a thin, sticky film, known as plaque, that coats the surfaces of teeth and the tongue, and they act mainly on certain carbohydrates in foods. Plaque eventually hardens into tartar, a hard mineral shell that forms around the gum line and erodes healthy gum tissue.

If you ignore proper dental care, gingivitis can quickly lead to a more serious dental problem, periodontitis (also called pyorrhea). Periodontal disease isn't painful in itself, but it is the leading cause of tooth loss in adults. In advanced periodontal disease, gums recede and pockets form under the gum line, where bacteria move in and erode the supporting bone that anchors the teeth. Gingivitis is the earliest stage of periodontal disease, and the only one that can be halted and even reversed with proper dental care.

What Causes It?

About one-third of the population is thought to have a genetic susceptibility to gum disease, and there is now a test available to detect this. But even if your test is negative, you can still develop gum disease and still need to take the same care of your teeth. A number of lifestyle factors also promote gingivitis. The most common one is improper or poor oral hygiene. A poor diet, especially a diet high in sugar, is a factor, as is smoking, since the chemicals in tobacco smoke have harmful effects on the gums and teeth.

Hormonal changes, particularly in women, can adversely affect the gums. Oral contraceptives may increase susceptibility to gum disease, and women may also find themselves more prone to gingivitis during puberty, pregnancy, menstruation, and menopause.

Because saliva helps wash away sugars as well as bacterial toxins, anything that decreases saliva production—which includes certain medications—can make gum disease worse.

Diabetes, HIV infection and AIDS, and other chronic diseases lower resistance to infection and can also play a role; the chronically ill need to be particularly careful about dental care.

New Treatment: Topical Antibiotics

▼

Using topical antibiotics—applied directly to the gums—is a new and promising treatment for gum disease, and your dentist may suggest it. But it is recommended only for people whose periodontal disease has not responded to conventional therapy or has recurred.

There are a number of ways to apply antibiotics directly to the gums: with floss-like cords impregnated with medication, with gels, or with liquids applied to periodontal pockets (the areas below the gumline that are most difficult to treat). Several studies have found that antibiotics can help, but no more so than scaling and planing the teeth (to remove tartar) as an initial treatment. That is, conventional treatments, including meticulous care at home, should precede the use of antibiotics.

If you are using topical antibiotics, you should be seeing your dentist frequently for scaling and planing. Topical antibiotics sidestep the potential adverse effects of antibiotics that you swallow. However, the treatment is not recommended for pregnant women, children, or in some cases people with compromised immune systems.

What If You Do Nothing?

Though gingivitis affects only your gums, ignoring it may lead to more serious dental problems, including eventual tooth loss. If the condition worsens, you may develop chronic bad breath and more bleeding. With severe periodontal disease, teeth may loosen, and you may notice gums pulling away from teeth.

Home Remedies

Once you discover symptoms of gingivitis, you should consult your dentist to determine the cause and extent of gum disease. In addition to whatever treatment your dentist recommends, good oral hygiene is crucial in halting or reversing the problem. Here are the basic points of gum care, which are described in more detail on pages 52-54.

• **Brush your teeth regularly.** Using a soft nylon-bristle toothbrush, brush at least twice daily. You can use a circular brushing motion or a straight, downward one. But to focus on the gum line, a back-and-forth scrub may be needed. Brushing teeth too vigorously may lead to an erosion of the gums and, eventually, sensitive teeth.

• **Brush your tongue.** It collects the same amount of bacteria that stick to your teeth.

• **Floss teeth and gums.** Each time you brush your teeth, be sure to floss afterward. Using a gentle sawing motion, ease the floss between the teeth, forming a crescent against one side of a tooth. Use your thumbs and index fingers to stabilize the floss. Lightly scrape up and down the tooth, from just under the gum line to the chewing surface.

• **Consider home dental devices.** Consult your dentist about an ultrasound toothbrush, a plaque removal device such as Interplak or Sonicare, or an irrigation device such as Water Pik.

Prevention

Good oral hygiene—most important, daily brushing and flossing—is the best way to protect against gingivitis. In addition, be sure to have regular dental checkups.

When To Call Your Doctor

Contact your dentist if you develop symptoms of gingivitis.

What Your Doctor Will Do

Following a detailed oral examination, your dentist will determine the extent of gum disease. Depending upon the stage of periodontal disease, you may need a prescription mouth rinse, oral irrigation with an antibiotic solution, general antibiotic treatments, more thorough removal of tartar under the gum line, or surgery. Your regular dentist will probably refer you to a periodontist. A wide range of treatments, including the use of topical antibiotics, is now available.

For More Information

• American Dental Association
• American Academy of Periodontology

Glaucoma

Symptoms

- Symptomless in early stages.
- In open-angle glaucoma, loss of peripheral vision, marked by blind spots; usually affects both eyes.
- In closed-angle glaucoma, sudden attacks that involve pain in one eye; blurring of vision; a halo effect around objects; a cloudy cornea; redness of the eye; and possibly nausea and vomiting.

Anyone with symptoms of closed-angle glaucoma should immediately seek medical help, since glaucoma of this type can quickly damage the optic nerve.

What Is It?

Glaucoma is a disease of the eyes marked by increased pressure within the eyeball that can ultimately damage the optic nerve. It currently affects about two million Americans. Glaucoma cannot be prevented, but it can be treated and sometimes cured by surgery or laser techniques. If it is caught early, glaucoma need not result in blindness.

Open-angle glaucoma, the most common type (accounting for 90 percent of all cases), produces almost no symptoms in its early stages; its earliest sign is a painless increase in eyeball pressure, which can only be measured by an eye-care specialist. Side or peripheral vision may be affected, but only gradually.

A rarer type—closed-angle glaucoma—typically manifests itself as a sudden attack. This form of glaucoma is sometimes mistaken for an upset stomach, since in addition to severe eye pain and reduced vision there may be nausea and vomiting. But in fact, closed-angle glaucoma is a medical emergency that should be treated immediately.

What Causes It?

The cause of open-angle glaucoma appears to be an increase in intraocular pressure (IOP)—that is, pressure within the eyeball. This rise in pressure may be due to a blockage of a spongelike network of connective tissue surrounding the lens. If the network becomes clogged, there is an excessive buildup of the aqueous humor—the clear fluid inside the eye that supplies nutrients and carries waste products away from the lens and cornea (which have no blood supply).

But researchers now know that there is more to glaucoma than IOP. Some people have IOP within the normal range and yet have glaucoma; others have high IOP and don't have the disease and won't go on to develop it. It's true, though, that high IOP is an important risk factor for developing glaucoma; if your pressure is above

> ### Who Should Be Tested?
>
> ▼
>
> There are no hard-and-fast recommendations about who should be tested for glaucoma and how often. When you see an optometrist or ophthalmologist, you'll usually get an eye-pressure test, as well as the test for peripheral vision and an exam of the optic nerve. Both the American Academy of Ophthalmology and the American Optometric Association recommend eye exams, including glaucoma tests, for all adults every three to five years, beginning at age 39.
>
> You may need screening more frequently if you are 65 or older, an African-American over 40, severely nearsighted, have diabetes, or are taking certain blood pressure medications or cortisone. Follow the advice of your eye-care professional about frequency of screenings.
>
> A family history of glaucoma is also a risk factor. And if you have been diagnosed with sleep apnea, you should also be tested for glaucoma.

normal, you need to be checked often.

Several suspected (but still theoretical) causes of glaucoma are insufficient blood supply to the optic nerve, low blood pressure, and sleep apnea.

Some people are at higher risk than others for developing glaucoma,

- anyone with a family history of the disease,
- African-Americans,
- the severely nearsighted,
- anyone with diabetes,
- anyone over age 65 (up to 3 percent of whom may have the disease),
- anyone taking certain blood pressure medications or cortisone.

Closed-angle glaucoma is caused by a sudden blockage near the iris that prevents aqueous humor from reaching the connective tissue, resulting in a rapid, extremely sharp rise in intraocular pressure that can cause permanent vision loss within a day or two.

What If You Do Nothing?

Glaucoma will worsen if not treated, and may lead to blindness through damage to the optic nerve. Early detection and treatment can help prevent or limit vision loss.

Home Remedies

Glaucoma requires diagnosis and treatment by a vision specialist.

Prevention

There is no way known to prevent glaucoma. But you can prevent or reduce the vision damage caused by glaucoma by getting tested and obtaining appropriate treatment if you have glaucoma.

When To Call Your Doctor

Studies have shown that a combination of screening procedures is more likely to uncover early glaucoma than the simple hand-held tonometer used by many primary-care physicians. Accurate screening for glaucoma is best done by an ophthalmologist or optometrist, and all adults should see one of these eye-care professionals for an exam, which should include testing for glaucoma.

What Your Doctor Will Do

An ophthalmologist can use a diagnostic procedure called tonometry to measure pressure within the eye. Other tests for glaucoma include dilating the pupil for a complete look inside the eye and carrying out measurements to detect subtle losses of peripheral vision.

Medications to reduce glaucoma come in pill or eyedrop form. These drugs are effective in preserving vision and must be taken for life. In some cases laser and surgical techniques may be helpful.

For More Information

- American Academy of Ophthalmology
- Glaucoma Research Foundation

290

Gonorrhea

Symptoms

- Painful urination.
- Green-yellow vaginal or penile discharge.
- Sore throat (if contracted through oral sex).
- Rectal pain or discharge (if contracted through anal sex).

What Is It?

Gonorrhea is a contagious bacterial infection that's been known since ancient times. It's estimated that 650,000 people are infected with gonorrhea annually in the United States. Following a 13-year decline in the number of cases reported to the Centers for Disease Control and Prevention (CDC), the rate of infection increased in 1998 and again in 1999, when 360,000 cases were reported. One reason for the increase may be that gonorrhea is becoming resistant to a wider variety of antibiotics used to treat it.

You can have gonorrhea without any obvious symptoms, especially if you're a woman. If any symptoms are noticeable, they generally occur within 2 to 10 days of infection. Gonorrhea is spread by direct contact with infected mucous membranes in the genitals, mouth, and throat. In women, the bacteria typically infect the cervix (the opening of the uterus), which becomes tender to the touch and inflamed. In about 15 percent of infected women, the infection travels to the fallopian tubes.

Men are usually infected first in the urethra, the tube that urine and sperm pass through.

What Causes It?

Gonorrhea is caused by a bacterium, *Neisseria gonorrhoeae,* that can grow rapidly in the body's mucous membranes. The infection is spread by sexual contact (vaginal, anal, oral). A baby can contract gonorrhea from an infected pregnant mother during childbirth, which may cause the infant to go blind unless promptly treated.

What If You Do Nothing?

Gonorrhea may be both chronic and progressive. If left untreated, it can result in arthritis, skin sores, and heart or brain infection. In women, the disease can cause pelvic inflammatory disease (PID), which can cause chronic pelvic pain and may also damage fallopian tubes, leading to ectopic pregnancy (potentially fatal to the mother). In men, gonorrhea can affect the prostate and also lead to scarring inside the urethra, making urination difficult. Gonorrhea can also cause permanent sterility in both women and men, and it can facilitate the transmission of HIV, the virus that causes AIDS. Infants born to infected mothers are at risk of becoming blind unless treated.

Home Remedies

Gonorrhea cannot be accurately diagnosed and treated without professional help. There are no home remedies, so see a doctor or another health-care professional if you get infected or think you might be infected. You should abstain from sexual intercourse until your physician is sure the infection is completely cured.

Prevention

- **Know your partner.** Get to know your sex partner before becoming intimate. Avoid anyone whose health status is questionable.
- **Use a condom.** Latex condoms effectively prevent the spread of gonorrhea.
- **Observe good hygiene.** Wash your genitals with soap and water before and after sexual contact.
- **Detect it early.** If you notice any symptoms, avoid sexual contact and see your physician or

other health-care provider immediately. Also notify all of your recent sex partners so that they can get tested and receive treatment, if necessary.

• **Get tested routinely if you are at high risk.** Individuals at high risk include young women (under the age of 25) who have had two or more sex partners within the past year and both men and women with a history of repeated episodes of gonorrhea. Also, be sure to get tested if you become pregnant and have had multiple sex partners.

When To Call Your Doctor

Contact your physician immediately if you have any symptoms of gonorrhea listed above or if you find that a sex partner has gonorrhea.

What Your Doctor Will Do

Following a thorough examination, your physician will diagnose the ailment with a smear or culture taken from the site of exposure, or with a nonculture blood test, specifically a DNA probe or an enzyme immunoassay (EIA).

The usual antibiotics, when taken as prescribed, can cure most cases of gonorrhea. Some strains of the bacterium are resistant to standard antibiotics and so newer medications must be used. Be sure to tell your doctor if your infection may have been acquired in Hawaii, the Pacific Islands, or Asia, where problems with resistance have been increasing recently (but are not confined to these areas).

For More Information
• American Social Health Association
• CDC National Prevention Information Network
• CDC National STD and AIDS Hotline

Groin Strain

Symptoms

- A sudden sharp pain in the upper inner thigh, typically after a quick, explosive movement or overexertion.
- Extreme tenderness in the area of the strain.
- Increase in pain and stiffness with movement or continued activity. In severe cases walking may be painful enough to warrant the use of crutches for several days.

What Is It?

Injuries to the adductor muscles—from microscopic ruptures to a major tear—are commonly called groin pulls or groin strains, even though the groin, technically an area at the junction between the abdomen and thigh, is usually not affected by this injury.

The adductors are five muscles that start at the top of the thigh at the pubic bone and extend along the inner thigh to the inside of the knee. These muscles act to pull your legs in toward each other, so that you can straddle a horse or perform a frog kick while swimming. These same muscles also stabilize the leg when you are running or moving from side to side, help you kick sideways in soccer and karate, and cut quickly in racquet sports and basketball.

What Causes It?

The adductor muscles may be strained when you make a quick turn, or anytime you're involved in explosive running, jumping, twisting, or kicking actions. Running on a slippery surface like wet grass can also result in a groin strain.

What If You Do Nothing?

A minor groin strain will heal itself within a few days. However, groin muscle pulls are not only painful but they tend to recur. Exercises to strengthen and stretch the inner thigh muscles can help safeguard against this.

Home Remedies

- **Stop the activity.** As soon as you feel pain in the inner thigh, stop exercising.
- **Apply ice.** Massage the sore spot with ice for 10 minutes and repeat four times daily for the next two to three days.
- **Support the muscle.** Wrap the injured thigh with an elastic support bandage.
- **Try over-the-counter NSAIDs for pain relief.** Nonprescription NSAIDs—aspirin, ibuprofen, and naproxen—may be taken according to label directions to relieve pain and also counteract inflammation.
- **Rehabilitate the muscles.** A groin strain can become a nagging, recurrent injury unless proper rehabilitation and strengthening are carried out. Rehabilitation can last from two weeks to as long as two years, depending upon your age, previous adductor injury, and previous injury to the area. Begin with the exercises that are described below.

Prevention

The best precaution against groin-muscle pulls is to make sure you are properly warmed up before beginning any exercise routine. Combining the following two strengthening exercises with some gentle stretching will also provide protective benefits. Don't do these exercises, though, until you are free of pain.

- **Butterfly stretch.** Sit down on the floor with your back straight and knees bent. Place the soles of your feet together and pull the ankles inward toward your crotch. Resting your elbows on the insides of your knees, lean forward from the waist so your elbows push your knees toward the floor.

Hold the stretch for 20 seconds and repeat 3 to 5 times.

• **Hurdler stretch.** Stand with the healthy leg bent at the knee, toes pointed forward. Stretch the injured leg straight out behind, flexing the foot so the toes point forward. Let your pelvis drop toward the floor as you bend the knee of the injured leg. Hold the stretch for 20 seconds and repeat 3 to 5 times.

When To Call Your Doctor

If the pain is severe to the point that you have difficulty walking, contact your physician. Also, if the self-care measures described here fail to relieve the pain after several days, contact your physician. In rare cases an inguinal hernia—a tender lump or bulge in the groin—may mimic groin pull symptoms; consult your physician to rule out this possibility.

What Your Doctor Will Do

A physical exam will be carried out. (X-rays are rarely useful.) If a groin strain is suspected, anti-inflammatory medication will be prescribed to relieve pain and a course of rehabilitation may be recommended.

For More Information

• American Academy of Orthopaedic Surgeons

Hair Loss

Symptoms

- **In men:** Receding hairline and progressively widening bald spot on the crown of the head (male pattern baldness).
- **In women:** Overall hair thinning.
- Sudden hair loss in sharply defined circular patches (a much rarer condition called alopecia areata).

What Is It?

Hair loss afflicts millions of people—and not just men, though their hair loss is often the most noticeable. Most women, too, experience some degree of hair loss as they grow older.

Hair is not living tissue like the skin but is composed of a protein called keratin, which is also the building block of fingernails and toenails. Each hair grows from a root enclosed by a follicle, a small pocket in the skin, that is nourished by blood vessels. Hair grows according to a genetic program (hormones are also involved), about half an inch a month; each hair grows for two to six years.

Part of your hair is growing and part resting at any given moment. After the rest period, the hair falls out. It's normal to lose from 50 to 100 hairs a day (not many out of 100,000 in the average youthful head). When a hair falls out, a new one presumably grows in, but the catch comes when it doesn't—when more falls out than grows back in. Genetic baldness is caused by the body's failure to produce new hairs. Nearly two-thirds of men develop some form of balding, and at least two-thirds of women have some form of hair thinning.

By far the most common form of hair loss is androgenetic alopecia, usually called male and female pattern baldness. (Alopecia is the medical term for hair loss.) About 35 million American men have male pattern baldness, the receding hairline that eventually turns into a bald pate (sometimes with very fine thin hairs replacing the original growth).

By age 50 half of all men of European origin will experience this kind of hair loss, which can begin as early as age 20. Some other genetic groups—Asians, some Africans and African Americans, and Native Americans—seldom or never get bald in this manner. Though the exact process that shuts down the hair follicles has yet to be explained, the male hormone testosterone plays a role.

Female pattern baldness usually begins at about age 30, becomes noticeable around age 40, and may be even more noticeable after menopause. The pattern of female hair loss is usually an overall thinning—two hairs where five used to be—rather than a bald area on top of the head, though women may have a receding hairline, too. It's thought that about 20 million American women have such hair loss. As in males, hair follicles simply shut down, with hormones playing some role in the process.

Not all hair loss is normal. Sudden hair loss can indicate a medical problem, so you should see a physician.

What Causes It?

Hereditary pattern baldness is determined by our genes and hormones. Sudden, dramatic hair loss, however, can have many causes. In women, contributing factors can be the hormonal changes of pregnancy and its aftermath. In both men and women, severe emotional stress, fad diets if pursued to the point of malnutrition, thyroid disorders, anemia, and various drugs and medications (particularly therapy for cancer) can cause hair loss. Large doses of vitamin A may also cause the problem.

Hair loss caused by constantly wearing tight-fitting wigs or hats is called friction alopecia. Trac-

295

Drugs to Treat Baldness

Many products promoted as hair-loss remedies don't work. These range from wheat germ oil and lanolin to vitamin supplements to scalp massage (sometimes along with electrical stimulation). Two medications may offer some help for baldness, though they are far from perfect.

Minoxidil

Now available over the counter, this medication (brand name: Rogaine) seems to stimulate hair growth in men suffering from male balding; it's also often effective for women with thinning hair. How the medication works is still not clear. It was originally developed as an oral drug to treat high blood pressure (it dilates blood vessels), and one unexpected side effect was that it stimulated hair growth. Then it was shown to promote new hair growth when applied to the skin.

It is available in two formulations, 2 percent and 5 percent. The 2 percent will promote hair growth in about 25 percent of men and 20 percent of women—and is the only formulation approved for women. There is disagreement about whether the 5 percent is actually more effective; it may also increase the incidence of side effects.

Minoxidil does have definite limits:

• It affects only the crown of the head, just one of the trouble spots in hereditary male pattern baldness. A receding hairline or baldness at the temples is rarely restored.

• New hair is usually thinner and lighter, like baby hair; only a relative handful of men will show what the drug's manufacturer has optimistically termed "dense" new hair growth. And many men who try minoxidil will not experience any significant hair growth.

• Side effects may include unwanted hair growth on the face, especially in women. Dizziness and increased heart rate have also been reported, along with skin irritation, especially on the scalp. But the drug does not appear to affect blood pressure or produce other serious side effects. Under no circumstances, though, should it be used by pregnant women.

• Minoxidil means lifetime commitment—at a cost of just under one dollar a day. Any new hair may vanish if you discontinue treatment, and the drug has not been shown to inhibit hair loss.

Finasteride

Marketed under the name Propecia for treating male-pattern baldness, finasteride is actually the same drug used in higher doses (and called Proscar) to treat an enlarged prostate (benign prostatic hyperplasia). Available only by prescription, Propecia works by blocking the hormone that shrinks hair follicles. It is not effective for men over age 60 or for those who are completely bald. It does promote hair growth, and slow hair loss, in younger men who are just beginning to lose hair. In one study, 60 percent of men showed new hair growth and more than 80 percent showed slowing of hair loss.

But keep in mind these drawbacks:

• Propecia may lower levels of PSA, a protein measured to detect prostate cancer, and so can distort test results, making it more difficult to detect prostate cancer or other prostate disorders. If you are using Propecia and about to have a PSA test, be sure to tell your doctor.

• It's not recommended for men with liver problems. It is also not approved for use by women, since it can cause birth defects and, in studies, has not restored hair on postmenopausal women.

• Reported side effects include reduced sexual drive and function (but these are rare).

• Like minoxidil, Propecia must be taken every day to sustain its benefit—at a cost of about $50 a month.

• No one has any idea of Propecia's long-term side effects. This is disquieting, given that the prime candidates are young men who could be taking the drug for many years.

tion alopecia is hair loss caused by pulling hair too tight in ponytails or braids, so that it falls out. In most cases hair begins to grow again once the underlying problem is corrected or corrects itself.

More serious is alopecia areata ("area baldness"), which causes loss of hair in patches and is thought to be an autoimmune disorder. It can proceed to complete hair loss and affects about 2.5 million people in the United States. This condition can sometimes be treated successfully, and anyone who suffers from it should see a dermatologist. In many cases, it simply goes away by itself and new hair grows back in.

What If You Do Nothing?

It's impossible to prevent male and female pattern baldness, and in most people the baldness will almost always become more noticeable as they age. For hair loss caused by illness, medication, radiation therapy, or hormonal fluctuations, hair will usually grow back when the condition or treatment has ended.

Home Remedies

You can find hundreds of hair-loss remedies offered on the Internet and in drug and health food stores. But if your hair loss is male or female pattern baldness, there aren't any nonmedical approaches that will halt hair loss or restore your hair. At the same time, there are hair-care practices and cosmetic remedies that can help you protect the hair you have and make the most of your appearance.

• **Choose your shampoos wisely.** Avoid alkaline pH shampoos. Use baby shampoo, and shampoo no more than once a day. "Revitalizing" shampoos or multi-product shampoo "systems" that promise to restore hair will not grow your hair back.

• **Dry your hair with care.** Avoid excessive toweling. If you use a hair dryer, keep it on a low setting.

• **Comb tenderly.** Always handle your hair gently, particularly if it is thinning. Combing is less injurious to hair than brushing.

• **Don't overbrush.** If you must brush, do so when your hair is dry. Grandmother's hundred strokes a day wasn't great advice, particularly if your hair is thinning. Be sure to disentangle the hair from the brush. Avoid hairbrushes and combs that pull your hair. Use either a natural bristle brush or a nylon brush with rounded edges.

• **Protect your hair.** Avoid bleaching, hot combs, excessive sun exposure, permanent waving, and straightening.

• **Resort to camouflage.** Especially for women, a short haircut and hair cosmetics such as sprays, gels, and mousses can hide thinning. Hair dyes can minimize the visual and psychological effects of hair loss. Permanent dyes, of course, can dry out the hair shaft if they are used over long periods, but they won't injure the root or promote additional hair loss. Whether using a dye at home or going to a salon, don't skip the patch test for possible allergic reactions. At home, follow package directions carefully.

• **Try cosmetic trickery.** Buy a powdered eye shadow the color of your hair and apply it lightly to your scalp in the thin spots. It's harmless and may make thinning hair less noticeable.

• **Be skeptical of products that promise hair growth.** Products containing lanolin, vitamins, or ingredients such as wheat germ are harmless when applied to the head, but they won't make hair grow or prevent it from falling out. Nor is there evidence to support any herbal products for hair growth. Products with large amounts of estrogen might stimulate hair growth (though the evidence for this is poor); unfortunately, there are almost always unpleasant side effects.

297

Surgical Solutions

▼

Certain surgical techniques for hair replacement provide varying degrees of hope for some people—though at considerable expense and with sometimes less than satisfactory results.

Hair Weaving

Also called "hair intensification" or "hair integration," hair weaving means adding to thin hair by weaving or braiding wefts of human hair or synthetic fibers into existing hair. Apart from the expense (anywhere from $50 to $2,500), this poses two problems: first, it may be difficult to keep your hair and scalp clean; second, it stresses existing hair and may cause it to fall out.

The American Hair Loss Council advises that only people with plenty of healthy hair should consider hair weaving—and even these people should plan to keep the "intensified" hair for only a few weeks.

Hair Implants

Hair implantation, or grafting, is a form of cosmetic surgery in which patches of skin with healthy hair follicles are transplanted into balding or bald areas. Usually, patches are taken from the back of the scalp and moved to the top of the head. The transplanted hairs always fall out, but new ones grow back in a few weeks. Another method is called scalp reduction—that is, the bald patch is partly excised and the areas of the scalp that still have hair are pulled closer together. Surgery works best to correct male pattern baldness rather than the overall thinning of hair that most women experience.

Hair transplants are better than they used to be. Doctors can now use micrografts instead of transplanting larger patches of hair, and they can place them in small incisions, feathering the hairline so that it looks like natural hair. There is also less risk of scarring using this technique. It is still a long, laborious, and expensive procedure requiring a series of office visits, sometimes at long intervals. Transplantation is not covered by most medical insurance, and the cost can easily run up to $10,000.

Unsatisfactory results are no longer as likely as they once were, but they are a real risk: a "doll's hair" look, scarring, and patches of thin transplanted hair over scalp sections that continue to grow bald. If you decide to go this route, choose a surgeon with care, and beware of seductive brochures showing "after" photos of men with thick, wavy hair. Ask to see some real clients. Also, confirm the doctor's credentials. Check with the department of plastic surgery at a nearby university medical school.

Prevention

It's impossible, at present, to prevent male and female pattern baldness.

When To Call Your Doctor

Any sudden hair loss is a reason to consult your physician, who after an examination may refer you to a dermatologist.

What Your Doctor Will Do

Your doctor will take a careful history, along with hair and scalp samples, if necessary, to identify the nature of the problem. Certain medications are associated with hair loss as a side effect, and if you are taking one of these, your doctor will try to find an alternative. If a scalp infection is the cause, specific treatment will be started. If alopecia areata—an autoimmune disorder that causes the immune system to destroy hair follicles—is suspected, therapy will be initiated with topical steroids.

For More Information
- American Academy of Dermatology
- American Hair Loss Council

Hammer Toe

Symptoms

- An uncomfortable clawlike deformity of a toe, usually the second toe next to the big toe.
- Corn formation on the top of a toe and a callus on the sole of the foot.

What Is It?

Hammer toe is a painful deformity wherein a toe bends unnaturally and becomes clawlike. This happens because the tendons of the toe contract abnormally, forcing the toe to bend downward and the middle joint of the toe to protrude upward. Although any toe may be affected, hammer toe usually affects the second toe. The toe assumes a clawlike position and cannot be straightened out.

When someone with hammer toe wears shoes, the toe is constantly rubbed, so walking may become especially painful if a callus on the sole of the foot or a corn on the top of a toe develops.

A hammer toe most often affects the second toe, giving it a clenched, claw-like appearance.

hammer toe

What Causes It?

It's thought that hammer toe may develop from wearing shoes that are too narrow or too short. This probably explains why women are far more prone to the condition than men: almost 9 out of 10 women wear shoes that are too small. Another cause is diabetes mellitus, which produces nerve damage in the feet that may lead to hammer toe.

What If You Do Nothing?

As long as hammer toe causes no pain or any change in your walking or running gait, it isn't harmful and doesn't require treatment. Seek medical attention if the toe becomes painful and you have difficulty walking. The condition is usually irreversible, but often its progression can be slowed or halted.

Home Remedies

• **Pad it.** Mild cases of hammer toe can be treated with corn pads or felt pads available in the pharmacy. Toe caps, the small, padded sleeves that fit around the tip of the toe, may relieve hammer toe pain.

• **Change your shoes.** Wear wide shoes with resilient soles. Avoid shoes with pointed toes.

Prevention

The key to prevention is to wear shoes that fit you properly and provide plenty of room for your toes. Here's how to get the right fit.

• **Have your feet properly measured.** The best way to do this is to get someone to draw the outline of your foot while you stand barefoot with your full weight on it, then measure the outline at the widest point.

• **Measure the soles of your shoes.** Ideally, they should be as wide as your feet, but certainly no more than half an inch narrower. Length matters, too, of course: your shoes should be half an inch longer than your longest toe.

Few people realize that their feet grow over the years: actually, the heel stays the same, but the front of the foot becomes wider and longer. The result: most women wear shoes that fit at the heel

299

but are much too narrow in the front.

• **Buy shoes that fit the longer foot.** For two out of three people, one foot is significantly bigger than the other. Have both feet measured whenever you buy shoes. Have your feet measured while you're standing, and buy shoes that fit the larger foot. Shop at the end of the day, when foot swelling is greatest. No shoe should feel tight.

• **Don't go by numbers.** You may think of yourself as a size 8B, but size varies from shoe to shoe. There is no standardization, so pick the shoes that fit best.

• **Limit high-heel use.** These shoes increase pressure on the front of the foot by at least 50 percent, so wear them only for special occasions. Flat shoes are more comfortable than high heels, but they, too, can be hard on your feet, especially if they are thin-soled.

• **Change your shoes.** If your shoes are too short or too narrow, get another pair. This is especially important for children going through periods of rapid growth. The toe area should be high enough so that it doesn't rub against the top of your toes—especially if hammer toes have started to develop.

When To Call Your Doctor

Contact your physician or podiatrist if you experience continuing pain because of a hammer toe or if a hammer toe interferes with your everyday activities.

What Your Doctor Will Do

Your physician will examine the affected toe. X-rays may be taken. Your physician may splint the toe and give you special exercises to perform. In severe cases surgery may be recommended to correct the problem.

For More Information

• American Orthopaedic Foot and Ankle Society
• American Podiatric Medical Association

Hangover

Symptoms

- Headache, sometimes severe.
- Dry mouth, thirst.
- Sour stomach, nausea, possible vomiting.
- Fatigue.

What Is It?

A hangover is a response to alcohol withdrawal. Compared to the delirium tremens (DTs) suffered by alcoholics, it is a relatively mild response, and typically it has no lingering health consequences. But it is a sign that you've had too much to drink.

Not everyone gets hangovers; individual susceptibility varies. The morning-after scenario depends not only on what and how much a person drinks but also on who that person is and his or her drinking history. Genetic makeup is a factor as well—for instance, some people process alcohol somewhat better than others. Some people rarely, if ever, get headaches, even after drinking.

Psychological factors are also involved—if a person expects to feel sick after drinking, he or she may be more likely to focus on symptoms.

What Causes It?

It takes the body about two hours to burn an ounce of pure alcohol (roughly the amount in one drink) in the bloodstream. Because alcohol is removed from the blood at this rate, even one drink per hour produces a steady increase in blood alcohol levels. Hence, people who are of average size don't have to get very drunk to suffer a hangover.

Some hangover symptoms are caused by the alcohol (or its breakdown products) remaining in the body. Other symptoms occur even after the blood alcohol level has returned to zero; these may be the after-effects of alcohol toxicity. One of the key factors behind a hangover is that alcohol acts as a diuretic: it stimulates the kidneys to pass more water than is being consumed. The dehydration that results contributes to dry mouth, sour stomach, and headache.

Some alcoholic beverages are more likely to produce a bad hangover. To a large extent, booze is booze: 12 ounces of beer, 5 ounces of wine, and 1.5 ounces of 80-proof spirits all contain the same amount of alcohol (ethanol). But some beverages, notably red wine and brandy, also contain small amounts of methanol (which is broken down much more slowly by the body) and other substances that may increase the severity of a hangover.

What If You Do Nothing?

A hangover improves as time passes. In fact, time is the only truly effective remedy for a hangover.

Home Remedies

No sure-fire remedy for the hangover has ever been found. Perhaps that's fortunate; if there were

---

Can't You "Sleep It Off"?

▼

You can't. Everyone knows that a person's judgment and performance are impaired when under the influence of alcohol—but they can still be impaired the next day, too. According to a Swedish study, after an evening of heavy drinking, your driving ability may be diminished by as much as 20 percent the next morning, even though your blood alcohol level may have returned to zero. And it didn't matter whether the subjects felt fine or awful—driving performance tended to be equally impaired. In another study, Navy pilots had impaired judgment up to 14 hours after drinking heavily (about five to seven standard drinks or a bottle of wine in an hour or two). Anyone who has overindulged should avoid driving or operating heavy machinery the morning after.

a cure, some people might drink more, with disastrous results.

• **Pain relievers can help.** NSAIDs—aspirin, ibuprofen, and naproxen—can help relieve a headache the morning after, as can acetaminophen. (However, pain relievers should not be taken while you are drinking in an effort to ward off a hangover. Combining alcohol with aspirin or ibuprofen may promote gastrointestinal bleeding, and alcohol combined with acetaminophen increases the risk of liver damage. All pain relievers will soon carry warnings to this effect.

• **Try ice.** Prepare an ice pack and apply it to the forehead (though for no more than 20 minutes at a stretch).

• **Drink plenty of water.** This helps counter dehydration caused by alcohol.

• **Drinking coffee may help a little—but not much.** Coffee and other stimulants won't speed the elimination of alcohol from the body or alleviate hangover symptoms. They may, however, perk you up.

• **Drinking more alcohol won't help.** In fact, it will only make things worse.

Prevention

Short of not drinking alcohol, no preventive measure is effective. Taking aspirin before drinking won't fend off a hangover. In one study, men who took two aspirin an hour before drinking ended up with alcohol levels 30 percent higher than without aspirin. Aspirin may interfere with the enzyme that breaks down alcohol, scientists theorized.

Eating (particularly fatty food) while or before drinking can slow the rate at which alcohol is absorbed into the bloodstream. But no matter what you eat with your drinks, don't drive.

Remember: if you're looking for a preventive or remedy for a hangover, you're probably drinking too much.

When To Call Your Doctor

For an ordinary hangover, you should have no reason to contact a doctor. However, habitual hangovers are one of the signs of alcohol dependence, and treatment for this may require medical help.

Hay Fever

Symptoms

For hay fever caused by grass, tree, and ragweed pollens, symptoms occur seasonally—typically from spring to mid-September. Other hay fever allergens are present year-round, in which case symptoms can occur anytime, indoors or out. Symptoms of a hay fever attack include.

■ Persistent sneezing, runny nose (usually with a clear discharge), and swollen nasal passages.
■ Red, itchy, watery eyes.
■ A dry itchy throat (or roof of the mouth), itchy skin, and wheezing.
■ Headaches also often develop, perhaps due to congested sinuses.

What Is It?

Hay fever is a misnomer: it's not usually caused by hay and does not produce a fever. Rather, it is an allergic reaction that occurs in your eyes, nose, and throat. The proper name is allergic rhinitis, and it's thought that more than 35 million people in the United States and Canada—people of all ages—are affected by it. According to the American Academy of Allergy and Immunology (AAAI), Americans lose 3.5 million workdays annually because of this condition.

Seasonal hay fever is generally caused by airborne pollens and outdoor mold spores that proliferate in warm weather, from spring to fall. Perennial hay fever, triggered by such allergens as household dust, animal dander, hair, fur, dog saliva, feathers, or mold spores, can flare up at any time of the year.

What Causes It?

It's your own immune system reacting to irritants, or allergens, that causes the runny nose and other symptoms of hay fever. It's not clear why some people are sensitive to specific allergens. But when an allergen enters the nose, throat, or eyes of someone who is susceptible to it, the body responds first by developing a sensitivity to it, then, upon further exposures, by releasing illness-fighting histamines and other inflammatory compounds (designed to fight off this foreign "invader") into the affected areas. The resulting inflammation of the mucous membranes produces the symptoms of hay fever.

A number of different irritants, or allergens, can trigger rhinitis—and they vary from person to person. Ragweed, grass, and tree pollens are the worst culprits, along with mold spores. Flower pollens are too heavy to be airborne (bees carry them), so they are seldom a cause of hay fever. Grass and tree pollens become airborne in spring—the first allergy season each year. Ragweed gets going in the late summer and early fall (except on the West Coast, where it is less common), followed by an upsurge of molds and fungi that live in decomposing leaves.

Many molds are present year-round, indoors and out. Some allergies are triggered by animal dander (actually a protein in the animal's saliva, which is transferred to the fur during grooming and then dries and sheds with the dander), feathers, cosmetics, cigarette smoke, and dust mites, as well as other indoor pollutants. Dust mites peak in warm, humid weather.

What If You Do Nothing?

As long as the allergens remain present, and you remain sensitive to them, you can have attacks.

Home Remedies

The most effective treatment is to eliminate the cause of your discomfort (see Prevention). If you can't, antihistamines may help. If your allergies are not severe, try one of the over-the-counter antihistamines, which may help control symptoms; a decongestant may also bring relief. The drawback is that most antihistamines cause drowsiness. Several effective nonsedating antihistamines are available by prescription only. These are less likely to cause drowsiness, but if you want to use them, be sure to talk to your doctor or pharmacist about possible interactions these drugs can have with other medications.

Try to avoid using over-the-counter decongestants; these products may provide temporary relief, but over the long haul cause the nasal passages to swell more than ever—a response known as the rebound effect.

Prevention

• **Pinpoint the allergy.** The first step in controlling, maybe preventing, hay fever is to find out what you are allergic to. Maybe you know already, from years of experience, that it's grass pollen in early spring or ragweed in the fall. If you don't know, you should see your physician to help diagnose the allergen that triggers your symptoms. If your problem is feathers, animal dander, or a cosmetic, you will probably be able to avoid hay fever entirely.

• **Stay informed about pollen counts.** If it's pollen that bothers you, you'll be interested to hear that the AAAI now sponsors a nationwide network that collects and broadcasts more accurate pollen counts. Various collecting stations all over the country do pollen and mold counts up to three days a week, which are then faxed to the AAAI, which in turn faxes them to radio stations and newspapers. The counts are given either numerically or described as "absent," "low," "moderate," "high," and "very high." According to the AAAI, there's no accurate way to forecast pollen counts. But if you hear that pollen

counts have risen, you can at least carry medication when you leave the house or postpone outdoor activity until things clear up.

• **Stay indoors on bad days.** When pollen counts are high, people with severe allergies should stay indoors if possible, especially between 5 am and 10 am, when pollens are most prevalent. Use an air conditioner if you have one. Be sure you keep the filters clean or you may end up blowing allergens around. You may be surprised to learn that a dog or cat that goes in and out of the house can carry pollen indoors, so try to avoid contact with pets if they have been outdoors.

Sorting Out Antihistamines

▼

Antihistamines come in many chemical classes, and are sold under scores of over-the-counter brand names and as generic "allergy pills." They are often combined with a decongestant, which may relieve symptoms temporarily. Single-ingredient products are usually the best choice, because you can take whichever you feel you need; if you find a combination drug that works best for you, that's all right, too.

All antihistamines available over the counter cause drowsiness, but the effect can be minimized by starting at low dosages and gradually increasing them. You can also use them at bedtime, when their sedative effect isn't a problem.

Read and heed the labels. Antihistamines are generally not recommended for pregnant or nursing women.

If you need stronger medicine or can't risk being sleepy, talk to your doctor about the newer prescription antihistamines. Most of these products work with just one dose a day, and they also don't cause dry mouth. Some are also nonsedating.

For more information on antihistamines, see page 573.

304

• **If you do go outdoors, wash your hair afterwards.** Washing your hair after spending time outside when the pollen count is high will remove pollen and thus may prevent a nighttime sneezing attack caused by pollen that falls from your hair onto the pillow.

• **Try the nasal spray Nasalcrom.** Available over the counter, Nasalcrom is considered a safe and effective medication for preventing hay fever symptoms (see box at right).

• **Check your car's air conditioner.** Just like home air conditioning, your car's AC system can help reduce your exposure to allergens. But if your car's air conditioner seems to be making you sneeze, the culprits are probably fungi that produce airborne spores and grow deep within the air-conditioning system. To minimize the problem, keep the car windows open part way for 10 minutes after you turn on the AC. Don't direct the vents toward your face. If these steps don't help, have your car treated with a disinfectant registered with the Environmental Protection Agency (EPA), available at car dealer service departments, some service stations, and most auto AC shops.

• **Most air purifiers aren't helpful.** The few controlled studies on air-purifying machines have found that they have little, if any, effect on allergens. Very small air cleaners cannot remove dust and pollen. Electrostatic precipitators, which electrically charge airborne particles and use polarized metal plates to pull them out of the air, can pollute indoor air with ozone, aggravating allergy symptoms. The best type of filter is the HEPA (high-efficiency particulate arresting)—effective but expensive.

• **Avoid smoke and other irritants.** In addition to not smoking, you should also avoid smoky environments. Insect sprays, fresh paint, and other households chemicals can also be irritating.

A Nasal Spray for Prevention
▼

Nasalcrom, containing cromolyn sodium, is safe and effective for preventing such hay fever symptoms as runny nose and nasal congestion—and both adults and children as young as six can use it. However, it won't help after the symptoms start. You need to spray before being exposed to the allergen, and you must spray four times daily. Nasalcrom may take a week or so to begin working. It blocks irritating chemicals (for example, histamines) that your own cells release when you are exposed to allergens. (It's your own immune system reacting to allergens that causes the runny nose and other symptoms.)

It's okay to use Nasalcrom with over-the-counter antihistamines. And unlike conventional decongestant sprays, Nasalcrom does not produce rebound congestion. For severe allergies, doctors sometimes suggest using it in combination with steroid nasal sprays, which are effective against allergy symptoms, but may produce unpleasant side effects such as soreness and nasal bleeding. (Nasalcrom does not work against cold symptoms.)

• **"Allergy-proof" your house.** If you're allergic to dust and dust mites, take steps to combat them (see page 155). Remove some or all carpets and soft furnishings. Keep floors and furniture dust-free. Get rid of feather pillows; use synthetic materials instead. Enclose your mattress in a plastic casing. Wash clothing frequently.

If you're allergic to your pet, the best remedy is to find another home for it. If that is out of the question, at least try to keep the pet out of your bedroom.

• **Get assistance.** If molds and fungi set you off, get somebody else to do your yard cleanup in the fall.

When To Call Your Doctor

In itself, hay fever is not a serious health problem and doesn't cause any permanent harm. But to alleviate it, you need to find out what you are allergic to. If you don't know, you should see a physician, who may be able to determine what triggers your attacks. You should also call a doctor if any type of secondary infection develops in your sinus cavities—signaled by pain, fever, a green or yellow discharge, or tenderness in the sinus areas or the teeth.

What Your Doctor Will Do

Your doctor will want a history of symptoms and a family history of known allergies, and will also ask about hobbies or work that may cause exposure to allergens. You may be referred to an allergy specialist. A physical examination of the upper respiratory tract will be made. If allergic rhinitis is suspected, skin tests will be made to confirm it. A blood sample may be taken and examined for antibodies, which in some cases can be helpful in determining treatment.

Your doctor may then prescribe antihistamines or other medications to initially treat the problem. Cortisone-based inhalants have proved effective against inflammation, and some doctors prescribe them. Atrovent nasal spray is sometimes effective at stopping a runny nose. Nasalcrom spray may be recommended to prevent the outbreak of hay fever symptoms.

If symptoms are severe, an allergy specialist may also recommend allergy shots. These desensitize you to specific allergens and eventually allow your body to tolerate them. Many people—children as well as adults—find the shots really do reduce symptoms. And it's not always necessary to repeat them annually.

For More Information

- American Academy of Allergy, Asthma & Immunology
- Asthma and Allergy Foundation of America
- National Institute of Allergy and Infectious Diseases

Headaches

Symptoms

- Tension headache: dull, steady pain that may be felt in the forehead, temples, or back of the neck, or throughout the head.
- Migraine headache: recurrent headaches characterized by throbbing, pulsating pain; often accompanied by visual disturbances, nausea, vomiting, lightheadedness, and a runny nose. Episodes can last 4 to 72 hours and occur one to four times a month.
- Cluster headache: steady, piercing pain located around or behind one eye or in one temple; usually strikes at night or in the early morning.

What Is It?

Headaches are one of the most common human ailments. For most people a headache is merely an infrequent annoyance, a passing discomfort that results from lack of sleep, sitting in a smoky room, or having an argument with someone. With aspirin, rest, and maybe a gentle massage, the pain goes away.

But for millions of others the pain does not go away; they suffer from chronic headaches. Americans spend upward of $400 million a year on headache remedies, leading researchers to estimate that as many as 45 million Americans suffer from chronic and/or severe headaches that seriously interfere with their lives.

Headaches are not completely understood by medical science, and researchers have advanced numerous theories to explain them. Tension, personality traits, heredity, and diet are a few of the factors that may play a role in chronic headaches. There appear to be various types of headaches, but any hard and fast classification is open to debate, in part because the types often overlap—both in their symptoms and in their response to medication. Moreover, triggering factors and modes of relief vary from person to person.

What Causes It?

The great majority of primary headaches (that is, those not caused by underlying disease) fall into three categories, according to the International Headache Society: tension (which includes depression headaches), migraine, and cluster. (Headaches can also be brought on by sudden exertion, as explained in the box below.)

• **Tension headaches.** These are also called muscle-contraction or stress headaches. Almost everyone occasionally gets a headache of this type. The pain is mild compared to migraine or cluster headaches. A feeling of tightness around the scalp is typical; muscles in the back of the upper neck may feel knotted and tender to the touch. It's not known whether it's the sustained muscle tension itself or the subsequent restricted blood flow that causes the pain.

Tension headaches are associated with stress

307

Exertion Headaches
▼

Some physical activities, including sexual intercourse and strenuous sports, have led to exertion headaches. Football players and joggers are the athletes most frequently struck by them. These attacks are probably vascular, caused by abrupt dilation or constriction of blood vessels, but researchers have not been able to pinpoint the exact cause of the pain. The headaches often hit just after exercise and are so painful that some sufferers have been rushed to hospital emergency rooms. This is a prudent precaution in sports such as football, where a head injury is possible. But in nearly all cases exertion headaches are neither harmful nor symptomatic of other ailments. With rest, the pain goes away.

(often the pain actually comes after the stress has ended), fatigue, or too much or too little sleep. Assuming a posture that tenses your neck and head muscles for long periods, such as holding your chin down while reading, can trigger these headaches; so can gum chewing, grinding your teeth, or tensing head and neck muscles during sexual intercourse. Men and women are about equally likely to suffer tension headaches.

Some people who have daily headaches have been found to be suffering from depression as well. Usually these are muscle-contraction headaches. Persistent headaches accompanied by lethargy, insomnia, or suicidal thoughts are signs of clinical depression.

Researchers do not understand the connection between depression and headaches, though some have suggested that the depression and the headaches may have a common biochemical cause. In some cases it may be the persistent headaches that cause the depression. And in some cases treating the depression makes the headaches go away.

• **Migraines.** The word migraine, derived from the Greek, means half a skull—an apt description of the pain, which often occurs in only one side of the head. However, the pattern of migraines is variable, and pain that starts on one side of the head can spread to involve the entire head.

Migraines appear to involve the abnormal expansion and contraction of blood vessels in and around the brain. In some people migraines start with an "aura"—neurological symptoms that typically include zigzag patterns of shooting lights, blind spots, and/or a temporary loss of peripheral vision. The pain of a migraine episode can be incapacitating and can last anywhere from a few minutes to several days; if it lasts longer than that, it's probably not a migraine. Migraine suf-

ferers may also experience nausea, vomiting, and sensitivity to both light and noise.

About 80 percent of migraine sufferers have a family history of the ailment; women are nearly four times more likely to be afflicted. The typical sufferer is young (under 35 years of age) and had her first attack during her teens or 20s. With age, attacks usually become less severe and less frequent. Hormonal changes can play a role: thus, susceptible women may have more attacks if they take oral contraceptives or it's around the time of menstruation; they may have fewer attacks dur-

Feeding a Headache

▼

Some researchers suspect that food plays a role in some headaches, especially migraines. But proving a definite link between diet and headaches has been difficult, and no single food seems to affect all sensitive individuals. Most of the suspect foods and beverages contain substances that may constrict or dilate blood vessels in the brain. One major culprit is tyramine, a chemical that occurs naturally in many foods. Nitrites, used in cold cuts and frankfurters, can also dilate blood vessels. A variety of foods may provoke headaches in sensitive people. The following foods have been most commonly implicated:

- Aged cheeses.
- Alcoholic drinks (especially red wine).
- Nuts and peanut butter.
- Yogurt.
- Sour cream.
- Cured or processed meats.
- Caffeine-rich drinks.
- Freshly baked yeast products.
- Chocolate.
- MSG (monosodium glutamate).
- Hydrolyzed vegetable protein.
- Aspartame (artificial sweetener).

ing pregnancy and after menopause. Attacks can also be triggered by certain substances in foods, by emotional factors, and environmental changes (like glaring light, strong odors, and changes in weather).

• **Cluster headaches.** These strike in a group, or cluster, for up to a few hours, and recur daily for days, weeks, or even months on end. Months of freedom may pass between attacks. Some researchers consider cluster headaches a variant of migraines, largely because the excruciating pain is centered on one side of the head, as in a migraine. But unlike the throbbing of a migraine, this pain is steady and piercing, it is centered in one area—usually behind one eye or in one temple—and it typically strikes at night or in the early morning.

Cluster headaches are about six to nine times more likely to strike men than women; the first attack usually comes in a person's 20s or 30s. They are sometimes misdiagnosed as a sinus disorder (because stuffy nose or sinus congestion is a common symptom) or even an abscessed tooth. There's no clear cause, though heavy smoking and drinking are possible contributing or triggering factors.

• **Other causes of headaches.** Many people assume that high blood pressure (hypertension) can trigger headaches. In fact, it's rare that high blood pressure actually causes a headache. If you suffer from frequent headaches, by all means get your blood pressure checked, especially if you are over 40. But in most cases, the two problems have to be treated independently.

Similarly, many people think first of a brain tumor as an important cause, but that is very rare. Of all the people who seek treatment for headaches, less than 0.5 percent have been found to have a brain tumor.

Eyestrain can cause a headache, but it will go away as soon as you rest your eyes. Poor lighting or poor posture may also lead to a headache, as can a hangover.

What If You Do Nothing?

Most headaches that aren't caused by some underlying disorder will clear up on their own—although tension headaches can last for days at a time. Because the pain, especially from migraines and cluster headaches, can be severe, most people will want to take steps to relieve symptoms.

Home Remedies

Many headache sufferers, and particularly migraine sufferers, find that it's essential to nip the pain in the bud—that is, to take medicine at the first sign of an attack. Unfortunately, the long-term frequent use of certain medications may actually result in drug-related "rebound" headaches. Many of the prescription drugs have unpleasant and sometimes dangerous side effects, so it's always best to rely on nondrug treatments when possible.

If you have recurrent headaches, try to discover what triggers them. Keeping a diary may help—it can show you that a certain activity, circumstance, food, or medication is associated with the attacks. Treatments like the following may allow you to get by without prescription medications.

• **For occasional headaches, start with over-the-counter pain relief.** The most common headache remedies are over-the-counter medications—nonprescription NSAIDs (aspirin, ibuprofen, or naproxen) or acetaminophen. If one type doesn't provide sufficient relief, try another the next time you have a headache. Remember that a drug is not harmless just because it is sold over the counter. No one should take a pain reliever for long periods without consulting a doctor.

• For migraines, an OTC combination may help. A combination of acetaminophen, aspirin and caffeine can relieve even severe migraine pain in some people, according to several panels of headache experts. You can find all three ingredients combined in Excedrin and other nonprescription headache formulations.

• Try to relax. Learning how to relax and cope with stress sometimes helps relieve headaches and other kinds of pain—in part by reducing muscle tension, in part by shifting attention away from the pain.

One common technique is progressive muscle relaxation. It calls for tensing and then relaxing specific muscle groups, working from the feet to the head, while focusing on deep, regular breathing. Another technique, called the relaxation response, is a form of meditation in which you repeat a word or phrase until your mind is free of distracting thoughts and your body relaxed.

One study published in the journal *Headache* found that migraine sufferers who were taught relaxation training had 30 to 40 percent fewer attacks over the course of three years. The 24 subjects in the study were also better able to cope with the attacks they did have and required less medication.

• Ice can help. Reusable gel packs—kept in the freezer and then wrapped around the neck during a headache—may provide relief in lieu of medication or as an adjunct to it. A study published in *Postgraduate Medicine* found that of 90 headache sufferers, 70 percent experienced some relief from such gel packs. Running cold water over your head may have a similar effect.

• Try heat for tension. You may find that heat, rather than cold, helps relieve some tension headaches. You can try a hot shower or bath, or moist heat applied to the back of the neck (use a wet towel wrapped around a waterproof heating pad—be sure to check heating pad directions).

• Massage. Many people find that massaging muscles in the neck, forehead, and temples promotes relaxation and offers some relief, especially for tension headaches.

• Apply headbands. A study published in *Headache* found that a headband (with two small rubber disks to apply pressure over areas of maximum pain) provided at least partial relief in 60 out of 69 migraine headaches. The band provides more consistent pressure on the temples, scalp, and forehead than finger pressure.

• Exercise. For some people regular exercise helps relieve tension and thus may prevent some headaches. Neck, back, and shoulder stretches may also be beneficial.

• Improve your posture. When working at a computer terminal, for instance, adjust your seat

An Herb for Migraines

For centuries feverfew, a member of the flower family that includes daisies, was relied on to treat headaches. The herb was somewhat forgotten, however, until the late 1970s, when migraine sufferers started talking about feverfew's potential to ward off these often debilitating headaches.

Since then, studies of feverfew as a migraine preventive have had confusing results. But the herb has been recognized by Canada's Health Protection Branch as a nonprescription drug for preventing migraines. If you suffer from migraines, you might want to try feverfew. In the United States, however, commercially available preparations usually have very little plant material in them. (In Canada, you can purchase standardized doses of the dried leaves). Also, feverfew may interact adversely with aspirin. (See page 619 for more information on feverfew.)

and table so that you don't have to bend your neck for long periods.

• **Consider biofeedback.** This high-tech relaxation method calls for hooking a subject up to a device that feeds back readings on a physiological variable—muscle tension, for instance, or skin temperature. The feedback supposedly enables the subject to gain some control over the variable. Biofeedback seems to help some headache sufferers.

• **Get to the source.** You may discover that your headaches disappear only when you resolve some underlying stressful problem in your life.

Prevention

Regular exercise and relaxation can help prevent headaches. If you are prone to migraines, avoid oversleeping, since this may lead to headaches. Also, keep a daily record to help identify possible activities as well as foods and beverages that appear to trigger headaches (see page 308). Avoid eyestrain and poor posture, both of which can trigger tension headaches.

When To Call Your Doctor

Most people who suffer from migraines or cluster headaches need to consult a doctor about treatment. In addition, in a small number of cases severe headaches may indicate a more serious disorder, such as very high blood pressure, stroke, bleeding in the brain, or even a brain tumor.

The following signs should send you to your doctor right away.

• A sudden onset of severe headaches, especially if they're your first ones.

• A headache with a fever and neck stiffness.

• A headache accompanied by confusion or loss of speech—especially after a blow to the head, even one that occurred several weeks earlier.

• A headache accompanied by inflamed, clogged sinuses. Occasionally, a severe headache results from infection and the buildup of pus in the sinus passages.

• Any increase in the intensity or frequency of headaches.

• A severe headache during or immediately after physical exertion or straining. Some activities, including sexual intercourse and strenuous sports, may lead to exertion headaches, which are usually harmless. But to rule out internal head injury, it's prudent to see your doctor.

What Your Doctor Will Do

In addition to taking a careful patient history and doing a physical examination, your doctor may order tests to rule out sinusitis, glaucoma, or other conditions that can produce headache symptoms.

If over-the-counter pain relievers haven't proved sufficient, you and your doctor will work to find the right prescription drug for you. A wide variety of such drugs is available—from narcotic pain relievers and antidepressants to beta-blockers, muscle relaxants, and drugs that relieve migraines by modifying specific neurotransmitters. Newer medications for treating migraines include "triptans" such as sumatriptan (Imitrex), zolmitriptan (Zomig), and rizatriptan (Maxalt).

Most of these medications are meant to get rid of the headache, but for people whose headaches are very severe or frequent, there are also drugs designed to prevent attacks.

Some migraine drugs are available as nasal sprays and/or self-administered injections, which are usually faster acting than oral tablets.

For More Information
• American Pain Foundation
• National Headache Foundation

Hearing Loss (Progressive)

Symptoms

- Progressive loss of hearing after exposure to loud noises or with age.
- Difficulty hearing high-frequency sounds.
- Difficulty distinguishing words during conversations, especially when in noisy or crowded circumstances.
- Difficulty hearing over the telephone.
- A need to turn up volume controls on televisions, radios, and other sound equipment.

What Is It?

A loss of hearing can strike people at any age, but most cases affect older people—in fact, it is the third leading chronic health complaint among older adults, after arthritis and high blood pressure. Even though the ear is a remarkable piece of sound-receiving equipment, designed to last for decades without repair or replacement parts, with age it inevitably grows less acute. The first sign of trouble is often difficulty hearing high-frequency sounds, like birds singing or children's voices.

At the same time, age-related hearing loss is occurring at younger ages these days because of exposure to sounds that have become a part of modern life—rock concerts, headphones, stereo equipment, jet planes, jack hammers, and dozens of other noisemakers that create decibel levels capable of wearing out the extremely sensitive receiving equipment in our ears.

It isn't easy to admit to hearing impairment; it's too often taken as an embarrassing sign of old age. But the truth is that most people suffer some degree of hearing loss after age 50—and for half of all men and a third of all women over 65, hearing loss is advanced enough to make social communication difficult.

Called presbycusis, from the Greek meaning

"old hearing," this age-related degeneration of the inner ear results in lowered sensitivity to high frequencies (you don't catch those high notes or the doorbell the way you once did) and a loss in the ability to discriminate among speech sounds (people seem to mumble). Or you may be aware of a persistent low hiss or ringing in the ears. Any one of these symptoms should send you to your doctor for advice. Some of this hearing loss is preventable, and much of it is modifiable.

What Causes It?

Damage to fine specialized hair cells and other sound-sensing structures in the ear underlie most cases of presbycusis. A common cause—or at least a common accelerator—of this damage is excessive noise. Medical conditions and certain medications can also contribute to hearing loss. Another cause of impairment is conductive hearing loss, which occurs when earwax or fluid builds up in the ear canal and interferes with the functioning of the outer and middle ear, or when an infection in the inner ear blocks sound wave transmission from the eardrum to the inner ear. Damage to the ear canal, eardrum, or tiny bones of the middle ear can also cause this type of hearing loss.

What If You Do Nothing?

Some cases of hearing loss are temporary—for example, the buzzing you may experience after attending a loud rock concert or being exposed to some other loud noise for several hours. In this instance, a night of rest usually restores normal hearing. But hearing loss due to presbycusis is permanent, as are other types of hearing loss, and these require a doctor or other specialist to identify and treat the underlying cause.

There are good reasons to get the problem treated. Hearing loss can isolate you, diminish your effectiveness at work, and detract from social and family life. It is a source of emotional stress to you and to everyone who deals with you. Also, if you get used to not hearing, you may find it harder to adjust to a hearing aid.

Home Remedies

Most hearing problems can be alleviated by a hearing aid (though only about one-third of those people who need hearing aids actually have them). Usually, having one device for each ear is most effective. Before you buy a hearing aid, see your doctor. In addition, take these steps to cope with difficulty hearing.

• **Don't be shy.** Ask people to repeat or slow down if you don't understand.

• **Cut out background noise.** Turn off the radio or TV during conversation.

• **Look for the quiet space.** In noisy places, station yourself near sound-absorbent surfaces (cur-

313

Hearing Aids: Many Choices

▼

If your doctor recommends a hearing aid, you'll need a written evaluation to buy one (unless you are over 18 and sign a form waiving an evaluation). You should also take your hearing test results along to a reputable dealer so that the dealer can match a hearing aid to your particular problem. Medicare will pay for an evaluation of your hearing loss if requested by a physician, but not for the hearing aid itself.

All hearing aids consist of a microphone, amplifier, a speaker to transmit sound, volume control, and battery. Three popular types are behind-the-ear devices; tiny in-the-canal models, which hardly show but are hard to adjust (and the batteries don't last long); and in-the-ear models, which have similar disadvantages to in-the-canal devices. Until recently, smaller hearing aids didn't amplify sufficiently and tended to distort sound. But new technologies, especially digital designs with microchips, have greatly improved hearing aids.

The audiologist you consult should be able to help you pick a model that suits your needs. Be sure to tell the person who is fitting you which environments and activities are most important to you. (Most audiologists also sell hearing aids—but be wary of one who sells only one model or brand.)

It pays to shop around. Look for a dealer who will give disinterested advice and reliable after-sales service. Don't assume that only the most expensive model will do.

Most dealers offer a 30-day free trial period for hearing aids. It may take a few visits and some patience to adjust an aid to your needs and to make sure it fits comfortably.

tains, books, or upholstered seating) and stay clear of echoing expanses of plaster and glass.

Prevention

There are many commonsense ways of avoiding hearing loss.

• **Turn down the headphones.** When wearing headphones, never use the music to drown out other noise. If you want to use headphones while your companion watches the ball game on television, perhaps you should move to another room rather than compete with the television noise. If you're on a bus that is making a deafening racket, lay your headphones aside. If you can't hear any sounds around you, you've got the volume too high.

• **Avoid excessive noise.** If background noise in any setting drowns out a normal conversational voice, you should try to escape or reduce the noise as soon as you can. If you have to shout to be heard, something is wrong.

If you must be exposed to high noise levels while you are working or commuting, give your ears a break during leisure time. Don't go to the noisiest restaurant or nightclub in town.

• **Use earplugs.** If you have to be in noisy environments frequently, carry a pair of earplugs and use them. They won't keep you from hearing a concert, for example; they'll just keep the decibels from damaging your ears.

When To Call Your Doctor

See your physician if you detect even mild hearing loss. Most hearing loss is correctable, but delay in dealing with the condition can only intensify it, sometimes irreversibly. It could also be a sign of another medical problem that needs attention.

What Your Doctor Will Do

An internist or another primary-care physician will probably do some simple preliminary testing. For more systematic testing, your doctor may refer you to an audiologist (a specialist in hearing problems) or an otolaryngologist (ear, nose, and throat specialist), who will take a complete history and perform hearing tests to determine the type and extent of the hearing loss. The specialist can also make recommendations about hearing aids. If an infection is present, your doctor may prescribe antibiotics. If damage to inner ear bones is responsible for your hearing loss, reconstructive surgery may be recommended to correct the problem.

For More Information

• American Academy of Otolaryngology-Head and Neck Surgery
• American Speech-Language Hearing Association
• Better Hearing Institute

Heartburn

Symptoms

Most symptoms of heartburn occur after you eat or when you are lying down.

- Painful burning sensation in the upper abdomen that moves up into the chest, often making its way to the neck and back of the throat.
- Belching and regurgitation of bitter gastric juices.
- Discomfort that worsens when you lie down (unlike chest pain due to heart attack, which is often associated with physical activity).
- In some cases, nausea.

What Is It?

Heartburn is a common stomach discomfort that affects approximately 60 million Americans annually and about 25 million adults daily. Heartburn gets its name from the chest pains that regularly accompany it—pains that can be so severe you may think you're having a heart attack. In fact, the pains have nothing to do with your heart. Rather, they are caused by stomach acid that washes up into the esophagus and produces a burning sensation and discomfort. The symptoms are most often caused by a condition known as gastroesophageal reflux disease, or GERD.

What Causes It?

The principal cause of this stomach distress, and of GERD, is the malfunctioning of your lower esophageal sphincter (LES). This muscle temporarily relaxes to let food pass into your stomach and then closes to keep stomach acids from splashing, or refluxing, into your esophagus—the food tube that runs from the throat to the stomach. When the LES doesn't close properly, stomach acids back up and irritate the lining of the esophagus, causing an uncomfortable burning sensation. This typically occurs after meals, when the stomach is secreting gastric juices and when pressure in the stomach is more likely to push stomach contents up through the LES.

If you are pregnant, overweight, or over the age of 40, the LES begins to weaken, increasing your risk of heartburn. (At least one-quarter of all pregnant women experience heartburn every day.)

What If You Do Nothing?

Mild occasional heartburn will usually resolve itself in a matter of hours and is no cause for concern. But if you have heartburn frequently, you should see your doctor, since persistent acid reflux can lead to inflammation and scarring of the esophagus, making it difficult to swallow. Chronic GERD can also lead to a precancerous condition called Barrett's esophagus. You will probably need to adopt some lifestyle and dietary changes in combination with medications to reduce or eliminate the problem.

Home Remedies

There are many over-the-counter preparations aimed at alleviating heartburn (see page 585). None is recommended for long-term use. Be sure to read warning labels carefully. Pregnant women, children, and people with ulcers or kidney problems should consult a doctor before using any type of heartburn medication.

• **Take an antacid.** If you have heartburn symptoms, don't try to "tough it out." The discomfort of occasional heartburn (once or twice a month) can be relieved by taking an over-the-counter antacid. These medications come in tablet, liquid, or foam, and in regular and extra-strength formulations.

Be aware that magnesium-containing antacids

may cause diarrhea, while those containing calcium most often cause constipation.

Antacids should remedy the situation almost immediately. A recommended dose taken one to three hours after eating should provide varying degrees of relief. If a single dose fails to bring relief, the problem could be more severe, and you should contact your physician.

Don't use antacids frequently or regularly. Not only may side effects worsen, but antacid use may mask symptoms that require medical attention. Antacids can also interfere with the absorption of other medications.

• **Consider an H2-blocker.** These over-the-counter drugs—which contain 50 percent of the minimum dosages in the prescription forms—are meant to be taken before heartburn strikes in order to prevent excess acid from being secreted (see page 587). If you already have heartburn, you will get faster relief from a conventional antacid. If you think you are going to get heartburn, H2-blockers may be worth a try.

• **Don't drink milk as a remedy.** Contrary to popular myth, milk is not a recommended antidote to heartburn. A glass of milk does provide immediate relief as it goes down, but milk lacks a buffering action, and will eventually stimulate even more acid production in the stomach. In less than 30 minutes you may develop heartburn that's more severe than the case you're treating.

Prevention

• **Don't overeat; instead, eat more frequent, smaller meals.** When you overeat, the excess food squeezes your stomach and forces digestive juices upward. Instead of eating a large lunch and large dinner, which cause the stomach to produce a lot of acid, eat four to six smaller meals and space them throughout the day.

Heartburn or Heart Attack?

▼

Heartburn and heart attack do have overlapping symptoms. But there are major differences. The following symptoms are more likely signaling a heart attack:

• pain that radiates up to the jaw or out to the arm.
• pain accompanied by sweating, nausea, dizziness, or shortness of breath.
• pain on physical exertion.

If these symptoms are present, call 911, or have someone take you to a hospital emergency room immediately.

• **Avoid fatty or acidic foods.** Certain foods regularly bring on discomfort or exacerbate symptoms in many heartburn sufferers. Included on the list are oranges and grapefruit, Bloody Mary mix, yellow onions, tomatoes and tomato-based sauces, and high-fat foods, especially greasy or fried meat. (Fat slows gastric emptying.) Red wine, after-dinner liqueurs, chocolates, and peppermints are also prime causes of heartburn.

• **Try to avoid becoming constipated.** Straining during bowel movements can increase abdominal pressure and encourage heartburn. Increasing your intake of dietary fiber and fluids is the safest, most effective way to promote more efficient elimination.

• **If you smoke, quit.** Smoking affects the lower esophageal sphincter and allows stomach acids to enter the esophagus.

• **Avoid caffeine.** The caffeine in soda, coffee, tea, and chocolate can increase the production of stomach acid secretions and lead to heartburn.

• **Limit your alcohol intake.** Many beverages containing alcohol relax the LES and may cause heartburn.

• **Loosen your belt.** If you eat more than usual,

loosen your belt after a big meal to keep it from squeezing your stomach and forcing acids upward.

• **Watch those midnight snacks.** Don't eat just before retiring, and don't eat a large meal less than four hours before bedtime. The combination of a large meal and the horizontal resting position will tilt digestive juices toward your esophagus. It's better to stay upright for at least several hours after eating.

• **Sleep on your left side.** If you often have heartburn at night, this position will keep the acidic contents of your stomach below the juncture with the lower esophagus, thus reducing acid backup into the esophagus.

• **Raise your bed.** Keeping your body at a slight upward-tilting angle will also help prevent stomach acids from moving into your esophagus at night. Put six-inch blocks of wood under the bed frame at the head of the bed, or buy a wedge that fits under your mattress.

• **Reduce daily stress.** If stress causes heartburn, find ways to reduce it through professional counseling, relaxation techniques, or regular exercise.

• **Check medication side effects.** Certain medications such as antihistamines, birth control pills, antihypertensives, sedatives, some heart drugs, and asthma medications may aggravate heartburn because they decrease the strength of the LES. If you are taking any drug regularly, ask your physician if it may be the cause of your heartburn.

• **If you're overweight, lose weight.** Extra pounds stress the LES and contribute to its weakening.

When To Call Your Doctor

Contact your physician if you have persistent heartburn and experience little or no improvement after two weeks of self-care measures, or if symptoms include wheezing, difficulty swallowing, vomiting blood that looks like coffee grounds, or passing black stools. Your symptoms may be caused by a problem other than gastroesophageal reflux, such as an ulcer, gallbladder disease, or other gastrointestinal problems.

What Your Doctor Will Do

A good medical history will help your physician make a diagnosis of heartburn. The doctor will first seek to rule out angina and heart attack, since the chest pain of these serious ailments is often indistinguishable from heartburn. If heartburn is then suspected, your diet will be reviewed to identify offending foods. Your doctor may also prescribe an endoscopy, in which an endoscope is inserted into your esophagus and stomach (gastroscopy) to determine your condition and, if necessary, obtain a tissue sample for biopsy.

For chronic reflux and heartburn, your doctor may prescribe medications that reduce acid in the stomach. These drugs include H2-blockers (such as Tagamet and Pepcid AC) and proton pump inhibitors (such as Prilosec, Prevacid, or Acip-Hex). There are also medications that reduce heartburn by speeding up the emptying of stomach contents.

In rare cases, severe reflux may require surgical treatment. But never opt for surgery until all other measures have been exhausted.

For More Information

• American Gastroenterological Association
• International Foundation for Functional Gastrointestinal Disorders
• National Digestive Diseases Information Clearinghouse

Heel Pain

Symptoms

- Discomfort in the heel first thing in the morning, when you put pressure on your foot.
- The pain may ease up as the day goes on, though it may worsen if you are running or walking.

What Is It?

Although runners and other athletes often get painful heels, it can happen to anybody. If the pain originates in the plantar fascia, which is the thick connective tissue under the skin on the bottom of your foot and the sides of the heel, then the condition is called plantar fasciitis. The plantar fascia, which acts as a kind of bowstring for the arch of the foot, can develop small, painful tears under repeated stress.

Other sources of pain may be minute breaks in your heel bone or a heel spur, which is a bony growth on the underside of the heel bone. Tendinitis or bursitis may also be part of the painful heel syndrome.

What Causes It?

Sometimes there is more than one contributing cause. More commonly, one of the following factors promotes the heel trouble.

- Bad biomechanics. This is another way of saying abnormalities in your walking or running gait that stress your heel bone and the tissues attached to it. Your heel should be the first part of your foot to hit the ground when you are walking, and ideally the arch distributes your weight toward the outside of your foot and then toward the ball of it. But if your feet roll inward (pronate) or outward (supinate) excessively, the weight isn't properly distributed, and the plantar fascia and heel bear too much weight.

- Being overweight. Excess pounds stress the heels, as does habitually carrying heavy loads.

- Growing older. Although no scientific study shows that older people are more prone to heel pain, it's probably true that they are. As you grow older, the pads that protect the heel from injury, like pads under a carpet, can wear down and thus fail to provide the shock absorption they once did.

- Frequent running, walking, or tennis playing. These vigorous weight-bearing activities stress the heel, especially if a person also has excessively pronating feet or other biomechanical problems.

What If You Do Nothing?

Heel pain will often clear up on its own—though it may take months to do so. However, if pain is severe and you begin limping, over time this can can put adverse stress on other body parts, including your ankles, knees, hips, and back.

Home Remedies

- **Rest.** If your heel does begin to hurt, rest is the first line of defense. Limit your activities for a few days.
- **Take over-the-counter anti-inflammatories.** Nonprescription NSAIDs (aspirin, ibuprofen, and naproxen) should help reduce pain, though they won't accelerate healing.
- **Apply ice.** Massage your heel with a small plastic jar or cup filled with ice, or do foot-rollers: roll your heel over an ice-filled plastic jar or a container of frozen juice. Afterward, pull your toes upward with your fingers.
- **Do some stretching stretches.** Tight calf muscles can tighten the fascia and contribute to heel pain. Try the stretches shown on page 319.
- **Cross train.** Cross train with non-weight-bearing activities such as swimming, water running

Plantar Fasciitis: Inexpensive, Effective Home Remedies

▼

According to two years of national research by the American Orthopaedic Foot and Ankle Society (AOFAS), involving 76 men and 160 women, a few simple exercises and over-the-counter shoe inserts are by far the most effective way to treat heel pain arising from the plantar fascia. Stretching and cushioning over a period of six to eight weeks are all it takes in most cases to cure a painful heel.

The first line of treatment consists of two simple exercises (see drawings) to stretch the Achilles tendon (at the back of the foot) and the plantar fascia.

These should be done several times throughout the day. Dr. Glenn Pfeffer, chairman of the AOFAS Heel Pain Study Group, has suggested 15-second stretches every waking hour.

Next, buy a silicon heel cushion at the drugstore, and wear it in a comfortable shoe with shock-absorbent soles. The Bauerfeind Viscoheel (silicon) was one brand used in the study; the Tuli heel cup (rubber) and the Hapad Comforthotic (the cheapest, made of felt) were also used. Silicon worked best of the three simply because it provided the most cushioning.

Some groups in the experiment only did the stretching exercises: 72 percent got better with just exercise. But the results for those who combined cushions with exercise were really impressive. From 80 to 88 percent of those using rubber or felt showed improvement, as did 95 percent with silicon. Surprisingly, all of these treatment methods worked better than a custom arch support, which was also tested. Other recent studies, too, have found that exercises and cushioning the foot constitute the first line of treatment for heel pain.

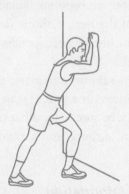

Calf stretch (achilles tendon). Standing two to three feet from a wall, place one foot near wall, keeping feet perpendicular to it. Lean forward and place forearms against wall, keeping rear knee straight (but not locked) and rear heel on floor. Hold for 10 seconds, feeling the stretch in calf. Repeat 10 times. Then switch legs and repeat. For a variation, keep the rear knee slightly bent during the stretch.

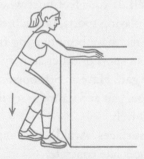

Heel stretch (plantar fascia). Stand near table or counter and lean forward on it. Slowly squat while trying to keep heels on floor. When heels just start to lift off floor and you feel the stretch across the bottom of feet, hold position for 10 seconds. Straighten up, then repeat 10 times.

in deep water, or bicycling in order to protect the heel while maintaining physical conditioning.

• **Gradually resume running or walking.** Once pain diminishes, slowly return to your previous level of physical activity. Reduce your training intensity if pain returns—you need to find a happy medium between rest and activity.

• **Be patient.** It can take months for the problem to go away. However, for nearly everyone, the prognosis is complete recovery.

Prevention

• **Buy shoes that offer support.** Make sure they have shock-absorbent soles, rigid shanks, and some extra padding in the heels. Good ankle counters are important, too, so your foot doesn't slip up and down.

• **If you are overweight, try to slim down.** This will take pressure off your tired and overtaxed feet.

• **Pace yourself.** If your feet hurt when you are exercising or playing sports, take a break. Try to judge if your feet have been hurting from over-doing it in your sport or other activity.

• **Check your gait.** Have an orthopedist or podiatrist check your gait and stance to see if your feet pronate excessively.

• **Check the surfaces.** Avoid exercising on non-resilient surfaces like concrete.

• **Switch shoes.** If you must wear dress shoes for work, wear athletic shoes to and from your place of employment, as well as at home.

• **Discard or repair any shoes with worn-down heels and soles.**

When To Call Your Doctor

If heel pain is severe enough to wake you at night and doesn't improve over time with self-care measures—heel pain often persists for several months—you may need the advice of a physician or podiatrist to figure out what's causing it. Also contact your physician if you suspect an infection, arthritis, gout, diabetes, or other ailment that could be a contributing factor to your heel pain.

If your heel pain is due to a biomechanical problem, your plantar fascia and heel may bear too much stress. A specialist in foot mechanics may be able to correct the problem with a custom-made orthotic device.

What Your Doctor Will Do

After a close examination, which may include an x-ray and blood tests, your doctor may recommend any of several options, including taping and strapping of the heel, orthotic devices, medication, and special exercise, depending on what your diagnosis is.

Surgery is seldom necessary, except in some cases for removal of a spur. If your physician suggests surgery, be sure to try other treatments first. As with any surgery, you should get a second opinion.

For More Information
• American Academy of Orthopaedic Surgeons
• American Orthopaedic Foot and Ankle Society
• American Podiatric Medical Association

Hemorrhoids

Symptoms

- **External hemorrhoid:** painful hard bump on the edge of or just outside the anus. May be accompanied by anal itching, bleeding, and pain upon defecation.
- **Internal hemorrhoid:** bright red blood on toilet paper, stool, or in the toilet after a bowel movement (often the first and only symptom). there may also be a discharge of mucus.
- **Prolapsed hemorrhoid:** an often painful, moist swelling of skin protruding outside the anal opening.

What Is It?

Hemorrhoids, also known as piles, are a familiar disorder, and usually not a serious one. It's thought that 75 percent of Americans will have them at some time in their lives. The word comes from hemo (blood) plus rrhoos (flowing or discharging), and indeed the first symptom of hemorrhoids is usually a spot or streak of bright red blood on toilet paper or in the stool after a bowel movement.

The tissue of the anus and rectum is a cushion of blood vessels, connective tissue, and muscle. A hemorrhoid is an inflammation or enlargement of the veins in this tissue, caused by excess pressure in the anal or abdominal area.

Most people can tell if they have external hemorrhoids. These develop from veins around the edge of the anus, and are often felt as hard, itchy, tender lumps that are likely to be painful at times. If the veins rupture, bleeding also occurs.

The majority of hemorrhoids, however, are internal, developing an inch or more above the anus. Usually they cannot be seen or felt, and so often go undetected until they bleed. In some cases, an internal hemorrhoid can also prolapse—it falls through the anal opening and forms a protruding mass that may be painful and itchy. A prolapsed hemorrhoid can slip back into the rectum or can be moved back in with gentle pressure from a finger. But persistent or permanently prolapsed hemorrhoids need medical attention.

What Causes It?

It used to be said that constipation was the chief cause. Now doctors are not so sure. A study published in the *American Journal of Gastroenterology* found that constipation and hemorrhoids were not linked; instead, diarrhea seemed to be a more likely cause.

Still, excess pressure in the anal area can promote hemorrhoids. That's why habitually straining while moving your bowels can promote or aggravate hemorrhoids. So can pregnancy, because the uterus puts additional pressure on the lower abdomen (though the hemorrhoids often disappear in the weeks following delivery). Other possible contributors to hemorrhoids include eating a low-fiber diet, being overweight, and being sedentary. It's also thought that genetics plays an important role.

What If You Do Nothing?

Hemorrhoids are more of a nuisance than anything else and are rarely a serious risk to health. With proper care, pain or bleeding from an external hemorrhoid resolves itself very quickly in most cases. If you can withstand the pain and itching, the hemorrhoids may eventually diminish so living with them becomes tolerable.

But when you do notice the bleeding for the first time, you should get a doctor's opinion. Probably it's only a hemorrhoid, but in a very small number of cases, rectal bleeding may be the first sign of serious gastrointestinal disease, including cancer.

Home Remedies

If a doctor has confirmed that you do have hemorrhoids, there may be no need for medical treatment. The following measures can ease the discomfort of hemorrhoids if you have them.

• **Don't strain or hold your breath on the toilet.** When possible, choose a time for defecating when you aren't rushed, and when the internal action of peristalsis can be helpful for you—perhaps after breakfast or soon after drinking a glass of water. Avoiding constipation also helps ease straining during a bowel movement.

• **Practice good hygiene.** Keep the anal area clean, but avoid using rough toilet paper. Gently wipe with wet paper or premoistened wipes.

• **Try frequent warm baths.** For painful hemorrhoids, try warm-water sitz baths two or three times daily, in a squatting position. (For convenience you can buy a plastic sitz-bath seat that fits over the toilet rim.)

• **Apply zinc oxide paste or powder or petroleum jelly to ease defecation and soothe itching.** Nonprescription cortisone cream (0.5 percent strength) or witch hazel (which has an astringent effect) may also help. Be careful of relying on certain over-the-counter hemorrhoid remedies such as Preparation H—these can be damaging to anal tissue, especially with prolonged use (see box).

• **Try cold compresses or ice packs several times a day.** These can help reduce both inflammation and discomfort.

• **Wear cotton underwear and loose clothing.** This helps avoid irritation.

• **Be careful of what you eat.** Some people find that certain foods and beverages aggravate hemorrhoids. Prime offenders may include nuts, red pepper, mustard, regular and decaffeinated coffee, and alcohol. You can try eliminating foods that seem to be making matters worse.

Over-the-Counter Remedies
▼

Many people rely on over-the-counter preparations to relieve inflammation and pain from external hemorrhoids. The most useful ingredients in many of these products are likely to be zinc oxide or petroleum jelly—both of which cost less if bought on their own. And generic products are just as good as brand names (and cheaper).

You can also get some pain relief from products ending in "caine," which are local anesthetics. These ingredients can irritate the skin, so pick a product specifically for hemorrhoids.

Products that claim to shrink tissue, such as Preparation H or Anusol, must carry certain cautions (people with heart disease and diabetes should not use them, for example), and they must also advise hemorrhoid sufferers to seek medical help if the condition worsens or fails to improve. Such products can also be damaging to anal tissue, especially with prolonged use.

Limit use of any over-the-counter product to seven days, and do not use any of these products on bleeding hemorrhoids. If symptoms persist, call your doctor.

Prevention

Though hemorrhoids may not be avoidable in all cases, you can do many things to prevent them from developing.

• **Eat a high-fiber diet.** This helps to prevent constipation. Fruits, whole grains, and vegetables form the base of a well-balanced diet, and this helps produce soft but formed, regular bowel movements. The increased fecal bulk is easily eliminated without straining the hemorrhoidal veins. To prevent painful gas, cramping, bloating, or diarrhea, increase your fiber intake gradually.

• **Drink plenty of water.** Drinking 8 to 10 glasses a day will help ease bowel movements.

• **Don't self-prescribe laxatives.** Laxatives frequently cause diarrhea, which can be as rough on the hemorrhoids as the straining associated with constipation.

• **Avoid sitting or standing for long periods.** If your job is sedentary and you must sit for long periods, stand up now and then and take a short walk. If you have to stand for long stretches of time, you may stress your rectal veins. Sit or lie down for brief periods whenever possible.

• **Reduce your weight.** Excess pounds increase pressure and cause hemorrhoids.

• **Exercise regularly.** Daily exercise improves circulation, prevents constipation, helps prevent hemorrhoids from developing, and aids in the shrinkage of existing hemorrhoids.

• **Be careful lifting.** Abdominal strain can increase pressure on the rectal-anal veins. Whenever lifting heavy objects, bend your knees first and pull up with your arms, straightening your legs simultaneously. Get someone to help with extremely heavy objects.

When To Call Your Doctor

Any of the following symptoms means you should consult a doctor: severe pain, throbbing, rectal bleeding that continues in excess of a week or is not associated with bowel movements, or blood that is dark rather than bright red. Throbbing pain and the formation of a lump near the anus may mean that an external hemorrhoid has "thrombosed" (formed a blood clot). Constant pain or persistent blood loss may mean that you have some condition other than a hemorrhoid, such as an anal fissure, fistula, or abscess. These maladies require their own forms of treatment.

What Your Doctor Will Do

A detailed history will be taken followed by an examination of the anus and rectum. A physical exam will reveal any external hemorrhoids. Using

---

Medical Treatments for Hemorrhoids

▼

When hemorrhoids are persistent and distressful despite self-care measures, your doctor may recommend removing them. There are several ways to do this, including ligation (tying them off with a rubber band); injection of a chemical solution that shrinks the vein; laser surgery; and in severe cases surgical removal in a hospital.

Surgery is the most invasive treatment, and you should consider it only if your primary physician advises it for external and/or internal hemorrhoids that bleed continually or are repeatedly swollen and painful. It's always wise to seek a second opinion before deciding to have surgery.

Don't let your first stop be a surgeon's office or a clinic that advertises quick-fix laser treatment ("In and out the same day!"). All of the above methods involve varying degrees of discomfort during recovery, and there may be complications to the procedures. Moreover, none of them guarantees that hemorrhoids won't recur (in fact, recurrence is frequent).

---

a gloved finger, a proctoscope, or an anoscope, the physician may detect internal hemorrhoids in the rectum. If no hemorrhoids are found, further tests may be recommended to find the cause of bleeding.

If hemorrhoids are found but home remedies don't bring relief, your doctor can prescribe suppositories, injections, and other therapies to soothe and reduce the swelling and pain. If these are ineffective, surgery may be recommended (see the box above).

For More Information
• American Gastroenterological Association
• National Digestive Diseases Information Clearinghouse

323

Hepatitis

Symptoms

During its acute phase, viral hepatitis is often mistaken for the flu and therefore often goes undetected. The most common symptoms include:

- General discomfort.
- Fever.
- Loss of appetite.
- Nausea and vomiting.
- Aching muscles or joints.
- Abdominal discomfort or pain.
- Dark urine and pale stools.
- Jaundice, indicated by a yellow tinge to the skin, the whites of the eyes, and in body fluids, in about half the cases.

Note: Sometimes there are no symptoms.

What Is It?

Hepatitis means inflammation of the liver, and one of the most common (and potentially serious) causes of liver inflammation is the infectious form of hepatitis, which is caused by one of five viruses, called hepatitis A, B, C, D, and E. Some forms of hepatitis are benign, but others can become chronic. This may result in chronic inflammation and scarring, and cause the infected person to become a permanent carrier, remaining infectious long after all symptoms have disappeared.

Hepatitis disturbs the ability of the liver to carry out its normal functions—secretion of bile, conversion of sugar to stored carbohydrate (and back again), and excretion of waste products—and may cause mild to severe flulike symptoms as well as jaundice and serious life-threatening ailments such as liver cancer and cirrhosis. There is also a noninfectious form of hepatitis that is caused by toxic substances—particularly alcohol, but also certain toxic chemicals—and by the excessive use of certain medications, especially if they are taken with alcohol.

What Causes It?

Viral hepatitis is contagious and is passed through human contact and contaminated water and food, as well as by unprotected sex and injection drug use. There are a variety of routes by which the different viral forms of hepatitis spread, and accordingly, certain groups are at greater risk for contracting each type of virus.

• **Hepatitis A.** A common form of the disease is hepatitis A, which can cause severe flulike symptoms but usually leaves no lasting effects and confers lifelong immunity. It is highly infectious and is most easily transmitted when an infected person handles food. An estimated 125,000 to 200,000 people are infected each year in the United States. Typically, the infection is passed through contaminated foods, water, and human feces. About 25 percent of all people infected with hepatitis A will experience no symptoms; those who do will have a fever of about 100°F, will feel exhausted, and will develop jaundice (yellow eyes

---

Hepatitis Prevention for Infants

▼

The U.S. Public Health Service, the American Academy of Pediatrics, and other physician groups have advocated that all infants be immunized routinely against hepatitis B. Like some other immunizations, hepatitis B requires three injections and confers long-term immunity. The cost can be as much as $100 for the three shots—though the cost would decline if the vaccine were more widely used. If you have children in your care or are expecting a baby, it's worth asking your doctor about the vaccine.

and skin). Some people with hepatitis A become seriously ill and require hospitalization. The infection can also cause liver damage. But people usually recover completely from hepatitis A.

• **Hepatitis B.** About 200,000 to 300,000 Americans, typically adults, are diagnosed with hepatitis B each year, and almost 6,000 die from the infection annually. Hepatitis B is spread by direct blood contact, sexual intercourse, the sharing of contaminated needles, and through blood transfusions in which the virus is present—much like HIV, the AIDS virus. The virus may also pass through cuts or scrapes in the skin, and it can be transmitted via saliva on a shared toothbrush. Many pregnant women with acute or chronic hepatitis B pass the infection to their babies, generally during delivery, potentially leaving them as chronic carriers of the disease.

Employment in the health-care field (doctors, nurses, laboratory technicians) increases the risk of infection, as does injection drug use and sexual contact. Although symptoms are generally mild—about half of those who become infected develop jaundice—a small number of patients for unknown reasons go on to develop a chronic carrier state with the potential to infect others. It's now estimated that there are one million such carriers currently in the United States. Chronic carriers are at risk for developing cirrhosis and/or liver cancer.

• **Hepatitis C.** This variant was known as non-A, non-B hepatitis until 1988. It's estimated that nearly three million Americans are chronically infected with hepatitis C, with about 36,000 new cases occurring each year. The majority of those infected have no symptoms, but many do develop symptoms, which can include nausea, extreme fatigue, fever, headaches, diarrhea, jaundice, loss of appetite, and abdominal pain. About 85 per-

cent of acute infections become chronic, which may lead to cirrhosis or liver cancer and which appears to be irreversible and ultimately kills thousands each year—more than types A and B combined. Hepatitis C is the leading reason for liver transplants in the United States.

As with hepatitis B, transmission is primarily by direct blood contact—usually via contaminated needles. Hepatitis C can also be sexually transmitted, but this is rare. While blood transfusions once posed a leading risk, the risk of getting either the B or C virus through transfusions is now minuscule (less than 1 in 3,300 units of blood), thanks to screening tests used by blood banks.

• **Hepatitis D.** Hepatitis D only occurs as a coinfection with hepatitis B, intensifying the severity of the hepatitis. In the United States most cases are contracted through frequent blood transfusions or from injection drug users who share needles.

• **Hepatitis E.** This infection only occurs in developing countries and is not considered a problem in industrialized nations. The virus causes an acute illness, but does not develop into a chronic carrier state.

What If You Do Nothing?

Most cases of infectious hepatitis resolve on their own within two to four weeks, though some may take two to three months. But a number of people with hepatitis B or C become chronic carriers who face potentially fatal complications, notably cirrhosis and liver cancer. If symptoms or laboratory tests indicate the possibility of chronic infection, drug therapy can be considered.

Home Remedies

Though drugs are being used to treat hepatitis, no known pharmaceuticals or other specific treatments provide a cure for the illness, so therapy

325

focuses on prevention and on relieving symptoms until the infection has run its course. Major objectives include getting appropriate rest, eating a proper diet, and controlling the spread of the virus.

• **Eat a hearty breakfast.** Hepatitis symptoms of nausea and vomiting typically get worse as the day goes on. Eating a substantial breakfast will help ensure that you maintain an adequate daily intake of calories. Eating several small meals during the course of the day, rather than a large lunch and dinner, may also help you cope with nausea.

• **Wash up.** If you have hepatitis A, it's important to wash your hands thoroughly after going to the bathroom.

• **Don't drink alcohol.** Alcohol can't be effectively metabolized by the damaged liver, so refrain from drinking during the course of the disease and for a month after all laboratory tests show normal results.

• **Check with your physician about over-the-counter and prescription drugs.** Acetaminophen, aspirin, birth control pills, and certain antibiotics are potentially toxic to the liver.

Prevention

• **Wash your hands.** Always wash with soap and water after using the toilet, after changing diapers, before preparing foods, and before eating. This helps stop the spread of many diseases, including hepatitis A.

• **Cook your foods.** You are at risk of contracting hepatitis A if you eat certain foods, such as shellfish, in a raw or undercooked state.

• **Practice safe sex.** Using condoms and avoiding multiple sex partners will significantly reduce your risk of hepatitis B and C.

• **Get inoculated against hepatitis A.** A vaccine is available for use against this virus. Formerly, the closest thing to a vaccine was gamma globulin for those who had been exposed or were likely to be, but it offers limited and short-term protection (lasting only about five months). The new vaccine provides protection for at least 10 years. You do need a booster shot after 6 to 12 months. The vaccine is safe and has few side effects. These are the people who need protection against infection from hepatitis A:

• Anybody over age two who will be traveling in Mexico and Latin America, Africa, Eastern Europe, the countries of the former Soviet Union, or in other areas where hepatitis A is common.

• Anyone who has oral-genital sex.

• People with chronic liver disease, for whom hepatitis can be very dangerous.

• Injection drug users who share needles.

• Children living in states or communities with a high rate of hepatitis A (twice the national average or higher).

• **Get inoculated against hepatitis B.** There is an effective vaccine with minimal side effects. Newborns should be routinely vaccinated, just as they are immunized against polio and other diseases (see box on page 324). Recently, an increasing number of state health departments have taken steps to require hepatitis B vaccinations for all adolescents, who are viewed as a high-risk group. Unfortunately, parents and physicians have been slow to accept the idea of immunization—perhaps because of the high cost and an unwillingness to believe that the disease is a real danger to people not designated as high risk.

Other high-risk groups include sexually active gay men, heterosexuals with multiple partners, health-care workers, injection drug users, children of immigrants from regions where hepatitis is common, such as Southeast Asia, and people who travel frequently to high-risk areas. The three-dose vaccine usually provides immunity for seven or more years.

• **If you are pregnant, have a hepatitis B blood test.** If it's positive, a physician can help protect the newborn with an injection at birth of a special type of gamma globulin. The infant should also be vaccinated against hepatitis B.

• **If you had a blood transfusion before July, 1992, get tested for hepatitis C.** Though it is now very rare for hepatitis C to be acquired through a transfusion, methods used to screen donated blood were less accurate before July, 1992, so the risk of acquiring the virus from a transfusion was greater.

• **Be careful with any needles.** If you are getting your body pierced or tattooed, or receiving acupuncture, make sure the needles are brand new or have been properly sterilized in an autoclave.

• **Don't use an injection street drug.** If you do use such drugs, never share needles.

When To Call Your Doctor

Contact a physician if you develop symptoms of viral hepatitis or if you already have hepatitis and symptoms persist despite treatment. Also contact your physician if you have been exposed to someone known to have acute viral hepatitis.

What Your Doctor Will Do

Along with taking a complete medical history, your doctor may feel the right side of the abdomen to check for any tenderness or enlargement of the liver and then take blood tests to look for the virus or antibodies to the virus.

Most people with hepatitis don't need extensive medical treatment. In more serious cases or if a diagnosis is still uncertain, a liver biopsy may be recommended to determine the extent of liver damage. Some people with progressive hepatitis may require prolonged treatment.

For More Information

• American Liver Foundation
• Centers for Disease Control and Prevention

Hiatal Hernia

Symptoms

■ Heartburn one to four hours after eating.
■ Belching.
■ Difficulty swallowing after eating.

What Is It?

A hiatal hernia develops when a portion of the stomach slides upward into the chest cavity through the esophageal hiatus (opening) of the diaphragm, the broad tough muscle that separates the chest from the abdomen. If this opening becomes increasingly weakened, powerful stomach acid flows backward from the stomach into the esophagus, irritating it and producing symptoms of heartburn. In severe cases (which are rare) the stomach may protrude upward into the lower chest.

Hiatal hernias may develop in people of all ages and both sexes, but the condition is most common in those over 50. Many people, in fact, have a small hiatal hernia but aren't aware of it until, complaining of chronic heartburn, they visit a doctor. Fewer than 20 percent of the individuals with hiatal hernias ever experience any symptoms. (Usually, the hernia shows up only incidentally on an x-ray.) Most hiatal hernias don't need treatment, though surgery may be necessary when the hernia is in danger of becoming strangulated (constricted in such a way that blood flow is cut off)—a complication that is quite rare. Severe esophagitis (inflammation of the esophagus) may also necessitate treatment.

What Causes It?

The most frequent cause of a hiatal hernia is muscle weakness due to normal aging, accompanied by increased pressure in the abdominal cavity produced by coughing, straining on the toilet, or any sudden overexertion. Pregnancy, obesity, and excess fluid in the abdomen can also contribute to a hernia.

What If You Do Nothing?

Small hiatal hernias are common and usually harmless. If you have been told by your physician that you have a hiatal hernia, you should take precautions to avoid episodes of heartburn, as described below. Otherwise, the hernia and associated heartburn can lead to inflammation, scarring, or narrowing of the esophagus.

Home Remedies

If hiatal hernia symptoms become troublesome, practice the following self-help measures (similar to those for heartburn).

• **Keep meals small.** Eat meals four to five times daily. Also, eat slowly and avoid lying down for

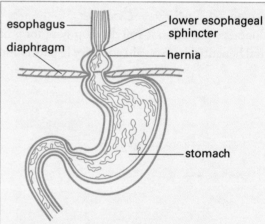

A hiatal hernia occurs when part of the stomach protrudes into the chest area through an opening in the diaphragm where the esophagus joins the stomach. This can prevent the lower esophageal sphincter from closing properly, allowing stomach acid to back up into the esophagus, causing heartburn and other symptoms.

two or three hours after eating—practices that help prevent heartburn.

• **Watch what you eat and drink.** Try to avoid high-fat foods, since they tend to slow gastric emptying. Likewise, alcohol can induce heartburn, so you should avoid it as well, along with citrus juices and caffeine, which can trigger or worsen symptoms.

• **Don't smoke.** Smoking helps increase the production of stomach acids, and the coughing caused by smoking can aggravate the hernia.

• **Don't wear constricting garments.** Tight trousers, pantyhose, girdles, or belts put undue pressure on the hernia.

• **Avoid straining during bowel movements.** The key to this is to avoid constipation.

• **If heartburn does strike, take antacids.** The discomfort of occasional heartburn—once or twice a month—can be relieved by taking an over-the-counter antacid, which should bring relief quickly (see page 585).

Prevention

There is no known way to prevent a hiatal hernia.

When To Call Your Doctor

Contact your physician if you have persistent symptoms of a hiatal hernia. Also contact your doctor if symptoms fail to improve after one month of treatment.

What Your Doctor Will Do

After taking a careful history and performing a physical examination, your physician may suggest various diagnostic tests to discover if there is any obstruction (for which you may be referred to a gastroenterologist). Your physician may prescribe antacids to prevent stomach acids from irritating the hernia. If constipation is a problem, a change in your diet may be recommended.

Persistent reflux (regurgitation of stomach contents into the esophagus) can lead to changes in the esophageal tissue (such as the development of esophageal ulcers and/or Barrett's esophagus) and so should be managed and monitored by a gastroenterologist.

For More Information

• American Gastroenterological Association
• National Digestive Diseases Information Clearinghouse

Hiccups

Symptoms

- Sharp, involuntary spasms of the diaphragm that produce a contraction and "hic" sound in the glottis—the area of the larynx containing the vocal cords.
- Hiccups typically follow rapid eating, overeating, or excessive alcohol consumption.

What Is It?

Hiccups occur when a sudden rush of air in the windpipe is abruptly cut off by an unexpected spasm of the diaphragm. Hiccupping involves a disturbance in the involuntary nerves that regulate the breathing process. When these nerves are triggered, a signal is sent and the diaphragm—the wall of muscle that separates the chest cavity from the abdominal cavity—goes into spasm. At the same time, there is a sudden and simultaneous closing of the glottis (the flap of skin at the top of the windpipe). The spasm causes a sudden inhalation, but with the glottis closed, air can't get into the lungs, and the blocked air produces the familiar sharp "hic" sound. Hiccups typically occur from 4 to 12 spasms per minute—though in severe cases, up to 100 or more per minute can occur.

Hiccups are involuntary, repeated over a short period of time, and normally disappear as suddenly as they appeared. Unlike a sneeze or a cough, however, a hiccup is a mystery ailment with no known purpose. It is also universal: even fetuses do it.

What Causes It?

No one is quite certain of the cause of hiccups, but they can be triggered by anything that irritates the nerves connecting the diaphragm, larynx, rib muscles, and breathing centers of the brain. Eating too quickly or too much, going from a warm environment to a cold one, and eating frozen treats too quickly are examples of circumstances associated with hiccups. Carbonated beverages often cause hiccups, perhaps because the carbon dioxide gas expands in the stomach. Shock, fear, or over-excitement are other causes, and abdominal surgery is also linked to hiccups. Liquor has been linked to hiccuping, too, possibly because alcohol relaxes the nerves that normally inhibit hiccups.

What If You Do Nothing?

Common self-help measures may shorten the duration of hiccup episodes, but if you're patient, hiccups should go away spontaneously in a matter of minutes once the diaphragm settles back into its normal rhythmic pattern.

Home Remedies

There are dozens of home remedies for short hiccup episodes, from the simple to the elaborate. None are backed with any scientific research, and even if one of them helps you combat one bout of hiccupping, there is no guarantee it will to work for you the next time. The remedies listed here are intended to get the diaphragm back in synch with your lungs or, at the least, to distract you from the hiccuping.

- **Plug your ears.** Stick your index fingers in your ears for about 20 seconds. This may short-circuit the nerves that control the hiccup impulse.
- **Try the ice cure.** Fill a glass with ice cubes, add water, and slowly drink it. The rapid change of temperature in the esophagus may shut down your hiccup response.
- **Inhale carbon dioxide.** Place the opening of a brown paper bag around your nose and mouth and seal it firmly in place with your fingers. Tak-

ing small breaths, rapidly breathe in and out about 15 times, then breathe in deeply. Count slowly to 10, then release. The elevated levels of carbon dioxide in the blood may cause the hiccups to end. Repeat the cycle until the hiccups disappear.

Prevention

Hiccups cannot be prevented.

When To Call Your Doctor

Hiccups are normally a minor annoyance. They clear up on their own and don't pose any medical problems. Contact your physician if hiccups last longer than a day, interfere with your work, eating, or sleep, or seem to be associated with a prescription medication you are taking.

What Your Doctor Will Do

Your physician will take your medical history and may perform a physical exam to determine if an underlying disease associated with hiccups might be the cause (which is rare). Pneumonia, heartburn, diabetes, and even a heart attack are sometimes accompanied by hiccups. Lung tumors or an infection or tumor in the stomach can also cause hiccups. If unrelenting hiccups are not related to any medical problem, your physician may administer prescription medication to control them.

For More Information

• American Gastroenterological Association

331

High Blood Pressure (Hypertension)

Symptoms

High blood pressure usually has no symptoms, which is why it's called the silent killer. Some patients with very high blood pressure complain of headaches, but most often high blood pressure is discovered during a routine physical exam or when there is a complication due to high blood pressure—for example, a heart attack or stroke.

What Is It?

High blood pressure, also known as hypertension, affects at least 50 million people in the United States and 4 million in Canada. It is probably the most common medical problem in the industrialized world, and the major treatable risk factor for heart attack and stroke. So it pays to be aware of the latest findings and recommendations concerning what to do about high blood pressure.

Blood pressure is created by the pumping of your heart. It is a variable force that moves blood through the circulatory system. When your heart contracts, blood flows into the arteries, and at the end of the contraction the pressure is at its high point. Then as the heart relaxes, blood flows from the veins into the heart, and the pressure reaches its low point. Thus a blood pressure measurement is expressed as two numbers: systolic (high point) and diastolic (low point).

About 70 percent of people with high blood pressure have what is now referred to as Stage 1 hypertension—systolic pressure between 140 and 159, diastolic pressure between 90 and 99 (see chart on page 333). Doctors used to talk about "mild" or "borderline" hypertension, but this language is falsely reassuring, since many cases of Stage 1 hypertension worsen over time if untreated. And many researchers believe that even slightly elevated blood pressure (85 to 89 dias-

tolic), or "high normal," can be a health hazard if it persists for years.

About two out of three people over 60 with high blood pressure have what is termed "isolated systolic hypertension"—that is, their diastolic pressure is normal. A study of data from the large-scale Framingham Heart Study shows that this form of hypertension is as health-threatening as high diastolic pressure among middle-aged and older people. This study has prompted the government to warn doctors and patients of the dangers of high systolic pressure—though the goal is still to keep both numbers in the normal range.

In addition to being a major risk factor for stroke and heart attack, untreated hypertension can harm the arteries, resulting in damage to the brain, heart, and kidneys. Yet in the United States only about half of the individuals who have hypertension know it, mainly because it seldom causes noticeable symptoms. This is unfortunate, since blood pressure can be controlled in most people through lifestyle changes and, when necessary, treatment with drugs.

What Causes It?

A complex bodily system regulates blood pressure, which fluctuates normally according to your activity level and many other factors. The main regulators of blood pressure are small blood vessels called arterioles, which widen and constrict, causing pressure to fall and rise. When the regulatory system goes awry, the arterioles stay constricted, and blood pressure stays chronically high.

In most cases the cause of this is unknown—and the condition is called "essential hypertension." In about 10 percent of cases, the elevated blood pressure is due to a specific underlying disorder, such as kidney disease.

We do know that, in western countries, the

major risk factors for high blood pressure are advancing age, high sodium and/or alcohol intake, being overweight, being sedentary, and a family history of hypertension. For reasons that are unclear, the incidence of hypertension is higher among African-Americans, poor people, and those with lower educational levels. But anybody in any walk of life can develop hypertension.

While hypertension that develops as people grow older is common in the industrialized world, it is almost unheard of among rural peoples in underdeveloped countries. But people who move from other cultures and adopt a westernized lifestyle tend to develop hypertension, too. Nobody knows exactly what causes this—diet, especially sodium intake, a lack of exercise, and

Evaluating Blood Pressure Levels

▼

The blood pressure classifications below, which were developed by the Joint National Committee on Detection, Evaluation, and Treatment of High Blood Pressure, apply to adult men and women who are not currently taking antihypertensive medications and who are not acutely ill.*

Blood pressure is indicated by two numbers, each referring to how high, in millimeters, the pressure of the blood in your arteries can raise a column of mercury (Hg). The first number, the systolic pressure, represents the force of blood during a heartbeat. The second number, the diastolic, indicates the

pressure between heartbeats.
When determining what category a person falls into, use the higher category indicated by systolic and diastolic readings. For example, someone with a reading of 140 mm Hg systolic and 100 mm Hg diastolic would fall into the Stage 2 (moderate) category.

333

CATEGORY	SYSTOLIC (MM HG)		DIASTOLIC (MM HG)	RECOMMENDED FOLLOW-UP
Optimal	≤120	and	≤80	Recheck in 2 years
Normal	<130	and	<85	Recheck in 2 years
High-normal	130–139	or	85–89	Recheck in 1 year**
Hypertension*				
Stage 1 (Mild)	140–159	or	90–99	Confirm within 2 months**
Stage 2 (Moderate)	160–179	or	100–109	Undergo complete medical evaluation and/or begin treatment within 1 month
Stage 3 (Severe)	>180	or	>110	Undergo complete medical evaluation and/or begin treatment within 1 week
Isolated systolic hypertension	≥140	and	<90	Confirm within 2 months**

*   Based on the average of two or more readings taken at each of two or more visits after an initial screening.
**   Applies only to initial blood pressure readings. Multiple readings at these levels may require more aggressive management.

becoming overweight may be part of it. So may the demands of modern life. Job stress can certainly contribute to hypertension, especially a job that demands careful attention to detail but offers little personal satisfaction or sense of control. Job insecurity can also contribute to hypertension.

Emotions, such as fear and anger, temporarily raise blood pressure, but then it drops to its prior level when the emotions subside. No personality type is more prone to high blood pressure, although one study did suggest that middle-aged men (not women) with high anxiety levels were more likely to develop hypertension than others.

Caffeine in teas, colas, or coffee can temporarily raise blood pressure, especially if you are not used to caffeine. But caffeine is not known to cause hypertension.

What If You Do Nothing?

In many people blood pressure increases with age—so if you are in your 30s, for example, and your blood pressure is slightly elevated, it may eventually rise into the Stage 1 category. In addition, if you have certain lifestyle risk factors for hypertension—if you smoke, are overweight, consume too much alcohol, or are sedentary—and you do nothing to modify these factors, your blood pressure is likely to increase over the years. For example, if your blood pressure is normal and you are sedentary, you have a 20 to 50 percent greater risk of developing hypertension than a person who's fit and active.

Home Remedies

Some of the risk factors associated with hypertension—heredity, race, and age—can't be altered. Nonetheless, there is increasing evidence that a number of dietary and lifestyle changes can often help reduce elevated blood pressure. Such changes

---

What About Supplements?

▼

A number of supplements are promoted as aids in controlling hypertension—but don't rely on them. High doses of fish oil, which contains omega-3 fatty acids, may lower blood pressure on a short-term basis in some people. But high doses have potential adverse effects, including an increased risk of stroke, so are not recommended. Moderate doses have no effect on blood pressure.

Garlic promoters have made countless claims about the health benefits of garlic—including its ability to lower blood pressure. However, the studies testing garlic's effects on blood pressure have been flawed and the results contradictory. Eating garlic can't hurt you—but it's also unlikely to be of help if you have hypertension.

Researchers are studying the effects of diet on hypertension, but it's difficult to isolate one nutrient from others and assess its effects on blood pressure. We know that calcium, potassium, and magnesium are important in blood pressure regulation—however, there is no evidence that high doses of them from supplements will lower blood presssure or help prevent hypertension. (Some people on certain high blood pressure medications may be advised by their doctors to take potassium supplements.)

What does appear to have beneficial effects on blood pressure is obtaining these vitamins and minerals from food—by increasing your intake of fruits, grains, and vegetables.

---

are the first step in treating people with high-normal or Stage 1 blood pressure, who may be able to avoid or postpone the need for antihypertensive medications. Even if you are prescribed such drugs, you should continue to modify your behavior, since this may help you get by on a lower dose and thus reduce any adverse effects the drugs may cause.

• **Maintain a healthy weight.** Losing even a few

pounds if you're overweight can reduce your blood pressure.

• **Don't smoke.** Smoking doesn't cause hypertension, but it does promote heart disease. A hypertensive who smokes is at serious risk.

• **Exercise regularly.** For one thing, exercise can help you lose weight. It can also lower your blood pressure somewhat, though it's not understood exactly how this happens. If you are sedentary and just beginning an exercise program to combat hypertension, remember that you may not see the effects for weeks.

• **Keep your sodium intake low (below 2,400 milligrams daily).** About 10 to 15 percent of the population is salt-sensitive, meaning that salt (sodium chloride) drives their blood pressure up. Since you can't know in advance whether you are in this group, you should moderate your salt intake in hope of controlling or preventing hypertension. Reducing sodium intake is always the first line of treatment for people who have developed high blood pressure.

• **Eat a diet rich in fruits, vegetables, and low-fat dairy products.** Diet, by itself, is seldom an adequate treatment for hypertension. But at least one study has shown that a diet emphasizing fruits and vegetables along with low-fat dairy products (and whole grains)—a healthy, well-balanced diet, in other words—can substantially lower blood pressure. Such a diet helps control weight, is low in sodium, and supplies good amounts of potassium. (A diet high in potassium has been shown to produce modest drops in blood pressure in some hypertensives.)

• **If you drink alcohol, do so in moderation**—no more than one drink daily for a woman, or two for a man. A drink is defined as 1.5 ounces of 80-proof spirits, 5 ounces of wine, or 12 ounces of beer, all of which contain the same amount of alcohol.

Who Needs To Do Home Monitoring?

▼

Generally, candidates for monitoring blood pressure at home include persons with "white-coat" or "office" hypertension (their blood pressure becomes abnormally high in a medical setting), or hypertensives trying to fine-tune their medication. In both cases, your doctor will advise you whether it's appropriate. Your doctor may also want you to measure at home if you have unusual risk factors. You'll need some training to do it accurately.

The instrument you'll have to purchase is a sphygmomanometer (SFIG-mo-man-OM-ater)—a mouthful and a handful.

Consider using the aneroid type of monitor (cuff, bulb, and gauge). It is less expensive and more accurate than the electronic-digital type; it is less awkward to use than the familiar mercury-filled column with cuff and bulb. All three monitors require a stethoscope, but with the electronic model, the stethoscope is built in. (Monitors that fit around your finger or wrist, though compact, are the least accurate.)

335

Prevention

The same factors that help control hypertension may help prevent it in the first place. There's no guarantee—but even if these measures don't work, they offer other potential health benefits, most importantly a reduction in risk factors for cardiovascular disease.

When To Call Your Doctor

If you're in good health and your blood pressure has been normal, you should have your doctor check it every two years.

If your blood pressure is above normal, see the chart on page 333 for guidelines. This advice may not apply to everyone, however. If you are sedentary or overweight, or if you have a family history of hypertension or heart disease or other risk factors, you may need to have your blood pressure monitored more frequently.

Remember that it's important to have your blood pressure evaluated both because of the health risks related to hypertension and because other conditions that might contribute to the problem must be ruled out.

You should also consult your doctor if you are taking antihypertensive drugs and you experience any unpleasant side effects. Never stop taking your medication without talking with your doctor.

What Your Doctor Will Do

Your doctor will measure your blood pressure, and if the initial reading is elevated, then your blood pressure will be measured on several different occasions over a week or longer.

Some people exhibit "white coat" hypertension—their blood pressure becomes abnormally high in a medical setting—and if that is the case, your doctor may also recommend that you monitor your blood pressure at home. If your blood pressure is normal outside the doctor's office, then

you are probably not at risk for the diseases associated with high blood pressure. However, if your pressure outside the office is within the high normal range (130-139/85-89), you should be retested within a year. (A few studies have found that white coat hypertension may be an early warning sign of chronic hypertension.)

If your hypertension is high normal or Stage 1, the first line of treatment is to adopt the healthy lifestyle measures listed above. These changes may produce the desired result. If not, or if your blood pressure is already at Stage 2 or Stage 3, your doctor will prescribe one or more safe and effective drug(s) for controlling hypertension. A wide range of drugs is available, so that therapy can be tailored to a patient's age, ethnicity, tolerance for different side effects, medical conditions, and other factors.

For More Information

- American Heart Association
- National Heart, Lung, and Blood Institute Information Center

HIV Infection/AIDS

Symptoms

Symptoms vary depending on how HIV affects a person's immune system. Milder clinical symptoms include the following:

- Persistent fatigue.
- Fever that can last a few days to a month or longer, with no other symptoms present.
- Night sweats.
- Unexplained weight loss.
- Diarrhea.
- Swollen glands.

Once HIV destroys a sufficient amount of the body's immune system, certain otherwise controllable infections, such as a specific type of pneumonia or cancer, can then gain a foothold.

What Is It?

HIV, or human immunodeficiency virus, is a bloodborne virus that causes acquired immune deficiency syndrome, or AIDS, the clinical name of a syndrome that was first reported in the United States in 1981 and is now recognized as a great pandemic.

AIDS is one of the most dangerous health problems of modern times. Because of the complexity of this disease, and the rapid development of new treatment strategies, treating AIDS should be carried on with the advice and care of an expert in this area. Preventing the spread of AIDS, however, is straightforward and a responsibility that each person can and should undertake.

HIV attacks the body's immune system and can eventually destroy it. A severely impaired immune system leaves the infected person increasingly unable to fight off invading bacteria and viruses, and thus susceptible to a whole host of "opportunistic" infections and diseases that are often debilitating and can eventually cause death.

The Centers for Disease Control and Prevention (CDC) has cited nearly 30 diseases and sets of symptoms associated with AIDS in the United States. These include Kaposi's sarcoma (a form of skin cancer), tuberculosis, pneumonia, and certain neurological disorders such as meningitis.

A diagnosis of AIDS is based on the type and severity of symptoms in the presence of HIV infection. Another criterion used to designate AIDS is a significant decline in a person's T-cells—white blood cells that are critical to a healthy immune system. In many infected people, AIDS can be slow to develop, and the full effects of the disease may not appear until 8 to 12 years or more after the initial infection. In children, the time between exposure to HIV and the appearance of symptoms can be measured in months if the infection goes untreated.

So far there is no cure, and no vaccine to prevent the disease. New vaccines are in various phases of testing, but making a successful vaccine has proved to be very difficult. The development and availability of new medications have allowed increasing numbers of HIV-infected people—both children and adults—to delay the onset of symptoms, for years in many cases. These treatments have also slowed the course of the disease for those who have developed AIDS, improving the quality of their lives and enabling them to live longer.

During 1996, the number of AIDS-related deaths in the United States decreased substantially for the first time since the epidemic began in 1981—a nationwide decline of about 25 percent from the previous year that Federal officials attributed to the success of drug therapies introduced in recent years, along with better access to care and increased financing for AIDS treatment.

This downward trend in AIDS-related deaths,

as well as a decline in new cases, continued for the next several years, but the numbers then began leveling off. The CDC estimates that, as of 1999, there were approximately 40,000 new cases of HIV infection occurring annually, 40,000 new cases of AIDS, and 16,000 AIDS-related deaths.

AIDS is more prevalent in many developing countries, particularly sub-Saharan Africa and parts of southeast Asia, than it is in the United States. Worldwide, approximately 36 million people are living with HIV or AIDS, with an estimated 15,000 new infections occurring each day. But even in the United States, some 650,000 to 900,000 residents are living with HIV infection—of whom more than 200,000 are unaware of being infected. And the CDC estimates that four to five million Americans are at high risk for becoming infected because of their sexual behavior and drug use practices.

What Causes It?

The HIV virus is an infectious agent known as a retrovirus, which has the ability to take over certain cells and interrupt their normal genetic functioning. Although there is much that we don't yet understand about HIV, there is a good deal we do know. The virus can be cultured in a laboratory, and scientists have devised reliable tests to detect its presence in blood samples. We also know that the virus is hard to transmit. This is because HIV dies very quickly once it is outside the body. Consequently, it is not transmitted through air or water, nor does it travel easily from person to person, as other infections may. It cannot penetrate intact human skin, and it cannot be spread by casual contact such as touching or hugging, sharing food or a drinking glass, using the same towel, or sharing bathrooms or toilets. Rather, the virus is carried in bodily fluids such

as blood, semen, vaginal fluids, and breast milk, and it can only be spread by the bodily exchange of these fluids with an infected person.

The most common path of HIV transmission is during sexual activity, when the virus in semen or cervical secretions enters cuts or small abrasions. The virus passes from one person to another during anal intercourse more efficiently than it can during vaginal intercourse, and it also passes—though rarely—during oral sex. The virus can also be spread via blood-contaminated hypodermic needles and syringes, and—if donated blood is contaminated—blood transfusions. In addition, an infected mother can pass the virus to her child in utero or during delivery. (Although the virus has been found in saliva and tears, scientists believe that transmission via these fluids is unlikely since the virus is present in very low concentrations.)

In Africa and Asia, AIDS is primarily a heterosexual disease. Worldwide, more than 80 percent of all adult HIV infections have resulted from heterosexual intercourse. During the 1980s in the United States, AIDS was confined primarily to certain well-defined risk groups—males who have sex with males, injection drug users, and people with hemophilia (because they need frequent transfusions). But the number of people infected by heterosexual intercourse began rising in the 1990s.

Of new infections among women in the United States, the CDC estimates that 75 percent were infected through heterosexual sex. And while the rate of infection by this route is still comparatively low among men (about 15 percent of new cases), for both men and women the risk increases with frequency of intercourse and especially with multiple partners.

Should You Be Tested?

▼

If you answer yes to any of the following questions, you should seek counseling and testing for HIV. (See page 340 for information about home testing.)

- Have you had unprotected sex (that is, without a condom) with someone whom you can't be sure is not infected with HIV?
- If you're a man, have you had unprotected sex (anal sex) with other men?
- Have you shared needles or syringes to inject drugs?
- Have you had a sexually transmitted disease?
- Have you had unprotected sex with someone who would answer yes to any of the above questions?

You should also consider the factor of blood transfusions. Did you receive a blood transfusion or clotting factor between 1978 and 1985? Some recipients of blood transfusions between the fall of 1978, when HIV first appeared in the United States, and May 1985, when blood-donor screening became routine, were at risk for infection, particularly if they received the blood in San Francisco or New York City or if they had multiple transfusions. People with hemophilia, who also were recipients of donated-blood products, may also have been at risk during those years. Since 1985 the risk of contracting an infection from transfusions or blood products has been minimized thanks to the rigorous screening of donated blood.

In addition, if you have had sex with someone and you didn't know his or her past behavior, or you have had many sex partners, you should consider testing. If you have any doubts about what to do, get counseling. If you are at risk and decide not to be tested, you should assume that you might be infected and take precautions to prevent transmitting the virus to others.

Where To Go For Testing

If you wish to be tested, contact your doctor, local health department, local AIDS organization, or the CDC's National AIDS Hotline (800-342-AIDS). You can be tested in your doctor's office or at publicly funded HIV testing sites, community health clinics, family planning clinics, hospital clinics, and drug treatment centers. The complete test is free at some public health clinics; other clinics charge a fee of $40 to $70, depending on where you live. Results are typically available in one to two weeks; to obtain results more quickly, or to have testing done at a private doctor's office, can cost anywhere from $100 to $250, depending on who does it and where you live. You can also do a home test.

Before being tested you should receive proper counseling about the test and HIV, as well as about the meaning and confidentiality of the results. Unless you are tested anonymously, your results may become part of your medical record and may become known to insurance companies, which could affect your future coverage. A counselor can tell you how to avoid this.

After the test, you should receive further counseling. If you test positive, you'll need to know what your medical options are, how to prevent spreading the disease, and what the psychological, financial, and social repercussions may be.

If you test negative, you'll need to know how to stay uninfected. Also, if you are in the "window" period (when you could be infected but can still test negative), and if your exposure to the virus is considered to have been high risk, you will be advised about repeating the test within six months from your last HIV exposure.

A new Web site for HIV testing information has been set up by the CDC (and maintained by the CDC National Prevention Information Network, or NPIN) at www.hivtest.org.

339

What If You Do Nothing?

If you think you may have been exposed to HIV infection or you have developed symptoms that might be AIDS-related, one of the quandaries is whether to be tested. But there are now clear benefits to diagnosing HIV infection early.

• Promising new drugs can slow the progress of HIV, and other drugs can prevent, delay, or treat opportunistic diseases that strike people with AIDS. There are also better ways to monitor the progress of the disease. For a pregnant woman who is infected with HIV, early treatment with antiviral drugs can reduce by two-thirds or more the chances that her baby will be infected with the virus.

• Testing has proved to be very accurate. The most commonly used test is a fairly simple blood test, and if it detects antibodies to the virus, it is followed by a confirmatory blood test. The Food and Drug Administration (FDA) has approved an accurate oral antibody test that uses a special pad to absorb material (not saliva) from the cheek and gum.

• The confidentiality of the test results is now easier to ensure. Not only are there clinics that offer anonymous testing, but accurate, anonymous home testing is available (see box).

Because of these benefits, anyone who might be at risk should know his or her HIV status. Yet as many as one-third of all HIV-positive Americans do not know they are infected. At the very least, each of us should be familiar with—and know when to use—safer sex practices and other measures for preventing transmission of HIV.

Home Remedies

There are no home remedies for AIDS. If you think you have HIV infection or AIDS, you should always consult a qualified practitioner, who can

Home Testing for HIV

For years, the Food and Drug Administration (FDA) and AIDS advocacy groups opposed home testing, largely because of fears that counseling via telephone would not be adequate. Indeed, people testing positive for such a terrible infection ideally should get face-to-face counseling and, if needed, crisis intervention. But after the FDA studied other forms of telephone counseling and crisis intervention, it decided that the potential benefits (easier access and greater privacy) of the home test outweighed the risks.

Recently, the only home test approved by the FDA has been the Home Access test (sold in drugstores and via a toll-free phone number: 800-HIV-TEST). More than a dozen unapproved tests are also on the market, but there's no guarantee that these are reliable or accurate. (If you have a question about an HIV home test kit, you can call the FDA's Office of Special Health Issues at 301-827-4460.)

The test simply involves pricking your finger and putting drops of blood on a card with an ID number. You mail the card to a certified lab and wait about a week, then call a toll-free number for the results, using your ID number.

If you test negative (that is, you are not infected), you'll get a recorded message that includes an explanation of the "window" period—the time when you may be HIV-infected but still have a negative antibody test. If you test positive, you'll get the news from a trained counselor, who can answer questions and supply detailed information, as well as referrals for counseling and treatment. Conversations are anonymous and confidential.

Testing and face-to-face counseling by a trained health-care professional are undoubtedly preferable to the home test, so if you're considering the test, it's a good idea to talk to your doctor or call the CDC's National AIDS hotline. But the home test is a decent alternative, provided the process helps educate people about HIV/AIDS and leads to medical treatment, if they need it.

advise you and help provide medical treatments that may be able to offset or delay symptoms.

Prevention

Until a vaccine can be developed, halting the spread of AIDS must depend solely on educating those at risk—which includes all sexually active people, particularly those who have not lived in strict, long-term monogamy. Though education may not be the ultimate weapon, it is an effective and powerful means of controlling the spread of the disease.

One common myth about AIDS is that it is a disease of male homosexuals and injection drug users; other people have nothing to worry about. It is true that the vast majority of reported AIDS cases in the United States continues to be homosexual or bisexual men or injection drug users. But while these two main risk groups remain for the moment well defined, anybody who has unprotected sex can get AIDS. When it is transmitted heterosexually, women appear to be at greater risk than men: the virus is far less likely to pass from woman to man during vaginal intercourse than from man to woman. Between 120,000 and 160,000 American adult and adolescent women have been infected, and the number is rising sharply, especially among low-income African Americans and Latinas. As of 1999, women accounted for 23 percent of AIDS cases reported nationally.

The frequency of sexual contact appears to be more important than the form. Though a single contact can spread HIV, people who have multiple sexual partners are in much more danger than those with fewer partners. Prostitutes, both male and female, are more likely to be infected by HIV and to transmit it, since in addition to frequent exposure, many use injectable drugs.

Ultimately, it is not who you are, but what you do and with whom you do it, that puts you at risk for contracting HIV. The following are known to be high-risk practices.

• *Sharing drug needles or syringes.*

• *Anal sex with someone who might carry HIV.* The virus is passed easily during anal sex.

• *Unprotected vaginal or oral sex (without a condom) with someone who might carry HIV.* Obviously, the more times you have unprotected sex, the greater your risk. Sex with prostitutes is particularly risky.

With that in mind, here are steps you should take to prevent AIDS.

• **Choose your sexual partners carefully.** Ask about the sexual history of a potential partner. Any person who has had multiple partners or has a sexual relationship with someone who has multiple partners may be at risk. Unless you and your sex partner are both sure you are not infected, you need to take precautions: use condoms, and avoid high-risk practices such as anal intercourse. Couples who have not been monogamous may wish to consider testing.

• **Always use a latex condom.** Used consistently and correctly (see page 58), latex condoms provide a highly effective HIV preventive: the virus cannot penetrate an intact latex condom. ("Natural membrane," or skin, condoms are not effective.) Adequate lubrication with a water-based lubricant (such as K-Y jelly) is important to prevent condom breakage. Unless you are certain that you and your sexual partner have not been exposed to AIDS, using condoms must be habitual for any and all episodes of sexual intercourse.

• **Don't rely on spermicide.** The evidence that spermicides protect against HIV and other sexually transmitted diseases is not conclusive—and spermicide use may actually increase the risk of transmitting HIV by causing inflammation in vaginal tissue. The CDC does not recommend using spermicides alone. Condoms are the first line of defense—but not lubricated with nonoxynol-9. Still, if all you have at hand is a condom with nonoxynol-9, it is better than no condom.

• **Don't inject recreational drugs.** If you do, never share needles.

• **Age is no barrier against infection.** The number of AIDS cases diagnosed in people over 50 has climbed steadily through the AIDS epidemic, reaching 78,000 through the end of 1999. Gay men represent the majority of the over-50 AIDS cases, but many cases are low-income women who contracted HIV through drug use or heterosexual partners.

• **Health-care workers should take precautions.** Accidental self-puncture with an HIV-infected needle is a possible danger for doctors, nurses, dentists, physician's assistants, and laboratory workers who give injections or handle blood. However, the number of infections acquired in health-care settings is quite small: from 1978 to 1999, only 56 cases of HIV infection due to exposure in a health-care setting were documented by the CDC. (In fact, health-care workers are at considerably greater risk of becoming infected with hepatitis B and C.)

• **If you are infected with HIV, follow these same preventive measures.** It is incumbent upon anyone who is infected to avoid exposing others to HIV. In addition, anyone who is HIV-positive and contemplating parenthood should be aware that there is a high risk—from one in three to one in two—of an infected mother transmitting the virus to a fetus or newborn (though early treatment with medications can help reduce the risk).

When To Call Your Doctor

You should call your doctor if you suspect you have been at risk for exposure to HIV, whether or not you have symptoms. If you wish, you can first take a home test. Be aware that the antibodies to the virus—which is what the blood test measures—can take six months to develop after the initial infection, so a negative result (indicating that the virus isn't present) is not reliable. If you have taken the test soon after possible exposure to HIV and tested negative, follow up with another test four to six months later.

If you do home testing and the result is positive (indicating you are infected), it is vital that you consult a physician or a counselor who specializes in HIV and AIDS.

If you have been diagnosed with HIV or AIDS and are undergoing treatment, discuss with your doctor what criteria to use for monitoring and assessing your condition.

What Your Doctor Will Do

Your doctor will examine you to determine the extent and possible cause of any symptoms, including taking a history to determine if you should be tested for HIV (or lab tested to confirm the results of a home test). The doctor will want to know when you think you were exposed to the virus, since there is a time lag, or "window," during which a person can be infected with HIV but will test negative.

Testing is fairly simple. A blood sample is taken from the arm and analyzed in a laboratory. What the test detects is not the presence of HIV, but rather the antibodies that the immune system produces after the virus enters the bloodstream. The first stage of the testing is known as ELISA (enzyme-linked immunoabsorbent assay). Should it prove positive, it may be repeated to confirm accuracy. After one or more positive ELISA tests, usually a more specific confirmatory test, called the Western blot, is performed. Other tests are also available, some of which don't involve drawing blood. You can discuss these with your doctor.

If testing confirms a diagnosis of HIV, your doctor will talk to you about treatment options, further testing to determine the extent of your infection, and methods to prevent opportunistic infections. If your doctor is not experienced in diagnosing and treating HIV/AIDS, he or she should refer you to an HIV/AIDS specialist. Efforts will also be made to treat existing symptoms, reduce the risk of infections, and maintain proper nutrition.

Your doctor can also help you find an AIDS support network to help provide emotional support and information.

For More Information

AIDS testing is conducted confidentially and, in many communities, anonymously. Check with your county health department if you are concerned about anonymity with regard to your insurance company or your employer. You can also call these resources for information about testing, counseling, and treatment.

- Centers for Disease Control and Prevention
- CDC National Prevention Information Network

343

Hives

Symptoms

- Sudden onset of itching of varying intensity, with swelling of the skin's surface into red or skin-colored welts or blisters.
- The welts may change shape, develop a white center, or suddenly disappear without cause in a matter of minutes or hours.

What Is It?

Hives, or urticaria, are red, extremely itchy areas of swollen skin called wheals that can range in size from pin-size dots to large patches. These wheals may be circular or irregular in shape, but with distinct edges.

Hives are common: up to 20 percent of the population is affected at some time, and the disorder is especially common for people who have had other allergic reactions, such as hay fever. Hives come without warning and may disappear in less than two hours, but they can last as long as a day or two, or recur on and off for months.

What Causes It?

Hives are an allergic reaction that can be caused by a variety of environmental factors. Tension and emotional stress can also trigger hives, as can something you've eaten, touched, or inhaled.

Antibiotics are a common cause. Penicillin is the classic trigger and can induce the condition even if someone has taken the antibiotic many times before without any problem. Aspirin is another offender, as is the coating used on multivitamins and other pills. Reactions to food additives, specific foods, cosmetic ingredients, and animal dander may be involved. Some people develop hives after taking a hot shower, bath, or Jacuzzi, while others develop them after being out in the sun, or exposed to cold wind or water.

Viral infections may cause hives, as can other infections. Many people are surprised to find that they develop hives after an exercise session. While you may search for an exact cause for your hives, remember that in more than half of the cases, an exact cause is never discovered.

What If You Do Nothing?

Hives generally will go away on their own within several hours.

Home Remedies

- **Try over-the-counter remedies.** Antihistamines are the mainstay of hive relief. The best way to relieve the itching and swelling of hives is to take an oral antihistamine such as Benadryl or Chlor-Trimeton. Remember, however, that most antihistamines will produce drowsiness, so follow package directions.
- **Ice them.** For temporary relief of itching and swelling of small hives, rub ice directly over the hives for several minutes. This will slow the release of itch-causing histamines.
- **Soak and soothe.** Add colloidal oatmeal to a tepid bath and soak in the water for 15 minutes to temporarily soothe your skin. Cold compresses and calamine lotion can also help relieve the itching.
- **Analyze your diet.** Temporarily remove or permanently eliminate foods from your diet that regularly cause hives to develop. Some of the prime offenders often include shellfish, dairy products, nuts, pork, strawberries, chocolate, tomatoes, and oranges.

Prevention

- **Find your allergen.** This may be easier said than done, and unfortunately, many people never find the exact cause of their problem because there are multiple trigger factors.

• **Avoid areas populated by bees.** If you are at risk for an allergic reaction to bee stings, you are a potential candidate for anaphylactic shock, a life-threatening situation that can lead to suffocation, loss of consciousness, and death. Be sure to carry a special anaphylaxis emergency kit with you at all times (see page 131).

When To Call Your Doctor

Contact your physician immediately if you develop hives in your throat and breathing becomes difficult. Also call your doctor immediately if you develop hives after taking a medication for some other condition—especially if you also experience dizziness, wheezing, and/or breathlessness. The next dose may bring on a more dangerous swelling in the throat and could lead to anaphylactic shock.

If you develop hives after being stung by a bee or other biting insect, contact your physician, who can determine if you are allergic to stings and can recommend appropriate treatment.

Also call your physician if the hives become uncomfortable, if the hives are severe, or if they do not respond to treatment after six weeks.

What Your Doctor Will Do

Your physician will analyze your diet, medication, and review any recent sickness. For chronic hives, laboratory studies may be performed. For itching hives, a prescription antihistamine may be given for rapid relief. Your physician may also prescribe corticosteroid drugs to treat severe hives.

For More Information

- American Academy of Allergy, Asthma & Immunology
- American Academy of Dermatology
- Asthma and Allergy Foundation of America

Impetigo

Symptoms

- A small group of red blisters that break, becoming a damp area which oozes fluid and pus. The blisters typically appear on the face, but may also be found on the legs and arms.
- Honey-colored crusted areas that form soon after the blisters break.

What Is It?

impetigo is a highly contagious bacterial *(Staphylococcus aureus* or *Streptococcus pyogenes)* infection that typically occurs after a cut, bite, or sting has been scratched and becomes infected. The infection most often occurs among infants and children, but can also affect adults.

What Causes It?

Physical contact with another person who has the infection is the usual cause. It is also possible to acquire the infection from dirty towels or clothing used by someone with impetigo.

What If You Do Nothing?

Impetigo rarely becomes a serious problem for adults and adolescents, but since it is highly contagious, it should be treated.

Home Remedies

If only a few small sores appear, the following self-care measures can help clear up impetigo.

• **Remove the scabs.** Dip a clean washcloth in warm water and gently rub the scabs until they come off. Then gently wash the entire area with soap and water.

• **Use an antimicrobial.** After washing, apply an over-the-counter antimicrobial ointment such as Betadine three times per day. Wash the affected area with soap and water before each application.

After applying the ointment, cover the entire area with gauze. Reapply the ointment three times daily for seven days. You can also ask your doctor about a more powerful prescription ointment called mupirocin (Bactroban).

• **Contain the infection.** To keep the bacteria from spreading, don't touch any part of your body after you have touched an area with impetigo. Wash your hands often. Also, do not let other people use your towel or washcloth.

Change bed linens daily, and wash them with bleach using the hot water cycle.

• **Take care when shaving.** Avoid shaving over facial impetigo sores. Germs may be harbored in razors, so be sure to change blades daily.

Prevention

• **Keep clean.** Wash your hands regularly with soap and water. Don't scratch insect bites or pick at scabs or skin irritations. Also, be careful not to share combs, towels, or hairbrushes. Wash all cuts and scrapes with soap and water.

When To Call Your Doctor

Contact your physician if you or your child develops an infection accompanied by a fever of 100°F or higher. Also contact your physician if impetigo covers an area greater than two inches in diameter, if the infection keeps spreading, or if the infection fails to improve significantly within three to four days despite home treatment efforts.

What Your Doctor Will Do

After an inspection of infected areas, an antibiotic cream or oral medication may be prescribed.

For More Information

• American Academy of Dermatology

Impotence (Erectile Dysfunction)

Symptoms

- Persistent difficulty achieving and maintaining an erection for a period long enough to engage in sexual intercourse.

What Is It?

Impotence is the inability to have and maintain an erection sufficient for sexual intercourse. Owing to the negative connotations and misconceptions surrounding the word impotence, the problem is now more commonly called erectile dysfunction, or simply, ED.

According to some experts, ED is the most widespread sexual problem among American men. Nearly all men experience occasional brief episodes of ED because of routine or temporary causes such as fatigue, emotional stress, or illness. For some people erectile problems become chronic. While ED may be connected to diminished sexual desire, in most cases it is not linked to libido (the emotional or psychic component of sexual desire), nor does it affect the ability to have an orgasm.

ED can occur at any age, but it's more common as men grow older. An estimated 5 percent of American men are impotent at age 40; among those over age 65, the proportion increases to 15 to 25 percent. However, the problem is not an inevitable consequence of aging. The causes are complex, combining physical and psychological factors. While the vast majority of men with ED can be helped, many experts believe that as many as 90 percent do not seek medical assistance because of fear of embarrassment and a belief that nothing can be done medically. This is unfortunate, because once underlying medical conditions and psychological factors are addressed, the frequency and duration of erections nearly always improves. Most men with erection problems don't have to live with them.

What Causes It?

Up until just a decade ago, more than 90 percent of all cases of ED were attributed to emotional causes. Now, however, experts estimate that only about 10 percent of cases are purely psychological in origin.

An erection depends upon many physical factors, including the blood supply and nerve tissue in the penis, as well as hormones. Circulatory problems, nerve disorders, heart disease, diabetes, and the side effects of certain medications (tranquilizers, blood pressure medications, antidepressants, and anti-inflammatory drugs) can contribute to impotence. Smoking, excessive use of alcohol, and low levels of the hormone testosterone may also come into play. Impotence can also result from prostate surgery or radiation treatment for cancer.

Psychological factors, including stress, depression, and performance anxiety, are now believed to play a limited role in cases of ED. When such factors are involved, it is mostly in men under age 40. But even in older men, emotions and sexual history may complicate physical factors.

What If You Do Nothing?

Frequent or chronic erectile problems are unlikely to improve without some form of intervention, particularly among men over the age of 50. There are now proven treatments for ED, but out of embarrassment and/or a lack of knowledge about medical solutions, many men choose to do nothing about their ED, which often leads to emotional distress.

347

Home Remedies

If you are having erectile problems, it's a good idea to seek a medical evaluation. If you have an underlying illness, early treatment may restore sexual potency.

Becoming more informed about sexual matters, undergoing treatment for physical problems, giving up smoking, and reducing excessive alcohol consumption can all contribute to restoring potency. If ED occurs only occasionally, some of the following measures may help address—and solve—the problem.

• **Exercise regularly.** In addition to improving blood flow, regular moderate exercise—for example, walking, swimming, jogging, bicycling, or resistance training—helps raise energy levels, boosts physical awareness, and stimulates sexuality. Be aware that bicycle riding carries with it a risk of crossbar injuries to the perineal nerves (located just behind the scrotum) that can lead to ED.

• **Limit alcohol intake.** ED among men in their late 40s and 50s is associated more often with excessive alcohol consumption than with any other single factor. There are plenty of other health-related reasons to avoid excessive drinking, so if it appears to be dampening your sex life, cut back or avoid alcohol altogether.

• **Reduce stress in your life.** Stress and other emotional difficulties can affect the brain and thereby decrease libido and the ability to achieve or maintain a suitable erection.

• **Stop smoking.** Smoking has not been found to be a direct cause of ED. However, research has found that when smoking is combined with other risk factors, such as heart disease, high blood pressure, and untreated arthritis, ED levels are consistent and extremely high.

• **Lose weight.** Obesity is not a direct cause of ED, but researchers know that being overweight is associated with the onset of diabetes and the buildup of fatty deposits on the interior walls of arteries, and both of these problems are certainly linked with ED.

• **Relieve your anxieties.** Not every sexual experience has to end with orgasm. Thinking that you must achieve a climax can make you anxious,

---

Medical Treatments for ED

▼

Several methods have been developed to treat impotence that is caused primarily by physical factors. If you decide to try any, talk to your doctor about starting with the least invasive—the oral prescription drug Viagra (sildenafil citrate). Viagra improves blood flow to the penis to allow an erection, and it is effective for most men: In one study, it relieved impotence in almost 70 percent of men. It may not be safe for some men with cardiovascular disease.

For these men, there are other treatment options for ED, though they are more invasive or cumbersome. One option is a penile suppository, which is inserted into the urethra 10 to 30 minutes before intercourse; a drug is dispensed that widens arteries in the penis, triggering an erection that lasts 30 to 60 minutes in about two thirds of men most of the time. The drug, called alprostadil, can also be administered by injection with an ultrathin needle into the base of the penis (which may produce infection or scarring as side effects).

A third option is a vacuum erection device (VED)—a pump that draws blood into the penis. It may seem awkward, but it has a very low failure rate and no serious side effects.

By contrast, a penile implant, consisting of a bendable rod or an inflatable cylinder connected to a tiny pump, has drawbacks that make it the least popular option. Not only does an implant require surgery, but implants may fail or become infected, and then must be removed. Be sure to get a second, or even third, opinion before getting an implant.

which can result in ED. Instead, you and your partner can agree to focus on caressing and kissing rather than having an orgasm. This may relieve performance anxiety.

Prevention
See the suggestions listed above.

When To Call Your Doctor
Contact your doctor if you are consistently unable to achieve or maintain an erection. Also contact your physician if new medications you are taking have caused a change in erectile function, or if work-related stress or other psychological factors are affecting your sexual abilities. (The side effect of many prescription drugs for depression, allergies, and heart disease is ED.) More than 200 medications currently on the market can seriously disrupt sexual performance.

What Your Doctor Will Do
The first thing your doctor should do is take a detailed medical and sexual history. If mild to moderate ED is diagnosed, your doctor may recommend a qualified urology specialist, who can perform tests to see if blood flow into the penis is adequate. The specialist may also check to see whether spinal cord problems might be involved

or if blood testosterone levels are low.

If your problem is largely psychological, your physician should counsel you or refer you and your partner to a therapist. (If you are awakening at night or in the morning with a full, firm erection, then the cause of the dysfunction is most likely psychological.) Sex therapy offers a cure rate of 60 to 80 percent for erectile problems caused by psychological causes. If counseling is in order, a referral from your doctor or from a psychologist is probably the best way to find a properly certified sex therapist, although some family practitioners may have training in sexual therapy.

If the problem is associated with medication you are taking, your doctor will talk with you about alternative medications that will not affect your ability to have an erection.

For impotence that cannot be treated by any other means, some medical solutions are available (see page 348). Be sure to try all nonsurgical options before considering a penile implant.

For More Information
- American Foundation for Urologic Disease
- American Urological Association
- National Kidney and Urologic Diseases Information Clearinghouse

Ingrown Toenail

Symptoms

■ Pain, tenderness, and red swollen skin around the margins of the toenail.
■ Pus (sign of infection).

What Is It?

An ingrown toenail is one of the most common foot afflictions, not to mention one of the most painful. The problem usually occurs on the big toe, with the sides or upper corners of the nail curling down and cutting into soft tissue, causing swelling and redness. Besides being painful, ingrown toenails can also lead to infection.

What Causes It?

Improper trimming of the toenail, and tight shoes, socks, or stockings that press the nail into the tissue, are the two major causes of ingrown toenails.

Trauma can also cause an ingrown toenail if you accidentally stub your toe or drop something on it. The impact can break the nail or force the nail into the nail bed, causing the toenail to become ingrown.

What If You Do Nothing?

If the problem goes untreated, the entire side of the nail can become embedded in the skin as the nail grows outward. Even without this complication, the condition can become quite painful, particularly if an infection develops. If the infection is severe, it can spread to the rest of the toe and even into the foot.

Home Remedies

• **Investigate the source.** If you have developed an ingrown toenail, try to determine the cause and then eliminate it.

• **Soak and pack.** Soak your toe in warm water for 15 to 25 minutes to soften the nail and drain out any inflamed material under the nail. If the nail is not extremely painful or infected, use clean tweezers to raise the nail and press a few strands of absorbent cotton or a piece of dental floss under the nail to keep it from further cutting the skin. Repeat this process daily, until the nail finally grows out past the nail fold.

• **Take pain relievers.** Take acetaminophen or nonprescription NSAIDs—aspirin, ibuprofen, or naproxen—as needed.

• **Don't cut in the middle.** Contrary to myth, making a V-shaped cut in the middle of your toenail won't make it grow toward the middle and thus won't prevent an ingrown toenail.

• **Consider changing your shoes.** If possible, switch to open shoes, shoes with a wider toe box, or sneakers while your nail is healing.

• **Be careful when you're on your feet.** Avoid running or other strenuous activities involving your feet while your toe heals.

Prevention

• **Trim your nails carefully.** When trimming toenails, follow these directions to keep them from becoming ingrown:

• **Cut the nail neatly.** Use heavy long-handled scissors or a nail clipper.

• **Don't tear.** Always trim the nail; never tear it away with your fingers.

• **Always trim the nail straight across.** The end of the nail should be square, not a half moon. Don't trim too close. Finish the edge with an emery board or nail file and clean the grooves with an orange stick.

• **Keep your feet clean and dry.** Daily attention to hygiene may help head off infection.

• **Wear comfortable shoes.** Shoes should be comfortable when you buy them. They should not rub, pinch, or bind the front of your feet in the area known as the toe box. Avoid high heels or tight-fitting shoes; these place abnormal pressure on your toes.

• **Protect your feet.** If you expect to be lifting heavy objects, be sure to wear sturdy shoes to protect your feet.

When To Call Your Doctor

Contact your physician if you suffer severe or increasing pain due to an ingrown toenail, if you cannot trim the nail, or if redness and swelling around the toe are accompanied by severe pain and/or a discharge. If you have diabetes, see a health professional for all foot problems.

What Your Doctor Will Do

Your physician will apply a local anesthetic and clean up the borders of your nail. Using a special tool, the physician may cut away the part of the nail growing into your flesh, instantly removing the pressure on the toe skin. Antibiotics may be prescribed, and daily soaking instructions will be recommended. Chemical or laser treatment may be needed to keep the nail from regrowing on that side.

For More Information

• American Podiatric Medical Association

Insomnia

Symptoms

- Difficulty falling asleep.
- Fragmented sleep—waking frequently during the night or waking earlier than desired.
- Fatigue, drowsiness, inability to concentrate, and mood shifts—all of which can result from insomnia.

What Is It?

An estimated 20 to 40 percent of all adults complain about insomnia—a general term that refers to difficulty falling or staying asleep. Insomnia is not really a disorder but a symptom with many causes. For example, temporary insomnia can be caused by jet lag, which upsets the body's biological clock, or by some specific, stressful situation like a divorce or change in job. Once these situations have been resolved, sleep returns to normal.

How alert and refreshed you feel, rather than how many hours of sleep you get, is a better sign of whether insomnia is a problem for you. Not everyone needs eight hours—the number often used as the benchmark for a good night's sleep. Some people feel well rested after only six hours of sleep a night—though research suggests that others who think they are doing fine on five or six hours would actually benefit from more sleep.

Age is a key factor in assessing insomnia. It's a sign of troubled sleep if a child or young adult has difficulty falling asleep or wakes up repeatedly. But in about 80 percent of people over the age of 60, sleep becomes more fragmented. People in this age group tend to wake up more often (and for longer periods) during the night, and earlier in the morning, with generally less deep sleep and more light sleep.

What Causes It?

Causes range from psychological and medical conditions to environmental factors like noise and room temperature. Medical problems linked to insomnia include depression, Parkinson's disease, urinary frequency, kidney failure, stomach ulcers, congestive heart failure, and asthma.

Insomnia can also be caused by specific sleep-related disorders, especially sleep apnea (a breathing malfunction that may interrupt sleep hundreds of times a night) and restless legs syndrome (an ailment marked by burning, prickling, and aching sensations in the legs at night).

Many medications can also disturb sleep—both prescription and nonprescription drugs, including over-the-counter sleep aids that are used improperly. Habitually using alcohol at night to induce sleep is linked to sleep interruptions and waking up feeling unrefreshed.

Many experts are convinced that in the majority of cases the original cause becomes secondary; instead, the insomnia persists because of behavioral factors that reinforce it, such as excessive time in bed, drug dependency, and napping. Also, the harder you try to fall asleep, the more anxious you become, which makes success all the more difficult.

What If You Do Nothing?

Occasional insomnia is nothing to worry about. And remember that there are wide individual differences in how much sleep people need to feel refreshed and alert. Some need nine or ten hours, others only six.

Also, don't worry that you have to "make up" every hour of lost sleep. One good night will usually repair the fatigue.

Home Remedies

If you have an underlying disorder, or if insomnia is the result of medication you are taking, you need to consult your doctor. But when there is no underlying cause, rather than reach for sleeping medications, try the following self-help measures. Several studies have shown that in many, if not most, instances of insomnia, such steps are more effective at treating the problem than prescription sleeping pills.

• **Don't drink alcohol before bedtime—and don't smoke.** Alcohol can disrupt sleep patterns and make insomnia worse. Nicotine makes you wakeful, too.

• **Avoid eating a heavy meal in the evening, particularly at bedtime.** Don't drink large amounts of liquids before retiring.

• **Eliminate caffeinated beverages, except in the morning or early afternoon**.

• **Unless you're older, try to avoid daytime naps.** It's all right to use a nap for catching up on occasional lost sleep, but naps shouldn't become a substitute for sleep, even if you're tired. Naps probably can be beneficial for older people whose sleep is fragmented—and certainly it's better to nap than to rely on sleeping pills.

• **Spend an hour or more relaxing before you retire.** Read, listen to music, watch TV, or take a warm bath.

• **Go to bed and get up on a regular schedule.** Get into bed at the appointed time even if you're not tired, and arise for the day on schedule no matter how much you haven't slept .

• **If you can't sleep, get up and do something.** If you've gotten into bed and after 20 minutes still can't sleep, get up and read or do some other quiet activity for a short time. However, don't bring work into bed with you; go somewhere else to do it. If you wake up in the middle of the night and can't fall asleep, try reading for a bit. Counting sheep (or flowers or whatever appeals to you) or reconstructing a happy event or narrative in your mind may also lull you to sleep.

• **Try to correct any stress that's keeping you awake.** If your sleeplessness arises from worry or grief, it may be hard to return to your regular sleeping schedule until you've done something to relieve the problem. If you can't do anything about the situation right away on your own, try confiding in a friend, joining a support group, or finding a qualified counselor.

Prevention

The measures described above will also help prevent insomnia. In addition, try to avoid taking sleeping pills. Not only can they produce daytime drowsiness and other side effects, but they lose their effectiveness if you take them every night.

353

Supplements That Promise Sleep
▼

Melatonin and valerian are two popular dietary supplements promoted as sleeping aids. Melatonin is actually a human hormone that seems to play a role in synchronizing circadian rhythms, and it is now widely marketed in health-food stores as a jet lag cure. There is evidence that melatonin helps people fall asleep faster, but it may not help them stay asleep. Like many prescription sleeping pills, it can also produce drowsiness the next day.

Similarly, a dose of valerian before retiring seems to reduce the time it takes to fall asleep. But it has yet to be shown in a well-designed trial that valerian improves the quality of sleep. And there is no method for standardizing doses of either of these substances.

If you decide to try valerian or melatonin, treat it like any sleeping medication—don't combine it with alcohol, tranquilizers, or barbiturates or take it for more than a few days.

When To Call Your Doctor

If chronic insomnia persists for more than a week or two after you have tried self-help measures, you should see a doctor or visit a sleep disorders clinic for a professional evaluation. Stress, an underlying medical condition, or a medication you are taking may be the cause of your sleep problem.

In addition, while increasingly fragmented sleep in many older people may be normal, it can also result from a specific sleep disorder such as sleep apnea, a potentially dangerous condition that requires medical diagnosis and treatment.

What Your Doctor Will Do

Your doctor will ask you about your sleeping routine and possible sources of stress in your life, and about medications or other substances (including alcohol) that might interfere with your sleep.

For short-term treatment, your doctor may prescribe a sleeping medication (see below). For elusive or persistent sleep disorders, you may be referred to a sleep disorders clinic, where a detailed evaluation of your sleeping and waking patterns can be obtained. Treatment may entail behavioral strategies such as relaxation training and restricting your sleeping time, and medication may also be recommended. Many major medical centers have such clinics; evaluation and treatment is often covered by health insurance.

For More Information

- American Academy of Sleep Medicine
- National Sleep Foundation

Medications for Insomnia

▼

Prescription sleeping pills—known as hypnotics—and other sleeping aids are among the most frequently taken medications in the United States. But how effective and safe are they—and what, if anything, should you take?

Over-the-counter sleeping pills. Most such drugs are antihistamines (just like many hay fever remedies, which may also induce drowsiness) and at the suggested dosage are probably harmless. It won't hurt to try them for occasional sleeplessness—they may work for a night or two—but studies show that they quickly lose their effectiveness.

Benzodiazepines (tranquilizers). Marketed under such names as Valium, Xanax, Dalmane, Restoril, and Halcion, these prescription-only antianxiety drugs act as sedatives and are widely prescribed for people suffering from insomnia. They are less likely than barbiturates (which are no longer used as sleeping pills) to be lethal in overdose or to create physical dependency. But long-term users of benzodiazepines do experience some dependency and will usually have withdrawal symptoms when they stop taking the drugs. Many side effects have been reported for all benzodiazepines—disorientation, confusion, "hangover" the next day, blurred vision, nightmares, and daytime depression.

Nonbenzodiazepines. Two newer medications, zolpidem (Ambien) and zaleplon (Sonata), belong to a class of medicines that have a shorter "half-life" than benzodiazepines—meaning the new drugs quickly dissipate in the body and the natural sleep cycle takes over. They are also are far less likely to produce next-day grogginess and other side effects associated with benzodiazepines.

If, for some reason, you and your doctor decide you need one of these drugs, try a low dose first, and don't take it for more than three or four nights in a row. Also, never combine it with alcohol. Your goal should be to reestablish normal sleeping habits without any drugs.

Irritable Bowel Syndrome

Symptoms

Symptoms vary from person to person and are often triggered by a particular food, stressful event, or bout of depression. The most common symptoms include:

- Moderate to severe abdominal cramps, pain, belching, and bloating. Pain is often relieved by a bowel movement.
- Constipation or diarrhea, sometimes bouts of both lasting for days, weeks, or months. Diarrhea, which occurs immediately after awakening in the morning or right after eating, sometimes has white mucus in it.
- Gas.
- A feeling that the bowels have not completely emptied.
- Nausea.
- A worsening of symptoms after eating a big meal, during menstrual periods, or when you are under stress.

What Is It?

Irritable bowel syndrome—also known as spastic colon, mucous colitis, nervous bowel, or simply IBS—is a common abdominal complaint, not a disease, and is probably the least understood but most common reason for visits to gastroenterologists. IBS usually develops in late adolescence or early adulthood and affects three times as many women as men. It's estimated 15 to 20 percent of the adult population in the United States has IBS to some degree, but only about half seek medical attention. It is also a major cause of absenteeism from work.

IBS does not require surgery, is not caused by any known physical abnormality, and is not the same thing as inflammatory bowel disease—a much more serious disorder that may produce ulceration of the intestinal wall. It's still a chronic disorder and is more difficult to cope with than the occasional bout of diarrhea or nervous stomach most people experience from time to time.

IBS is linked with digestion. After partly digested food leaves the stomach, it is moved along through the small and large intestine by a gentle synchronized wavelike contraction and relaxation (peristalsis) of the intestinal wall muscles. In IBS sufferers, the muscles go into spasm for unknown reasons, causing residue to move either too quickly (causing diarrhea) or too slowly (leading to constipation).

When you have IBS, you have no fever or bleeding, and you can't think of anything you've eaten or done to have brought on these gastrointestinal problems. Mysteriously, the diarrhea may give way to constipation, but you may still have abdominal pain and a lot of gas. The condition may correct itself and then return suddenly when you least expect or want it—for example, before an important occasion about which you already feel tense.

What Causes It?

No one is sure what causes IBS. Some doctors attribute it to an as-yet-undetermined physiological disorder, and emotional stress and anxiety are certainly associated with it—though there is no evidence that irritable bowel syndrome itself is a psychological disorder. Rather, stress, anxiety, and/or depression may be a result of having the disease. Current research is being conducted to investigate the possibility of a lower pain threshold for people with IBS, which then triggers the disorder.

Certain foods may cause sudden flare-ups. Common triggers include high-fat foods, such as bacon, vegetable oils, and margarine, as well

355

as gas-producing foods like beans and broccoli. Lactose intolerance—the inability to digest lactose (milk sugar), caused by an enzyme deficiency—can also produce the same symptoms.

What If You Do Nothing?

It's estimated that half of the people with IBS don't seek medical attention and choose instead to live with their "nervous stomach" because their IBS symptoms aren't that bothersome.

Although the disorder can cause much discomfort, it does not lead to serious disease. If you can learn to control the chronic flare-ups and relieve the often bothersome symptoms of IBS yourself, you can probably keep the condition from interfering with your everyday activities.

Home Remedies

The challenge of IBS comes in trying to treat symptoms without having a clear idea of the causes. IBS usually responds to one or a combination of self-care measures, but it may take some time and trial-and-error to notice results. Depending on your specific symptoms, your doctor can suggest a number of treatments that may help (see What Your Doctor Can Do).

• **Watch your diet.** Though no food or category of foods is a known or even suspected culprit, there's no harm in watching your diet, because certain foods may make your symptoms worse. Keep a food diary and if certain foods seem to set off symptoms, try avoiding them for a while. Don't eliminate them unless they cause problems more than once.

• **Add fiber.** A high-fiber diet (fruits, vegetables, and whole grains, taken with plenty of fluids) is known to promote normal bowel function as well as to reduce bloating and other symptoms of IBS. Some people find that the constipation of IBS

can be managed by including wheat or oat bran in their daily diet. But bran may not work for some people, and in others it can actually worsen symptoms. If you try bran, start with one teaspoon daily, and slowly increase the amount—up to 9 or 10 teaspoons spread over the course of the day. Be sure to drink plenty of water any time you consume bran.

• **Eat smaller, more frequent meals.** Four to six smaller meals eaten throughout the day may be easier to digest than three large ones.

• **Try eliminating gas-forming foods.** If your predominant symptom is gas, eliminating beans, peas, lentils, broccoli, cauliflower, onions, cucumbers, and leafy vegetables may help. If symptoms improve, gradually reintroduce these foods and see what happens.

• **Don't delay.** If you feel the urge to move your bowels, do so. Any delay may contribute to becoming constipated.

• **Exercise regularly.** This can help reduce stress, stimulate the digestive process, and relieve symptoms.

• **Avoid sorbitol.** This artificial sweetener found in candy, gum, and other sugarless products may cause diarrhea.

• **Don't abuse laxatives.** You may become dependent on them and this can eventually weaken your intestines.

• **Don't assume that you're lactose-intolerant.** Many people with IBS diagnose themselves as lactose-intolerant and stop eating dairy products. But in fact, lactose intolerance doesn't put you at increased risk for IBS. In any case, it's easy to find out if you are lactose-intolerant with a simple breath test ordered by your doctor.

• **Reduce daily stress.** If you think psychological problems or emotional stress are the chief cause of your symptoms, try relaxation techniques like yoga or meditation. Exercise may also help. You may benefit from talking with a counselor. Or you and your doctor may decide to try antidepressants.

Prevention

There is no known way to prevent irritable bowel syndrome. Nonetheless, by learning how to minimize occasional episodes of IBS with modifications in your diet and with stress management, you may help reduce incidences of the ailment.

When To Call Your Doctor

If you frequently suffer from the symptoms of irritable bowel syndrome and they interfere with your normal activities, you should make an appointment with your doctor. A physician can also check for more serious disorders such as gallstones, diverticular disorders, bowel diseases like colon cancer, and ulcers. Your doctor will also want to make sure you are not suffering from bacterial or other infections. Some medication you are taking could also be the culprit.

What Your Doctor Will Do

A detailed patient history will be taken, and a physical examination will be performed. A stool sample may be required to eliminate the possibility of a more serious ailment or infection. A sigmoidoscopy may also be performed. For this procedure a slender, flexible, lighted telescope is inserted into the colon to check the walls of the bowel and rule out inflammatory bowel disease. If necessary, a barium enema or colonoscopy will be performed to further examine your colon.

Once other ailments are precluded and IBS is suspected, your doctor may quiz you about your diet and advise against certain foods. For painful attacks, medications may be prescribed that address the major symptoms: for example, sedatives can help calm anxiety, antidiarrheal medication may be helpful for watery stool, bulk laxatives (high in fiber) can relieve constipation, and antispasmodic drugs may be recommended to reduce the pain of cramping. There are also drugs that partially block the parasympathetic nervous system to decrease cramping; Robinul and Bentyl are the two most commonly prescribed for this purpose. When it comes to treatment, though, irritable bowel syndrome is poorly understood, and the therapies currently available are not known to have lasting success.

357

For More Information

- International Foundation for Functional Gastrointestinal Disorders
- Intestinal Disease Foundation
- National Digestive Disease Information Clearinghouse

Jet Lag

Symptoms

- Extreme fatigue.
- Daytime drowsiness.
- Insomnia.
- Irritability.
- Gastrointestinal disturbances.
- Headaches.
- Decreased mental alertness, athletic ability, and strength.

What Is It?

Jet lag can be defined as a disorientation in sleep patterns and disturbance of normal body rhythms experienced after flying across several times zones. As anybody who has ever suffered from jet lag knows, it's no fun. If you travel between the United States and Europe, for example, your body functions for a day or longer according to the clock you left behind, depending upon how many time zones you've crossed. This has the effect of putting you out of synch with your new sleeping, waking, and eating schedule.

Westward journeys are less stressful than eastward: it's easier for a person's biological clock to set itself back than forward. Thus, adding a couple of hours to the day may not disrupt sleep patterns, but losing a couple of hours almost always does. Flying north to south has no effect.

Jet lag affects not only travelers but shift workers, people in the military, and others who keep odd hours—in particular, flight crews who are repeatedly subjected to this kind of stress and yet must turn in high-level performances.

What Causes It?

The phenomenon of jet lag is linked to the fact that human beings operate according to an inborn circadian rhythm (circadian is derived from *circa* and *dies,* the Latin words for "around the day"). This inner body clock regulates practically all physiological functions, including hormone levels. Scientists now believe that the hormone melatonin, which is triggered in the brain by darkness and suppressed by light, influences these daily rhythms.

Researchers believe that jet lag is caused by upsetting the body's circadian rhythms that regulate sleep. Traveling from one time zone to another, the particular rhythm that the body has for daytime and nighttime is suddenly thrown out of synch by the new daytime and nighttime. The more time zones that have been crossed, the worse the jet lag.

Moreover, the circadian day is actually 25 hours, not 24—and thus it is easier to lengthen our days than to shorten them. This explains why we may feel all right after a plane flight westward across two or three time zones, but can feel exhausted after flying the same distance eastward.

What If You Do Nothing?

Jet lag symptoms will clear by themselves in a matter of hours or days, depending on your age, distance traveled, and how well you prepared for your trip.

Home Remedies

• **Change your sleep time.** If it's possible, try going to bed and getting up an hour earlier for three days before a long eastward trip. For a westward trip, go to bed and get up an hour later. Of course, not everybody can change sleep time so easily. You don't want to have jet lag before you even depart.

• **When traveling, try not to do anything that's likely to cause sleep problems.** On the plane, avoid or go easy on alcohol and caffeine, which can disrupt sleep patterns. Drink plenty of fluids to prevent the unpleasant effects of dehydration. Heavy meals can interfere with a good night's sleep, so it's smart to avoid them. Though the jet lag diet (alternating large high-protein meals with lighter ones for three days before traveling) has had its advocates, there's little evidence that any diet can forestall jet lag.

• **Prepare for resting on board.** On a night flight, try a sleep mask, wrap-around dark glasses, a neck pillow, a blanket, earplugs, or any device that may help you get a little more shut-eye. Stretch out if you're on an uncrowded flight.

• **Make quick adjustments.** When you reach the new time zone, try to adjust as quickly as possible to new eating and sleeping times, even if it means staying up when you're tired or eating breakfast when your body says it's dinnertime.

• **Try to expose yourself to daylight after a long trip.** This doesn't mean you should get sunburned, of course. But exposure to light may be the means for resetting a lagging or confused biological clock. Indeed, small studies have shown that proper exposure to light can reset circadian rhythms by as much as 12 hours, backward or forward.

According to a report in the *Journal of Biological Rhythms,* some studies of light exposure as a cure for jet lag have had encouraging results, but others have not. Maybe it will help some people, but so far nobody knows what the optimal times or optimal amounts of light might be. (One report in *Nature* found that low light, not necessarily sunlight, is probably the synchronizer of our biological clocks.)

• **Reschedule meetings.** Jet lag can wipe out even the best-laid business plans. If you have any business meetings at your new destination, try to schedule them 24 to 48 hours after you arrive there, so you'll be acclimated to your new environment, bright and alert.

• **Melatonin may—or may not—help.** Though thousands of travelers use melatonin supplements to combat jet lag, the evidence is still out on whether the supplements are at all effective. For one thing, it's difficult to measure and compare jet lag symptoms. Moreover, like other dietary supplements sold in the United States, dosages of melatonin are not standardized and the purity of products isn't regulated, so different brands can vary considerably. (You can find more information on melatonin on page 631.)

Prevention

Jet lag cannot be entirely prevented, but you can reduce its severity with the home remedies outlined above.

When To Call Your Doctor

Jet lag symptoms don't ordinarily require medical attention. However, if you travel frequently and jet lag consistently interferes with your sleep and causes chronic fatigue or other problems, consider consulting a specialist who deals in circadian rhythm disturbances.

For More Information

• National Sleep Foundation

Jock Itch

Symptoms

■ Itchy, scaly, red patches on the genitals, groin, buttocks, and inner thighs.
■ Pus-filled blisters.

What Is It?

Jock itch, or tinea cruris, is a common fungal infection that affects the groin area of men. Women rarely contract jock itch.

What Causes It?

Moisture is the critical factor with jock itch because it allows fungi to thrive. Since people wear clothing for most of the day, the groin is usually moist and dark, creating a perfect breeding ground for the microscopic fungi that live on the skin to multiply and cause trouble. People who exercise regularly and wear an athletic supporter (jock strap) are susceptible to jock itch if they don't bathe after exercise or don't wash the undergarments they wear for exercise before working out again.

Jock itch may also develop on people who perspire heavily, or when overweight individuals walk and their thighs rub against each other.

What If You Do Nothing?

If jock itch isn't treated, the infection tends to become chronic and can quickly spread to the buttocks and trunk.

Home Remedies

• **Daily cleansing.** Use plain water and clean the area daily. To avoid irritation, do not put soap on the rash.
• **Use antifungal cream.** Twice daily, apply a light layer of an antifungal compound (such as clotrimazole), available without a prescription in any pharmacy. You should see results in three to five days. Continue to use the medication an additional one to two weeks after the rash has cleared up to make sure the fungus doesn't return.

If you have recurrent bouts of jock itch, use the medication for several weeks after the rash has disappeared.

Prevention

• **Stress dryness.** Use cornstarch-free powder after bathing to keep the groin region dry. (Cornstarch can encourage fungus growth.)
• **Stress cleanliness.** Wear clean workout gear every time you exercise.
• **Lose weight.** If jock itch is caused by your inner thighs rubbing against each other, begin a program of regular exercise to reduce your weight and therefore the size of your thighs.

When To Call Your Doctor

Contact your physician if there is no improvement within a week after trying the self-help measures outlined above.

What Your Doctor Will Do

After taking a careful case history, your physician will scrape off scales or pustules and examine them under a microscope. A more careful hygienic regimen and/or a powerful oral antifungal medication may be recommended.

For More Information

• American Academy of Dermatology

Kidney Stones

Symptoms

A kidney stone is usually asymptomatic until it is dislodged from the kidney and migrates into the ureter, a narrow tube connecting the kidney to the bladder. When that occurs, the primary symptom is pain, which typically begins in the back, just below the ribs. Waves of sharp pain occur every few minutes, and over the first few hours (or days) the pain will follow the path of the stone through the ureter. Men may experience pain in the testes and penis as the stone passes. Once the stone is passed, the pain stops. The following symptoms may also occur.

- Bouts of nausea and/or vomiting.
- An urge to urinate but an inability to pass normal amounts at one time.
- Blood in the urine.
- Fever and chills (if a concomitant infection is present).

What Is It?

Kidney stones (which doctors refer to as renal calculi) are one of the most common disorders of the urinary tract—and also one of the most painful. The stones themselves are small, solid lumps composed of minerals and crystallized salts that separate from urine and build up in the urinary tract.

Stones can form anywhere in the urinary tract but typically develop on the inner surfaces of one or both kidneys over a period of time. Once formed, the stones sometimes travel into and through the ureter—and it is this passage through the ureter that can cause the intense pain.

Stones vary greatly in size—as minuscule as a grain of sand to as large as a golf ball. Tiny stones may cause no symptoms when they pass through the ureter. But when a larger stone (whole or broken into pieces) moves out of the kidney and enters the ureter, it produces pain (renal colic) caused by the ureter contracting in order to squeeze the stone and urine through the tract. This singular distress—marked by frequent episodes of crescendoing pain—continues until the stone eventually makes its way along the ureter to the bladder, at the front of the body.

It's estimated that 1 in 10 adults in industrialized countries will develop kidney stones at least once in their lives, with men outnumbering women four to one. White people are more prone to kidney stones than African-Americans, and most stone attacks affect people over the age of 30. At least half of those suffering a kidney stone attack will have a recurrence within five years if there is no medical intervention.

What Causes It?

All kinds of waste products are filtered out of the blood by the kidneys and excreted in urine. Stones are mixtures of mineral substances—chiefly calcium, magnesium, and phosphate, along with oxalic acid (mostly produced in the body, but also found in some foods), uric acid (an end product of metabolism from nucleic acids in animal products), and, rarely, the amino acid cystine. If these substances accumulate without enough fluid to carry them away, stones may form in susceptible people.

The most common stones are almost pure calcium oxalate; others are formed from a combination of calcium oxalate and calcium phosphate. A core has to form first, and then crystallization can begin. But why stones crystallize in some people and not others isn't clear. A family history of stones has something to do with it. Also, certain disorders are linked to an increased risk. Recurrent urinary tract infections may create a chemical environment conducive to kidney stone development. High uric acid levels, sometimes associated with symptoms of gout, may also lead to the formation of uric acid stones. People with inflammatory bowel disease are also at increased risk of developing kidney stones. Bacterial infections in the kidney account for about 10 percent of cases.

Living in a hot climate may also be a factor. It's thought that hot weather causes increased sweat loss and reduced urine production; thus the urine contains a higher concentration of stone-producing mineral content.

What If You Do Nothing?

Most stones are small, and are passed out in the urine without notice or pain. Large kidney stones may stay in the kidney and cause no problems. When a large stone does enter the ureter, it can cause pain that may last up to 72 hours or more and that sends many people to the emergency room. The pain stops once the stone passes into the bladder. While you may need medication to combat the pain, a stone usually passes without causing any complications.

If a large stone can't pass, however, it can block the flow of urine and cause eventual kidney damage. To prevent this, the stone may need to be removed.

Home Remedies

Since 90 percent of all kidney stones are less than 5 millimeters in diameter, self-treatment typically consists of measures to promote their natural passage out of the body. But if the stone is large, you will probably need to contact your doctor to prescribe medication for pain relief, since over-the-counter pain relievers are rarely helpful. In addition, take the following measures.

• **Flush the stone out.** Drink at least three quarts of water a day to flush the small stone into the bladder. Drink even more when it's hot outside. To be sure you are drinking enough, your urine should be almost colorless.

• **Walk.** If possible, go for a walk. This movement may speed up the passage of the stone.

• **Trap the stone.** The key to effective treatment and prevention is diagnosing the kind of stone you form. Each time you urinate, do so through a piece of gauze, cheesecloth, or strainer with a fine mesh to trap the stone when it passes. Give it to your physician for analysis to find its cause, which will help with more specific treatment. Most stones are made of complex salts of sodium or calcium, but stones composed of uric acid indicate you have a treatable metabolic disorder.

Prevention

Since the exact cause of kidney stone formation is not known, avoiding them is practically impossible. If you have a history of stones, talk to your doctor about the preventive measures you should take. Kidney stones are a complex problem, and no single piece of advice is appropriate for all sufferers. The following measures may help prevent or reduce painful incidences in many people predisposed to this malady.

• **Drink two to three quarts of water daily.** Make sure your urine is pale yellow or almost colorless. Increase your intake of fluid in hot and humid weather.

• **You probably don't have to avoid calcium.** A few stone formers do reduce their risk of recurrence when they cut down on calcium. But recent research suggests that getting the recommended amounts of calcium may actually help prevent stones in some people. This is good news, because eliminating calcium can harm bones and general health. And a low calcium intake may lead to higher oxalate levels. At the same time, don't consume excessive amounts of calcium. Because treatment of stones should be individualized, you should consult your physician about this and other dietary measures if you have a history of stones,

- **Consider limiting oxalate-rich foods.** It's well known that some stone formers reduce their likelihood of a recurrence by cutting back on certain foods. If you have too much oxalate in your urine (determined by a urine test), your physician may recommend that you lower your intake of spinach, rhubarb, black pepper, cheese, peanut butter, nuts, beer, tea, and chocolate. These contain oxalic acid—salts that bind with calcium ions and promote stone formation.

- **Consider reducing your intake of animal protein.** Some stones are specifically linked to certain kinds of protein in the diet, which leads to too much uric acid and calcium stone formation. Again, consult your physician. Changing the diet to help the body utilize calcium more efficiently or taking medicine to reduce uric acid may help prevent this type of stone.

- **Keep your sodium intake low.** A low-sodium diet—less than 2,400 mg a day—can reduce calcium in the urine. Avoid fast foods, as well as canned soups and other processed foods.

- **Avoid crash weight-loss diets.** Some fad diets, high-protein diets, and other plans for quick weight loss can cause a condition called ketonuria, which may increase uric acid production and thus tend to promote kidney stones. Habitual use of stimulant laxatives is also particularly bad for stone formers.

- **Treat underlying urinary tract infections.** People with chronic urinary tract infection often develop stones composed of struvite, which is a combination of magnesium, ammonium, and phosphate. Preventing urinary tract infection will prevent these struvite stones.

- **Talk to your doctor about drug therapy.** One type of medication, called thiazides, can keep calcium out of the urine. Allopurinol, another drug, can keep uric acid from forming. Medication to alter the acidity of urine may also be prescribed.

When To Call Your Doctor

Contact your physician if you have symptoms of a kidney stone—especially if you have never had a stone. Also, contact your physician if you have blood in your urine, you begin to have a stinging or burning sensation when urinating, you have a frequent urge to urinate, or you develop a fever along with these symptoms.

What Your Doctor Will Do

Following a thorough history and physical examination, your physician may take specimens for urinalysis and blood studies to rule out kidney disease and to help diagnose kidney stone presence. The urinary tract may be x-rayed, or an ultrasound scan may be used to monitor the stones. Your doctor may prescribe pain medication or antibiotics and send you home until the stone passes. If a stone is blocking the ureter, the physician may recommend ultrasound shock wave treatment (lithotripsy, a non-invasive procedure) or laser surgery (an invasive procedure) to break the stone into smaller pieces.

After removal of a stone, your doctor will assist you in developing a program to prevent further stone formation.

For More Information

- National Kidney and Urologic Diseases Information Clearinghouse

Knee Injuries

Symptoms

- Pain, swelling, tenderness, and/or discomfort in your knee.
- Difficulty moving your knee joint; possibly a cracking sound when you bend your knee.
- An inability to straighten your leg.
- Discomfort or pain while walking or running.

What Is It?

Your knees are put under a lot of stress, whether you're running, playing basketball, dancing, or simply cleaning house. Just climbing stairs can put pressure on each knee equal to four times your body weight. The result is that an estimated 50 million Americans suffer at some point from knee pain or injuries. At least one out of every four sports injuries involves the knee. In addition, for millions, the knee is affected by chronic, age-associated ailments such as arthritis.

The knee is the largest joint in the body. Functioning simultaneously as a hinge, lever, and shock absorber, the knee is the key to your ability to stand up, walk, climb, and kick. Yet it depends almost entirely on soft tissue—ligaments and tendons—for stability. Because of its complexity and the great forces to which it is routinely subjected, the knee is susceptible to a host of injuries, which can take weeks, if not months, to heal, even with proper rehabilitation. Here are the most common problems and their causes.

• **Sprain (torn ligament).** The knee connects the thigh bone (femur) to the shin bone (tibia), and the only things holding these two large bones together are four ligaments, which are strong but not very flexible. If these are stretched beyond a certain point, one or more of the ligaments can be sprained.

The sprains can range in severity from minor tears to complete ruptures, in which the ligament tears away from the bone and snaps (often with an ominous popping sound). Most seriously, the anterior cruciate ligament can rupture when you twist the knee in a fall, typically while downhill skiing. Other ligaments in the knee can be injured by a violent blow to the knee or sudden wrenching or twisting, as in hockey or soccer.

• **Runner's knee (chondromalacia patella).** This overuse injury is due to degeneration of the shock-absorbing cartilage (called the meniscus) under the kneecap and covering the ends of the femur and tibia. It is characterized by dull, aching pain under or around the kneecap and is usually most noticeable when you are descending stairs or hills. Nearly 30 percent of runners eventually develop this disorder. Skiers, cyclists, soccer players, and people who participate in high-impact aerobics classes are also susceptible to it.

• **Tendinitis.** The tendons above or below the kneecap (patella) can become inflamed, usually through overuse—for instance, from dancing, hiking, or cycling. One frequent complaint is jumper's knee, a form of tendinitis that afflicts basketball and volleyball players and weight lifters in particular.

• **Iliotibial band syndrome.** If the tendon that runs down the outer side of the knee is tight, repetitive motion (as in running or cycling) can cause the tendon to rub against the bony area at the end of the thigh bone and become irritated.

• **Torn cartilage.** This injury to the cartilage in the knee typically occurs when you twist the joint while putting weight on it. Over the years frequent squatting can weaken the knee to the point where something as minor as getting out of the car can tear the cartilage.

• **Arthritis.** The knee is a common site for osteoarthritis, which involves the degeneration of cartilage at the joint and subsequent inflammation. It is the result of normal wear and tear over the years.

What Causes It?

Most overuse injuries such as runner's knee and tendinitis (which are the problems most amenable to self-care) are linked to the muscles of the thigh, particularly the quadriceps. This large four-part muscle group on the front of the thigh, along with the hamstrings (located behind the thigh), provides the muscular support system for the knee. In addition to helping power movement, the quadriceps also stabilizes and guides the kneecap in its groove at the end of the thighbone. Weak or inflexible quadriceps may lead to improper tracking of the kneecap and instability of the supportive tendons, contributing to both runner's knee and jumper's knee.

What If You Do Nothing?

Any persistent knee pain (beyond mild discomfort) shouldn't be ignored, since it may lead to chronic pain, stiffness, and swelling. Moreover, the surest way to speed recovery is to treat a recurring ache or pain right away, even if you're able to continue the exercise or activity associated with it. If you feel pain, at the very least stop and rest.

Knee Strengtheners

Staying fit through physical conditioning is the best way to avoid the stiffness and muscle weakness that can contribute to an injury to your knees. The three basic exercises shown here will help restore and maintain knee strength.

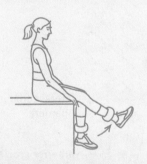

Knee extensions. Sit on a desk or counter and hold onto the edge. Slowly straighten one leg, extending the knee completely. Hold for five seconds, then lower it slowly. Repeat 10 times, then switch legs. You can also do this with a light weight.

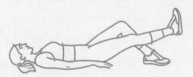

Straight leg lifts. Lie on your back and bend one knee, keeping your foot on the floor. Slowly lift the straight leg about 12 inches off the floor; keep hips and lower back on the floor. Hold for five seconds, then lower it slowly. Repeat 10 times, then switch legs. You can also do this with a light weight around your ankle. Avoid this exercise if you have back problems.

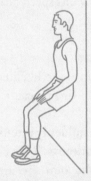

Wall sit. Lean your back against a wall and squat until your upper legs are at a 45-degree angle to the wall. Hold for one minute, while tightening your buttocks. This exercise strengthens your quadriceps and gluteal muscles. Be sure to keep your knees aligned with your feet.

Bear in mind, though, that rest alone isn't likely to eliminate the cause of the problem. To avoid reinjury, you should not only actively treat the problem but take preventive measures such as those described below.

Home Remedies

For knee pain stemming from overuse injuries like runner's knee or tendinitis, you can reduce aches and pains and speed recovery with the following measures.

• **RICE the injury site.** Stopping any activity and resting is the first step in RICE, an acronym for rest, ice, compression, and elevation. Apply ice as soon as possible (see page 453 for icing tips). Use an elastic wrap for compression, and then keep your leg elevated to reduce pain and swelling.

• **Take over-the-counter pain relievers.** Nonprescription NSAIDs (aspirin, ibuprofen, and naproxen) will help reduce pain and swelling, though they won't speed healing; acetaminophen will help with pain.

Prevention

You can reduce the likelihood of a knee injury with the following precautions and conditioning exercises.

• **Beware of suddenly intensifying or lengthening your workouts.** This can create additional friction in the joint and increase the risk of an overuse injury.

• **Run on the right surface.** Avoid running on very hard, very soft, or hilly terrain, all of which put added stress on knee joints.

• **Check your exercise shoes.** If they are worn or don't fit well, they may put your knees at risk.

• **Check your feet.** The knee sometimes pays the price for foot abnormalities (such as flat feet), overpronation (the feet roll inward too much), or poor leg alignment (such as knock-knees), which can put greater stress on the joint. An orthotic device—a custom-made arch support—may help correct some foot or alignment problems. Make sure your knee is always aligned with your foot while exercising.

• **Minimize knee stress when cycling.** To accomplish this, set your seat to the proper height and don't pedal in high gears.

To gauge seat height, check your knee position at the bottom of the stroke: your knee should be only slightly bent.

Cycling in high gear—which increases tension on the pedals—also increases the pressure on your knees. Stay in low gears, which means faster, easier revolutions on the pedals. You'll get more aerobic exercise with less stress on your knees.

• **Stretch your leg muscles before and after exercise.** Maintaining flexibility allows you to attain

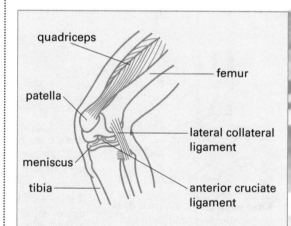

The intricate arrangement of components in the knee include the kneecap (patella), which protects the front of the knee joint, and the meniscus, a pad of cartilage under the kneecap that absorbs shock. Ligaments along the sides and back reinforce the joint and connect it to the leg bones (the tibia and femur).

maximum range of motion for your knees.

• **Strengthen your leg muscles.** It's especially important to condition the quadriceps. If you are a runner or walker, your quadriceps are probably much weaker than your hamstrings, so it's a good idea to alternate cycling (an excellent way to strengthen the quadriceps) with running. Walking up stairs or hills also helps strengthen these muscles.

• **Be kind to your knees.** If you have knee problems, hills and stairs can put too much stress on your knees, so you need to take it easy on these inclines or avoid them if they cause you pain. Also don't kneel or do full squats, which can greatly increase stress on the knee. And avoid "knee-unfriendly" sports such as football, running on concrete, soccer, squash, tennis, and skiing.

When To Call Your Doctor

Call your doctor immediately if you hear a popping sound when you injure your knee. Also call if your knee is swollen, stiff, and painful, or if you have any knee discomfort that interferes with your everyday activities.

What Your Doctor Will Do

After a careful physical examination to determine the cause of the knee pain, discomfort and/or instability, your doctor may recommend magnetic resonance imaging (MRI) to help make a more definitive diagnosis. For chronic or severe overuse injuries, physical therapy may be advised. For acute injuries such as a torn ligament, damage to the meniscus, or loose bodies floating in the knee cavity (which cause the knee to "lock"), surgery may be recommended. Much knee surgery is now done by arthroscopy, in which tiny optical and surgical instruments are inserted through small incisions. Because it avoids opening up the knee, arthroscopic surgery substantially reduces the time a patient needs to stay in the hospital and can also speed up recovery time

For More Information

• American Academy of Orthopaedic Surgeons
• National Institute of Arthritis and Musculoskeletal and Skin Diseases Information Clearinghouse

Knock-Knees

Symptoms

■ Knees that touch when you are standing (but ankles don't touch).

What Is It?

As a child matures and begins to walk, knock-knees can develop as he or she tries to maintain balance on weakened legs. When a knock-kneed child stands up, his or her knees touch each other, but the ankles do not. As the legs gain strength and start to mature, they generally straighten out and the condition disappears. Knock-knees may continue after the age of three or four, but by age five most legs straighten.

For adults, being slightly knock-kneed is a normal variation in alignment; many adults are somewhat knock-kneed. This is rarely a problem, and surgery or physical therapy is seldom undertaken to correct it. But severe knock-knees in adults can lead to problems: in a study of army recruits, for example, those with severe knock-knees were more likely to be injured in the intense activities of basic training.

What Causes It?

Knock-knees are common, often developing as part of the childhood growth process.

What If You Do Nothing?

In children the legs usually will straighten out as the child grows. However, if a case of knock-knees is severe or if it is still present at the age of five, medical attention is needed to prevent permanent problems.

Home Remedies

• **In children, wait and watch.** Knock-knees are common among children, and in most cases the legs will eventually straighten out. Medical treatment is seldom required.

• **Use orthotics.** For adults with severe knock-knees, orthotics—foot supports, made of foam, leather, plastic, fiberglass, graphite, or some combination, that fit in your shoes—can reduce the increased risk of exercise-related injury by correcting the structural imbalance.

Prevention

In most cases knock-knees can't be prevented.

When To Call Your Doctor

Contact your physician if a child's legs don't straighten out or if a knock-kneed appearance develops in a child six years of age or older. Adults with knock-knees should consult an orthopedist or podiatrist if the condition is so pronounced that it causes pain or interferes with movement.

What Your Doctor Will Do

A careful examination will be performed to rule out conditions that tend to cause knock-knees such as juvenile arthritis and rickets. X-rays may be taken to determine the severity of the condition. For severe knock-knees your physician may recommend braces to be worn at night and special shoes.

Surgery may be a corrective option after the age of 10 for girls and 11 for boys if the braces and shoes aren't able to straighten the legs. For adults the doctor may fit the patient with orthotic devices for the shoes to keep the feet from rolling inward excessively (pronating).

For More Information

• American Academy of Pediatrics

Lactose Intolerance

Symptoms

- Abdominal pain, cramps, and bloating within a few hours of consuming milk or milk products.
- Excessive gas.
- Diarrhea.
- "Grumbling" abdomen and bowel.

What Is It?

Lactose is a sugar found in the milk of humans and other mammals. The ability to digest milk occurs because lactase, an enzyme that's produced in the small intestine, breaks down lactose into two simple sugars, which are then used by the body. When there is an insufficient amount of lactase, unabsorbed lactose moves to the colon where the bacteria cause it to ferment, leading to bloating and gastrointestinal discomfort.

Virtually all human infants depend on milk for survival and digest the nutrients in it, including lactose. But early in childhood, most people start producing less lactase and consequently cannot digest more than a small amount of milk. In these people, who are termed lactose intolerants or lactose maldigesters, drinking milk (especially drinking it in the absence of food) can produce uncomfortable symptoms—such as gas, stomach cramps, and diarrhea—within 30 minutes to two hours. (A few people, including infants, may be allergic to the protein in milk, but that's not lactose intolerance.)

There are degrees of tolerance and intolerance for milk; in fact, not all lactose intolerants have to give up milk consumption. Although the ability (or loss of ability) to digest lactose is an inherited trait, drinking habits also depend on custom and preference.

Many Americans who believe they are lactose intolerant are mistaken: The prevalence of lactose intolerance is overestimated, according to a review in the *Journal of the American Dietetic Association*. But the extent of the problem varies widely among different racial and ethnic groups. Only 15 percent of white Americans are affected by some degree of lactose intolerance; the proportion of African-Americans affected is significantly higher at 60 to 80 percent. The problem occurs with varying severity in about 90 percent of Asian-Americans, 65 to 100 percent of Native Americans, and about 50 percent of Mexican-Americans. Up to 75 percent of adults worldwide may be affected.

What Causes It?

While some infants are born with the ailment, lactose intolerance usually develops in childhood beginning at three to five years of age. The production of lactase then steadily decreases until adolescence and remains at low levels throughout life. The ailment can also develop later in life because of chronic digestive disorders such as irritable bowel syndrome, Crohn's disease, or celiac disease. In both adults and children, a temporary form of lactose intolerance may occur owing to illness (such as gastroenteritis) or side effects of medication (such as antibiotics or NSAIDs like ibuprofen) that affect the intestinal lining and stop lactase production for a few weeks.

What If You Do Nothing?

Lactose intolerance is not a health risk. But if you are truly lactose intolerant, symptoms can occur whenever you consume milk and other dairy products high in lactose. (However, the amount that you consume makes a difference in how much discomfort you experience.)

Home Remedies

Lactose intolerance cannot be cured, but once

lactase deficiency has been diagnosed, there are strategies you can use to avoid or control its symptoms. The most obvious step is to eliminate all dairy products from your diet. However, this is not only difficult for most people but also often unnecessary. Instead, first follow the measures below (including turning to nondairy sources of calcium in your diet if you do reduce your consumption of dairy products).

• **Be sure you are truly lactose-intolerant.** Bloating, flatulence, and stomach cramps aren't always caused by lactose intolerance; it's not a condition that develops suddenly.

You can do a simple test for lactose intolerance at home. Drink two glasses of skim milk on an empty stomach and see if symptoms such as bloating, gas, and diarrhea occur during the next three to four hours; this suggests lactase deficiency is probably the cause. If so, repeat the test using lactase-treated milk. If you then experience no symptoms, you probably have lactose intolerance. But if you have chronic gastrointestinal discomfort, see a doctor for further testing.

• **Consume small portions of milk and milk products.** You can eliminate dairy products from your diet, but not only is that difficult, it often isn't necessary. While many people can't tolerate large portions of dairy products, they have no problems with smaller servings. In fact, studies have shown that many true lactose maldigesters (classified as such by laboratory tests) can consume moderate amounts of milk and dairy products without symptoms, particularly if the milk is part of a meal. Whole milk causes fewer problems than skim, because its fat slows the rate of stomach emptying.

• **Eat dairy products along with food.** This will slow the emptying of the food from the stomach into the intestine, where lactose is digested, and decrease or eliminate symptoms. This strategy allows more time for the available lactase to act upon the lactose-containing food.

• **Try active-culture yogurts.** Fermented milk products such as yogurt with active cultures are usually easier to digest than milk. Most yogurt is low in lactose anyway, and the bacteria in it help break down what milk sugar there is. But as much

Lactose-Intolerant Children

▼

Lactose intolerance, an inability to break down and absorb sugars found in milk and milk products, is common in infants. A few are born lactase-deficient, but at ages three to five, the incidence increases and about 75 percent of all children worldwide have decreased levels of lactase; an estimated 15 percent of all American school children are thought to be lactose-intolerant. When milk or milk products are ingested by lactose-intolerant children, symptoms develop within eight hours and include explosive watery diarrhea, abdominal distention, and flatulence.

To find out if your child is lactose-intolerant, a physician will first perform a physical examination. The child may then be asked to consume specific foods and the subsequent stool will be analyzed for unabsorbed substances.

Once lactose intolerance has been confirmed, the physician will recommend a reduction of milk and milk products in the child's diet, along with some of the measures described on these pages—including giving the child soy protein formula, milk products with added lactase, or special lactase supplements that you add to the milk products to aid in digestion.

You can also try adding yogurt and cheese to the child's diet. These fermented foods are lactose-reduced and consequently may have no negative effects, while offering an excellent source of calcium, vitamin B_2 vitamin D, and protein.

as 30 to 70 percent of the lactose originally in the milk may remain in the yogurt. For lower lactose, look for yogurt that states "Live and Active Cultures" on the label—or just experiment until you find a brand that agrees with you.

• **Cheese is all right.** There should be no problems with cheese, especially hard, aged cheeses like Swiss, Parmesan, and Cheddar, since most lactose is removed along with the whey when the cheese is made.

• **Give soy milk a try.** This product made from soybeans may be poured on cereal, used for cooking, and consumed as a beverage by infants and adults. Acidophilus milk or buttermilk may not be any better for people sensitive to lactose; the degree of fermentation is variable, and so lactose content also varies.

• **Consider using lactose-reduced and lactase products.** If the other strategies don't work for you, try lactose-reduced milk, which is available in most markets. This type of milk contains about 70 percent less lactose and tastes sweeter than regular milk. You can also buy lactase tablets or liquid in drugstores or grocery stores and add them to the milk yourself; five drops per quart can break down over 70 percent of the milk sugar in about 24 hours (for greater reduction, let the treated milk stand for 48 to 72 hours). If you add drops to commercially treated milk, you can eliminate nearly all the lactose.

You can also swallow lactase tablets or capsules just before you consume a milk product, but that's usually much less effective than adding drops to the milk itself.

• **Read labels carefully.** The Food and Drug Administration (FDA) doesn't require food companies to label their products "lactose free." Limit or avoid foods containing milk (nonfat milk as well), lactose, whey, dry milk solids, and milk curds.

Lactose may be added to prepared and processed foods, including baked goods, breakfast foods, luncheon meats, salad dressings, and soups. Some artificial sweeteners may also contain lactose.

• **Increase the calcium in your diet.** If you eliminate or drastically cut back on dairy foods, you must compensate for the lack of calcium and other essential nutrients. (For a list of additional calcium sources, see pages 23 and 24.)

Prevention

There is no way known to prevent the condition of lactose intolerance, but the self-care approaches discussed above can prevent symptoms.

When To Call Your Doctor

Contact your physician if self-treatment measures don't provide relief for you (or for your child) and you continue to experience gastrointestinal discomfort. For infants, call your doctor if your baby fails to gain weight or refuses food or formula. If the infant is on a doctor-recommended milk-free diet, be sure to contact the doctor if the diet does not relieve symptoms.

What Your Doctor Will Do

After taking a history, your physician may order a breath hydrogen test to confirm lactose intolerance. Based on the findings, your physician will make recommendations to reduce or eliminate certain foods.

For More Information

- American Academy of Allergy, Asthma & Immunology
- Asthma and Allergy Foundation of America
- National Digestive Diseases Information Clearinghouse

Laryngitis

Symptoms

- Hoarseness (ranging from mild to severe loss of voice) and increasing difficulty in producing normal sound.
- Scratchy throat, sometimes a sore throat, and a dry cough.
- A frequent need to clear the throat.
- Fever (occasionally).

What Is It?

Laryngitis is an inflammation of the larynx, or voice box—the part of the windpipe containing your vocal cords. To create speech, the vocal cords open and close. When they become swollen, the sounds become distorted or faint, or the ability to produce any sound may be lost.

What Causes It?

Acute laryngitis usually is caused by an infection, mainly viral and very occasionally bacterial. The other principal cause is overusing your voice. As the noise around you increases, you tend to shout over it and thus alter the quality of your voice. In addition, more people these days work in jobs requiring heavy telephone use. Trying to sound authoritative, people sometimes unconsciously pitch their voices lower than is really comfortable. Your vocal cords react just like any other tissue strained by overuse—they resist, causing inflammation that results in hoarseness. Teachers, singers, public speakers, and others who use their voices a great deal or must speak loudly are at risk.

The causes of chronic laryngitis include smoking; exposure to fumes, chemicals, dust, or other irritants; mouth breathing; frequent upper respiratory problems such as allergies, sinusitis, or bronchitis; and heartburn, or GERD (gastroesophageal reflux disease).

What If You Do Nothing?

Acute viral laryngitis is rarely serious and usually clears up within a few days. Persistent hoarseness, therefore, is a sign that something else may be the problem—a more serious bacterial infection, small benign growths (known as nodes or polyps) on your vocal cords, or a malignancy.

Home Remedies

• **Rest the voice.** If you are hoarse or if your voice is squeaky, it's important to rest your vocal cords. This means that for two or three days you should speak only when it is absolutely necessary.

• **Don't whisper.** That puts more pressure on your vocal cords than speaking softly. Instead, speak in a soft, breathy voice. Also, try not to clear your throat—swallow a few times or cough gently.

• **Keep your vocal cords well lubricated.** First, increase your fluid intake—drink at least 8 to 10 glasses of water daily, which will help thin the mucus around the vocal cords. In addition, increase the humidity in your surroundings to 40 to 50 percent relative humidity. (If you use a humidifier or vaporizer, be sure to clean the device and any filters regularly).

Avoid alcohol and cigarettes, which dry out the vocal cords. A glycerin throat lozenge may be helpful, but avoid cold pills containing decongestants or antihistamines, which may dry out your throat.

Prevention

Here are some of the rules professional entertainers follow to protect their voices.

• **Be aware of voice pitch.** Don't pitch your voice unnaturally high or low.

• **Avoid talking over background noise.** Wait until the hubbub subsides so you don't have to raise your voice unnecessarily.

• **Get some phone support.** If you have to be on the telephone for long periods, a phone rest or a headset may lessen the strain on muscles in your face, throat, and neck, thus relieving some vocal cord tension. Try to rest your voice between telephone calls.

When To Call Your Doctor

If hoarseness, voice change, or discomfort lasts more than two weeks (and you don't have a cold or allergy), check with your doctor—a bacterial infection could be present. Your doctor may also refer you to an otolaryngologist, a throat specialist who may prescribe medication.

For children: Call a doctor immediately if hoarseness is accompanied by difficulty swallowing or breathing, gasping for air, drooling, and/or high fever. This may signal a serious bacterial infection—epiglottitis—that requires prompt medical attention.

What Your Doctor Will Do

Using a special mirror, your doctor can examine the larynx to check for redness, inflammation, possible bleeding, and other signs of laryngitis. If a bacterial infection is diagnosed, the physician may prescribe a course of antibiotics. For severe or chronic hoarseness, your doctor may refer you to a throat specialist to determine if nodes or polyps or other lesions are causing the trouble.

Many chronic voice problems can be solved with the help of a speech-language therapist. Such therapists are usually certified by the American Speech-Language-Hearing Association and licensed by the state; your throat specialist should be able to refer you to one.

When all other measures fail, surgical treatment for polyps may be an option.

For More Information

- American Academy of Otolaryngology-Head and Neck Surgery
- American Speech-Language-Hearing Association

Lice

Symptoms

Head lice

- Extremely itchy scalp.
- Presence of nits (eggs) on hair near the scalp.
- Presence of tiny insects, usually at the base of the neck or behind the ears.
- Enlarged lymph glands at the back of the scalp (severe cases.

Pubic lice (crabs)

- Uncomfortable itching and scratching in the groin area, often intense.
- Presence of tiny nits in the crotch area.

Body lice

- Red bites on the skin, particularly the buttocks and trunk.
- The presence of nits in clothing, particularly the underwear. When they need to feed, lice leave clothing for the body.

What Is It?

Lice are flat, wingless parasites the size of a sesame seed that live on the body and cause skin inflammation by biting and by sucking blood. Three types of lice affect humans. Head lice *(Pediculus humanus* var. *capitis)* live on and suck blood from the scalp, causing severe itching. These lice pose a major public health problem in the United States, especially with school-age children. It's estimated that about 16,000 new cases of head lice—the most common lice infestation—occur every day.

Pubic lice *(Phthirus pubis),* also known as crabs because of their crablike shape, live in the pubic area. These tiny parasites are passed through sexual contact or lice-infested bedding or clothing. They attach firmly to the hair follicles in the pubic area and feed off human blood, causing an unrelenting itch.

Body lice *(Pediculus humanus* var. *corporis)* live in the seams of clothing, usually on people who don't change their clothes often enough. The lice attach to the body to feed, typically causing lesions on the shoulders, buttocks, and abdomen.

What Causes It?

Lice are often transmitted in overcrowded or unhygienic environments. But even good hygiene doesn't ensure protection against head lice infestation. Head lice seem to prefer feeding on clean scalps, for example. An outbreak can start merely by one infected individual coming into close contact with others or sharing with them a hat, hairbrush, comb, or clothing.

Female lice lay approximately six eggs daily. These eggs, or nits, are tiny translucent specks that look like dandruff and cling firmly to hair shafts. They hatch in 8 to 10 days and reach maturity in 18 days. To survive, lice pierce the skin and feed off human blood. This leads to skin inflammation and intense itching for the victim.

What If You Do Nothing?

If lice are not treated, they can spread quickly. The itching can also be intolerable.

Home Remedies

• **Apply a medicated shampoo or lotion—with care.** For head lice and pubic lice, several over-the-counter products are available—among them Nix (which contains permethrin) and Rid and A-200 (which contain insecticides called pyrethrins). If your child has asthma or allergies, consult your physician before using any lice shampoos.

It's important to follow label directions precisely. Do not repeat a treatment simply because itching doesn't stop immediately. The itching from extant lesions may persist for a few days after treatment, even though the lice have been eliminated.

• **Remove the nits.** Nits glue themselves to hair shafts so securely that ordinary washing and brushing will not remove them. A fine-tooth comb must be used to pull out the dead nits from the hair. To loosen them from the hair shafts, use a mixture of half vinegar and half rubbing alcohol and massage it into the hair before combing.

Part the hair in one-inch sections and begin removing all nits. Most are found in the hair behind the ears and at the base of the neck. It's a time-consuming task, but you must be thorough; nits are not always killed with topical medications, and any survivors that aren't removed may reach maturity and start the reinfestation.

• **Clean thoroughly.** Wash all sheets, blankets, and pillowcases in extremely hot, soapy water. Dry at high heat for 20 minutes or longer. If possible, iron all clothing and linen. For clothing or toys that can't be washed, put them in plastic bags and seal them securely for three weeks. Thoroughly vacuum all rugs, furniture, and mattresses; don't forget your car.

• **Sanitize.** Soak all hairbrushes and combs in rubbing alcohol for 10 minutes.

• **Keep checking for lice.** Everyone living in the home should be inspected daily for lice. Anyone who develops scalp sores or itching should receive a dose of medicated shampoo, even if lice or nits are not seen in the scalp.

Prevention

• **Don't share combs or hairbrushes.** Sharing grooming items is a quick way to transmit lice.

• **Wash often.** Bathe and shampoo daily, and put clothes in the laundry after a day of wear.

• **Inspect children regularly.** Check especially for head lice. The nape of the neck and behind the ears are prime spots for nits and lice.

• **Notify others.** If you or your child have lice, notify parents of school children that lice have been found. Adults should also inform sexual partners and co-workers.

• **Avoid sex with infected people.** Lice are quickly spread by sexual contact—and while the use of a condom can prevent sexually transmitted diseases caused by bacteria or viruses, it won't prevent lice from spreading.

• **Be alert to other sources of infection.** Lice are often found in car seats, headrests, theater and airline seats, and stereo headphones.

When To Call Your Doctor

Contact your physician if itching interferes with sleep, if the rash has not cleared up one week after treatment, if new nits appear in the hair or eyebrows, or if sores appear infected. Also contact your physician if you or your sexual partner has symptoms of lice.

If an over-the-counter treatments fail to eradicate lice, talk to your doctor.

What Your Doctor Will Do

After a close examination your doctor will remove any lice from the eye area. If nonprescription products don't eliminate the lice, your doctor may recommend a prescription product. Prescription shampoos containing two powerful insecticides— lindane (usually sold under the name Kwell) and malalthion (brand name: Ovide)—are effective, but are also highly toxic, especially for young children. Directions for using them must be followed very carefully.

For More Information

• American Academy of Dermatology

Lyme Disease

Symptoms

Lyme disease is hard to diagnose because its symptoms can vary greatly from person to person. Early symptoms are usually mild and often overlooked. No single symptom appears in all cases, and there's no predictable time frame or sequence of symptoms.

- Red raised bull's-eye rash at the site of the tick bite that expands over several days and can last for weeks (about 75 percent of cases).
- Flulike symptoms, including chills, fever, headache, lethargy, and muscle pain.
- Stiff neck.
- Inflammation in large joints, especially the knees, if the disease is untreated and allowed to progress over months.

What Is It?

Lyme disease is a tickborne infection that can cause flulike symptoms and joint inflammation. First identified as a form of arthritis in 1975 in the woodlands around Lyme, Connecticut (hence its name), cases are known to have occurred in most states, predominantly in the Northeast and upper Midwest, and on the Pacific coast. The ticks tend to thrive in those areas where suburban lawns meet woodlands. Deer, whose population has grown in the East in recent years, help spread infected ticks to new areas. Migratory birds have brought Lyme disease to the South. Even city dwellers may develop Lyme disease. All it takes is a weekend excursion to the countryside for you—or your dog—to meet up with an infected tick.

Although this disease has received the most publicity in the United States, it has existed in Europe at least since the beginning of the twentieth century (though its assorted symptoms were often not attributed to a single disorder). Lyme disease is found today on all continents except Antarctica. While the peak periods may vary from region to region, this is primarily a summer disease. You're most likely to be bitten by a deer tick between May and September, when immature ticks, or nymphs, are active. That's also when people are outdoors the most. The risk of being bitten is lower in April, October, and November, and lowest from December through March.

Even if you're certain you've been bitten by a deer tick and that the tick was infected, it's unlikely that you'll develop Lyme disease. The chance of infection is very low (less than 1 percent), even in areas where Lyme disease is prevalent. A tick has to feed on a human for 24 to 48 hours before the disease can be transmitted.

What Causes It?

Lyme disease, caused by a corkscrew-shaped bacterium known as a spirochete (*Borrelia burgdorferi*), is transmitted primarily via certain species of deer ticks. These are smaller than the common dog tick, though it is often difficult to tell the two types of ticks apart. A deer tick, before it becomes engorged with blood, looks like a mole or a blood blister. While the eight-legged adults are less than one-tenth of an inch long, the nymphs are about the size of a pinhead, and the larvae are nearly invisible. The male is black and the female is dark red and black. When filled with blood, the tick becomes gray and increases in size three- to fivefold.

Although deer can become infected, in the eastern United States white-footed field mice serve as the main host for both the bacteria and the young ticks. The adult ticks usually feed and mate on deer, then drop off to lay eggs. These in turn hatch into minuscule larvae, which become infected by feeding on white-footed mice. The larvae molt and become infected nymphs. (In the West, the culprit is the closely related black-legged tick, also carried by wood rats.)

Both nymphs and adult ticks feed on a variety of animals. The nymphs are the chief threat to humans—about 70 to 90 percent of all cases are caused by nymph bites. Adult ticks are generally less of a threat to humans because they're large enough to be seen and removed before they transfer the bacteria.

The nymphs and adults wait on low vegetation in wooded areas and adjacent grasslands and transfer themselves to whatever brushes by; they don't fly or jump. Dogs and cats can carry the ticks to your home and property. (Horses and household pets can get Lyme disease but cannot transmit it to humans; rather, they bring ticks close to humans.)

Ticks prefer dark, moist areas on people, typically the back of the knees, the groin area, and under the arms.

What If You Do Nothing?

Without treatment, Lyme disease runs its course, which can last anywhere from a few weeks to years. However, ignoring or delaying treatment can lead to chronic arthritis or heart problems, as well as skin and nervous system abnormalities that may be difficult to treat successfully. It's clearly better to get yourself properly diagnosed and attend to the ailment as early as possible.

A New Vaccine For Lyme Disease

▼

A three-part injectable vaccine called LYMErix was approved by the FDA as the first Lyme disease vaccine. Vaccination costs $50 to $100. The most common side effect appears to be a little redness and soreness at the injection site.

Who should be vaccinated:
- Anybody aged 15 and over who lives where Lyme disease is common, particularly those who hike or spend time outdoors in wooded areas, should consider it. Risk of infection is highest in the Northeast, upper Midwest, and in a few counties of northern California.
- If you aren't sure about the incidence in your area, call your local health department and ask. There's no need to be vaccinated, obviously, if you are not in danger.
- Those who've already had Lyme disease should consider vaccination. Unlike such infections as chicken pox, Lyme disease does not confer immunity. You can get it twice. But you should not be vaccinated if you still have any acute or chronic symptoms of the disease.

There are some drawbacks:
- Children under 15 were not included in clinical trials, and no one knows if the vaccine is safe and effective for them. Pregnant women should not be vaccinated.
- There have been reports of severe adverse reactions, including cases of arthritis and even Lyme disease, in some people. The FDA is investigating the reports; in the meantime, ask your doctor about possible reactions.
- You need two shots a month apart, and then a third one a year later. It may be hard to remember to get the third shot, but it significantly boosts immunity.
- No one knows how long immunity lasts and when a booster shot might be needed. Future research may clarify this.
- For those over 60, the efficacy of the vaccine declines.
- If you've been vaccinated, this can affect the accuracy of certain blood tests for infectious diseases. Tell your health-care provider before taking tests.

Home Remedies

There are no home remedies for Lyme disease. If you think that you've been bitten by a tick in an area where Lyme disease is present or that you've developed symptoms, you should see a physician for diagnosis and treatment.

Prevention

There is now a three-shot vaccine for Lyme disease that has been shown to prevent disease in anywhere from 68 to 92 percent of people—though without the third shot, this drops to about 50 percent (see page 377). But it is still better to avoid being exposed to the disease, since the vaccine is not perfect. (The vaccine does not protect against other tickborne diseases.)

To lessen your risk of contracting Lyme disease, take these precautions:

• **Wear long trousers and a long-sleeved shirt with buttoned cuffs.** Tuck the shirt into your pants and your pants into your socks or boots. Wear hard-finished, light-colored fabrics. It's easier to spot ticks on white or tan trousers than on black ones.

• **Apply insect repellent to your pants, socks, and shoes.** Repellents containing the substance called DEET are approved for warding off ticks. Be careful if you put any on your skin, since DEET can be hazardous if too much of it is absorbed through skin, which can happen if you apply high concentrations.

Most states permit the sale of permethrin, which is an excellent tick repellent. Permethrin should be applied only to clothing.

• **Avoid tick habitats.** Try to stay near the center of trails in overgrown country.

• **Check occasionally for ticks when you're in underbrush or wooded areas.** Later do a thorough check of your entire body. Have someone look at your back and head if possible. Remove ticks promptly and properly (see page 137). The sooner you remove a tick, the better your chance of avoiding infection. If an infected tick is on you for less than 24 hours, you probably won't develop the disease.

• **Check your pets.** When pets come indoors, inspect them closely for ticks.

When To Call Your Doctor

Contact your physician if you think you may have contracted Lyme disease. You will also need to see your doctor if you want to be vaccinated against Lyme disease.

What Your Doctor Will Do

Lyme disease is difficult to diagnose because its symptoms mimic other illnesses. And while some people get a rash after they are infected, as many as 25 percent do not. Current tests remain poor at best. The results of the tests vary from lab to lab, and the meaning of the results is not standardized. This greatly compounds the problems of diagnosis. Newer, more reliable tests are in the experimental stage, but it will probably be several years before they are available for clinical use.

Lyme disease is treatable and almost always curable, especially in its early stage. If you have—or had—the characteristic rash, your doctor will probably prescribe a course of antibiotics. Similarly, if you live in an area with a high incidence of the disease and find a tick on you that your doctor or the local health department identifies as a deer tick, or a western black-legged tick if you live in California, you'll probably be put on antibiotics.

For More Information

• American Lyme Disease Foundation

Menopausal Problems

Symptoms

For many women the only sign of menopause is the end of menstrual periods, preceded by irregular periods and changes in the amount of blood flow. Other common signs or symptoms that some women experience include the following.

- Hot flashes, or hot flushes, often accompanied by profuse sweating.
- Vaginal dryness.
- Stress incontinence.
- Mood swings, depression, and sleep problems are reported by some women, but there is widespread disagreement as to whether emotional changes and sleep disturbances are the result of menopause.

What Is It?

Menopause is part of a gradual biological process (except when surgically induced), culminating in the cessation of ovulation and menstruation. In the three- to five-year period preceding a woman's final menstrual period (known as the perimenopause), her ovaries produce less and less estrogen and progesterone, the two major female hormones. (Together with two other female hormones, known as follicle-stimulating hormone and luteinizing hormone, estrogen and progesterone orchestrate ovulation, menstruation, and if fertilization occurs, pregnancy.) During perimenopause, menstrual periods may become irregular or unusually light or heavy. Ovulation (the monthly release of an egg) becomes less frequent and eventually stops.

The cessation of menstruation usually occurs at approximately age 50. Menopause is considered complete when a woman has been without a period for a year. Some women reach this point in their early 40s, others not until their late 50s.

Neither is abnormal. (If a woman ceases to menstruate before the age of 40, it's not considered true menopause, but premature ovarian failure, though the results are the same.)

Although menopause is clearly associated with a number of physiological symptoms, it's a myth that menopause causes clinical depression or psychosis. Some women do feel angry and depressed, of course, and do experience mood swings. Those suffering from night sweats and other troublesome symptoms may be irritable from lack of sleep. At midlife, too, women may be coping with professional and marital problems, may be dealing with adolescents, or may be assuming responsibility for the care of grandchildren or older relatives. All this might contribute to depression. But the influence of hormone deficiencies on emotions is a matter of debate. A number of studies suggest that women with young children are more likely to be depressed than menopausal women.

When it comes to health, more important than the immediate symptoms of menopause are its long-term consequences. Today, once a woman enters menopause, she can expect to live almost another 30 years—years that can be productive and rewarding. Yet once her supply of estrogen decreases markedly, her risk of two serious diseases increases dramatically. One of these is heart disease. Before menopause, few women die of heart attacks. After menopause, women begin to catch up with men in rates of heart disease; by age 75, rates become similar. At age 65 the same number of women die of heart disease as of cancer, and after age 75, heart disease is the chief cause of death among women.

Postmenopausal women also find themselves at increasing risk of osteoporosis, the bone-thinning disorder that can eventually result in disabling fractures. Women begin life with less bone mass than men, and after menopause, bone loss among women is more rapid than it is among men. That is why, after age 65, so many women suffer from osteoporosis.

Women need to be aware of these increased risks and to take steps—ideally, well before menopause—to prevent them.

What Causes It?

Natural menopause is a normal biological shift that probably starts in a woman's mid- to late 30s, when estrogen and progesterone levels begin a very gradual decline—a process that accelerates at some point after age 40. (Estrogen production does not completely stop. The ovaries still produce a little, as do fat cells and the adrenal glands.)

Women who have never had children tend to reach menopause earlier. Ethnicity, marital status, genetics, and geography don't seem to influence menopause. Smokers, however, experience menopause, on average, two years earlier than nonsmokers, though no one understands why.

Women who have hysterectomies (surgical removal of the uterus) experience an abrupt cessation of menstruation, though their ovaries continue to produce hormones. If their ovaries have also been removed, they experience an abrupt menopause, which may cause more-severe symptoms than a naturally occurring one.

What If You Do Nothing?

Menopause is a natural transition in a woman's life, not a medical condition or a health problem. But estrogen and progesterone play many roles in a woman's body, affecting many tissues, including the breasts, skin, vagina, bones, blood vessels, and digestive system, in addition to the reproductive organs. When production of these impor-

tant hormones declines, many changes, both short- and long-term, are to be expected. However, menopausal symptoms vary considerably from one woman to another. Many women have occasional and/or mild symptoms that are largely tolerable without any sort of intervention. Other women experience symptoms that are so severe that medical advice or treatment is required (though symptoms usually diminish over time).

About 75 percent of American women experience hot flashes—sudden feelings of intense heat, accompanied by a flushed face and, often, sweating, and followed by a clammy feeling. Sometimes an aura precedes the flash—you sense that you're going to have one. Heart rate increases, and your body temperature fluctuates. All this is caused by a shortage of estrogen, which is somehow involved in regulating body temperature (though no one understands how).

By day, hot flashes can be embarrassing and disconcerting, and they can result in sweat-soaked clothing. By night, hot flashes or night sweats (hot flashes accompanied by sudden sweating) can disrupt sleep. A woman may awaken several times a night in sweat-soaked sheets and feel exhausted the next day.

But even in one woman, hot flashes vary in intensity, frequency, and the span over which they occur. Because estrogen production fluctuates as it diminishes, hot flashes can come and go. Some women have them for a month and never again. It's also possible to have hot flashes for months, then have them disappear for months, only to recur. But hot flashes do subside over time: only 20 percent of women experience them four years after menopause.

Another common consequence of menopause is vaginal dryness—a reduction in vaginal lubrication (usually accompanied by thinning of the vaginal walls) that may lead to pain during sexual intercourse. This, rather than the decline in estrogen, is a primary reason for reduced sexual desire in menopause. A decline in testosterone levels also plays a role.

The decline in estrogen can cause the cells lining the urinary tract to thin and the muscles that control urine flow to weaken. Consequently, some women experience urinary incontinence. Some women are also more prone to urinary tract infections because of changes in urinary tract mucosa and vaginal bacteria.

Home Remedies

If hot flashes are disrupting your life, you should certainly see a doctor. Hormone replacement therapy (HRT) can put a stop to hot flashes and night sweats, and can correct vaginal dryness. However, it isn't appropriate for everyone (see page 382).

Medical science knows little about nondrug or dietary remedies for hot flashes, vaginal dryness, and other menopausal symptoms. The herb black cohosh is promoted as a menopausal remedy, but its effectiveness is questionable and can also have side effects (see page 613). The following self-care measures may prove helpful and they are certainly safe.

• **Dress in layers.** Start with a porous fabric like cotton next to your skin. Avoid woolens. If a flash starts, take off the top layer. Try drinking a glass of cold water or juice if a flash is beginning.

• **Sleep comfortably.** Sleep on cotton sheets, and keep your bedroom cool. Layer your sheets and blankets so that you can remove a layer if you have a flash.

• **Monitor your diet.** Alcoholic beverages and highly spiced foods seem to induce hot flashes in some women.

• **Exercise.** Some women have found that regular exercise helps ease hot flashes. Exercise can also help you sleep better.

• **Try tofu—it can't hurt.** Plants contain estrogenic compounds that resemble (but are not identical to) human estrogens. One estrogen "family," called isoflavones, occurs in high concentration in soybeans and the soybean product tofu. Whether isoflavones in soy or plant estrogens in other foods are effective against hot flashes isn't proved, but certainly tofu is a good addition to a healthy diet. If you want to try it as a hot-flash remedy, get the real thing, rather than soy drinks, which are not as high in isoflavones.

Supplements containing soy isoflavones are not recommended, since it's hard to be sure what they actually contain and what their hormonal effects are. Large doses of isoflavones might cause hormone imbalances that increase the risk of certain cancers.

• **Be patient.** The problem won't last forever. Hot flashes are worse right at menopause. They usually subside and may go away entirely within three to five years.

• **Treat vaginal dryness.** A seeming loss of sexual desire may in fact be due to this condition, which can make intercourse painful. Vaginal creams containing estrogen or nonestrogenic water-soluble lubricants can alleviate vaginal dryness (see page 489). Many women, happy to be liberated from birth control and worries about pregnancy, report an increase in sexual pleasure in their 50s.

Although ovulation may occur less regularly as a woman approaches menopause, she may still be able to get pregnant. If you are certain you don't want to become pregnant, it's important to use a reliable method of contraception until you are clearly past menopause.

HRT: Points to Consider

▼

Millions of women age 50 and older now take take some form of hormone therapy—either estrogen replacement therapy (ERT) or hormone replacement therapy (HRT), a combination of low-dose estrogen and progestin. It's been known for some time that replacing estrogen after menopause can help relieve symptoms of menopause. In addition, there has been persuasive evidence that estrogen replacement can also reduce the long-term risk of osteoporosis (thinning bones) as well as heart attack and other forms of cardiovascular disease.

But the results of recent and ongoing studies have left researchers—and the public—with a nagging feeling of uncertainty about the cardiovascular benefits of hormone therapy. Studies have generally shown that hormone therapy has positive effects on HDL ("good") cholesterol levels in postmenopausal women—but the benefit has varied. In one study, HRT had positive, but lesser, effects than ERT—yet far more women take HRT because ERT increases the risk of endometrial cancer, while HRT does not.

In addition, there continue to be concerns about whether long-term hormone therapy (10 years or more) increases the risk of breast cancer.

Therefore, hormone therapy for healthy postmenopausal women continues to be controversial. What does seem clear is that no one solution is right for all women—and that many women do very well without hormone therapy.

Only you, in consultation with your doctor, can decide if HRT (or ERT) is appropriate for you. Here are some points you should both consider:

- Are you having severe hot flashes or other menopausal symptoms? Taking hormones can relieve them. If your symptoms are mild, however, you may prefer to manage without medication.

- Do you have a family history of osteoporosis or other risk factors for the disease? (See page 397.) Hormone therapy is known to reduce the risks for this crippling disease, or at least to help delay its onset.

- Do you have a family or personal history of breast cancer? If the answer is yes, you may be advised not to undertake hormone therapy, although its effect on breast cancer risk is by no means clear. Short-term use of hormones (five years or less) does not appear to raise breast cancer risk—nor does it offer benefits against heart disease and osteoporosis. If you decide on long-term therapy, you might wait to begin until you are in your sixties: You could still get the benefits and then stop after 10 years in order to limit your breast cancer risk.

- Do you have varicose veins, or a history of blood clots or of gallbladder or liver disease? Are you obese? If so, you may not be a candidate for hormone therapy.

- Are you willing to tolerate possible side effects of hormone therapy such as spotting, monthly bleeding, or breast tenderness? (Some combinations of estrogen and progesterone administered continuously may not produce bleeding.)

- Are you willing to be on a regimen of medication for many years? (You can take hormone therapy for a short period, but when you stop, you cease to receive its benefits.)

- If you are taking hormone therapy for the long term, the cost can be an issue.

If you are at risk for heart disease, this may be another reason to consider hormone therapy. However, the actual benefit isn't clear. Moreover, whether or not you take hormones, it's vital to live a healthy life if you want to lower your risk of any chronic disease. Our recommendations for preventing a heart attack (page 64) and preventing osteoporosis (page 398) offer additional ways to protect yourself.

Prevention

Menopause is a normal consequence of aging. But some of the troubling symptoms and health consequences (such as osteoporosis) associated with menopause can be prevented or delayed with hormone replacement therapy.

When To Call Your Doctor

When you first experience changes in your menstrual patterns—either irregular periods or unusually light or heavy blood flow—it's a good idea to see your doctor to make sure the changes are related to menopause and not caused by a medical problem. (You still need to have regular gynecological checkups that include a Pap smear). Also see your doctor if you miss a period or you experience vaginal bleeding between periods.

What Your Doctor Will Do

To rule out medical problems associated with abnormal menstrual bleeding, your doctor will perform a pelvic exam. A Pap test may show the effect of low estrogen levels on the vaginal lining (mucosa). There are also tests and measurements designed to reveal hormone levels in the blood and urine. If you are at risk for osteoporosis, your doctor may also recommend testing your bone density. You and your doctor will also evaluate your personal and family histories to decide whether or not you would benefit from HRT.

For More Information

- American College of Obstetricians and Gynecologists

383

Menstrual Cramps

Symptoms

Irregular, sharp, cramping pain in the uterus, lower abdomen, or lower back, sometimes with pain that shoots down the thighs.

- Backache, nausea, vomiting, or diarrhea.
- Hot and cold sensations.
- Fatigue.
- Occasional headache.
- May or may not be accompanied by PMS (premenstrual syndrome).

What Is It?

For most women, menstruation creates no medical problems: even the most uncomfortable symptoms are not permanent, nor do they usually indicate any serious underlying condition. But for some women the pain is severe enough to interfere with everyday activities.

The Greek-derived word dysmenorrhea, meaning painful menstrual flow, is a term for what most women call cramps. Besides pain in the lower abdomen or back, women may also experience nausea, diarrhea, vomiting, and occasional headaches. When it occurs, pain always comes at the beginning of a menstrual period and may last up to three days. It chiefly affects women 25 years of age and under; for reasons not well understood, dysmenorrhea tends to vanish as women grow older, especially after the birth of a child. However, for some it can continue until menopause.

What Causes It?

Although it can cause emotional distress, dysmenorrhea is not psychological in origin. The discomfort comes from uterine spasms, which are most powerful at this time and temporarily deprive the uterus of oxygen. These spasms are triggered by prostaglandins, hormonelike sub-

stances that the body sometimes releases in excess during menstruation. The high level of progesterone is what triggers the prostaglandins. Thus, cramps are a fairly sure sign that ovulation has taken place.

In some instances painful menstruation may also be the result of an underlying gynecological disorder, such as uterine fibroids, pelvic inflammatory disease, a pelvic tumor, or endometriosis.

What If You Do Nothing?

For most women, cramps are not severe and vanish within a day or two of the start of the menstrual cycle. Home remedies can help provide relief. If cramps are incapacitating, you should seek treatment from your doctor.

Home Remedies

For centuries women have relied on home cures for cramps—hot drinks, massage, stretching exercises, keeping warm. No specific exercise for relieving dysmenorrhea exists, and there is no scientific evidence that any of the old tried-and-true remedies really work. Yet personal experience cannot be discounted; different things work (or don't work) for different people. Here are some common self-help measures.

- **Take a bath.** The hot water may help relax the uterus.
- **Apply heat.** Placing a heating pad or hot water bottle on the lower abdomen may relieve the discomfort of cramps.
- **Exercise several times daily.** Walking, swimming, running, bicycling, and other aerobic activities may help diminish cramping symptoms by inhibiting prostaglandin release and contributing to the release of endorphins, the body's own natural pain relievers.
- **Take a pain reliever.** Acetaminophen may be

effective in relieving the mild to moderate headache and the backache that often accompany menstrual cramps. Researchers aren't sure if acetaminophen affects prostaglandin production, but if it does, it is a milder drug than NSAIDs (aspirin, ibuprofen, or naproxen), which are also effective. If acetaminophen doesn't provide relief, you may want to try one of the NSAIDs, which suppress prostaglandins. Follow label directions.

If you usually have menstrual cramps, you may want to begin taking an NSAID (as an antiprostaglandin) the day before you expect a period and to continue for a day or two. The medication may help relieve pain by decreasing the severity of uterine contractions. People respond differently to each medication, so you may need to try different types to find one that works best for you.

See if there is a dietary connection. Some women complain that certain foods and beverages—including coffee and tea, chocolate, and soda—induce or intensify cramps. There is no scientific evidence for this, but you can see if avoiding any of them helps.

Prevention

Get plenty of rest. If you find that you are prone to regular cramping during menstruation and you become unusually tired or nervous, napping occasionally during the day and maintaining regular sleeping patterns may prevent or help reduce the severity of cramping.

When To Call Your Doctor

Contact your physician if you don't achieve appreciable relief after trying the various self-treatments. Also contact your doctor if you experience painful cramping that lasts longer than three days, or if any cramping occurs in between your menstrual periods.

What Your Doctor Will Do

A detailed history and pelvic exam may uncover a possible cause of recurrent, painful menstruation. Your doctor may prescribe a more powerful antiprostaglandin medication or an oral contraceptive. Oral contraceptives are a highly effective treatment for cramps, since they prevent ovulation and hence high levels of progesterone and prostaglandin production. They are available only by prescription and must be taken on a regular basis, not just when symptoms appear. (Smokers and women over 35 must consider other risks in taking oral contraceptives.)

If your doctor suspects secondary dysmenorrhea—when painful periods are caused by a disease or disorder such as endometriosis or pelvic inflammatory disease—appropriate treatment for the disorder will be recommended.

For More Information

• American College of Obstetricians and Gynecologists

385

Mononucleosis

Symptoms

Mononucleosis produces flulike symptoms.
- Severe fatigue.
- Fever and chills.
- Sore throat, sometimes severe.
- Swollen glands (usually a day or two after the symptoms listed above) and enlarged spleen (in about 50 percent of cases).
- Nausea and vomiting (occasionally).
- Jaundice (in about 5 percent of cases).
- Measles-like rash on the face or body (in about 15 percent of cases). If amoxicillin, an antibiotic, has been taken, rash occurs in 90 percent of cases.

What Is It?

Often referred to as mono, mononucleosis is an infectious disease with initial symptoms—fever, sore throat, and swollen glands—that feel like a bad case of the flu (influenza). The condition is most common in teenagers and young adults in developed countries. (When it strikes young children, it is so mild that it usually goes unnoticed.) Over half of all college students have antibodies to the virus that causes mono, which means they have been infected with the virus previously.

Because mononucleosis may affect the liver, some people with the disease develop jaundice, a yellowing of the skin caused by an increase of bile in the blood. A skin rash similar to German measles (rubella) can also develop, and the rash can be aggravated if a physician prescribes amoxicillin—an antibiotic often used to treat severe bacterial infections of the throat—before mono has been diagnosed.

Mono is usually not a serious condition, and most people who come down with it generally feel better within several weeks. The sensation of fatigue can sometimes persist for two months or longer, which has in the past led some experts to think that the virus that causes mono is also linked to chronic fatigue syndrome. But research has shown no such link. Major complications from mono are rare. About half of all mono patients get an enlarged spleen, and one of the most potentially serious complications is for the spleen to rupture—a rare circumstance that requires emergency surgery.

What Causes It?

The Epstein-Barr virus, a common member of the herpes family of viruses, is the cause of most cases of mononucleosis. The virus is communicable, but only through direct contact with the saliva of an infected person, which can occur through sneezing, coughing, and—perhaps most commonly—kissing. (Mono has been referred to as the kissing disease.) The virus remains active in an infected person's saliva for six months or more after symptoms have subsided. Some people, however, are able to come in contact with an infected person and not get sick, presumably because their immune systems are able to resist the virus.

What If You Do Nothing?

Mono is self-limiting; most people will recover on their own, typically in two to four weeks, though fatigue may last longer.

Home Remedies

There is no current treatment for the virus that causes mononucleosis, but you can take these steps to relieve symptoms.

• **Try to rest.** Resting yourself physically is helpful during the acute, feverish phase of the illness. If you have an enlarged spleen, you need to be especially careful about resuming physical activity until your spleen has returned to normal; otherwise, you risk rupturing it.

• **Drink plenty of fluids.** Even if a sore throat makes it uncomfortable to swallow, help yourself to ample amounts of water and fruit juices, especially while you have a fever.

• **Take nonprescription pain relievers.** To relieve headache, sore throat, and fever, you can use an NSAID (aspirin, ibuprofen, or naproxen) or acetaminophen. Children 19 or younger should avoid aspirin, which carries a risk of Reye's syndrome when taken by children with flu or chicken pox (and symptoms of mono are similar to flu symptoms). Instead, take acetaminophen or ibuprofen (though the latter won't reduce fever).

• **Ease up on work and activity.** Along with resting, it's helpful to postpone difficult projects (such as lengthy papers or final exams if you are a college student) until after you've recovered.

Prevention

Mono can't be prevented. Nearly all adults over 35 have antibodies to the virus, so they aren't at risk. You can reduce the risk by avoiding direct contact with people known to be infected, but the virus can be carried in saliva long after symptoms have disappeared.

When To Call Your Doctor

It's best to check with your doctor if you develop symptoms of mono, particularly if you have a severe sore throat; your doctor can rule out other possible infections, including hepatitis and strep throat, which call for different treatment measures. Also contact your doctor if you develop severe abdominal pain, which may indicate a ruptured spleen. And call your doctor if symptoms from mono last longer than 10 days.

What Your Doctor Will Do

After checking for signs and symptoms of mono (including an enlarged spleen), your doctor can confirm a diagnosis with blood tests for the Epstein-Barr virus.

For More Information

• Centers for Disease Control and Prevention

Motion Sickness

Symptoms

- Paleness.
- Perspiration.
- Pallor.
- Nausea and vomiting.
- Dizziness.
- Spinning sensation.
- Loss of appetite.

What Is It?

Motion sickness is a loss of equilibrium that occurs when people travel in a car, bus, boat, train, airplane, or amusement park ride. The problem is common among children between the ages of 2 and 12. Though adults can also get motion sickness, their more mature nervous systems are better able to deal with the effects of movement. Some children are especially susceptible, so that they usually become motion sick each time they travel in a vehicle.

What Causes It?

What causes motion sickness is mixed signals to the brain—a discrepancy between what the eyes see and what the body senses. The problem resides in the inner ear, which has fluid moving in its semicircular canals to monitor the directions of motion. Certain movements, such as the rolling of a ship or air turbulence in a plane during a flight, stimulate these fluids, while at the same time the eyes are focused on rapidly moving scenery instead of a stable horizon. The brain receives messages from nerves affected by this imbalance, and in turn the brain sends a message to the stomach, resulting in nausea and possibly vomiting.

What If You Do Nothing?

While motion sickness isn't usually a health prob-lem, it is often uncomfortable and can interfere with a trip. If you (or a child) are susceptible, the likelihood of motion sickness during travel is high. So it's best to focus on preventing symptoms before you set out.

Home Remedies

Once you begin to feel ill, there is not a lot you can do for relief from motion sickness, apart from getting to solid ground.

- **Take care of the nausea.** Lie down in a dark room with a cool cloth over your forehead and eyes. Have a pan handy in case you vomit.
- **Replace fluids.** If you have vomited, you want to avoid becoming dehydrated. Take sips of clear fluids until your stomach settles down.
- **Herbal remedies may help but are unproven.** Ginger is the herb most touted to ease motion sickness. There is little solid scientific evidence that it works, but at least it won't make you sleepy or dry out your mouth. You can buy ginger capsules at the store, or eat candied ginger.

  Peppermint is also popular—and pleasant. But keep in mind that large doses of raw ginger or peppermint oil can irritate the stomach lining as well as the mouth.

Prevention

It's easier to prevent motion sickness than to treat it once it begins.

- **Start with medication.** If you always suffer from motion sickness, the best plan is to try medication. Some over-the-counter antihistamines have been approved by the Food and Drug Administration (FDA) for motion sickness. The active ingredients are antihistamines: cyclizine (Marezine and generic brands); dimenhydrinate (Dramamine and generics); diphenhydramine (Benadryl and generics); and meclizine (Bonine and generics). In studies, these drugs have been similarly effective in preventing overall symptoms of motion sickness.

Start taking your chosen drug 30 to 60 minutes before you leave. Remember that each of these drugs may cause drowsiness.

• **Be vigilant concerning food and drink.** Eat something before your trip, but don't eat a lot. Fruit juice and toast, for example, may be all that you need. Avoid eating heavy meals and drinking alcohol before traveling.

• **Sharpen your focus.** In a boat or in a car, be sure to focus on the horizon or some other fixed point in the distance. In a plane, sit by a window and look outside. This way your eyes will see the same motion that your body and inner ears feel.

• **Choose your spot wisely.** In a car, van, or train, be sure to have a seat that gives you a clear view of the road ahead; do not sit in a seat facing backward. In a plane, choose a window seat over the wings, where you will experience the least motion. At sea, stay amidships and topside.

• **Avoid strong odors from food, tobacco, or perfume.** Such smells can induce or increase nausea.

• **Choose amusement park rides carefully.** Avoid rides that spin.

• **Don't read.** Trying to focus on the page or on the screen of a laptop computer while your inner ear is jiggling may be enough to trigger motion sickness.

• **For severe motion sickness, consider the Relief-Band.** This is a device approved by the FDA for combating nausea. You strap it to the inside of your wrist, and it delivers mild electrical stimulation to nerves in the area, which in theory controls nausea. No one knows exactly how it works, and it may not work for everyone, but some pilots have used the product against airsickness. Models can cost from $85 to $100, and are sold over the counter in drugstores as well as on the Internet.

When To Call Your Doctor

Motion sickness is usually an inconvenience rather than a health problem. However, if you travel regularly and are often disturbed or incapacitated by it, contact your physician.

What Your Doctor Will Do

Your doctor may prescribe an antinausea medication called scopolamine (Transderm Scop). Administered by a dime-size skin patch that's placed behind the ear a few hours before beginning a trip, the medication is highly effective. It can have such side effects as dry mouth, blurry vision, and drowsiness. The drug is not recommended for children. You can also ask your doctor or pharmacist about the ReliefBand (see Prevention).

For More Information

• American Academy of Otolaryngology-Head and Neck Surgery

Muscle Cramps

Symptoms

■ A sharp, painful spasm or contraction (tightening) in a muscle. The affected muscle may feel hard to the touch (a knot).

■ With more severe cramps a visible twitching of the muscle beneath the skin can occur.

What Is It?

Though they are harmless and do not involve injury, few things are as painful as common muscle cramps. A cramp, also called a spasm, is a sudden involuntary painful shortening of a muscle. Cramps can occur in any muscle at any time, but they most often occur in the thigh, calf, or foot and usually while you are lying in bed, playing sports, or exercising.

Nighttime calf cramps usually strike in bed at night as a result of contracting the calf muscles by suddenly pointing your toes or by lying with your feet in that position. (Swimmers, who kick with their toes sharply pointed, can suffer calf spasms similar to nocturnal leg cramps.) One study showed that 70 percent of people over the age of 50 get this nocturnal variety. In general, as you age you may find that you experience leg cramps more frequently.

What Causes It?

Cramps remain something of a mystery, and it's seldom possible to pinpoint why they happen. Inactivity and activity can both cause cramps.

Athletes' cramps occur for a number of reasons. An imbalance in the blood of minerals called electrolytes (potassium and sodium), which often results from excess sweating and dehydration, may cause muscles to cramp. Another common cause is overexertion or muscle fatigue, marked by excessive tightening of the muscles and/or a buildup of lactic acid in them. Poor conditioning may also contribute to cramps.

If you exercise strenuously during in the day, your muscles may tighten while you sleep and thus cramp. Similarly, if you're not accustomed to them, wearing high heels may cause cramps. Also, certain medications, notably diuretics taken for hypertension, may promote cramps.

What If You Do Nothing?

Ordinary cramps, which typically occur in the leg or foot, do no permanent harm, nor are they signs of serious underlying problems. Cramps usually last just a few minutes and clear up on their own.

Home Remedies

• **Stop the cramp.** For calf cramps, flex your foot by pointing your toes upward. Lying down and grabbing the toes and ball of your foot and pulling them toward your knee may help. At the same time, massage the muscle gently to relax it fully.

For hamstring cramps, extend your leg straight out, gently stretching the hamstring muscles. Massage the sore area with your fingers.

• **Ice the muscle.** Ice packs can reduce blood flow to the muscles and thus relax them.

• **Walk it off.** Putting your full weight on your heels may help stop cramping in your leg.

• **Drink up.** Drinking water helps correct any fluid loss from excessive sweating, a common occurrence during a long athletic event in the heat. If a mineral imbalance—too little potassium or sodium, for instance—is contributing to the cramping, an electrolyte-replacing sports drink may help. Most people, though, can get adequate sodium and potassium from their diet; supplements are not necessary.

• **Quinine is questionable.** For years quinine sulfate pills have been a staple of treating nocturnal leg cramps—but with little evidence they are effective or safe. One study did show that prescription quinine reduced the frequency of leg cramps. However, the drug can also have serious, sometimes fatal, side effects, and the Food and Drug Administration (FDA) at one point asked the manufacturer to take it off the market.

Chloride pills and vitamin E supplements also have their proponents—but again, there is no proof of their effectiveness.

Prevention

• **Change your sleep habits.** If you seem predisposed to nocturnal leg cramps, don't point your toes while stretching, and try not to sleep with your toes pointed. Sleep on your side, and don't tuck in your blankets and sheets too tightly, since these can bend your toes downward. An electric blanket will keep your muscles warm and may prevent cramping.

• **Get into a stretching routine.** Sometimes cramps are unavoidable, but a regular program of calf-stretching exercises to lengthen the muscles that have shortened may help if you're prone to have calf cramps. Stand about three feet from a wall and lean into it for 15 to 20 seconds, keeping your forearms against the wall and your heels on the floor (see the calf stretch on page 319). Placing the ball of your rear foot on a book and slowly lowering your heel will add to the stretch.

Do these stretches daily or as often as necessary. Good stretching times are before and after exercise and before going to bed.

• **Drink before and during exercise.** In hot weather, drink at least 16 ounces of fluid two hours before exercising and four to eight ounces every 10 to 20 minutes while you exercise.

• **Check your medicines.** Recurrent cramps may be due to a medication you're taking. Diuretics commonly prescribed to lower blood pressure are typical offenders because they deplete the potassium in your muscles. Talk to your physician about switching to another drug and/or taking potassium supplements. Also ask about the advisability of increasing your daily intake of potassium-rich foods like bananas, oranges, and potatoes.

• **Don't take salt tablets.** These may be counterproductive because they cause excessive amounts of water to be drawn into the stomach, which can cause dehydration, nausea, and vomiting. If you don't get enough sodium in your diet, add some extra salt in your cooking, sprinkle it on your food, or eat salt-rich snacks such as pretzels or crackers to help restore any imbalance in your body.

When To Call Your Doctor

Contact your physician if you continue to be bothered by recurrent muscle cramps despite trying self-care measures. If you experience cramping or muscle spasms in the lower back or neck, accompanied by pain that radiates down the leg or into the arm, seek medical help immediately, since these may be signs of a serious heart or abdominal condition.

What Your Doctor Will Do

In cases of recurrent cramping, your physician will first rule out more serious underlying circulatory, neurologic, and metabolic disorders. For severe cramping that causes neck and back pain, medications may be prescribed.

For More Information

• American Academy of Orthopaedic Surgeons

391

Osteoarthritis

Symptoms

For some people, symptoms remain mild or nonexistent, while for others, symptoms worsen to the point of becoming disabling.

- Stiffness in the morning or after exercising.
- Joint stiffness and pain that is aggravated by movement, relieved by rest.
- Limited movement and loss of flexibility in the joints.
- Audible crackling noises when an affected joint moves.
- Redness, warmth, or swelling of a joint (rare).

What Is It?

Osteoarthritis (OA), also known as degenerative joint disease, is the most common form of arthritis—the medical term for a wide variety of disorders that involve inflammation of a joint. OA results from the gradual destruction of cartilage, the smooth lining of a joint that reduces friction and absorbs shock. As the disease progresses gradually over the years, the cartilage cracks and flakes off, leading to subsequent pain and sometimes deformity whenever the underlying and now exposed bones rub together. All joints may be affected, but it is most common in the fingers, ankles and feet, knees, hips, neck, and the spine.

About 90 percent of people over the age of 40 show x-ray evidence of OA—typically a gradual loss of the soft, smooth cartilage at joint surfaces and frequently compensatory overgrowths of bone at the joints, called spurs. These spurs may grind against each other as the joint moves. But most people do not experience symptoms until later in life. More than 20 million Americans currently have symptoms of the disorder.

There are two types of OA. Primary osteoarthritis, resulting from normal wear and tear, most commonly affects thumb joints and the end joints of other fingers, as well as the hips, knees, neck, and lower spine. Secondary osteoarthritis can occur after injury to a joint; from disease; or as a result of chronic trauma (due to obesity, posture problems, or occupational overuse).

In some people symptoms of OA remain mild or even fade away. In others, symptoms grow progressively worse until they are disabling. Because the joints become stiff and painful, a person's natural tendency is to minimize movement. Unfortunately, this can simply lead to a wasting of the muscles and to stiffer joints—and consequently more pain—since inactivity weakens the muscles that stabilize joints.

What Causes It?

The exact cause of osteoarthritis is still unknown, but it appears to be a combination of several factors, most notably a breakdown of the cartilage, the cushioning material of the joints. Time and use may wear it away, but OA is now known to be not simply wear and tear but a disease that prevents the cartilage from repairing and renewing itself normally. Genetic factors are also probably involved—OA appears to run in families.

Obesity seems to increase the risk of developing arthritis in the back, hips, and knees. Poor posture and being sedentary may also promote OA. Also, a broken bone or overuse of a joint—common among athletes—may speed up the development of osteoarthritis.

What If You Do Nothing?

For occasional mild joint pain and stiffness, there is no cause for concern since the symptoms typically clear in a matter of days. This is especially so if arthritis occurs in the fingers. However, if symptoms become more severe, especially if they affect your weight-bearing joints and therefore your daily activities, you may need to seek professional help.

Home Remedies

First, see a doctor to make sure your problem really is osteoarthritis. There is no cure at present that can stop or reverse OA. You can, though, help slow the disease's progress, decrease joint pain, and improve function with the following measures.

• **Heat and cold can bring relief.** Cold packs, warm compresses, heat lamps, and warm baths or showers may bring periods of relief from the throbbing pain or stiffness associated with arthritis. Experiment with both cold and heat to see what works best. Apply the heat or cold to the painful joint for 20 minutes three times a day.

• **Support the joint.** A splint, brace, neck collar, crutches, or a cane may provide the support you need, eliminating or reducing stress on a painful affected joint.

• **Exercise.** A regular exercise program designed by your physician or a physical therapist is one of the few effective therapies recommended to slow down the development and progression of arthritis. The program should be aimed at restoring, maintaining, and increasing flexibility, muscle strength, and overall fitness. Excellent activities include swimming, water aerobics, walking, and bicycling as well as strengthening and stretching exercises.

• **Lose weight.** Increasing evidence indicates that extra weight damages the weight-bearing joints and speeds up the course of arthritis. Reducing your weight to acceptable levels may help stop or reverse the process.

• **Capsaicin can help.** Capsaicin creams can be beneficial for arthritis pain. Capsaicin, the sub-

stance that makes hot chili peppers hot, is an ingredient in some nonprescription salves and lotions. Capsaicin acts partly as a counterirritant and partly as a suppressant of pain impulses. Capsaicin creates a little diversionary pain that masks the real one, but it also blocks substance P, which is present in aching joints as part of the body's

---

"Miracle Cures": Be Skeptical

▼

Two nutritional supplements—glucosamine and chondroitin sulfate—are promoted as nothing less than "miracle cures" for arthritis. Both substances, produced naturally in the body, reputedly not only relieve pain, but can even, in some cases, bring about a complete reversal of the disease. For most people, there is probably no harm in trying the supplements for possible pain reduction—and one promising controlled study showed that glucoasamine can also help slow deterioration of cartilage as well as relieve pain in some cases. But no studies have shown these supplements are effective at reversing arthritis, and little research has been done regarding their long-term safety. Glucosamine can have adverse effects on blood sugar levels and so might pose risks for people with diabetes. In the United States the supplements are also unregulated, so that you can't be sure of what you are getting or how much to take.

MSM and SAM-e are two other supplements that are supposed to help alleviate arthritis pain. There is no scientific evidence to support the use of MSM, though there is some preliminary research showing that SAM-e may provide relief.

If you decide to try a supplement—or any other unproven arthritis treatment—always talk it over with your doctor, to be sure you're not doing anything that can harm you. (For more detailed information on what is known about the supplements mentioned here, see pages 628 and 632.)

393

Arthritis and Exercise

▼

If you have OA, it need not limit your mobility—at least not if you exercise and keep moving. But many of the 40 million Americans who suffer from OA don't exercise because of pain and stiffness in their joints. Thus, the muscles grow weaker and the joints become more painful.

Many people with osteoarthritis can maintain flexibility, and even restore it to some degree, through a well-designed exercise program that is implemented gradually and followed regularly. Specialists have devised scores of exercises to stretch muscles or strengthen important joints. Exercise may cause you some pain at first, but the discomfort should diminish.

The exercises illustrated here are a way to begin, and fall into two categories.

Range-of-motion exercises relieve stiffness, restore flexibility, and help with joint movement. If you haven't yet lost your full range of motion, an exercise like the shoulder stretch can help prevent such loss as well as help minimize joint stiffness. Tai chi, the gentlest form of martial arts training, offers an excellent range-of-motion exercise.

Strengthening exercises are particularly important because weak muscles add to joint problems. Many studies have found that strength training

can relieve knee pain, improve strength, and boost physical functioning. With isometric exercise, you contract the muscle without moving the joint. Isotonic exercises, using bands, weights, or machines, require you to move the joints and can result in greater strength gains. Water workouts, free weights, or weight machines can be useful.

Aerobic exercise is also beneficial. Continuous movement for 10 minutes or longer, such as walking, swimming, and cycling (at low pedal resistance, over level surfaces at first) can definitely reduce pain and improve physical functioning. Rowing, water walking, aqua aerobics, and ballroom or other low-impact dancing are also excellent choices.

Generally, it's wise to avoid high-impact activities like tennis, aerobic dance, or running, which can overload sore joints.

Before You Start

Exercises must be individualized, depending on the joints involved and the degree of pain. Your doctor or physical therapist will help you develop an exercise program that focuses on your most painful joints and takes into consideration your overall level of fitness. Whatever exercises you do, there are some general rules.

Start gradually and never overdo it. Follow the instruc-

tions of your doctor or physical therapist. There will probably be some pain or discomfort, but stop a particular exercise if there's unusual or severe pain. Cut back if necessary, but don't stop exercising entirely.

Always warm up first. After walking in place for a few minutes, do some gentle stretches. Gently massaging stiff joints may help, as may heat (a warm bath or shower, or an infrared lamp). Wear a sweat suit, or leg or arm warmers.

Vary your exercises, so that you work different muscle groups. Don't rely on one long, strenuous (and painful) session a week. Begin with as few as three repetitions of an exercise. Over the course of several weeks try to work up to 10 repetitions, or as many repetitions as your doctor recommends.

Gentle exercise should be a daily routine. And it's a long-term project—you shouldn't stop for more than a few days.

Note: Remember, unless you know you are healthy and have only mild osteoarthritis, talk to your doctor before attempting any of these exercises.

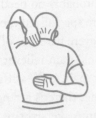

Shoulder stretch. Reach one palm over shoulder and place back of other hand on lower back. Slide hands toward each other, trying to touch fingertips (many people can't reach that far). Alternate arms.

Leg strengthener. Stand in front of chair. Slowly bend at hips and knees as if to sit down, but don't go all the way down to the seat. Lower your hips as far as you can without sitting. Keep your upper body upright. Then slowly straighten up.

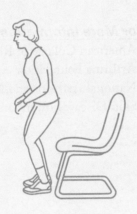

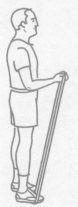

Arm curl. Hold one end of an elastic band in fist, palm up, the other end securely under arch of foot. Start with arm extended downward (but elbow not locked). Slowly curl forearm toward shoulder, keeping elbow close to side. Then lower slowly; repeat. Switch arms.

pain-and-inflammation chemistry. You may need to use the cream three or four times daily, and you may not notice any improvement until you've applied the cream for a week or more.

• **Medications may be most effective.** A number of drugs, including over-the-counter pain relievers, can ease arthritis pain. You may need to experiment to find the most effective drug and dosage. Any of these drugs can cause problems such as gastrointestinal bleeding, however, so if you are taking any painkiller on a long-term basis, you need a physician's advice and supervision (see What Your Doctor Will Do).

Prevention

Osteoarthritis can't be prevented, but you may be able to slow the progress of the disease by following the self-care measures outlined above. Losing weight (if you are overweight), gradually starting an exercise program, and avoiding any repetitive activities that can cause wear and tear on joints are the most helpful measures.

When To Call Your Doctor

If joint pain or stiffness begin to interfere with daily activities, call your physician.

What Your Doctor Will Do

Your doctor will take a history and perform a thorough exam of your joints to determine the presence and extent of arthritis. X-rays may be taken and, in rare cases, fluid may be drawn from an affected joint through a needle for analysis in a laboratory.

If you need pain relievers on a daily basis, you and your doctor should discuss the risks and benefits of different medications. The first line of treatment is usually acetaminophen (such as Tylenol and generics), which does not cause stom-

395

ach upset or bleeding, but can affect liver and kidney function over the long term. Nonsteroidal anti-inflammatory drugs (NSAIDs)—aspirin, ibuprofen (such as Advil and Motrin), or naproxen (Aleve)—are the next option if acetaminophen doesn't work or stops working. Because NSAIDs can cause gastrointestinal bleeding and/or ulcers when used over the long term, you should take them under medical supervision. Be sure to consult your doctor about using these drugs if you have high blood pressure or diabetes mellitus, since they may cause problems with your kidneys.

As an alternative, your doctor may suggest that you try one of the new prescription NSAIDs known as COX-2 inhibitors. They are designed to have the pain-relieving effect of NSAIDs with a lower risk of gastrointestinal bleeding. These heavily-promoted drugs are expensive, and are so new that the long-term effects are not completely known. Other medications are also available that your doctor can prescribe to reduce NSAID-related stomach problems. But if you have arthritis and are doing well on nonprescription pain relievers, there is probably no need to switch.

Stronger or more specialized medications can be prescribed for severe flare-ups of arthritis pain if more conventional pain relievers aren't effective. When joint pain and stiffness become severely debilitating, there is a range of surgical procedures that can make arthritis more tolerable. Each has its own benefits and limitations, and you should always be sure that the surgery is your best option. But fortunately, most people who have osteoarthritis will never need to have surgery.

For More Information
- American College of Rheumatology
- Arthritis Foundation
- National Arthritis and Musculoskeletal and Skin Diseases Information Clearinghouse

Osteoporosis

Symptoms

- Lower-back pain.
- A gradual loss of height; a stooping posture.
- Sometimes no obvious symptoms until a bone breaks, typically the hip, arm, or wrist.

What Is It?

Meaning porous bones in Latin, osteoporosis is a thinning of the bones, which makes them fragile and brittle so that they fracture easily.

Bone tissue constantly "remodels" itself—lays down calcium and then releases and replaces it—but for most of adult life there is an equilibrium: calcium is laid down and released without apparent change in bone density. However, at about age 35 for women and slightly later for men, bone density begins to decrease. This doesn't mean that the bone is diseased or abnormal. It just means there's less of it: when new bone forms, it's less dense. The body continues to remove calcium from the bone storehouse, but as people age some of this calcium is not replaced.

Although osteoporosis can affect men (see page 399), it's about eight times more common in women. For both men and women, the chief risk factor is age: the disease usually becomes detectable in people in their 60s, 70s, and beyond. About 1.5 million older Americans suffer fractures each year owing to osteoporosis. It can also result in a decrease in height because of the compression of the vertebrae, and it causes the stooped posture known as dowager's hump. It's a major cause of disability among older women.

Like hypertension, osteoporosis has been called a silent disease: you may not be aware of it until you fall and fracture a bone. Today, there are medications that can halt the course of the disease, and may even reverse it to some extent. But prevention is the best line of defense.

What Causes It?

Gender may be the most important factor in bone maintenance. The sex hormones (testosterone in men, estrogen in women) are a major influence on calcium uptake by bone tissue and thus skele-

---

What Puts You at Risk: A Checklist

▼

Of the risks listed here, the more you have, the greater your chances of developing osteoporosis.

- ✔ Increasing age.
- ✔ Being female. By age 65, the average man still has 91 percent of his bone mass, but the average woman only about 74 percent.
- ✔ Being chronically underweight or having a slight frame.
- ✔ Being white or Asian (usually small-boned).

- ✔ Having osteoporosis in the family.
- ✔ Eating a poor diet, low in vitamins and minerals, especially calcium.
- ✔ Being sedentary, and failing to get enough weight-bearing exercise.
- ✔ Smoking. In women smoking cigarettes lowers the estrogen content of the blood, thus weakening the bones. Smoking is particularly dangerous for women who have other

risk factors for osteoporosis.
- ✔ Heavy drinking. It's not known why heavy drinking weakens the bones—perhaps because heavy drinkers often eat a poor diet.
- ✔ Long-term use of certain medications. Some people with asthma and rheumatoid arthritis take glucocorticoid medications for long periods, which can diminish bone strength. So can long-term use of excessive thyroid hormone.

tal strength. Other hormones aid in the release of calcium and the breakdown of bone mass. In this respect women are at a disadvantage. They begin life with less bone mass, on average, than men. Then at menopause, usually around the age of 50, a woman's supply of the hormone estrogen decreases, and her bone loss becomes more rapid than a man's.

Nutritional factors—the intake of calcium and vitamin D, as well as other nutrients whose function in bone building is not fully understood—also play an important role in formation and loss of bone mass.

Another factor is physical activity: a lack of it can hasten the onset of osteoporosis. Bones respond to mechanical stress by becoming denser and stronger. Without the stress that comes primarily from weight-bearing activity such as walking, in which your legs support your body, and from strength-building activity (such as weight lifting), your bones will eventually grow weaker.

Another influence on bone is genetics. Asian and white women tend to be small-boned, which makes them susceptible to osteoporosis. African and many African-American women tend to have more bone mass throughout life (which is a protective genetic trait), though that does not mean they never develop osteoporosis.

Certain lifestyle habits, such as smoking and alcohol consumption, have also been identified as risk factors. The long-term use of certain medications, including antiseizure drugs and glucocorticoids (which are used to treat a wide range of disorders), can also lead to bone loss.

What If You Do Nothing?

If you have osteoporosis and do nothing to stop the loss of bone, the condition will worsen and can have serious implications for your health.

Home Remedies

There is no cure for osteoporosis nor are there any remedies, but you can take steps to slow down and even reverse some of the bone loss. These include exercise and dietary measures as well as medication. You should discuss available options with your doctor.

Prevention

Unfortunately, many women think they don't have to start worrying about osteoporosis until menopause. This a myth. Recent research shows that certain lifelong habits are the best preventive for osteoporosis. You can't do much about small frame size or hereditary factors that put you at risk—but that's all the more reason to take preventive steps.

It's best to begin a prevention program in childhood or early adulthood, when bone density is on the increase. The more bone you build early in life, the better you will be able to withstand bone loss later in life. But even if you've waited until your 40s, 50s, or 60s, there is still plenty of reason to follow a preventive program.

• **Consume enough calcium.** Besides building strong bones and maintaining bone density and strength, calcium also plays a role in regulating your heartbeat and other vital functions. Adults up to age 50, including pregnant or lactating women, are advised to consume at least 1,000 milligrams daily. The goal for postmenopausal women should be 1,200 to 1,500 milligrams. Similar increases in calcium consumption for men are important as well, especially for men over 65, who should also try to consume 1,200 to 1,500 milligrams of calcium daily.

Many dark green leafy vegetables are rich in calcium. But the favorite food source of calcium for most Americans remains low-fat or nonfat dairy products. The vitamin D added to milk and the lactose naturally in milk and dairy products are thought to aid in the absorption of calcium. Many people may also need to take calcium supplements to meet the daily recommended amounts (see page 24).

If you're a woman on hormone replacement therapy, calcium is still important: estrogen enhances bone strength, as does an adequate calcium intake, but the beneficial effect of the two combined is greater than the sum of the effects of each alone. That was the conclusion of a review of 31 studies on the subject in the *American Journal of Nutrition*.

• **Include other bone-building nutrients in your diet.** Many vitamins and minerals—including vitamins C, K, and D, magnesium, and potassium—either contribute directly to bone formation or help bones retain and utilize calcium. You can find these nutrients in a diet rich in fruits, whole grains, and vegetables as well as in dairy products and fortified cereals. A daily multivitamin/mineral is also recommended for most people (see pages 26-27).

• **Make weight-bearing exercise part of your daily life.** That means walking, running, dancing, or weight lifting—or activities such as housework or mowing. Swimming and yoga are not weight-bearing exercises and thus don't build bones, though they have other benefits.

• **If you smoke, stop.** Do so not only for the strength of your bones but for your general health and well-being.

• **If you drink, do so moderately.** Light to moderate drinking is defined as an average of no more than one drink a day for women, two a day for men. One "drink" is 5 ounces of wine, 12 ounces of beer, or 1.5 ounces of 80-proof liquor (all contain about half an ounce of pure alcohol).

Men Need Strong Bones, Too

Most people think of osteoporosis as a disease affecting only women, but in fact men do suffer from bone loss as they age. In the United States, one-quarter of all hip fractures—about 80,000 per year—occur in men, usually at advanced ages.

The bone loss is linked to decreased testosterone production, which occurs gradually in men, but since they generally have denser bones to begin with, bone loss in men is not sudden or dramatic compared to the loss in women. By age 70, men will have lost, on average, one-seventh of their bone mass, but the loss does not usually produce symptoms in men until age 75 and older. About one in every eight men will suffer some kind of bone fracture caused by bone thinning, and such injuries can lead to disability or even death in the very elderly. Occasionally osteoporosis occurs early in men—those in their 50s and 60s may develop brittle bones, depending on various factors.

The men most likely to suffer bone loss include white men and those who eat a diet deficient in calcium; advancing age and a family history of osteoporosis are also significant risk factors. Those with chronic low levels of testosterone (impotence and the lack of erections during sleep may be signs of low testosterone) are also at risk.

Following the preventive steps on these pages should help ensure the preservation of strong bones in men. Some doctors are prescribing testosterone replacement therapy for men. However, virtually nothing is known about its long-term effects, including whether the therapy will actually halt bone loss.

• **If you are menopausal, consider hormone replacement therapy (HRT).** This consists of low-dose estrogen and progesterone treatments that can unquestionably slow bone loss and prevent fractures as well as reduce hot flashes and other menopausal problems. The added progesterone also reduces the risk of endometrial cancer. Estrogen probably protects against heart disease, though the evidence is controversial.

HRT, if used to prevent osteoporosis, should be started at menopause—when bone loss greatly accelerates—for maximum effect. But it can still have a beneficial effect even if started years later.

Only you, in consultation with your doctor, can decide whether HRT is appropriate for your health (see page 382). Some women do very well without HRT, which has its downside, too. If you have one or more risk factors for osteoporosis, you should consider HRT.

• **Consider nonhormonal medications for osteoporosis.** A number of prescription drugs that slow or stop bone loss or increase bone density have been approved by the Food and Drug Administration (FDA) for both treatment and prevention of osteoporosis. These provide alternatives to HRT, and some have been approved for use by men (see What Your Doctor Will Do).

Whether you opt for one of these medications or for HRT, don't neglect modifying other risk factors such as exercise and calcium intake.

When To Call Your Doctor

Contact your doctor if you develop chronic pain in your spine, ribs, or feet after a strain or other injury. The doctor needs to rule out a bone fracture and can evaluate you for osteoporosis.

What Your Doctor Will Do

After a careful examination, your physician may recommend any of several techniques available for measuring bone density. A noninvasive 10-minute test called DEXA (for dual energy x-ray absorptiometry) can be used to measure the bone density of your hips and spine. Generally, the test—which delivers a very small radiation dose—is a good idea for women at high risk. Nobody recommends that all women be tested.

A newer test, called Sahara, uses high-frequency sound waves, rather than radiation, to measure bone in the heel, and from the measurements estimate fracture risk in other locations. The test is both cheaper and easier to perform than DEXA.

If test results indicate evidence of osteoporosis, your doctor will begin more aggressive steps to slow down or stop the loss of bone mass. A calcium-rich diet and/or supplements will be recommended, as will a weight-bearing exercise program, including walking, jogging, dance, or weight training.

If you are through menopause, HRT may be recommended. If you decide against, or cannot undertake, HRT, long-term daily use of a prescription medication such as raloxifene (Evista), alendronate (Fosamax), or risedronate (Actonel) may be recommended to promote bone density and rebuild bone. Alendronate and risedronate have been approved for prevention and/or treatment of osteoporosis in some men as well as in women. When used for prevention, these medications are intended only for people who are at high risk for osteoporosis. Make sure you understand the risks and benefits of any medication and that your physician monitors your progress.

For More Information

• National Osteoporosis Foundation
• NIH Osteoporosis and Related Bone Diseases–National Resource Center

Pinworms

Symptoms

In many cases, there are no symptoms. When symptoms do occur, they include:

- Persistent, often severe, nighttime itching of the anal area, causing insomnia and irritability. Girls may also experience vaginal itching.
- Less frequently, loss of appetite, restlessness, abdominal discomfort.
- Occasionally, worms may be visible in stool or near the anus.

What Is It?

Infections from worms (helminths) are parasitic conditions that can produce major health problems, particularly in tropical and underdeveloped countries. Though helminthic infestations can occasionally be serious in the United States and other developed countries, usually the symptoms they produce are an annoyance rather than a health threat, and most cases clear up within a week or so with proper treatment. Unfortunately, symptoms are often so similar to other ailments that the helminthic infection may be initially mistaken for constipation, diarrhea, or irritable bowel syndrome.

Pinworms are the most common helminth infesting people in the United States, and most of those infected are children. At any given time, between 10 and 40 percent of children under age 12 are estimated to have pinworms.

Members of a class of helminths called nematodes, pinworms are tiny: an adult pinworm, *Enterobious vermicularis*, is barely half an inch long, with the diameter of a strand of a thread (pinworms are also called threadworms). The worms live in the large intestine (colon) of humans. When male and female pinworms mate, the female produces about 10,000 eggs. After migrating through the colon and crawling out of the anus, she deposits sticky masses of the eggs on the skin near the anal opening of the host. Within six to eight hours, the eggs mature.

Reinfection often occurs when an infected child touches or scratches the rectal area—the adult worms as well as the eggs can cause intense itching—and later puts the finger or thumb (to which the eggs cling) in his or her mouth. The pinworms eggs are swallowed, subsequently hatch in the small intestine, and later move to the large intestine. The entire cycle takes four to six weeks.

What Causes It?

Most commonly, pinworms reinfect their human hosts when they become trapped under fingernails and directly reenter the host either through the mouth or through food that has been touched and contaminated. Close contact between infected and uninfected people can also help transfer pinworms.

In addition, some pinworm eggs may be dislodged from the body, landing in house dust, clothing, bedding, and even the fur of house pets, where they can survive for two to three weeks. If the pinworm eggs are airborne, the eggs can be inhaled and swallowed.

Unlike many helminthic infections, which include tapeworms and hookworms, pinworms are not limited to rural and poor areas but occur in most geographic areas and among all socioeconomic groups.

What If You Do Nothing?

Mild worm infections can often clear up without treatment. Nevertheless, if you notice symptoms of pinworms, you should not let them go untreated since infections can easily spread to uninfected people.

Home Remedies

There are no home remedies to treat pinworms. They need to be treated immediately with medication to keep them from spreading to uninfected people, so you should contact your physician. In the meantime, follow the preventive tips to avoid reinfestation.

Prevention

• **Practice good hygiene.** Wash your hands with soap and water after using the bathroom and before eating—and make sure a child does the same. Scrub the fingernails clean and cut them short.

• **Change bed linens and clothing.** Sheets, pillow cases, towels, and underwear used by each household member should be changed after each treatment for pinworms. Launder all clothing and linens in hot water.

• **Check pets.** Have your cat and dog treated for worms regularly.

• **Cook food thoroughly.** High heat will kill any live worms present in food. Avoid dishes with raw meat or fish, such as steak tartare or sushi.

• **Clean all utensils used with raw meat.** Wash them thoroughly in hot, soapy water.

When To Call Your Doctor

Contact your physician if you or a child has any symptoms of pinworms. Anal itching is a symptom of a many conditions, including eczema, seborrheic dermatitis, and body lice, and the condition should be diagnosed by a doctor.

What Your Doctor Will Do

Your doctor will take a history and perform a thorough physical exam. If pinworms are suspected, your doctor may ask you to apply a strip of clear adhesive tape or a special "pinworm paddle" with an adhesive surface to the anal region at home. The tape can then be examined under a microscope (in a lab or in your doctor's office) to see if pinworm eggs are present. Your doctor will then determine what treatment, if any, is required. Usually an oral antiparasite medication will be prescribed. Because pinworms spread so easily, everyone in the household of the infected person should usually be treated as well.

For More Information

• American Academy of Pediatrics
• Centers for Disease Control and Prevention

PMS (Premenstrual Syndrome)

Symptoms

PMS, or premenstrual syndrome, is associated with both physical and psychological symptoms that include the following.

- Depression or feeling of hopelessness.
- Anxiety.
- Significant mood swings.
- Irritability leading to interpersonal conflicts.
- Decreased interest in normal activity.
- Difficulty concentrating.
- Fatigue.
- Changes in appetite.
- Sleeping too much or too little.
- A feeling of being out of control.
- Physical symptoms such as breast tenderness, headache, joint and muscle pain, bloating, and weight gain.

What Is It?

One-fourth of menstruating women have no premenstrual symptoms at all. The rest have some symptoms (breast tenderness, bloating, headaches, heightened awareness of emotions), usually mild, that signal the onset of a period. For most women, such symptoms can be annoying, but they are not disabling. However, 5 to 10 percent of women have severe, disabling symptoms known as premenstrual syndrome, or PMS.

PMS refers to a variety of physical and psychological symptoms that often appear one to two weeks before the start of a menstrual period, a time known as the luteal phase. For many women the tension evaporates in a burst of energy and feeling of well-being just before a period starts. Others find premenstrual symptoms minor nuisances that vanish after a few days. But for some women the problems remain and may intensify over a two-week period.

Scientists first began studying PMS in earnest in 1931, when it was termed "premenstrual tension," and there's been no lack of research since then. Nonetheless, there's still no widespread agreement about what causes PMS or how to treat it. Even the definition remains in dispute. One difficulty in diagnosis is that some of the more disturbing emotional symptoms (irritability, depression, fatigue) may, in some cases, not be tied to the menstrual cycle at all.

In an effort to help doctors in dealing with this potentially perplexing ailment, the American College of Obstetricians and Gynecologists recently issued new guidelines on diagnosing and treating PMS. Another set of guidelines is provided by the Diagnostic and Statistical Manual of Mental Disorders (DSM-IV), the bible of the psychiatric profession, which calls severe PMS premenstrual dysphoric disorder, or PMDD, to distinguish it from nondisabling PMS.

To be diagnosed with PMDD, a woman must have 5 or more of the 11 symptoms listed above during the week between ovulation and the onset of menstruation. The symptoms must decrease and begin to disappear shortly after menstruation begins; they must not be present before ovulation. They must markedly impair a woman's ability to function and must persist for at least two cycles. Also, the diagnosing physician must rule out other psychiatric and medical conditions (thyroid problems or depression, for example) that might be involved.

What Causes It?

The cause of PMS is unknown, according to the latest statement from the American College of Obstetricians and Gynecologists (ACOG). One theory is that the brain chemical serotonin (which regulates mood) is somehow adversely affected by hormonal activity in women with PMS. About all that can be said is that it's related to the menstrual cycle. Symptoms always cease when a woman experiences surgical or natural menopause. It may be that some women are more vulnerable than others to the hormonal shifts of the menstrual cycle.

What If You Do Nothing?

PMS symptoms should clear up within a day or two after the onset of menstrual bleeding. If symptoms are so severe that they interfere with normal life and interpersonal relationships, contact your physician.

Home Remedies

Remedies and treatments for PMS abound. A study published in the 1980s reported that more than 327 treatments had been proposed. A combination of some of the following measures may help, but claims for most remedies are unproved and few have proved worthwhile.

• **Keep a diary.** Since there are no specific tests for PMS, charting your daily physical and emotional symptoms may help. Keep a daily diary of your cycles for a minimum of three months, noting what the symptoms are, their severity, and exactly when they occur and disappear. Such a record will give you a sense of control, as well as assist in the diagnosis and treatment of the disorder if you decide to seek medical advice. (If these symptoms do not fall within the two weeks preceding a period, they are probably not connected with your menstrual cycle.)

• **Try exercise.** As with menstrual cramps, no specific exercise will relieve PMS. Nevertheless, regular aerobic exercise like walking, running, swimming, bicycling, in-line skating, and aerobic dancing can help elevate mood, reduce fluid retention, and relieve stress. Try to exercise several times a week for at least 20 to 30 minutes.

• **Reduce stress.** Learn specific relaxation techniques such as yoga, meditation, or progressive muscle relaxation.

• **Eliminate caffeine.** Some people have found this helpful.

• **Don't count on vitamins and minerals (except possibly calcium).** Many dietary supplements have been promoted to curb PMS symptoms. Vitamin B_6 for example, has been widely touted, even though it has not been shown to have any value for PMS. But according to an article in the *Journal of the American College of Nutrition*, there is convincing evidence that calcium can help reduce symptoms such as breast tenderness, bloating, headaches, and mood disorders. Studies suggest you need to take 1,000 to 1,200 milligrams a day to get this benefit; don't exceed 2,500 milligrams total from food and supplements.

About PMS Clinics

▼

These clinics have sprung up everywhere. If you decide to try one, be careful when making your choice.

Be wary of a clinic that
• Insists on expensive preliminary lab work.
• Charges high fees payable in advance.
• Pushes one treatment (such as progesterone suppositories) for all patients.
• Offers a fast diagnosis and quick fix.

Choose a clinic that
• Is run by a reputable gynecologist or primary-care physician, preferably one recommended by a physician you trust.
• Offers psychiatric counseling or can refer you, if necessary.
• Understands the psychological and medical aspects of PMS.
• Tailors the treatment to the patient.

• Think twice about PMS herbal products. Many herbal remedies and "formulas" that promise to relieve PMS are promoted in health food stores, supplement catalogs, and on the Internet. Typically, part of their pitch is that they contain only "natural substances." Some products are composed of 15 or more herbs and vitamins, including dong quai, wild yam, chasteberry, borage oil, and alfalfa. There is no convincing evidence that any of these remedies work. Nor can you even be sure they contain what they say they do, since their contents aren't standardized or monitored by the Food and Drug Administration (FDA) or any other regulatory agency.

Prevention

There is no way known to prevent PMS.

When To Call Your Doctor

Contact your physician if PMS symptoms are severe or worsen and prevent you from carrying out daily activities.

What Your Doctor Will Do

No specific laboratory test is available for detecting PMS. Your doctor should thoroughly review your symptoms and may ask you to keep a daily "symptoms diary" for several months if you have not already done so. Based on this information, you and your doctor can determine if your symptoms are due to PMS or if some other disorder is involved.

Your doctor may first recommend lifestyle changes if you haven't tried them. If these don't prove helpful, or if your symptoms are especially severe, medications will probably be prescribed. These may include oral contraceptives, which have been widely prescribed for PMS and which may help with physical symptoms, but may not be effective at relieving mood-related symptoms. Various antidepressant drugs may help with mood changes. A diuretic called spironolactone may be prescribed if severe bloating due to fluid retention is a primary symptom.

For More Information

• American College of Obstetricians and Gynecologists

405

Pneumonia

Symptoms

- Fever (over 100°F, may reach 105°F).
- Chills.
- Cough, sometimes with bloody sputum; this cough may last as long as six weeks after the initial infection has cleared.
- Chest pain on inhalation and shortness of breath.
- Rapid pulse, rapid breathing.
- Weakness and fatigue.
- Muscle pain, sore throat, and headache.
- In severe cases extreme breathing difficulty, blue tinge to fingernails, lips, or other skin areas, mental confusion.

What Is It?

Pneumonia is a general term for a range of acute infections that attack the tissues lining the air spaces—the alveoli—of one or both lungs. The tissues become inflamed, making it difficult for oxygen to reach the bloodstream, impairing breathing. The inflammation that pneumonia causes may be limited to a single area (lobar pneumonia) or may occur in patches throughout the lungs (bronchopneumonia).

Pneumonia can strike people from infancy through old age, though those over 65 are at higher risk. Until the development of antibiotics, pneumonia caused by bacterial infections was the leading cause of death in the United States. It is now the sixth most frequent cause of death, but in developing countries the mortality rate from bacterial pneumonia can be much higher, particularly among young children.

Symptoms of pneumonia can range from very mild to severe—in fact, the illness can be so mild that some people may not know they have it. Infants and the elderly are at the greatest risk of developing serious complications from pneumonia. Healthy adults usually can be cured within two weeks, though aggressive medical treatment may be required.

One of the more serious forms of infection is hospital-acquired pneumonia, which strikes a patient who has been hospitalized for some other condition. It occurs most frequently in patients in intensive care units and/or those who are on ventilators. Though less common than pneumonia that develops outside a hospital (called community-acquired pneumonia), it is the second most common cause of infections acquired in hospitals and has mortality rates as high as 50 percent.

What Causes It?

Pneumonia has many causes, but viral or bacterial infections are the most common—often as a complication of a lingering cold, or a bout with the flu or bronchitis. Nearly half of community-acquired pneumonia cases are believed to be viral, about 30 percent are bacterial, and roughly 20 percent are thought to be caused by mycoplasmas (organisms that have both viral and bacterial characteristics). However, in 40 to 60 percent of cases, the specific agent causing the infection isn't identified. Most cases of hospital-acquired pneumonia are bacterial infections.

Pneumococcal pneumonia, the most common form of bacterial pneumonia in adults over 30, is caused by *Streptococcus pneumoniae*. This bacterium is found in the throats of many healthy people. When body defenses are weakened—by illness, old age, or impaired immunity, for example—the bacteria can work their way into the lungs and multiply. An estimated 150,000 to 570,000 cases of pneumococcal pneumonia are diagnosed in the United States each year, and they account for most pneumonia-related deaths.

Fortunately, a vaccine is available to help prevent pneumococcal pneumonia (see box).

Both bacterial and viral pneumonia can strike year-round, but the autumn and winter months, when colds and influenza proliferate, are major times for the disease, in part because people spend more time indoors, where bacteria and viruses can spread rapidly from one person to another.

Other risk factors for developing community-acquired pneumonia include smoking, recent surgery, and the use of chemotherapy or other immunosuppressive medications. Being in a nursing home or other long-term care facility can also put you at high risk.

Medical conditions that can increase the risk for developing pneumonia include sickle-cell anemia, heart disease, asthma or other chronic lung diseases such as emphysema, poorly controlled diabetes mellitus, alcoholism, chronic kidney disease, and many types of malignancies. In many people with AIDs, pneumonia caused by *Pneumocystis carinii,* an organism believed to be a fungus, is a common cause of pneumonia.

What If You Do Nothing?

Most cases of viral pneumonia are relatively mild and clear up within one to two weeks. In fact, if the infection develops slowly, you may be unaware that you have pneumonia—a condition known as walking pneumonia.

Bacterial pneumonia, on the other hand, is more serious. Left untreated, it can lead to scarring of lung tissue or the infection can spread to other vital organs. The earlier a diagnosis is made and treatment started, the less damage will be done to the lungs. Recovery may take anywhere from 10 days to three weeks.

Vaccines for Adults and Children
▼

Many people are surprised to hear that a vaccine is available to protect adults against strains of the pneumococcal bacteria, which are responsible for most cases of bacterial pneumonia in this country. That may be one reason why only about 45 percent of those who should get the shot, do.

Unlike flu shots, which must be given each year to cope with the newest strains of virus, a single pneumonia vaccination confers immunity for many years. But the Centers for Disease Control (CDC) recommends a booster dose five or more years after the first dose. As with the flu shot, the vaccine has few side effects, usually nothing more than a sore arm.

Anyone who is age 65 or older should get the shot, as well as anyone over age two who is at high risk for serious or life-threatening complications from pneumonia (such as people with chronic kidney disease, diabetes, heart disease, and other disorders that may lower resistance to infection). The vaccine does not protect against viral pneumonia or the type of pneumonia *(Pneumocystis carinii)* that people with AIDS are prone to develop.

If you're 65 or older or in a high-risk group, talk to your physician about getting the pneumonia shot if you haven't had it, or if your previous shot was more than five years ago. (Medicare, by the way, covers the cost of the shot.)

The CDC also recommends that a recently-approved children's vaccine be administered to all children under the age of 5. A child may need as many as three doses of the vaccine as well as a booster shot.

Children ages two to five who are at high risk of contracting pneumococcal illnesses, such as those with HIV infection or chronic illness, may be advised to receive single doses of the older and new vaccines (see page 524 for more information).

407

Home Remedies

Pneumonia, whether bacterial or viral, should be diagnosed and treated by a physician. In either case, though, you can do certain things to help ease symptoms and speed your recovery.

• **Get plenty of rest.** Rest is necessary until the fever and shortness of breath subside.

• **Lower your fever and reduce pain.** Over-the-counter pain relievers—aspirin, ibuprofen, naproxen, or acetaminophen—will help do both when taken according to label directions.

• **Take an over-the-counter cough suppressant.** Look for a product containing dextromethorphan if you have a dry, painful, and persistent cough. Don't use a suppressant if you are coughing up sputum. Suppressing the cough may encourage mucus accumulation in the lungs, which can lead to serious complications.

• **Loosen lung secretions.** Inhale steam, use a humidifier, take hot showers, and drink at least eight glasses a day of water or other nonalcoholic, noncaffeinated fluids to make lung secretions easier to cough up and expel.

• **Get some relief from chest pain.** Use a heating pad on a low setting and place it over your chest for 10-minute intervals.

Prevention

• **Get a flu shot.** An annual flu vaccination may reduce your risk since pneumonia is a common complication of severe flu among those in high-risk groups.

• **Don't smoke.** Tobacco byproducts weaken your ability to battle infection.

• **If you're at high risk, get immunized.** If you're over 65, contact your physician for a pneumococcal pneumonia vaccine. Other candidates for pneumonia vaccine are people who have heart, lung, or kidney disease, have a weakened immune system, or are alcoholics. The vaccine provides long-term protection.

• **A new vaccine is now available for use in children.** If you have a child under age 5, check with your doctor.

When To Call Your Doctor

Contact your physician whenever you have symptoms of pneumonia.

Call for an ambulance if you experience severe difficulty in breathing or if you develop a blue tinge to your skin.

What Your Doctor Will Do

After reviewing your symptoms and examining you, your physician may take a chest x-ray to confirm the diagnosis. If the pneumonia is bacterial, antibiotics may be prescribed. Cases of viral pneumonia are generally treated with medications to relieve the primary symptoms. Depending on the severity of your pneumonia and your age, hospitalization may be recommended.

For More Information

• American Lung Association
• Centers for Disease Control and Prevention

Posture Problems

Symptoms

- Slumped, hunched, or rounded shoulders, protruding abdomen, swayback (an excessive forward curve in the lower back), caved-in appearance of the chest.
- Back and neck pain, headaches.

What Is It?

Sitting and standing put considerable pressure on the lower back; standing exerts five times more pressure than lying down, and sitting, surprisingly, is even more strenuous. In fact, researchers now believe that poor sitting posture is a major contributor to low-back pain. Poor standing and lying posture aren't good for your back either.

In addition to helping prevent back and neck problems, good posture is important in positive ways. It improves your appearance and helps you project self-confidence and self-assurance. It can help you mentally and emotionally. And certainly it is worth achieving just for the aches and pains it may prevent.

As long as people aren't actually in pain, they tend to forget how delicately their backs are engineered. The three spinal curves (neck, upper, lower) need to be kept in balanced alignment, and to do this, strong, flexible muscles are important. Poor posture can strain both muscles and ligaments, making you more vulnerable to injury—as well as complicating such everyday tasks as carrying groceries or even sitting at a desk. An improperly aligned spine may narrow the space between vertebrae, thereby increasing the risk of compressed nerves.

Posture is not simply what happens when you are sitting or standing still—it's also dynamic, and includes your posture when you move. Poor posture may include many elements—rounded shoulders, protruding buttocks and abdomen, overly arched lower back, and the head pushed forward into an exaggerated position.

What Causes It?

Poor posture may be caused by many factors, including previous injuries, disease, poor muscle tone, and emotional stress. A sedentary lifestyle can reduce muscle tone and strength and lead to bad posture. Sore, aching feet have a negative effect on posture, too. Foot pain may mean simply that you're choosing the wrong shoes. Or you may need special supports—orthotic devices—in your shoes and an evaluation by a podiatrist. One very important factor is habit. Contrary to what some people believe, straightening up now and then isn't enough: you need to be aware of—and to practice—other strategies to improve standing and sitting.

What If You Do Nothing?

In itself, poor posture isn't a health problem. But it won't improve without some effort on your part, and in the meantime it can have an adverse impact on your musculoskeletal system. If you don't take steps to improve your posture, you may eventually limit your lung expansion—which means less energy available to your body and brain—and develop chronic muscle aches, including headaches and back pains.

Home Remedies

- **Standing.** Take a look in the mirror for these signs: a protruding abdomen, slumped or rounded shoulders, or swayback (an excessive forward curve in the lower back). Any of these could be putting extra pressure on the muscles and ligaments of your spine. A slight hollow in the lower back is natural and desirable; in fact, good stand-

Some exercises to improve posture

These simple stretching and strengthening exercises target muscles (such as the hamstrings and abdominals) essential to good posture. Try to do these in the morning and again at night.

Lower-back and abdominal workout. Lie on your back with arms out to your sides. Bend your knees and raise them toward your chest. Slowly lower both knees to the floor on one side. Hold for 15 seconds. Bring knees back to starting position, keeping arms and shoulder blades on floor, then lower to other side. Repeat 5 times on each side.

Thigh stretch. Lying flat on your stomach, grasp left ankle with left hand. Press the bent leg back against your hand's resistance. Hold for 20 to 30 seconds. Then pull that leg upward so that the heel touches your buttocks. Hold for 20 to 30 seconds, then lower your leg part way. Repeat 5 times with each leg.

Hamstring stretch. Working with a partner, sit on the floor with legs straight and hands behind you for balance. 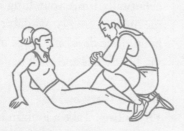 Put one leg on partner's shoulder and press down 20 to 30 seconds. Then ask partner to press down gently just above your knee while he rises up slightly to create a passive stretch. Hold for 20 to 30 seconds. Repeat 5 times with each leg.

Neck stretch. Sitting on a stool or chair, and holding the seat with your right hand, put your left hand on the rear right side of your head. Gently pull your head down while rotating your chin to the left. Hold for 20 to 30 seconds. Change hands and repeat on the opposite side. Repeat 5 times on each side. You can also stretch your neck by gently pulling head down toward shoulder without rotating head.

Shoulder and upper back workout. Sit on a straight chair, but without touching the back. (1) With hands clasped behind your head, raise your shoulders toward your ears, then press down. (2) Press the back of your head into your hands, so that muscles along your upper spine tighten; hold for 5 seconds. (3) Press your elbows back 10 times, so that you feel the movement in your shoulder blades.

Back stretch. Hold the rim of a sink to brace yourself, with your arms straight but not locked. Place our feet hip-width apart, right under your shoulders, with knees slightly bent. With your head hanging slightly and neck muscles relaxed, let your hips sink back as if you were about to sit down. Feel the stretch down the length of your spine. Hold position for 10 seconds. Gradually straighten up. Repeat 5 times.

410

ing posture maintains this and the two other natural curves that are visible from a side view—a gentle forward curve in the neck area and backward curve in the upper back.

The goal is to avoid exaggerating these curves. The military stance, with chest thrust forward and shoulders and derriere pushed way back, isn't desirable, since it creates a swayback.

• **Think tall.** Simply stand with your head held over your shoulders, your chin parallel to the floor, and your neck straight. Your shoulders should be level without any slumping, and in front your chest, waist, and hips should all line up.

• **Practice tightening your abdominal muscles and flattening your stomach.** Clasp your hands and press against the abdomen as you slowly draw in the muscles, flattening them as much as possible. Hold the position for a few seconds, then relax. Repeat three or four times, and also on occasion throughout the day. Without the hand movement, this is an almost invisible exercise that you can do anywhere.

• **When standing for long periods, minimize stress on the lower back.** Put one foot on a low stool or another stable object. Frequently shift your weight from one leg to another. To relax, bend over and let your head, neck, shoulders, and arms hang down briefly. Don't stand too long in one position.

• **Sitting.** The extra pressure that sitting exerts on your lower back comes from the upper body shifting forward, forcing the back muscles to strain to hold you upright. Slouching increases the pressure on your lower back to about 10 to 15 times as much as when you're lying down. Hunching over tenses the muscles in the neck and upper back. Good sitting posture involves the same slight forward curve in your lower back that's also the key to good standing posture. The following steps can help improve your sitting posture.

• **Choose a chair that firmly supports your lower back.** For long periods of sitting, choose a straight chair. The chair shouldn't be heavily padded, since that can cause excess curving of your back. It should fit under your desk or table so that you maintain your upright posture. Chair armrests are a plus, too, since you can support some of your weight on them, especially when you shift positions in the chair. Propping up reading matter also helps.

• **Sit firmly back in the chair.** Don't sit on the edge. Keep your shoulders against the chair back, your chest lifted, and your upper back straight. A rolled up towel or small lumbar pillow can provide extra support. When working at a desk or table, bring your chair close enough that you needn't lean over. Your feet should touch the floor comfortably—if they don't, rest them on a small stool or telephone book.

Sitting with your knees slightly higher than your hips can reduce excess curvature in your

411

Standing Tall

▼

A simple test can make you more aware of what constitutes good posture and can help improve your spinal flexibility. Stand in a normal, relaxed posture with your back against a wall—upper back and buttocks touching it. Slip your hand into the space between your lower back and the wall; it should slide in easily and almost touch both your back and the wall. If there's extra space, you may have a swayback. To correct it, imagine that a string is tied to the top of your head and is pulling you straight up; then tuck in your abdomen and tilt your hips so that the space between your lower back and the wall is lessened. When you walk away from the wall, try to maintain the stance and the mental image of the string.

lower back. Crossing your legs occasionally can be a good idea, too. Change sitting positions frequently, and get up to stretch and move around every half hour, if possible.

• **Adjust for work.** If you're typing or working at a computer, make sure any work you're copying is at a comfortable level. Looking up or down for long periods can put stress on your neck, shoulders, and upper-back muscles.

• **Maintain driving posture.** Position your seat so that you can easily reach the wheel and get your foot on the brake and accelerator. Many seats adjust for height, so try to have your knees slightly higher than your hips. Change the seat position occasionally (tilting slightly forward or back) if you're driving for long periods. Avoid slumping forward or sitting in a twisted position (for example, with your elbow resting heavily on the windowsill or armrest). Stop every couple of hours and stretch or walk around.

If your seat provides inadequate support for your lower back, try a rolled up towel or lumbar roll. A seat pad may also help. Frequently repositioning your hands on the wheel can take some strain off upper back and neck muscles.

Prevention

All of the self-care measures for standing and sitting suggested above can help prevent poor posture. Here are some additional tips.

• **Choose a firm mattress to support your spine.** Try to avoid sleeping on your stomach—it's better to be on your side with your knees bent. If you do sleep on your stomach, choose a large pillow that gives your shoulders some support. Whatever your customary sleeping posture, make sure

your pillow supports your neck in a straight position. This may prevent neck pain and the sore muscles that can interfere with good posture when you're awake.

• **Maintain a healthy weight.** Obesity is hard on the muscles in your back and abdomen and can cause bad posture.

• **Avoid high heels and platform shoes.** Use them only for short periods. For daily wear, especially when you're on your feet, make sure your shoes fit and offer good support. For exercise, including walking, invest in a shoe that not only fits but supports your foot. High heels throw the back out of line and adversely affect posture.

• **Get regular exercise.** Besides promoting weight loss and better general health, exercise tones and strengthens the muscles that are important to good posture. Walking is one of the best ways to improve posture.

When To Call Your Doctor

Contact your physician or an orthopedist if you have chronic neck or back pain caused by poor posture, or when your own efforts to correct bad posture don't succeed.

What Your Doctor Will Do

After taking a careful history, your doctor may prescribe a course of physical therapy or recommend an exercise program. Many kinds of sports, exercise, and movement therapies can help improve posture.

For More Information

• American Academy of Orthopaedic Surgeons
• American Osteopathic Association

Presbyopia

Symptoms

- Blurred vision at normal reading distances.
- Headache, eye fatigue, stinging, burning, or gritty sensation in the eyes after doing close work.

What Is It?

Most people over the age of 45 begin to need glasses to read small print, even those who still have excellent distance vision. This condition is called presbyopia, a Greek word that literally means "old vision."

The changes are very gradual, and you won't notice the loss until one day you find yourself squinting at a newspaper that's held at arm's length and still appears to be blurred, or you have trouble reading anything in a dimly lit room. Threading a needle becomes a marathon task. By the time people reach their 50s and 60s, most of them will need some type of assistance with their vision.

What Causes It?

Presbyopia is a condition that occurs when the lens of the eye becomes less flexible and thus less able to change shape and focus on close objects, especially in dim light or when a person is tired.

What If You Do Nothing?

Presbyopia will gradually get worse as you age, and you will find that it's more difficult to read small print unless you begin using corrective lenses.

Home Remedies

- **Get some drugstore reading glasses.** These can cost $100 or more if prescribed by a specialist; yet over-the-counter glasses, which cost around $20 or less, may be just as effective. These glasses must meet the requirements of the American National Standards Institute (ANSI) and of the Food and Drug Administration (FDA), including passing impact resistance tests.

There's an important caution, however: over-the-counter reading glasses won't correct near-sightedness, astigmatism, or other refractive defects, and buying a pair of them is no substitute for an eye exam. When you pick out non-prescription reading glasses, be sure you have the time to try on several pairs and to read the test cards provided. You might also carry along a book or newspaper for testing.

Glasses will usually be marked with a number ranging from 1.00 to 4.00, indicating the magnifying power. (Low magnification would be 1.25 or 1.50; high would be 3.00 and above.) Start at the low end and work your way up, holding the card at a comfortable reading distance.

- **Increase the amount of light—especially for reading and other close-up activities.** Go from 60- to 100-watt bulbs whenever possible.

Prevention

There is no way to prevent presbyopia.

When To Call Your Doctor

Contact your eye doctor when the signs of presbyopia begin to interfere with daily activities. Many eye specialists advise glaucoma testing at age 40 or 50—when signs of presbyopia often start to appear. If your vision is changing rapidly, consult an optometrist or ophthalmologist to make sure that magnifying glasses for reading are all you need.

What Your Doctor Will Do

You will be given an eye examination. After you

explain to your eye doctor all the various tasks you do on and off the job that require clear vision, the doctor will use the information to help determine and fit the corrective lenses that will be best for you. (Eye surgery for correcting focusing problems—such as PRK and LASIK, two newer techniques that utilize laser beams to reshape parts of the cornea—cannot be used to correct or halt presbyopia. If you have presbyopia, you will still need glasses for reading even if you have surgery for near-sightedness, far-sightedness, or astigmatism.)

Depending on your existing vision problems, you may need bifocals or trifocals—glasses with two or three kinds of vision correction, as the name implies. A progressive-lens type of bifocal —which is manufactured to provide a gradual change in correction from top to bottom—is another option. Progressive lenses are more expensive than conventional bifocals and have a smaller field for reading. Progressives are also harder to prescribe and fit than regular bifocals, so buy them from someone who is experienced in fitting them.

If you wear contact lenses, you can consider bifocal contact lenses, though these won't work for everyone. Another choice is monovision—wearing a near-vision contact lens in one eye and a distance-vision one in the other, so that you see with one eye at a time. If you decide to investigate either of these options, discuss your needs with an experienced professional. Remember, too, that you may need new lenses every 12 to 18 months for a time to correct for worsening presbyopia.

For More Information

• American Academy of Ophthalmology
• American Optometric Association

Prickly Heat (Heat Rash)

Symptoms

- Pink, itchy rash that often develops in folds of skin that are covered—the neck, upper back, armpits, and, in babies, the diaper area. The rash is sometimes accompanied by tiny bumps or fluid-filled blisters.
- Rarely, intense itching or burning (when rash is severe).

What Is It?

Prickly heat, also known as heat rash or miliaria, can occur during childhood or adulthood, but is most common in infants and very young children. The rash appears when sweat builds up under the skin and can't escape properly—usually in areas where skin surfaces overlap, such as the neck, underarms, or groin. Prickly heat usually occurs in hot and humid conditions, but fever or being dressed too warmly can also trigger it.

What Causes It?

When sweating is profuse, the pores leading to the ducts of the sweat glands can become blocked. This prevents the skin from releasing sweat, which is the body's natural way of cooling off. The sweat is held within the skin, and subsequently, the rash forms.

Infants are most at risk for prickly heat because their sweat glands are still developing.

What If You Do Nothing?

By keeping your child (or yourself) cool, clean, and dry, the rash should clear up completely within two to three days.

Home Remedies

- **Use calamine lotion.** Apply it to the worst areas to ease itching.

- **Take frequent cool or lukewarm baths.** This will help cool overheated skin. Use mild soap and dry the skin thoroughly with a soft towel.

Prevention

- **Stay cool.** In hot and humid conditions, avoid direct sun. Try to stay in the shade or indoors during the hottest periods. If possible, put a child in an air-conditioned room; otherwise, use a fan.
- **Dress appropriately.** Clothing made of cotton or other breathable fabrics should be worn to facilitate cooling and the evaporation of sweat. In cold weather, don't overdress; dress in layers of clothing that can be removed or added to avoid overheating.
- **Keep the skin dry.** Avoid greasy ointments. They can hold moisture in and further clog the pores. They also tend to keep the skin warmer. If an infant is perspiring heavily, applying a cornstarch powder can help. Put the powder into your hand first and apply sparingly to prevent inhalation, which may cause lung injury.

When To Call Your Doctor

If the rash has not cleared up after three or four days despite appropriate at-home measures, or the rash has worsened or spread, or other symptoms such as fever or irritability develop, call your doctor or pediatrician.

What Your Doctor Will Do

Your doctor will check for other conditions—such as measles or chicken pox—that produce rashes and/or determine whether the rash is the result of an allergic reaction to a skin product, detergent, or new food.

For More Information

- American Academy of Pediatrics

Psoriasis

Symptoms

- Distinct rashlike patches of dry, reddened, raised and inflamed skin with white flaking scales (usually appearing on the scalp, lower back, elbows, knees, or knuckles).
- Itching.
- In severe cases cracked and blistered skin, often painful, and ultimately disfiguring.
- In some severe cases pitted, crumbly, and loosened fingernails.
- May be associated with arthritis.

What Is It?

Psoriasis is a noncontagious but persistent skin disorder that occurs when the normal cycle of skin cell growth and replacement is disrupted. Normally, new skin cells rise from the deepest layer of skin to the top layer—the epidermis—and replace dead skin cells, which are shed. This process ordinarily takes about 28 days. In areas marked by psoriasis, the process has been accelerated, taking place in only three or four days—and as a result excess cells accumulate, causing the characteristic scaly patches.

Eruptions of psoriasis tend to first appear between the ages of 10 and 30 and may continue the rest of a person's life. The rashes can increase and decrease in severity, often for no apparent reason, although they are often more severe during the winter (perhaps because of drier air) and prolonged periods indoors. Psoriasis cannot be cured, and it can be painful and unpleasant to live with, especially in severe cases when skin can crack and blister and nails may become pitted and deformed.

What Causes It?

No one knows what causes psoriasis. Strong evidence points to a genetic component (32 percent of patients have a family history of the condition). There are several things that can trigger psoriasis or make symptoms worse. These include alcohol, obesity, stress, sore throat from a strep infection, anxiety, certain medications, and sunburn. Contrary to popular belief, there is no link between diet and psoriasis.

What If You Do Nothing?

There is no cure for psoriasis. Since this chronic ailment is often painful and unpleasant to live with, some treatment is recommended to relieve the symptoms.

Home Remedies

Psoriasis is not curable, but it can be controlled. It's best to consult a doctor initially. The following home remedies can complement any treatments your doctor recommends. Only trial and error will determine which treatments are most effective for you. Improvement can take a few weeks or as long as several months.

• **Get some sun.** Most people should guard against too much exposure to the sun. But to minimize the effects of psoriasis, regular sunbathing offers some benefit. Proceed cautiously, staying in direct sunlight for 15 to 30 minutes a day. About 80 percent of people with psoriasis will see improvement in three to six weeks. Since sunburn on healthy unaffected areas of skin can aggravate the psoriasis or make it resistant to future treatment, apply sunscreen to those areas a half hour before sunbathing. Use a sunscreen with a sun protection factor (SPF) of at least 15.

• **Moisturize your skin.** Apply moisturizing skin creams liberally to your skin to keep it moist and less likely to crack. Avoid alcohol-based preparations, which can dry the skin; also avoid lanolin-based products if you are allergic to lanolin. When used regularly, petroleum jelly and lactic-acid-based moisturizers can keep the skin from drying.

- **Take a soak.** Special bath solutions containing either oatmeal, various oils, or coal tar may offer symptomatic relief for psoriasis. Soak for 15 minutes in warm bath water to soothe the skin and encourage healing. Moisturize when you get out.
- **Remove skin scales.** Nonprescription creams and ointments that contain salicylic acid help to soften and remove scales. Coal-tar gels, also available in the pharmacy without prescription, can slow down the rate at which skin cells are produced, thereby improving psoriasis.
- **Get some scalp relief.** For psoriasis plaques in the scalp, a special softening gel that contains salicylic acid is available over the counter. Apply it to the scalp at night according to directions, and wash it out in the morning with a medicated dandruff shampoo.
- **Be careful with your hair.** When combing your hair, don't comb too vigorously. Anytime you scratch or scrape your scalp with a comb or brush, you increase the risk of having psoriasis come back worse than before.
- **Avoid scratching.** If you have an itch and feel like scratching, reach for moisturizer instead.
- **Reduce stress in your life.** If stress makes your psoriasis worse, take steps to reduce it. Stress reduction exercises such as yoga, biofeedback, or meditation may work well for you.

Prevention

There is no way to prevent psoriasis. However, avoiding alcoholic beverages and minimizing your exposure to cold temperatures, preventing skin injuries, and reducing stress may prevent any psoriasis flare-ups.

When To Call Your Doctor

Psoriasis may be confused with seborrhea or atopic dermatitis. Certain types of skin cancer may also look like psoriasis. For this reason contact your physician, who will make the correct diagnosis and prescribe the proper course of treatment. Also contact your doctor if psoriasis symptoms fail to respond to self-treatment.

What Your Doctor Will Do

After taking a complete history and performing a skin examination, your physician may prescribe corticosteroids and/or other medications to control and alleviate your symptoms. Many new drugs are being developed for treating psoriasis; your dermatologist should be acquainted with them and know which ones might be of benefit to you.

For More Information

- American Academy of Dermatology
- National Psoriasis Foundation

Restless Legs Syndrome

Symptoms

- Irresistible urge to move the legs or other affected body parts.
- Unpleasant crawling and/or aching sensation inside the calf muscles while lying down. Similar sensations may also be felt in the thighs, feet, and arms.
- Involuntary jerking movements of the legs during sleep.

What Is It?

Restless legs syndrome (RLS), a physical malady that affects as many as 12 million Americans, is an unusual sensation in the leg muscles that creates an irresistible urge to move the legs for relief. The feeling has been described as a fidgeting, pulling, or itching sensation—or, more graphically, as worms crawling in the muscles. Symptoms may last for an hour or more, generally starting at night or during rest. Typically, symptoms start within 5 to 30 minutes after lying down, just prior to the onset of sleep.

People of all ages can experience RLS, although the problem occurs most often in older people, especially women. RLS often runs in families, and it worsens in times of stress. Since RLS can wake people from a sound sleep or prevent them from getting to sleep in the first place, it often results in insomnia.

What Causes It?

The exact cause of restless legs syndrome is unknown. People with RLS also sometimes have a condition called "periodic limb movement disorder," which involves an involuntary jerking of the legs. Some research suggests that the symptoms of RLS are related to lower-than-normal levels of the neurotransmitter dopamine in the brain. Pregnancy is linked with higher incidences of RLS (it generally clears up after delivery), as are iron-deficiency anemia, rheumatoid arthritis, diabetes mellitus, lung disease, and kidney disease. Emotional stress, and the regular use of tobacco or caffeine, may trigger or aggravate symptoms.

What If You Do Nothing?

RLS is extremely unpleasant and if left untreated can bring on an exhausting chronic insomnia. But if you're healthy, as most people with RLS are, simple changes in lifestyle may be enough to bring some relief from a condition that can last for years. It's also worth talking to your doctor about RLS, since some medications are being used to successfully treat the problem (see When To Call Your Doctor).

Home Remedies

- **Exercise your legs before bedtime.** Walk around for 10 to 15 minutes prior to going to bed. This will stretch the leg muscles and can help promote restful sleep. Massaging your leg muscles before bedtime may also help relieve symptoms.
- **Start walking.** If RLS strikes while you're in bed, get up and walk around. Try doing a few simple exercises.
- **Wear long, heavy socks.** Keeping your feet and legs warm in bed may help relax your muscles.
- **Try the cold approach.** Some people may find relief by soaking their feet in cold water. A cold compress applied to the shins and calf muscles may also help. You can leave your legs uncovered in bed.
- **Try sleeping on your side with a pillow between your knees.** This may help relax leg muscles.
- **Reduce emotional stress.** Stress management

Restless Legs Syndrome *continued*

techniques or psychological counseling may help relieve anxiety that triggers restless legs.

Prevention

Nicotine and large amounts of caffeine may trigger RLS in some people. Consequently, avoid products containing caffeine, and if you smoke, stop.

When To Call Your Doctor

Contact your physician if restless legs syndrome is severe and/or regularly interferes with sleep.

What Your Doctor Will Do

Little is known about restless legs syndrome, and it can be extremely difficult to diagnose and treat. A thorough physical examination will first be performed to exclude other disorders.

Some medications such as antihistamines may cause restless legs syndrome as a side effect; if that applies to you, your medication may be changed to prevent RLS. Some RLS patients have an iron deficiency, so the doctor will also check iron levels and prescribe iron supplements when needed.

After a diagnosis is made, various tranquilizers (benzodiazepines) may be prescribed for more severe cases. Doctors have also been prescribing anti-Parkinson drugs with some success.

For More Information

• Restless Legs Syndrome Foundation
• National Sleep Foundation

Rheumatoid Arthritis

Symptoms

- Early symptoms (prior to obvious joint involvement) are generally nonspecific and include fatigue and weakness; low-grade fever; loss of appetite and weight loss.
- Red, swollen, painful joints, most often those of the fingers, wrists, knees, ankles, and toes on both sides of the body. (This symmetrical pattern and inflammation differentiates it from osteoarthritis. Also, rheumatoid arthritis, unlike osteoarthritis, usually spares the joints nearest the fingertips.)
- Tender joints, warm to the touch.
- Stiffness, especially after awakening in the morning; usually improves during the day.
- Red, painless skin lumps (rheumatoid nodules) on the elbows, ears, nose, knees, toes, or back of the scalp.
- Bent and gnarled joints (with long-term rheumatoid arthritis).
- Chest pain, breathing difficulty (advanced cases).

What Is It?

Rheumatoid arthritis (RA) can be a very severe form of arthritis. It is a chronic, disabling disorder that can cause a multitude of physical woes, including inflammation and eventual destruction of the joints and cartilage throughout the body. It can also affect the lungs, muscles, blood vessels, skin, and heart.

Fortunately, not everyone who has this disease is severely affected. Many people with RA experience only minor symptoms, and in some cases the disease simply ends, or "burns out."

Less common than osteoarthritis, rheumatoid arthritis affects upward of 2 percent of the population, with three times more women than men suffering its effects. Although the disease typically manifests itself in people between the ages of 20 and 40, it can start at any age.

Many doctors and researchers consider the disease an autoimmune disorder. Disorders of this nature result when the body initiates an immunological response to protect itself against something mistakenly recognized as foreign.

The joint damage caused by RA begins with inflammation of a layer of tissue called synovium that lines the joints. The inflammation leads to a thickened synovial membrane owing to an overgrowth of synovial cells and an accumulation of white blood cells. The release of enzymes and other substances by these cells can erode the cartilage that lines the ends of joints, as well as the bones, tendons, and ligaments within the joint capsule. As the disease progresses, the production of excess fibrous tissue limits joint motion. Inflammation of tissue surrounding affected joints can also contribute to joint damage.

What Causes It?

The exact cause of RA is unknown, but a susceptibility to develop it is inherited. Since the ratio of women to men with RA is three to one, some experts believe hormonal factors may play a role. The disease is generally progressive, and early treatment is important to slow or stop the progression and any accompanying disability.

What If You Do Nothing?

A small number of patients diagnosed with RA (about 10 percent) experience a complete remission in one year, and roughly 40 percent go into remission within two years. But if the disease progresses and is not treated, it may severely restrict the range of motion of some joints, or worse, destroy the joints altogether.

Home Remedies

There is no cure for RA at present. The best chance for relieving symptoms requires seeing your doctor to develop a treatment plan—and then taking an active role in your treatment. This means maintaining a medication schedule, exercise program, and other therapy recommended by your physician. Educating yourself about the disease is also very helpful. In addition, the following self-care measures can bring relief.

• **Try hot or cold packs.** Depending upon which temperature feels better, apply a hot or cold pack to a stiff or painful joint.

• **Get plenty of rest.** Sleeping 8 to 10 hours a night is optimal. Resting during the day is also helpful. When your joints feel warm, swollen, and painful, cut back on physical activity.

• **Perform range-of-motion exercises.** To maintain joint mobility, perform light exercises that will help preserve the mobility in the painful joint.

• **Exercise gently and regularly.** The gentle movement of regular exercise is an effective therapy for RA. Walking and swimming are excellent activities to help maintain joint flexibility and strengthen supporting muscles (but let your physician or physical therapist outline your program). The key to a successful program is to find a balance between exercise and adequate rest.

• **Ease the strain on painful joints.** Make use of devices (such as an electric can opener, larger pens, grab bars in the shower, and other assistive devices) that lend support and/or minimize joint involvement. A special splint for the hand or wrist can be useful in protecting an injured joint and relieving pain (check with your doctor).

Prevention

At present, there is no known way to prevent rheumatoid arthritis.

When To Call Your Doctor

Contact your physician if persistent joint pain or stiffness develops, especially if it begins to interfere with daily activities. Also contact your physician if you have RA and new symptoms develop.

What Your Doctor Will Do

There is no specific diagnostic test for rheumatoid arthritis. Your doctor will take a careful history and then perform a physical examination of the joints, heart, and lungs. Blood tests may be done and x-rays may also be taken; synovial fluid may be drawn from affected joints and analyzed. If your medical history or the tests are positive, treatment will begin immediately.

A range of medications is available that can slow the destructive aspects of RA. Aspirin to reduce pain and inflammation is the cornerstone of therapy for many patients—but to be effective, aspirin is taken in doses higher than commonly used, which can cause stomach problems. If aspirin is ineffective or causes serious side effects, your doctor may prescribe another nonsteroidal anti-inflammatory drug (NSAID).

If NSAIDs don't adequately control symptoms, other drugs can be tried, including corticosteroids and disease-modifying antirheumatic drugs (DMARDs).

Your doctor or a physical therapist will also advise you about an exercise program. For severe cases physical therapy may be prescribed, and surgery may be recommended for people with severe joint damage.

For More Information

• American College of Rheumatology
• American Pain Foundation
• Arthritis Foundation

Rocky Mountain Spotted Fever

Symptoms

- Severe headache.
- Chills, with fever that often reaches 104°F and can stay elevated for weeks if untreated.
- A pink rash that appears within two to six days of the fever, typically on the wrist and ankles, and spreads to the rest of the body and the face within 24 hours. This rash is one of the few that appear on the palms and the soles of the feet. (About 10 percent of patients never get the rash.)
- Nausea, vomiting, diarrhea, abdominal pain.
- Muscle aches.
- Heightened sensitivity to light.

What Is It?

First common in the Rocky Mountain region of this country in the 1940s, Rocky Mountain spotted fever (RMSF) is a serious microbial illness caused by the bite of a tick that now primarily inhabits the southern Atlantic states—North Carolina, Virginia, and Maryland—as well as Oklahoma. More than 90 percent of the cases occur between April 1 and September 30, the time of year when the ticks are most active. The illness can last two to three weeks.

What Causes It?

The bite of an adult dog tick or wood tick infected with the organism *R. rickettsii* is the primary cause of the illness. The organism invades and multiplies in the cells lining the arteries and veins throughout the body.

What If You Do Nothing?

If left untreated, mild cases of RMSF may disappear within two weeks. Severe cases require medical attention and usually hospitalization, since the illness can result in heart failure, pneumonia, kidney problems, and other serious complications. Between 20 and 30 percent of the cases of RMSF end up being fatal if untreated. Most of those who die are elderly.

Home Remedies

There are no home remedies for RMSF, which should be diagnosed and treated by a physician.

Prevention

- **Minimize contact.** Stay out of tick-infested terrain, typically mountainous, heavily wooded, or sagebrush areas.
- **Protect yourself.** If you are in known tick areas, wear protective clothing and use insect repellent on exposed skin and clothing.
- **Look for ticks.** Once you arrive home, inspect your body for ticks.
- **Remove any ticks.** Use tweezers to pull or pinch off any tick attached to your skin (see page 137); if you must use your fingers to touch the tick, cover them with tissue.
- **Wash thoroughly.** Wash the area of the bite with soap and water or an antiseptic.

When To Call Your Doctor

Contact your physician for diagnosis and treatment if you develop telltale symptoms.

What Your Doctor Will Do

After diagnosing the condition, your physician will begin antibiotic drug therapy.

For More Information

- Centers for Disease Control and Prevention

Rosacea

Symptoms

- Areas of the face appear to blush for a few minutes to a few hours.
- In some cases, outbreaks can leave a permanent sunburned appearance.
- Blood vessels in areas with rosacea enlarge and become more visible through the skin.
- Pimples appear in some cases.
- In about half of the cases a burning and gritty sensation is experienced in the eyes.

What Is It?

Rosacea (rose-AY-sha) is a chronic inflammation of the skin of the face that causes redness and swelling. Characterized by enlargement of blood vessels in the skin, the condition—which affects 13 million Americans—typically affects the forehead, chin, cheeks, and nose. It often begins with brief periods of facial flushing that may not even be noticed. In time, rosacea leads to the appearance of small spidery blood vessels (telangiectasia) and tiny pimples in and around the reddened area (which is why it was once known as adult acne). In some cases rosacea may be accompanied by oily skin and dandruff.

In more advanced cases, thick red bumps may develop on the lower half of the nose and spread to the cheek. This condition, called rhinophyma, is more common in men than women, with its victims often mistaken for alcoholics, thanks to the comedian W.C. Fields, who had rhinophyma and rosacea and regularly referred to his nose bumps as "gin blossoms." But teetotalers can certainly get rosacea.

Rosacea is sometimes called the curse of the Celts because so many people who develop it are of Irish ancestry. In fact, it can also afflict other ethnic groups. Still, those most likely to develop rosacea are adults with fair hair and skin, typically women between the ages of 30 and 60. When it strikes men, rosacea is often more severe.

What Causes It?

Some experts believe a vascular disorder is the cause. Since rosacea can affect several family members, researchers think there is a genetic component to the disease. The actual cause of rosacea is still unknown, but a number of diverse factors can aggravate the condition, including stress, spicy foods, smoking, alcohol, temperature extremes, humidity, exercise, hot drinks, wind, excessive sunlight, and skin products that contain irritating ingredients.

What If You Do Nothing?

Rosacea rarely reverses itself and may last for years, worsening without treatment.

Home Remedies

Rosacea can't be cured, but it can be treated with several medications prescribed by your physician. In addition, the following measures may help.

- **Try to avoid direct sun.** Sunlight is a common aggravating factor. When you must be in the sun, wear a hat and be sure to apply sunscreen.
- **Keep a trigger diary.** One way to help control rosacea is to avoid anything that you think makes your face flush. Keeping a diary of such triggers may help. These might include alcoholic beverages, alcohol applied to the skin, hydrocortisone creams, sun exposure, hot baths, hot or very cold weather, vigorous exercise, heavy lifting, straining on the toilet, chronic cough, menopause, or emotional upset. Hot spices and peppers, hot drinks, chocolate, yogurt, and tomatoes may aggravate rosacea. So can certain drugs, such as niacin in large doses (for lowering cholesterol) and blood

pressure medications. Most over-the-counter "remedies" aggravate rosacea rather than help it.

• **Check your cosmetics and medications.** Certain medications may dilate blood vessels and worsen rosacea. Instead of using oil-based products, switch to less irritating water-based cosmetics.

• **Reduce stress in your life.** Do your best not to suppress anger, fear, or other strong emotions.

• **Avoid rubbing your face.** This can irritate your skin.

• **Switch to an electric shaver.** Razor blades can irritate the skin. Avoid aftershave lotions containing alcohol, menthol, witch hazel, or peppermint.

• **Apply a cold compress.** Soak a cloth in ice-cold water and apply it to the flushed areas of your face for 10 minutes. This will help constrict dilated blood vessels and slow down the inflammatory process.

• **Avoid extremes of temperature.** When it's very hot or cold, rosacea symptoms can intensify.

Prevention

There are no specific preventive measures for rosacea, but you can help control it by avoiding anything that makes your face flush.

When To Call Your Doctor

Rosacea can be treated and controlled if it is diagnosed early and treatment begins immediately. At first, rosacea usually appears, disappears, and then reappears a short time later. When you notice that the skin doesn't return to its normal color after an outbreak, and when you develop other symptoms such as pimples and enlarged blood vessels, you should contact your physician, who may refer you to a dermatologist. You may also see an ophthalmologist if your eyes and eyelids are involved.

What Your Doctor Will Do

After a careful examination and diagnosis, your physician may prescribe topical medications or oral antibiotics to reduce the facial redness and inflammation and to heal the bumps—a process that requires patience, since it can take weeks or even months. For severe cases laser treatment and/or surgery may be recommended. Rosacea can recur for years or even over a lifetime, and each recurrence should be treated.

For More Information

• American Academy of Dermatology
• National Institute of Arthritis and Musculoskeletal and Skin Diseases Information Clearinghouse

Rotator Cuff Injury

Symptoms

- Sharp or dull pain in and around the shoulder joint; often worse at night.
- Pain aggravated by rotating or lifting the arm, especially raising it to shoulder level or higher.
- Shoulder weakness.
- Loss of shoulder mobility.

What Is It?

Shoulder pain is often linked to the rotator cuff, a group of four delicate muscles (subscapularis, infraspinatus, supraspinatus, and teres minor) and their tendons. The rotator cuff stabilizes the upper arm in the shoulder socket and allows it range of motion.

Injuries to the rotator cuff vary in severity, ranging from rotator cuff tendinitis (a microscopic tear and inflammation of the rotator cuff) to rotator cuff tear, a rupture of a tendon.

Golfers, swimmers, tennis players, volleyball players, and baseball pitchers may all have trouble with their rotator cuffs, as may people who install high shelves, work with hand tools, or do anything with a lot of shoulder movement. Luckily, when caught early, a mild case of rotator cuff disease can be treated fairly easily.

What Causes It?

Sports with a repetitive overhead movement (swimming, baseball, or tennis, for example) can gradually strain the rotator cuff tendons, as can manual labor such as painting, plastering, or even housework. A more acute injury can occur from lifting heavy objects or falling onto your shoulder or upper arm.

The pain that results may be caused by what's known as an impingement syndrome. This means that because of exertion or overuse, one or more of the rotator cuff muscles and tendons are impinged upon—that is, compressed and irritated—by the shoulder bone, resulting in inflammation and possibly microscopic or even larger tears. The bursae, small fluid-filled sacs that protect the muscles and tendons from irritation by the bone, are usually inflamed as well. (Shoulder pain that occurs suddenly without an obvious acute injury or overuse activity may be bursitis.)

What If You Do Nothing?

Rotator cuff pain is unlikely to heal on its own; at the very least you need to rest the shoulder and avoid activities that may be causing the problem. If you have rotator cuff pain, the important thing is to treat the injury so that it does not become chronic and interfere with everyday activities.

Home Remedies

The first stage of this condition may be tendinitis or bursitis, which is common not only in athletes but in nonathletes—typically those 45 years and older—as well. A mild case of shoulder tendinitis or bursitis can be treated with the following self-care measures.

- **Rest.** If you suspect that a certain activity has caused the pain, stop it for a while.
- **Take over-the-counter pain relievers.** Nonprescription NSAIDs (aspirin, ibuprofen, and naproxen) will help reduce pain and swelling; acetaminophen will help with pain but not inflammation.
- **Reduce inflammation.** Apply ice during the first day or two; then try heat.
- **Condition your shoulder.** Do some gentle exercises, such as those shown on page 426, to restore range of motion and strengthen the rotator cuff. These exercises will help get you started, but first discuss them with your doctor. Do not continue

any exercise that causes pain.

For chronic rotator cuff pain, you'll need professional advice from a doctor or physical therapist in designing an exercise program.

Prevention

If you are a golfer or swimmer or you have other risks for rotator cuff injuries, the same exercises, when performed regularly, can help strengthen your rotator cuff muscles and tendons and make them less susceptible to injury.

When To Call Your Doctor

If you often have pain when raising your arm above your head, or with any activity, it's a good idea to get medical help. Your doctor may send you to a physical therapist or another specialist in body mechanics. Rotator cuff tendinitis usu-

---

Exercises for Preventing Shoulder Pain

A good way to prevent shoulder problems is to strengthen the muscle groups that you underuse and stretch all shoulder muscles involved in your activity.

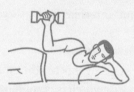

Shoulder strengthener 1. Lie on your side with your sore shoulder up and your head supported. Holding a light weight, bend your arm at a 90-degree angle and position your forearm parallel to the floor. Keeping your elbow against your side, lift the weight toward the ceiling, then slowly lower the weight forward. Repeat 10 times.

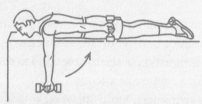

Shoulder strengthener 2. Lie on a table or bed, with the arm of your sore shoulder hanging down. Hold a light weight, and with your hand rotated outward, swing the arm straight back. Hold for 2 seconds, then lower slowly, and repeat 10 times. Variation: Rotate your hand inward and lift the weight forward, almost parallel to the floor; hold, lower, and repeat.

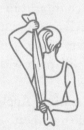

Towel stretch. Grasp a towel behind your back with one arm behind you and the other arm raised over your shoulder. Pull the towel upward, but not to the point of discomfort. Hold for 10 seconds, then switch arms.

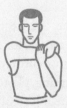

Shoulder stretch. Stretch the back of the painful shoulder by reaching with that arm under your chin and across the opposite shoulder. Gently push the arm back with the other hand. Hold for 15 seconds. Repeat 5 times.

ally responds well to moist heat, ultrasound, and gentle exercises, especially stretching.

What Your Doctor Will Do

After a careful physical examination, your physician will check your shoulder for pain and loss of motion. To exclude a possible fracture or bone spur, an x-ray may be taken. Other tests may be ordered for further evaluation of your injured shoulder, including magnetic resonance imaging (MRI).

Your doctor may prescribe medications to control pain and exercises to help restore full range of motion and use of the shoulder. In advanced cases of rotator cuff injury, surgery is sometimes recommended. However, a controlled study of 125 people with severe rotator cuff injuries (ages 19 to 66) found that a supervised exercise program produced the same improvements as surgery. Conducted at University Hospital in Oslo, Norway, and published in the *British Medical Journal,* the study showed that even in patients whose condition resists treatment, an exercise program is worth trying before any surgery is considered.

For More Information

• American Academy of Orthopaedic Surgeons

SAD (Seasonal Affective Disorder)

Symptoms

- Depressive periods during fall and winter seasons. Accompanying symptoms include sleeping more than usual; less energy; tendency to eat more, especially sweets and starches; social withdrawal.
- Nondepressed periods during spring and summer.

What Is It?

The short dark days of winter cause some people to experience a distinctive type of depression and malaise. SAD, or seasonal affective disorder, as it is now known, is cyclical. In winter, SAD sufferers tend to sleep more, be less productive at work, have less energy for recreation, lose interest in sex, and feel down in the dumps for no particular reason. They tend to eat more (especially sweets and starches). That, together with a low activity level, generally leads to winter weight gain. They may have trouble getting up in the morning, be irritable, and withdraw from friends and family. Children with SAD may do poorly in school.

From roughly April to the end of October, however, SAD sufferers feel better. Nobody knows how common SAD is, but researchers at the National Institute of Mental Health estimate that it may affect anywhere from 10 to 25 million Americans; at least 80 percent of them are women. Symptoms most commonly start during early adulthood. SAD is thought to be a disorder of the northern latitudes. Oddly, though, Alaskans and Canadians don't have higher rates of the disorder than those at lower latitudes. SAD seems to run in families, so there may be a genetic link.

The fact is, SAD symptoms are vague, hard to pin down, and very hard to distinguish from other forms of depression. A definition of SAD has been added to the *Diagnostic and Statistical Manual of Mental Disorders* (the psychiatric bible): you may have the disorder if you have had fall and winter depression for at least two years, alternating with nondepressed periods during spring and summer; at least one disabling depressive episode; no other major psychiatric disorder; and no other possible explanation for the change in mood.

What Causes It?

Logically enough, many researchers think that lack of sunlight is at the root of SAD. In general, research has shown that humans have emotional and physiological reactions to changes in the length of the solar day. Daylight is a crucial environmental cue by which humans, like other animals, adapt to the changing seasons and shorter or longer days. Daylight in large part helps to set our circadian rhythms, or biological clocks.

But how the lack of light disturbs us remains a mystery. Bright light apparently affects the production of the hormone melatonin, which may influence both our physical and emotional well-being and may set our sleep patterns. Light deprivation may also disturb the secretion of so-called stress hormones, such as cortisol, which influence how we react to physical and psychological stress.

The belief that light deprivation is behind SAD has led to the development of "light therapy" as one method of treating the condition. Bright, artificial lights are set to emit measured doses of light at a specific distance in order to redress the deprivation.

However, some recent findings have led researchers to question whether lack of light is indeed the cause of SAD. In fact, according to Dr. Norman Rosenthal, a researcher at the National Institute of Mental Health (and a pioneer in this field as well as a SAD sufferer himself), "neither the etiology of SAD nor the mechanism of the antidepressant effects of light is well understood."

What If You Do Nothing?

Because SAD symptoms seem vague and inconsistent, it's not clear how they evolve over the long term. In some people, symptoms gradually improve over time, while in others they remain the same or get worse. Certainly if you don't feel better, it's worth trying the measures suggested below.

Home Remedies

If you think you suffer from SAD or some milder form of seasonal depression, here are some commonsense steps you can take during the winter.

• **Make your house bright.** Trim bushes around your windows and keep the curtains open. Use bright colors on walls and upholstery.

• **Try to sit near a window if you work in an office and this is an option**.

• **Maximize your daylight time.** Get up early.

• **Get away in winter.** Try to take part of your vacation in the winter rather than all of it in the summer. Choose a sunny destination.

• **Exercise outdoors.** Skiing, for example, is an excellent way to get lots of light. If you exercise indoors, try to do so near a window.

• **If you try light therapy, be cautious.** A whole industry has sprung up to produce and sell battery-powered visors, portable light boxes, special light bulbs, and dawn simulators (lamps that switch on before dawn and gradually light your room, like the sun rising). The Food and Drug Administration (FDA) has warned the manufacturers of light-therapy equipment not to make medical claims for their products—that is, claims that the products can alleviate SAD or winter depression. But many people swear by the benefits of light therapy, despite the lack of strong clinical evidence or well-established guidelines for using it.

Keep in mind that, if the light is too concentrated, as in a halogen lamp, it is more likely to cause headache, eyestrain, or other side effects. Also, tanning lamps and plant lights are not appropriate, since they emit ultraviolet rays and can cause serious eye damage.

When To Call Your Doctor

If you suffer from severe winter depression, consider consulting a psychologist or psychiatrist.

429

What Your Doctor Will Do

A qualified doctor or other specialist will interview you to assess if your mood problems and other symptoms are seasonally related or have some other cause. The doctor will then help coordinate your anti-SAD efforts, which can range from psychotherapy and stress-management techniques to antidepressant drugs and perhaps light therapy. Some medical insurance covers light therapy after a diagnosis of SAD.

For More Information

• American Psychological Association
• National Mental Health Association

Scabies

Symptoms

- Small, red, itchy blisters or pustules that develop in soft skin areas such as between the fingers, around the wrists, and on the lower abdomen, genitals, and buttocks.
- Severe itching that is often worse at night and following a hot bath or shower.
- In some cases dotted thin lines of raised red skin—typically between the fingers, along the belt line, on the penis, and around the nipples in women—indicating where scabies mites have burrowed.

What Is It?

Scabies is a common contagious disorder caused by a microscopic burrowing mite, which digs under the uppermost layer of skin and lays eggs. The mite cannot jump or fly but is passed from host to host by direct personal contact. Generally, within two to three weeks after the eggs have been laid, the infected person develops a fierce allergic reaction characterized by an itchy rash that can eventually become inflamed. Scratching itchy areas may trap the mites and eggs under the fingernails, and they then get transmitted to other parts of the body.

In some people the symptoms are relatively mild, but in others the itching can be quite intense. Adults and older children seldom develop eruptions above the neck; in infants and small children, however, eruptions can occur over the entire body.

What Causes It?

Scabies is caused by the female human scabies mite *(Sarcoptes scabiei)*, a microscopic eight-legged creature that burrows into the upper layer of skin. If undetected and untreated, the mite will lay up to three eggs daily for up to 60 days. At any one time an infected person may have 10 to 15 female mites on the body.

Scabies can be picked up through skin-to-skin contact with an infected person, contact with contaminated clothing, or by sleeping in bedding that is contaminated. Children under the age of two are most at risk, followed by mothers and other family members who have frequent, close physical contact with the youngsters. Older Americans living in long-term-care facilities are also at greater risk of being exposed to infection, and any unsanitary and overcrowded living conditions increase the risk of contracting scabies. But the mites can thrive in all sorts of communities.

What If You Do Nothing?

Though not harmful, scabies is uncomfortable. Moreover, if you don't take steps to eradicate the mite that causes the ailment, the condition will worsen and you could easily contaminate others.

Home Remedies

Dried chrysanthemum flowers have been used since the late nineteenth century for scabies treatment. The active ingredient of the flowers is pyrethrum, which is still used in several nonprescription medications.

Unfortunately, these low-strength formulations frequently aren't strong enough to treat scabies effectively. Several prescription medications are available that eliminate the mites, generally within two weeks (see When To Call Your Doctor).

When treating scabies, close family members should also be treated preventively with one application of the scabies medicine, as should any other individuals who are in close contact with the infected person.

In addition to applying a prescription scabicide, follow these measures.

- **Decontaminate.** All bedding, towels, and any clothing used for the three days prior to treatment should be washed in extremely hot water to kill the mites. Vacuum all mattresses, chairs, rugs, and floors and then discard the vacuum cleaner bag. Place all shoes in plastic bags and keep them sealed for seven days before wearing them again.
- **Get rid of the itch.** Significant itching may continue for several weeks after the mites are eliminated, owing to an allergic skin reaction to the creatures. Take frequent cool baths and don't use strong soap. For temporary relief, use 1 percent hydrocortisone cream or calamine lotion on all itchy areas.

Prevention

- **Be scrupulous about personal hygiene.** Bathe regularly and wash clothes and bedding often.
- **Avoid the infection.** Refrain from physical contact with persons, clothing, or bedding that may be infested with scabies mites.

When To Call Your Doctor

Contact your physician if you think you (or a child) may have scabies, or if the condition persists for more than two weeks after being treated.

What Your Doctor Will Do

After performing a careful physical examination, your doctor will inspect the burrows and sores. A skin scraping will be viewed under a microscope for confirmation. The physician will probably recommend Elimite, a 5 percent permethrin cream that is the treatment of choice. Available by prescription, it will eliminate the scabies mites, usually within two weeks. You apply the medication from your neck to the soles of your feet, preferably after bathing at night, and leave it on for a minimum of eight hours, then wash it off with soap and water. A single overnight dose has been proven effective in more than 90 percent of cases.

Your doctor may also prescribe antihistamines for the itching and antibiotics for any secondary infections.

For More Information

- American Academy of Dermatology
- American Social Health Association

431

Sciatica

Symptoms

- Pain—which can be dull or intense—that often starts in the hip or buttock and radiates down through the leg, sometimes reaching the foot. The pain is frequently only on one side, and often becomes worse at night.
- Pain may also be aggravated by laughing, sneezing, straining on the toilet, and coughing.
- Weakness and numbness in the leg.

What Is It?

Sciatica is a back disorder that involves the sciatic nerve—which is actually a group of nerves (the body's longest) bound in one nerve sheath that runs from the lower back through the buttock and thigh to the knee, where it branches, and down into the foot. When pressure is placed on this nerve, pain may be felt from the lower back to the toes. The pain from sciatica most often strikes people in their 40s and 50s, but may occur at any age.

What Causes It?

It's not age that causes sciatica but probably a combination of other factors: work that requires repetitive lifting, sudden strain in lifting a heavy object, or constant exposure to mechanical vibrations (for example, long hours behind the wheel of a car or truck). Severe low-back pain, including sciatica, also shows a high correlation with job dissatisfaction and depression—though whether depression aggravates the back pain or is the result of it is hard to determine. Some studies have also suggested that cigarette smoking may be a risk factor.

You can also have sciatica without any of these risk factors. You may be a healthy, happy person who never lifts anything and yet, for no apparent reason, suffer a sudden attack when you bend or turn slightly.

Some experts blame slipped, or herniated, disks for irritating the sciatic nerve. Disks are the fibrous padding between the vertebrae; when a disk "slips," or herniates, it bulges and can press on the sciatic nerve. Other researchers blame the piriformis muscle in the buttocks—the muscle that allows you to lift your leg sideways. If inflamed by injury or overexertion, the piriformis muscle can press against the sciatic nerve.

What If You Do Nothing?

In about half of all cases, the pain from sciatica resolves spontaneously within four weeks.

Home Remedies

Sciatica often improves with only the simplest self-care measures. As the pain diminishes, it's all right to sit up and begin to move around as long as you avoid bending or any strenuous activity. Let your own discomfort level be your guide.
- **Relieve the pain.** You may want to try an over-

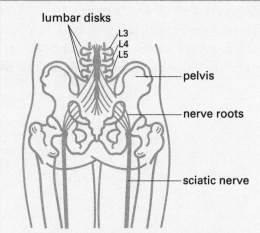

Nerve roots emerging from the spinal cord join to form the sciatic nerve, which extends down each leg. Sciatica commonly occurs when a herniated ("slipped") disk presses sciatic nerve roots against the backbone.

the-counter NSAID—aspirin, ibuprofen, or naproxen—or acetaminophen for five to seven days.

• **Rest.** If the pain is severe, a day or two in bed may bring welcome relief by helping calm down an angry nerve root. Two days in bed, studies have shown, will usually do as much good as a week. Lie on a firm mattress with your unaffected side facing down and your legs slightly bent. Place a pillow or two between your knees to support the affected leg.

• **Try heat.** Apply a heating pad to the affected buttock. A hot bath, shower, sauna, or whirlpool may also provide some relief.

• **Try cold.** Apply an ice pack to the sore buttock for 15 minutes several times a day.

• **Avoid heavy lifting.** When your back is sore or painful, avoid lifting anything heavier than 10 pounds. When you do lift, make sure your knees are bent and that you lift with your arms, not with your back muscles, keeping the object close to your body.

Prevention

• **Strengthen your muscles.** Though poor posture is not known to cause sciatica, strong abdominal and back muscles—which can be developed through exercise—can help keep your back healthy.

• **Exercise regularly.** A regular exercise routine might be particularly important if your job puts you at risk for back pain.

When To Call Your Doctor

Contact your physician if the pain is severe, or if it doesn't start to improve after several days of self-care measures. In addition, contact your doc-tor if you develop any leg or foot numbness. This may indicate a more serious problem.

What Your Doctor Will Do

Typically, after diagnosing sciatica, the first step a physician will try is bed rest and painkillers. Your doctor may prescribe a painkiller stronger than aspirin or ibuprofen.

If you don't get better, your doctor may need to determine whether your problem comes from a herniated disk, an inflamed piriformis muscle, or other causes. X-rays may be needed if the diagnosis is uncertain, but since they don't show soft-tissue problems, magnetic resonance imaging (MRI) may be ordered. An MRI reveals spinal architecture accurately and in great detail, though it is usually only useful if surgery is being considered.

Surgery may be an option in some persistent cases, but it is expensive, requires a long period of recuperation, and may not produce a cure. Before you consider back surgery, you should exhaust all other forms of treatment.

If your doctor suggests surgery, always get a second opinion. Whatever the diagnosis, ask for the most conservative treatments first—rest, exercise, painkillers, and physical therapy. And be patient.

For More Information

• American Academy of Orthopaedic Surgeons
• American Osteopathic Association

433

Seborrhea (Seborrheic Dermatitis)

Symptoms

- Redness and oily dandruff-like scaling around affected areas—typically the scalp, eyebrows, creases from the sides of the nose to the mouth, skin behind the ears, and the chest.
- Mild itching (rare).

What Is It?

Seborrhea, which is also called seborrheic dermatitis, is a common chronic skin disorder in which oily areas of the scalp, face, and chest start to flake. Other areas, such as the skin folds under the arms, breasts, groin, buttocks, and navel, may also be affected by this form of eczema.

Seborrhea can occur at any age but is common in the first three months of life, when it appears on the scalp as cradle cap. It then can reoccur between the ages of 30 and 60. Some people appear to be born with a tendency for seborrhea and are affected on and off by it throughout life, although regular treatment can help keep it under control. The condition is more common among men than women.

What Causes It?

No one is certain what causes seborrhea. Some researchers think it may be linked to a yeast that grows in oily, hairy areas of the body, or caused by hormones, which would explain why it appears at birth and disappears before puberty. Seborrhea in infants may actually be a separate disorder from the ailment that afflicts adults.

Seborrhea is also common in people taking antibiotics and in those recovering from stressful cardiac episodes. People with suppressed immune systems (such as those with HIV infection) and those confined for long periods to hospitals or nursing homes are also at higher risk.

What If You Do Nothing?

Seborrhea may subside without any treatment, although it usually shows a temporary improvement with medication. If the rash is a cosmetic problem, or if itching becomes a nuisance, it should be treated.

Home Remedies

Several over-the-counter remedies are often successful at alleviating seborrhea.

- **Hydrocortisone.** This is one of the more effective treatments. Apply low-strength (1 percent) hydrocortisone cream to the affected areas of skin until the condition clears up.
- **Dandruff shampoo.** Seborrheic dermatitis of the scalp (dandruff) can be treated with frequent use of nonprescription shampoos containing one of the following ingredients: selenium sulfide, coal tar, zinc pyrithione, salicylic acid, or ketoconazole (the latter is an antifungal shampoo sold under the brand name Nizoral). Follow label directions.

Prevention

No way has been established to prevent the development or recurrence of seborrhea.

When To Call Your Doctor

If self-care measures don't work, or if your condition worsens, contact your physician.

What Your Doctor Will Do

The diagnosis of seborrhea is usually obvious. If nonprescription hydrocortisone isn't strong enough, your doctor may prescribe stronger topical prescription medications or shampoos.

For More Information

- American Academy of Dermatology

Sensitive Teeth

Symptoms

■ Persistent, sometimes disabling pain in a tooth or several teeth.

What Is It?

Hypersensitivity is a common dental ailment, especially as people age. As gum tissue starts to recede, a tooth's root surface is exposed. It is made of a substance called dentin, which is thinner and softer than tooth enamel. The exposed dentin allows stimuli such as hot and cold drinks, sweet and sour foods, and even your toothbrush to trigger a temporary but acute toothache. Fortunately, dental hypersensitivity can be treated and cured.

What Causes It?

You may simply have what's called dentin hypersensitivity, a common problem. The cause of it is uncertain, but one theory proposes that the movement of fluids deep inside the tooth stimulates the nerves. Whatever the mechanism may be, wear and tear on the teeth—for example, overzealous brushing or constant teeth grinding, which causes enamel to thin—is usually responsible. Acidic foods, such as citrus fruits and juices or wine, may cause sensitive teeth to ache.

What If You Do Nothing?

Hypersensitivity may persist, but can suddenly disappear on its own.

Home Remedies

• **Switch your toothbrush.** Using an extrasoft toothbrush will prevent the wearing down of root surfaces.
• **Change your brushing technique.** Avoid brushing horizontally. This will help minimize tooth abrasion and the exposure of tooth roots.

• **Try a special toothpaste.** Specially formulated desensitizing toothpastes such as Sensodyne or Denquel can help bring relief. (Be sure to buy a brand with the seal of the American Dental Association.) These contain compounds, such as strontium chloride and potassium nitrate, that can reduce the painful nerve response, though it often takes a month or so of regular use for this to occur.
• **Schedule regular dental visits.** A thorough cleaning will reduce dental plaque and lessen the sensitivity.
• **Avoid foods that seem to aggravate the condition.** Hot coffee, ice cream, wine, and grapefruit juice are often prime offenders.

Prevention
See the recommendations listed above.

When To Call Your Doctor
Contact your dentist if the recommended self-care measures don't bring relief.

What Your Doctor Will Do
After a careful examination your dentist will make sure no underlying problem needs treatment—a cavity, nocturnal teeth grinding, a dying root, or a fractured tooth. Your dentist may recommend fluoride treatments. Although expensive, they can help reduce sensitivity. Sealants and resins, applied to sensitive areas, may also be useful. If nothing else works, root canal therapy may eliminate the problem.

For More Information
• American Dental Association

Shin Splints

Symptoms

■ Persistent pain—from mild tenderness to severe aching—in the front or side of the lower leg. The pain generally starts during exercise, but sometimes begins several hours later.

What Is It?

The catch-all term "shin splints" refers to a family of overuse injuries causing inflammation of muscles and tendons of the lower leg—usually the tissues surrounding the tibia, or shin bone. Characterized by pain in the lower leg, this condition, also referred to as medial tibial stress syndrome, is the most common overuse injury among runners.

During exercise, the muscles in the lower leg enlarge and press against the compartment formed by the two bones of the lower leg (the tibia and fibula). Repeated stress and pressure can cause irritation of the muscles, tendons, ligaments, or bones. Most commonly, the result is tendinitis. Initially, the pain often starts during exercise, then after days or even weeks it may disappear during exercise but occur later and then continue during daily activities.

Shin splints are referred to as "posterior" or "anterior," depending on the location of the injury. A posterior shin splint is characterized by aching pain on the inner side of the calf due to inflammation of the muscles that roll the foot inward and support the arch. People with flat feet are the likeliest candidates for posterior shin splints. An anterior shin splint causes pain along the outer side of the calf.

What Causes It?

The pain from shin splints is caused by damage to the soft tissue that typically results from repeatedly pounding the feet on hard surfaces while running or jumping. Seasoned athletes as well as beginners can develop the problem, and the shin splints can be compounded by such factors as running on concrete (rather than a softer surface such as grass) and wearing poorly cushioned shoes. Poor posture and gait can also contribute to shin splints.

What If You Do Nothing?

At the very least, you will probably need to stop the activity and rest the muscles and connective tissue in the lower leg. Otherwise, the condition is likely to grow progressively worse.

Home Remedies

For mild cases of shin splints, self-treatment measures can usually alleviate the problem. But if you haven't had this type of pain before, it's a good idea to consult a physician to get an exact diagnosis, since the cause could also be a stress fracture (see page 466).

• **Rest is essential.** Refraining from running and/or jumping for three to six weeks will allow the damaged tissue to heal.

• **For pain, use ice and NSAIDs.** Applying ice several times a day—for no more than 20-minute intervals—can help reduce pain and inflammation. A good way to ice shin splints is to use a paper or Styrofoam cup that has been filled with water and then frozen. Place the open end of the ice cup directly on the skin over the sore areas and gently massage with circular or back-and-forth movements. As the ice melts, peel away a strip of the cup to expose more ice.

Over-the-counter anti-inflammatories such as aspirin, ibuprofen, or naproxen can also help relieve pain and swelling.

• **Wear shoes that are well cushioned.** The shoes should provide good support and have plenty of impact-absorbing material to cushion the ball and heel areas of your feet.

Prevention

These precautions can help you safely return to a full complement of activities—and lessen your risk of reinjury.

• **Switch to low-impact activities.** Engage in activities such as bicycling, swimming, and pool running until you can resume running or jumping without pain.

• **Don't run in worn-out shoes.** If you run regularly, consider replacing shoes every three to six months. Studies have shown that regardless of brand, price, or construction, running shoes lose about 30 percent of their ability to absorb shock after approximately 500 miles of use.

• **Don't run on hard surfaces.** Try to avoid cement and concrete, and instead run on grass, school tracks, well-cleared paths, or boardwalks.

• **Take it easy.** Keep in mind that running more than 20 miles a week doesn't greatly increase your fitness, but it does increase your chance of injury. Don't suddenly increase the intensity of your workout. Also avoid excessive downhill running, which places additional stress on the front part of the lower leg. And be sure to warm up carefully before you work out.

• **Stretch and strengthen your calf muscles.** Do toe raises and foot rolls several times a day; lie on your back and flex your feet; sit on the edge of a table and flex your foot with a weight attached to it.

Also, be sure to stretch your calf muscles thoroughly when you warm up before running. (See the calf stretch illustrated on page 152.)

When To Call Your Doctor

For a first case of shin splints, especially if the pain grows worse or the shin muscles are inflamed and swollen, call your doctor. You should also get medical evaluation if the pain is concentrated in a small area along the inside part of the tibia, rather than extending to the surrounding tissue. This may mean you have a stress fracture—a microscopic break in the shin bone itself. An x-ray or bone scan may be used to diagnose a stress fracture.

Also, see your doctor if symptoms persist for more than seven days after self-treatment measures or if pain occurs when you resume running or jumping. You may have tendon or muscle damage that needs additional treatment.

What Your Doctor Will Do

In diagnosing the problem, your doctor will exam your feet and legs to see if an anatomical problem, such as flat feet, might be a factor. You may be referred to a podiatrist, who can see if an orthotic device (a specially fitted shoe insert) would improve your posture and gait. If so, you should wear it in all your shoes.

In persistent cases, a physical therapist may help alleviate the problem by strengthening any affected muscles.

For More Information

• American Academy of Orthopaedic Surgeons

437

Shingles (Herpes Zoster)

Symptoms

- Burning pain, tingling, and extreme sensitivity in one area of skin; the pain may last for one to three days before the skin reddens at the pain site.
- Mild chills and fever, malaise, headache.
- A rash of small fluid-filled bubblelike blisters that breaks out on reddened skin. The rash forms along a band, most commonly on the torso and buttocks, but also on the arms, legs, and face. In nearly all cases the rash occurs only on one side of the body.
- Within about 10 days, the blisters form scabs.

What Is It?

Herpes zoster, more commonly known as shingles, is a painful viral infection caused by varicella zoster, the same virus that causes chicken pox. After a childhood attack of chicken pox, the virus lies dormant in the nerve cells that extend from the spinal cord or the brain. In adulthood, the virus can be reactivated, resulting in a second eruption of chicken pox. (Therefore, you cannot develop shingles unless you have had an earlier case of chicken pox.) The blistery rash characteristic of shingles follows a line on one side of the body or face in an area supplied by a particular spinal nerve.

Shingles strikes about one in five adults who have had chicken pox as children. While young people do develop shingles, the ailment most often occurs after age 50, with the incidence increasing with age. The chance of developing shingles is greatest for people whose immune system is weakened—for example, people infected with the HIV virus or cancer patients undergoing drug or radiation treatment.

You cannot "catch" shingles from someone who has it. The virus can be transmitted to others, but only to someone who has never had chicken pox and only if that person is exposed to the rash—in which case the person may develop chicken pox, not shingles. If you have shingles, you should avoid contact with small children, pregnant women, and any adults who have never had chicken pox. (In the United States, 95 percent of adults have had the disease; those who have not should be immunized, since many adults with chicken pox have more complications than children.)

The prognosis for shingles is generally good, unless the virus spreads to the brain or eyes. For most healthy individuals, the lesions heal and pain diminishes within three to five weeks.

However, some shingles sufferers—including as many as 50 percent of the sufferers over age 50, according to some estimates—will have debilitating pain that persists for more than one month (sometimes for many months) after lesions have healed. This pain, called post-herpetic neuralgia, or PHN, is not from shingles but from nerve cell damage caused by the viral infection.

What Causes It?

No one is certain what triggers an attack of shingles. Researchers believe that the virus is reactivated when the immune system becomes too weak to keep the virus in a dormant state. This is probably why older people are more likely to get the infection. Stress and illness may also weaken the immune system, as does the use of immunosuppressant drugs. The immune system factor may also explain why people with HIV infection or AIDS, Hodgkin's disease, and other cancers—whose immune systems are suppressed due to illness or treatment for illness—are at increased risk of developing shingles.

What If You Do Nothing?

In most cases shingles is self-limiting—the body's immune system is ordinarily able to fight off the infection. However, the pain can be severe, and many people need medication for pain relief. Early treatment with antiviral drugs can also be important in bringing relief.

Medical intervention is critical, however, for people with damaged or suppressed immune systems. Not only are they vulnerable to shingles, but if they develop symptoms, there is a danger that the disease will spread and reach vital organs like the lungs, with results that are fatal.

Home Remedies

Shingles can't be cured, so home remedies are aimed at relieving discomfort.

• **Relieve the pain.** For minor discomfort, take over-the-counter NSAIDs (aspirin, ibuprofen, or naproxen) or acetaminophen. For severe pain, your doctor can prescribe stronger medication.

• **Cool it.** Apply cool, wet compresses or ice packs to reduce pain. Calamine lotion may also feel soothing if applied after removing the compresses.

• **Relieve the itch.** Soak in a bath to which you've added colloidal oatmeal.

• **Rest.** If you are overly fatigued or develop a fever, rest in bed.

• **Try deep heat.** Capsaicin cream, an extract made of hot peppers, has been used in pain clinics to reduce the pain of PHN victims by interrupting the transmission of pain impulses to the brain. This over-the-counter remedy is sold for treating muscular aches and pains; consult your physician before using it. Be sure not to apply it until the lesions caused by your shingles have completely healed.

• **Don't scratch.** Although it is hard to resist scratching, you increase the risk that the blisters will become infected from dirt on fingernails.

• **Clean regularly.** Use soap and water to keep the rash area clean. This will prevent any bacterial infections from developing.

Prevention

There is no way to prevent shingles. However, to be on the safe side, if you've never had chicken pox, it's best to avoid contact with the active rash of anyone with shingles or chicken pox.

When To Call Your Doctor

Contact your physician as soon as you develop symptoms of shingles—and particularly if you have any illness that compromises your immune system. *The earlier the symptoms are treated, the less severe the ailment may be.* Be sure to contact your physician immediately if you develop shingles on your nose or forehead—this signals possible eye involvement—or if you experience any eye pain. Eye damage from shingles can lead to blindness.

What Your Doctor Will Do

After a close examination to confirm shingles, your physician may prescribe the antiviral medication acyclovir or newer agents such as famciclovir to minimize the pain of shingles, speed healing, and help prevent any complications. A combination of acyclovir and corticosteroids may be even more likely to reduce the severity of PHN.

Other medications, including antidepressants, are sometimes effective for relieving PHN, and some alternative treatments (such as acupuncture) for chronic pain may also help people cope.

For More Information

• American Pain Foundation
• National Institute of Neurological Disorders and Stroke

Side Stitch

Symptoms

■ A sudden sharp pain during exercise that occurs below the bottom of the ribcage, usually on the right side, and fades once exercise stops.

What Is It?

While running or walking briskly, nearly everyone has experienced the sharp pain in the side known as a stitch. Side stitches are muscle spasms of the diaphragm, and they occur occasionally during strenuous exercise. Most people experience stitches on their right side, immediately below the ribs.

What Causes It?

No one is quite certain why stitches occur, though there's no shortage of educated guesses. One theory is that the diaphragm (the large dome-shaped muscle that separates the chest cavity from the abdominal cavity) sometimes fails to receive enough blood during its contractions, and much like a leg cramp, this results in spasm and pain.

What If You Do Nothing?

Side stitches will go away on their own.

Home Remedies

• **Stop or slow down.** Then bend forward and push your fingers into the painful area. These actions will force the diaphragm to relax and ease the spasm by increasing blood flow.
• **Breathe deeply and exhale slowly.** This should help relax the diaphragm.
• **Stretch the abdominal muscles.** Reach overhead and hold your arms in this position until the stitch disappears.

Prevention

• **Don't eat and run.** If stitches seem to hit you after a meal, wait 30 to 90 minutes after eating before you exercise.
• **Decrease the intensity and increase the duration of workouts.** This is especially true if you are just starting an exercise program. Stitches are more common in untrained exercisers than in well-trained athletes. If you increase your fitness level gradually, you can sidestep stitches.
• **Warm up before exercising.** Begin with five to 10 minutes of gentle jogging or calisthenics.
• **Avoid shallow breathing.** Shallow breathing uses only a small portion of your total lung capacity. When this occurs as you run, the diaphragm doesn't descend far enough to allow the connective ligaments of the liver to relax, possibly causing a stitch.
• **Practice deep breathing exercises.** Lie down on the floor and place a hand on your abdomen. Breathe in deeply. You are "belly breathing" if you feel your hand rise slightly. If only your chest moves up, you are not breathing deeply enough.
• **Try forced exhalation.** As you run, periodically pretend you are blowing out candles. To do this, purse your lips while exhaling. This causes you to breathe deeply.

When To Call Your Doctor

This is a minor inconvenience that does not need medical attention.

Sinusitis

Symptoms

- A feeling of fullness and head congestion.
- Headache pain or pressure around one or both eyes or cheeks that is worse in the morning or when the sufferer bends forward.
- Swelling in the upper eyelids.
- Yellowish green nasal discharge.
- Difficulty breathing through the nose following a cold or flu.
- Fever and chills.

What Is It?

Your sinuses are air pockets—eight of them—that are located above, behind, and below the eyes and are connected to the inside of the nose. Sinusitis is an inflammation of one or more of these cavities, usually because of a bacterial or viral infection or owing to allergies. Sinusitis typically starts off as an acute condition, but it can become chronic, lasting for months or even years if not treated adequately.

One function of the sinuses is to produce mucus, which helps pick up and flush out invading particles, bacteria, and air pollutants. When you're healthy, the mucus flows from the sinus cavities to the nose; it then flows backward into the throat and down into the stomach, where stomach acids destroy any dangerous bacteria.

However, once a cavity becomes irritated—because of a cold, flu, or an allergy attack—the mucous membrane that lines the sinus typically swells abnormally, blocking the drainage channels that permit normal mucus flow. (The mucous membrane in the sinuses is the same as that of the nose—so whenever the nose is infected, the sinuses are also generally involved.)

This subsequent buildup in pressure often results in headache, nasal congestion, and pain in the forehead or at various points around the teeth, eyes, ears, cheeks, and neck, depending on which sinuses are affected.

If the cause of the swelling persists, the sinuses also allow bacteria to breed and thrive. A bacterial infection can then develop, signaled by mucus that has a bad taste and accompanied by pain and pressure that can become severe.

What Causes It?

Sinusitis is caused by either a viral or bacterial infection that spreads to the sinuses from the nose. An upper respiratory infection such as the flu or the common cold are the most frequent causes of sinusitis. There are other possibilities as well: swimming in contaminated water; spread of infection from abscesses in the upper teeth; or irritation from air pollutants, dust, or tobacco smoke. Some people with structural problems, such as a deviated nasal septum or polyps in the nasal cavities, may also be prone to recurring sinusitis.

What If You Do Nothing?

Without treatment, sinusitis can last for weeks or months, often with pain, congestion, and fatigue. If bacteria travel from the sinuses to the lungs, bronchitis can result. The ears can also be affected, causing balance problems.

Home Remedies

- **Inhale steam from a basin of hot water.** Take deep breaths. This will help relieve sinus congestion and pain. Inhaling the vapors in a hot shower or bath may have similar effects.
- **Use a nasal decongestant.** Over-the-counter oral or nasal decongestants may help reduce swelling when used sparingly. Don't use a nasal decongestant for more than two days or you risk a rebound effect in which the nasal tissues swell

back up, often worse than before. Follow label directions carefully. (Be aware that the Food and Drug Administration has requested that decongestant products containing the ingredient phenylpropanolamine, or PPA, be taken off the market—see page 576 for more information.)

• **Avoid bending over with your head down.** This movement increases sinus pain.

• **Try exercising.** For some people vigorous exercise has a powerful decongesting effect—though for others, it can aggravate congestion. Try performing an aerobic exercise at a light intensity. Stop if you feel the congestion worsen.

Prevention

• **Control your allergies.** Sinusitis can be a complication stemming from a seasonal allergy. If allergies are the source of your sinusitis, find out what triggers them. Limit your exposure to the allergens that affect you and use antihistamines when necessary.

• **Keep hydrated.** Drink plenty of liquids each day—a minimum of 8 to 10 glasses—to loosen nasal secretions. Using a cool-mist humidifier in your home and sleeping with your head elevated can also help promote optimal drainage.

• **Reduce alcohol consumption.** When you have sinusitis, alcohol can dehydrate the body and make mucus dry and thick, leading to possible blockage of the opening of a sinus cavity.

• **Minimize your exposure to people with colds or known infections.** Practice sanitary health habits when you must be around such people; wash your hands frequently and avoid shared towels, napkins, and eating utensils.

• **Avoid chlorinated swimming pools.** If chlorine irritates your nose and sinuses, plan to do your swimming in a freshwater lake or saltwater bay or ocean.

• **Take care when flying.** The changing air pressure in a plane can force mucus into the sinuses. Consider using a nasal spray before taking off and shortly before landing to keep your sinuses open.

• **If you smoke, quit.** Tobacco smoke, like other pollutants, aggravates sinusitis symptoms.

When To Call Your Doctor

Contact your physician immediately if you develop any redness or pain in an eye, bulging of an eye, paralysis of eye movements, or nausea and vomiting in association with other sinusitis symptoms. Also contact your physician if symptoms persist longer than two weeks or are accompanied by bloody nasal discharges.

What Your Doctor Will Do

Your physician will examine your mouth and throat and look at your nasal passages. A computed tomography (CT) scan of your sinuses may be performed. If allergies are suspected, a skin test will help the physician determine whether you are allergic to dust, mold, or other common allergens. A course of prescription oral antibiotics and a decongestant may be recommended to keep the sinus drainage passages open and to reduce obstruction. In cases of severe or chronic sinusitis, surgery may be recommended to drain and clean the sinuses.

For More Information

• American Academy of Otolaryngology-Head and Neck Surgery
• National Jewish Medical and Research Center

Skin Cancer

Symptoms

General signs

- Any change in the size, color, shape or texture of a mole or other skin growth.
- An open or inflamed wound that won't heal.

Signs of basal cell carcinoma

- A sore that doesn't heal. Have it checked if it hasn't healed after three weeks and it crusts, bleeds, or oozes.
- A persistent reddish patch. It may be painful or may crust and itch; or it may not bother you at all.
- A smooth bump indented in the middle. The borders will be rolled, and as it grows you may notice blood vessels on the surface.
- A shiny, waxy, scarlike spot. It may be yellow or white with irregular borders.

Signs of squamous cell carcinoma

- Small, firm lump or patch, initially painless, that develops on the face or back of the hand. May be raised or flat, with a scaly or crusted surface.
- Slowly grows to take on a wartlike appearance; may become painful.

Signs of malignant melanoma

- A mole that begins to enlarge, thicken, or change color. (Some 70 percent of early-state lesions are identified because of recent changes in size, color, border contours, or surface texture.)
- A mole that suddenly begins to grow, or one that bleeds or ulcerates.
- A mole that has irregular rather than round borders.
- A mole with irregular pigmentation—some portions light colored, others almost black.

What Is It?

Skin cancer is the most common of all cancers.

The skin changes that result in cancer develop cumulatively and irreversibly in an individual over the years, and so may take decades to produce a malignancy. Men get skin cancer more frequently than women, and it usually shows up in older people, but no one is exempt. In fact, Americans are developing skin cancer at ever-younger ages because of the increasing amounts of time spent in the sun. Prolonged sun exposure is the principal cause of skin cancer.

Exposure to the sun's ultraviolet radiation is known to promote three kinds of skin cancer.

Basal cell carcinoma is the most prevalent type, striking one out of every eight Americans, including people in their 20s and 30s, women as well as men. The most common site for basal cell carcinoma is the face, especially the nose or ears, but it can appear anywhere. It is painless and slow-growing, and rarely spreads to other parts of the body.

Squamous cell carcinoma typically develops on the face, lips, the rim of the ear, and the back of the hands. If not treated, the lesions can grow in size and spread to other parts of the body, including internal organs.

About 1.3 million new cases of these two types of cancer are reported annually in the United States alone. Fortunately, both basal cell and squamous cell skin cancers have a 95-percent cure rate when detected and treated early.

Melanoma, the least common of the three (47,000 cases annually), is also the most dangerous, though early treatment can result in a cure. Melanoma develops from melanocytes—cells located in the epidermis that produce melanin, the dark pigment that helps protect the skin from ultraviolet radiation. Melanocytes are scattered throughout the epidermis and can also collect and form benign moles, or nevi. Melanoma occurs when melanocytes begin reproducing uncontrollably to form malignant tumors.

Once rare, the incidence of melanoma has increased five- to sixfold worldwide over the past four decades. Since 1973 the incidence of melanoma has risen about 4 percent a year, even as the use of sunscreen has increased. In 1996 alone the incidence rose by 6 percent and the mortality rate by 2 percent. And whereas melanoma was once a disease of the aging, now half of all those who develop it are between the ages of 15 and 50. Many scientists attribute some of this increase to the gradual destruction of the stratospheric ozone layer, which is allowing more ultraviolet radiation to reach the earth's surface.

What Causes It?

It is clear that the risk of basal and squamous cell carcinoma rises in proportion to the cumulative amount of time people have spent in the sun. But the sun's role in the development of melanoma is less clear, and in fact surprisingly little is known about what causes melanoma. People who spend lots of time in the sun (such as farmers) do not have elevated rates of melanoma, though they do have higher rates of squamous and basal cell carcinoma. And melanoma often turns up on parts of the body rarely exposed to the sun (such as the buttocks and soles of the feet).

Genetic factors—including skin and hair color and the number of moles—clearly play a role. But genetics can't explain the huge increase in melanoma incidence over the past three generations. Some researchers believe that intermittent sun exposure and severe, blistering sunburns, especially early in life, rather than simply years of sun exposure, cause melanoma. However, studies have been inconsistent about the role of sunburn.

The people at highest risk for melanoma are fair skinned—notably people with red or blonde

---

Steps to Early Detection

▼

Self-examination is the key to early detection of skin cancer. It isn't difficult—certainly no harder than the examination for breast cancer many women have learned to do. And it is vital: in many of the most successfully treated cases of malignant melanoma, the patients themselves brought the melanoma to their doctors' attention early on.

Pay special attention to areas of your body that are habitually exposed to sunlight: your face, neck, and hands. Don't forget your scalp and the back of your ears. Also check body parts not exposed to sunlight, such as your buttocks and underarms, since melanoma can occur in those places as well. Use a mirror to check areas you can't easily see or have a partner check them. (See page 60 for more details.)

Self-examination should be performed once a month. Don't forgo the procedure even if you now habitually stay out of the sun. While it's certainly protective to avoid excess sun exposure, you cannot undo damage from past exposure, which is cumulative, starting in childhood. In fact, some experts believe that by age 20 the average American has already received 80 percent of the damaging ultraviolet rays that may lead to cancer in later years.

In addition to self-examination, ask your doctor to include a total skin exam as part of your routine checkup. A study in the *Journal of the American Medical Association* found that physicians were much likelier to find thin, early melanomas, which are most treatable.

---

hair, who freckle (especially on the upper back), and/or who have rough red patches on their skin (actinic keratoses) as a result of sunning. If, in addition, you have a family history of melanoma or have had three or more blistering sunburns as a child or teenager, your risk also increases.

What If You Do Nothing?

If untreated, all these forms of skin cancer will ultimately become destructive. Basal cell carcinomas are slow-growing, but it is important that they be found and treated early because they can ultimately invade and destroy nearby tissues. Melanoma that goes untreated may quickly spread to other parts of the body, which is why it is the most dangerous form of skin cancer. Of the nearly 10,000 deaths from skin cancer each year, almost 80 percent are from melanoma.

Home Remedies

Skin cancer requires evaluation and treatment by a physician.

Prevention

Even if the only risk factor you have is fair skin, you still need to be cautious and to protect yourself. One of the major steps you can take to prevent all forms of skin cancer is to reduce your direct exposure to sunlight, use adequate sunscreens, and wear protective clothing. (For more detailed tips on protecting yourself from too much sun exposure, see page 55.)

When To Call Your Doctor

Contact your doctor if you develop any of the symptoms listed above. Any new growths, changes in the size or color of existing growths, any sore that doesn't heal, or any persistent patch of irritated skin are reasons to see your doctor.

If you have had skin cancer, you should be sure to have your skin checked regularly.

What Your Doctor Will Do

Your doctor (or a dermatologist) may perform a biopsy—that is, remove all or part of a growth that doesn't appear normal. To check for cancer, this sample of tissue is examined under a microscope to detect cancerous cells.

If cancer is detected, the doctor will determine what stage it is in: local (affecting only the skin) or metastatic (spreading beyond the skin). You may need to have additional tests, such as x-rays, to find out whether cancer has spread to other parts of the body and to help plan the best treatment.

When caught in time, basal cell carcinoma can often be removed by a doctor on an outpatient basis, leaving only a minor scar. Once malignant melanoma is detected, you should see a doctor with special expertise in melanomas. The treatment is prompt surgical removal and microscopic examination of a sample.

If melanoma is removed in the early stages, the 5-year survival rate is 95 percent; the 10-year rate, 90 percent. If removal is done during a later stage, when a tumor has begun to invade the surrounding tissues or other areas of the body, the survival rate drops sharply.

For More Information

- American Academy of Dermatology
- American Cancer Society
- National Cancer Institute
- The Skin Cancer Foundation

445

Sleep Apnea

446

Symptoms

- Intense snoring pattern that ends in a loud gasp or snort.
- Waking up abruptly at night.
- Headaches upon waking.
- Feeling lethargic during the day for no apparent reason.

What Is It?

Sleep apnea is a serious disorder in which breathing stops or becomes very shallow during sleep, causing oxygen levels in the blood to fall. The throat muscles contract, there is a gasp for air, and breathing starts again. This pattern may be repeated hundreds of times a night.

A person with sleep apnea actually wakes up briefly and falls asleep again without being aware of having awakened. Heavy snoring is often a symptom of the condition. The soft tissues of the mouth vibrate during snoring, but with apnea the tongue and other soft tissues periodically fall back and collapse the airway, sometimes totally, sometimes only partially.

Sleep apnea affects anywhere from 2 to 10 percent of adults, yet the condition is still rarely diagnosed. Family members may tell you that you stop breathing at night and snore explosively. If you sleep alone, you may not even know that you snore, and you may not link the possible consequences of apnea to the disorder. Since apnea prevents you from sleeping restfully, and robs you of restorative REM (rapid eye movement) sleep, it can lead to daytime drowsiness, irritability, faulty memory, and lack of ability to concentrate.

Because of daytime drowsiness, those with sleep apnea are seven times more likely than average to be in traffic accidents. Apnea may also increase the risk of hypertension, stroke, heart attack, and other cardiovascular hazards. (For example, half of those with the disorder are found to have hypertension—though the connection between sleep apnea and hypertension remains controversial.) In rare cases, especially among the elderly, apnea may lead to severe respiratory failure and death.

What Causes It?

There are two types of sleep apnea. Obstructive sleep apnea is specifically caused by a temporary blockage of the breathing passages. Central sleep apnea, another form of the disorder, is caused by a brain dysfunction, but the results are the same.

Excess weight and age are associated with sleep apnea, since the excessive relaxation of muscles at the back of the throat that triggers apnea is a consequence of getting older or gaining extra weight. Men, people over 65, and especially the seriously overweight are particularly prone to the condition. Consuming alcohol before bedtime and using sedatives can also promote sleep apnea.

What If You Do Nothing?

The snoring and other symptoms associated with sleep apnea are unlikely to improve without some form of intervention—at the very least weight loss for those who are overweight.

Home Remedies

If you suspect that you have sleep apnea, tell your doctor. If you're diagnosed with the disorder, there is no simple solution, but these self-help measures should help. Some are the same techniques used for stopping snoring (see page 448).

- **Lose weight.** This is the one measure that may have the most benefit; even a 10-percent reduction should help.
- **Cut back on alcohol.** Don't drink alcoholic bev-

erages in the evening. Also try not to eat heavy meals in the evening.

- **If you smoke, stop**.
- **Elevate the head of your bed.** Use bricks or fat telephone books under the bed frame to lift it about 10 inches.
- **Avoid sleeping on your back.** This helps keep the tongue from falling back and pressing against the airways.
- **Reposition your lower jaw.** There are various "mandibular advancement" devices that reposition the lower jaw as you sleep. A little like the mouthpieces worn by football players, the devices sell for about $50. Sleep clinics and many doctors can offer advice about these.

Prevention

The measures above, especially losing weight, may also help prevent sleep apnea.

When To Call Your Doctor

Contact your doctor if you or family members become aware that you are showing signs of sleep apnea, especially if you are overweight and/or hypertensive.

What Your Doctor Will Do

There are now kits available that allow you to test for sleep apnea at home; your doctor may rec-

ommend one of these. You may then be advised to lose weight if you are overweight or obese, and take other preventive measures. If these don't help alleviate symptoms, the next step is to visit an ear, nose, and throat specialist or a sleep clinic (found in many hospitals) for further testing and to discuss treatment options.

The primary treatment for sleep apnea is a device called a continuous positive airway pressure, or CPAP, machine, which pumps air through a tube into a patient's nasal passages via a mask the patient wears while sleeping. The device is cumbersome and inconvenient, and about 40 percent of patients who try it eventually stop using it. But patients who can tolerate it are usually very pleased with the results.

New surgical techniques have been used to treat sleep apnea, but they are drastic and are intended only for cases of the disorder that are life-threatening. If surgery is recommended, be sure to get a second opinion.

447

For More Information

- American Academy of Otolaryngology-Head and Neck Surgery
- American Sleep Apnea Association
- American Academy of Sleep Medicine
- National Sleep Foundation

Snoring

Symptoms

- Guttural intermittent noise when breathing during sleep.
- Episodes of stopped breathing.
- Daytime fatigue.
- Irritability.

What Is It?

Millions of people snore, but except for keeping someone else awake at night, is snoring a problem? It may or may not be. For some, snoring may only be additional noise. But if the snoring is chronic and loud—some snores can exceed 90 decibels, the government limit for noise in the workplace—the snoring may signal obstructive sleep apnea, a serious medical condition.

Anywhere from 25 to 45 percent of Americans snore at least occasionally. It is largely adult men who snore, but children between the ages of 3 and 13 can snore when they have large tonsils and adenoids, or when they have a bad cold. As they mature, most will stop snoring.

Men typically start to snore in their late 30s and 40s, and the snoring intensifies after the age of 50. Among older people there may actually be more snorers than nonsnorers. People who are overweight are also more likely to snore.

What Causes It?

Snoring occurs mostly during periods of deep sleep and is caused by the rattling of the walls of the upper air passages, which can happen when nasal passages dry out (such as when you sleep in an overheated room) or when you sleep on your back. A nightcap before bed can also bring on snoring by relaxing muscles in the throat.

In some cases a medical condition is responsible. Nasal polyps, enlarged tonsils or adenoids, and a deviated septum can all cause snoring, a can the congestion brought on by a bad cold Obesity is another cause.

What If You Do Nothing?

In most cases habitual snoring doesn't disappea on its own. If you have a bedmate who can tolerate it, and if you are getting a good night's sleep then there is no need to correct it. However, i loud snoring or aborted breathing is part of you snoring pattern, and if you find that you are drowsy during the day, you may have sleep apnea which requires treatment (see page 446).

Home Remedies

If snoring annoys your bedmate, try these techniques to stop it.

- **Avoid heavy meals and alcohol within three hours of bedtime.** Eating heavily before turning in, or drinking alcohol causes greater-than-normal relaxation of the throat muscles, which may cause a nonsnorer to snore.
- **Avoid tranquilizers, sleeping pills, and antihistamines before bedtime.** Most of these medications suppress throat-muscle tone, just like alcohol, and can cause snoring.
- **Lose weight if you are obese.** No one is certain why weight gain causes snoring. It may be linked to increased fat in the structures around the throat, which diminishes the size of the air passages. If you have a tendency to snore, it will ge worse when you gain weight.
- **Avoid sleeping on your back.** This position may lead to snoring because the tongue falls back and presses against the top of the airways. The bes positions are the stomach and the side. However for heavy snorers, sleep position has no effect they will snore in all positions.
- **Try the tennis ball treatment.** Tape a tennis

ball to the back of your pajamas. (A rolled-up pair of socks will also do the trick.) Every time you roll over on your back, you'll become uncomfortable and will roll back on your side.

• **Tilt the head of your bed upward.** Place telephone books or bricks under the head of the bed. This may help relieve chronic snoring.

• **Seek treatment for problems that cause nasal obstruction.** Congestion due to allergies and colds causes air passages to narrow, making air flow more turbulent, which causes the throat tissues to vibrate. Contact an allergy specialist for testing and treatment. If you have nasal congestion due to a cold, use a decongestant.

• **Freshen bedroom air.** When the room is hot and dry, nasal passages become clogged during sleep, and this often leads to snoring. Keep your windows open and, if necessary, use a humidifier

to keep the nasal passages moist while you sleep.

• **If you smoke, quit.** Along with its many destructive consequences, smoking has an irritant effect that causes mucus buildup, inflammation, and swelling of the pharynx, as well as bronchial congestion, all of which can contribute to snoring.

Prevention
See the home remedies listed above.

When To Call Your Doctor
If you are told that you snore loudly and that your snoring is punctuated by quiet intervals of a few seconds to two minutes, followed again by a snort and loud snoring, contact your physician. You may have sleep apnea. Also contact your doctor if the self-help measures fail to stop you from snoring and if the snoring is regularly interfering with the sleep of a bed partner.

449

What Your Doctor Will Do
After a complete physical exam to rule out a physical obstruction, your physician may recommend a sleep study, especially if sleep apnea is suspected. Continuous positive airway pressure, or CPAP, may be recommended for chronic snoring or if sleep apnea is diagnosed. Corrective surgery may be an option in some extreme cases. As with all surgical procedures, get a second opinion.

For More Information
• American Academy of Otolaryngology-Head and Neck Surgery
• American Academy of Sleep Medicine
• National Sleep Foundation

Snoring Cures

▼

Antisnoring devices have become a growth industry. Nasal dilators, over-the-counter jaw retainers and mouthpieces, and even herbal pills, contoured pillows, and nasal sprays are being touted as cures. Which of these works? Who knows? For sure, forget the pills, pillows, and sprays. As for the nasal dilators, some of them may help if your snoring is due to certain types of nasal obstruction. Just don't invest a lot of money in any device.

It sounds silly, but Breathe Right, a small adhesive strip placed across your nose at night, may help you snore less. Available in drug, grocery, and discount stores, it has a springlike action that pulls the nostrils open slightly, thereby reducing resistance in the nasal airways. Certainly it won't help all snorers—and there's no evidence it will relieve sleep apnea—but it may help those whose snoring is due to some types of nasal obstruction, which can encourage breathing through the mouth during sleep.

Sore Throat

Symptoms

- Burning, scratchy sensation in the back of the throat.
- Visible redness and swelling.
- Discomfort when swallowing and talking.

What Is It?

A sore throat, or acute pharyngitis, is one of the most common winter complaints and ranks as one of the top reasons for visiting a doctor's office. It's also the cause of more than 100 million days of absence from work each year as well as countless days of missed school for children. Sore throat is usually a symptom of an infection—typically viral but in some cases bacterial—or an irritation of the pharynx, the back column of the mouth behind the tongue.

It's not surprising that the throat is the site of pain. Along with the nose, the throat is the first defense the body has against invading viruses or bacteria. As a rule of thumb, sore throats caused by a virus develop gradually over a period of time. They are often accompanied by the flu or a cold, and if a fever is present, it will generally be 101°F or below.

A bacterial sore throat usually comes on fast, lymph glands in the neck often swell and become tender, and a headache develops. Fever is typically 102°F or higher. The throat may appear to be extremely red and have either white or yellow spots on the back.

Strep throat, or streptococcal infection, is the most common bacterial throat infection. Strep is less common than virus-linked sore throats, but if not properly treated with antibiotics, it can lead to complications such as glomerulonephritis (kidney inflammation) or rheumatic fever, which may be associated with serious problems of the heart, brain, skin, and joints.

What Causes It?

Most sore throats are caused by a virus, primarily those associated with the common cold. Less than 15 percent of all sore throats are caused by *Streptococcus pyogenes,* the bacterium that produces the illness known as strep throat.

Irritation may result from a local throat infection or from postnasal drip, which is often a symptom of sinusitis, colds, or various allergic reactions. Allergy-related sore throats are typically accompanied by itchy eyes and a congested or runny nose.

Flu is a common viral infection that's accompanied by high fever, fatigue, loss of appetite, cough, and a sore throat. Infectious mononucleosis, which is usually brought on by the Epstein-Barr virus, also has sore throat as a common symptom. Dental procedures can sometimes cause throat pain, while some sore throats are caused by eating spicy foods. Overenthusiastic cheering at sporting events can also leave a throat sore and painful. Other minor causes of sore throat include dry heat, smoking, and breathing polluted air.

A sore throat may also be an early sign of a more serious disorder such as aplastic anemia.

What If You Do Nothing?

Sore throats caused by a cold or flu virus are usually self-limiting and will clear on their own in a few days as your body builds up defenses against the virus. Viral sore throats don't respond to antibiotics, but symptoms can be diminished with self-help measures. Sore throats from bacterial infections require treatment with prescription antibiotics. Going without treatment can allow an infection such as strep to lead to rheumatic fever or other serious complications.

Home Remedies

• **Try pain relievers.** Adults and children can take over-the-counter pain relievers such as ibuprofen or acetaminophen according to label directions. (Since a sore throat may be due to flu, children age 19 or younger with a sore throat should not take aspirin because aspirin use and flu in children is associated with a risk of Reye's syndrome, a rare but potentially fatal disorder.)

• **Use a home gargle.** Gargling several times a day with a mixture of one teaspoon of salt stirred into eight ounces of warm water may temporarily soothe a sore throat and also help to break up any congestion.

• **Have a hot drink.** A cup of herbal tea or chicken soup can help relieve a sore throat by warming and flushing the irritated membranes.

• **Use a humidifier or cool-mist vaporizer.** This will add extra moisture to the air and help keep your nasal membranes and throat lining moist.

• **Suck on hard candy.** This will help stimulate saliva production, thereby keeping your throat moist.

Prevention

• **Practice sanitary measures.** The best ways to avoid catching or passing the microorganisms that trigger sore throats are to wash your hands regularly, avoid touching your nose, eyes, and mouth, and cover your mouth when coughing and sneezing.

• **Don't smoke.** Avoid cigarette smoke and other throat irritants.

When To Call Your Doctor

Contact your doctor if the sore throat lasts longer than one to two days and you have a fever over 102°—you may have a bacterial infection. Also see your doctor if you develop an earache.

Contact your physician immediately if, in addition to your sore throat and a high fever, your voice becomes muffled and/or your tongue and throat swell. These developments may indicate that an abscess has formed in the throat and that pus is collecting beyond the wall of the tonsils. Such an infection requires early treatment with antibiotics and possibly surgery.

What Your Doctor Will Do

After taking a careful medical history, your doctor may obtain a throat culture if bacterial infection is suspected. If the diagnosis is positive, antibiotics may be prescribed. If mononucleosis is suspected, a special blood test will be done.

If you have recurrent sore throats and the cause is tonsillitis (an infection of the tonsils, which are located on each side of the throat), your physician may recommend a tonsillectomy to remove the tonsils. As with all surgical procedures, be sure to get a second opinion.

For More Information

• American Academy of Otolaryngology-Head and Neck Surgery

451

Strains and Sprains

Symptoms

Strain
- Muscle stiffness, soreness, and generalized tenderness several hours after the injury.
- Swelling of the injured muscle.
- In some cases, skin discoloration appearing several days later.

Sprain
- Mild to severe pain when the injury occurs.
- Joint tenderness and possible swelling.
- Bruising that can be noted immediately or up to several hours after the injury.
- Inability or difficulty moving the injured joint.

What Is It?

These are the most common types of acute injury—that is, an injury that usually results from a single, abrupt incident causing sharp pain, often accompanied by swelling. Strains and sprains are especially common among eager weekend athletes who don't know the limitations of their unconditioned muscles and joints.

• **Strains.** When a muscle is overstretched, some of its fibers may tear. This is often called a pulled muscle. Mild strains are usually only a nuisance; the tears are microscopic and, with rest, repair themselves easily. More severe strains involve a greater degree of fiber destruction and produce sharp pain with loss of power and movement.

• **Sprains.** Whereas strains occur to muscles, sprains damage ligaments (the bands connecting bones) and joint capsules. Like strains, sprains can range from minor tears to complete ruptures. But sprains tend to be more serious than strains: not only do they often take longer to heal, but a torn ligament can throw bones out of alignment, causing damage to surrounding tissues.

Any joint can be sprained, but because of its construction and the fact that it must support your body weight, the ankle is the most frequently sprained joint—in fact, an ankle sprain is probably the most common sports injury. The knee, too, is vulnerable because it must absorb twisting stress every time the body rotates from the hips (see Knee Injuries, page 364).

What Causes It?

Strains occur when muscles or their tendons are stretched to the point that their fibers actually start to tear. This can happen when you lift a heavy weight or suddenly overextend a muscle—for instance, when swinging a golf club, sprinting to catch a bus, or stretching to catch a Frisbee. The most common sites for strains are the hamstring and quadriceps muscles in the thigh and the muscles in the groin (see Groin Strain, page 293) and shoulder—all large muscles that are used for sudden powerful movements. Strains also occur to a muscle that has been previously injured—even slightly—and never properly rehabilitated. Cold, fatigue, or immobilization in a cast reduces blood flow to the muscles and lessens muscle elasticity, increasing the risk of strains.

Sprains are most often the result of a sudden force, typically a twisting motion, that the surrounding muscles aren't strong enough to control. As a result the ligaments, which usually wrap around a joint, get stretched and torn.

What If You Do Nothing?

In most cases recovery from a minor muscle strain requires nothing more than rest. However, if you are active and exercise regularly, strengthening and stretching will usually be necessary after recovery to prevent a recurrence of the injury. Sprains usually require attention (see Home Remedies) to reduce swelling and lessen pain. When severe pain or swelling occurs, you need to consult a doctor; the injury may turn out to be a severe sprain or a fracture, either of which require medical attention and possibly a splint or cast.

Home Remedies

Minor sprains or mild to moderate muscle strains can usually be self-treated at home with these measures.

• **RICE the injured area.** The acronym RICE—rest, ice, compression, and elevation—is the key to treatment. These steps reduce swelling, slow internal bleeding, and reduce pain.

With most injuries, swelling starts immediately; to reduce it, apply ice right away to the injured area. Wrap an elastic bandage snugly over the ice and around the injured site. Leave the ice and bandage in place for 20 minutes, then remove the ice, rewrap the injury, and elevate the injured part above the heart to help drain excess fluid from the damaged part.

Depending on the severity of your injury, continue with the ice therapy every two hours for up to 24 hours. At that point, you can begin heat treatments (heating pad, compress, shower, or bath) to increase circulation and accelerate healing. If any swelling develops, stop the heat and continue with the cold.

• **Take OTC pain relievers.** Nonprescription NSAIDs (aspirin, ibuprofen, or naproxen) will alleviate minor pain symptoms, though they won't promote healing.

• **Start gentle exercise.** Once pain and swelling have stopped, you can begin gentle stretching

453

Ice for Pain Relief

▼

Ice is the most effective, safest, and cheapest form of treating a muscle ache or pain. Not only does ice relieve pain, but it also slows blood flow, thereby reducing internal bleeding, inflammation, and muscle spasm. This in turn helps limit tissue damage and hastens healing.

With acute injuries such as torn ligaments, muscle strains, and bruises, the key is to start icing as soon as possible. Even if you go to the doctor immediately, icing an injury promptly will help speed your recovery.

Follow these tips:

• Plain ice is fine: simply put ice cubes or crushed ice in a heavy plastic bag or hot-water bottle, or wrap the ice in a towel. You can also immerse an injured hand or foot in ice water.

• Ice massage is the quickest way to cool an injury: move the ice pack gently over the injured area.

• Apply the ice on the injured area for 10 to 20 minutes, then reapply it every 2 to 3 waking hours (or more frequently if necessary) for the next 24 to 48 hours. Be careful not to go over 20 minutes; longer than that may damage skin and nerves. Stop icing once skin is numb.

• Be careful with refreezable gel packs and self-freezing chemical packs, which may be colder than regular ice. Don't leave them directly on skin; either keep moving the pack, or wrap it in a thin towel. And beware of punctures in the pack, since the chemicals can burn.

• Don't use ice on blisters or open wounds, or if you are hypersensitive to cold or have a circulatory problem.

• Never put an unwrapped ice pack over the elbow or the outside of the knee, where the nerves are near the surface and can be damaged by prolonged exposure to cold.

Icing is not a substitute for seeing your doctor in case of a serious injury and/or an injury that doesn't respond to self-treatment in 24 hours.

exercises to restore flexibility. Gradually add strengthening exercises with light weights to strengthen muscles and connective tissues around the affected joint.

Prevention

• **Exercise regularly.** Participate in regular, moderate exercise to keep your muscles and joints strong and flexible. Stretch your muscles before and after exercise. Strong muscles are also an injury safeguard. Include several weekly strength-training sessions focusing on your major muscle groups.

• **Warm up sufficiently.** Warm up, then stretch all the muscles involved in your upcoming activity. Activities such as jogging in place or stationary cycling for 5 to 10 minutes increase blood flow and raise the temperature of large muscle groups. You can also warm up by slowly rehearsing the sport or exercise you're about to perform. A light sweat usually indicates that you've warmed up sufficiently.

• **Consider taping or wrapping a weak joint.** Good taping can add stability to an injured joint and make it less likely to be reinjured. (If the sprain is severe, consult your physician or a physical therapist.)

When To Call Your Doctor

Contact your physician if you are in great pain or if the injured area becomes severely swollen and/or badly discolored. Also contact your doc-

tor if pain or swelling persists or increases more than two or three days after the injury despite your self-care measures.

What Your Doctor Will Do

A careful assessment will be done for a mild to severe muscle tear. The physician will feel the injured site and compare it with the uninjured side to determine the degree of damage. Treatment will be based on the severity of the injury.

For a moderate to severe sprain, an x-ray of the injured area may be taken to rule out a broken bone. A cast may be applied to a severely sprained joint; surgery may also be recommended, though this is rare.

In less severe cases pain medication may be prescribed and crutches or a sling may be recommended until the injury heals. After the pain has subsided, your physician or a physical therapist can help develop an appropriate program of exercise to regain mobility and strength.

For More Information

• American Academy of Orthopaedic Surgeons

Stye

Symptoms

■ Tender, red bump at the base of an eyelash on the upper or lower eyelid.

What Is It?

Like hair elsewhere on your body, eyelashes grow from follicles, which lie just under the skin—in this case along the eyelid—and are composed of the hair root and connective tissue. A stye is a common, often painful, bacterial infection that occurs either in one of the many follicles or in an oil gland on the eyelid margin. The stye usually appears as a small red pimple or boil with a whitish head, though when it occurs deep in an oil gland it won't have any head at all.

Styes can be very painful when touched. Even with treatment, styes will frequently recur because the bacteria that infect the first follicle will spread to infect others; this can happen if you touch the eyelid, use contaminated washcloths, or squeeze the stye.

What Causes It?

A stye develops when one of the eyelash follicles or glands becomes clogged with oil or dirt. Having chronic blepharitis increases the risk of developing styes, and styes are also especially common in people with fair complexions, particularly those of Irish, English, and Scottish descent.

What If You Do Nothing?

Styes are generally harmless. Several days after a stye forms, it will usually burst and drain, relieving the pain in the process. The stye should subside completely within a week or so.

Home Remedies

• **Apply warm compresses.** Wash the eyelids twice daily with a mild soap. Apply a warm washcloth to the eye for 10 minutes four times a day to increase blood circulation, which brings more infection-fighting white blood cells to the area helping the stye form a head. Once the stye opens and releases the pus, you will feel pain relief.

• **Continue to cleanse the eyelid several times daily.** Cleaning the lid even after the stye drains will help prevent the bacteria from spreading.

Prevention

• **Don't rub your eyes.** Rubbing can spread the infection to other eyelashes.

• **Don't share washcloths or towels.** Infection can be spread from contaminated bath linens.

When To Call Your Doctor

If the stye doesn't heal, or if it becomes unusually large, contact your physician. Also see your doctor if you develop many styes or if they occur frequently.

What Your Doctor Will Do

After a careful examination your doctor may prescribe antibiotics. A troublesome stye may be lanced and drained at your physician's office.

For More Information

• American Academy of Ophthalmology

Sunburn

- **First-degree:** reddish skin that feels hot and tender.
- **Second-degree:** small, fluid-filled blisters that may itch and eventually break.
- **Third-degree:** severely red to purplish skin discoloration, blistered skin accompanied by chills, mild fever, nausea, headache, or dehydration.

Note: A sunburn becomes most evident 6 to 24 hours after sunning.

What Is It?

Sunburn is an inflammation of the skin caused by overexposure to the ultraviolet (UV) rays of the sun—in particular UVB, or ultraviolet B, radiation. UVA, or ultraviolet A, penetrates more deeply than UVB but is less likely to cause an immediate burn. Rather, it causes wrinkling and leathering, damages connective tissue, and may be crucial in the development of melanoma, the most deadly of skin cancers.

Sunburn is not only painful—it also speeds up the aging of your skin and significantly increases your chances of developing skin cancer. If you have fair skin, blue eyes, or red hair, you're at greatest risk for sunburn, but even if you have a dark complexion, you need to be careful in the sun. Most sunburns are first-degree burns, but extreme overexposure—especially if you are fair-skinned—can result in second- or even third-degree burns.

What Causes It?

Exposure to the sun thickens the skin while encouraging the production of melanin, a pigment that absorbs UV rays. This is the skin's defense against the sun. African-Americans and other people with comparatively dark skin probably need less sun protection than light-skinned people because their higher concentration of melanin protects them from UV rays. They seldom develop skin cancer and are less susceptible to sun-induced wrinkles.

But in people who are not genetically dark-skinned, repeated exposure to UV rays can result in the destruction of elastic fibers in the skin, which causes it to sag and wrinkle and damages blood vessels. Even though people who tan easily appear to be less susceptible to skin cancer, they still need protection against UV rays.

What If You Do Nothing?

Although very painful, a sunburn eventually heals as the skin renews itself, generally taking from one to four days for a first-degree burn that reddens the upper skin layer (epidermis) to four to seven days for a more severe second-degree burn that affects underlying layers.

Home Remedies

Virtually everyone is susceptible to some degree of skin damage from the sun's rays given sufficient exposure. If you inadvertently get burned

Using the UV Index

▼

The UV Index indicates the amount of UV radiation reaching earth at noontime. The index is based on a scale of 0 to 10+. It is determined for 58 major U.S. cities as well as for smaller towns and cities within a 30-mile radius of each city. The higher the index number, the greater your UV exposure when you go outdoors. The index appears in local newspapers, is regularly reported on TV and radio weather reports, and is available at many Internet weather sites.

by the sun, the following tips will help minimize any pain and swelling.

• **Soak the affected area for 15 minutes in cold water (but not ice water), or apply cold compresses.** This provides some immediate relief from the pain, conducts heat away from your skin, and reduces swelling.

• **Get some pain relief.** If your sunburn is very painful, take an over-the-counter pain reliever such as aspirin, ibuprofen, or acetaminophen. Aspirin and ibuprofen will both relieve pain and help reduce inflammation.

• **Try cooling lotions.** Products that contain menthol or camphor may provide temporary relief by affecting the nerve endings and constricting superficial blood vessels in the skin. Be careful: they can be irritating and can cause allergic reactions, especially in children.

• **Don't apply greasy creams or lotions such as petroleum jelly or baby oil.** These types of oily products act to seal in the heat.

• **Spray on first aid.** If the burn is very painful, you may want to consider a first aid spray containing benzocaine, a topical anesthetic that also acts on the nerve endings in the skin. Be careful, as this may sensitize the skin and lead to an allergic reaction upon subsequent applications of other medications in the "-caine" family. Don't use other "-caine" anesthetics for sunburn: they are readily absorbed into the bloodstream if the skin is broken and may cause immediate toxic or allergic reactions.

• **Powder your sheets.** Sprinkle cornstarch powder on your sheets to minimize chafing.

• **If you are sunburned all over your body, try an oatmeal bath.** The oatmeal soothes the skin and reduces inflammation. You can buy oatmeal bath products (such as Aveeno) in drugstores, but these tend to be expensive. Make your own oatmeal soak at home by finely grinding a cup of dry instant oatmeal in a blender or food processor. Scatter the oatmeal in a tub of cool water and soak for a while. (Cornstarch works equally well.)

Prevention

Sunburn is easily avoidable if you take some simple precautions. These include using an effective sunscreen with a sun protection factor (SPF) of 15 or higher and avoiding long sun exposure, even if you are wearing a sunscreen. Also make sure that children, especially infants, are well protected.

You will find more detailed information on protecting yourself from the sun on page 55.

When To Call Your Doctor

Most sunburns are first-degree burns that affect the outer skin layer, cause no blistering, and can be treated readily with home remedies. However, contact your physician if:

• You develop a fever or experience chills, nausea, or disorientation.

• Fluid-filled blisters form. Secondary infection is a possibility.

• The pain is especially severe. This could be a severe second-degree or a third-degree sunburn that has not only damaged the epidermis but the underlying nerves and subcutaneous tissue as well (see Burns, page 109).

What Your Doctor Will Do

After an examination, your doctor may remove the fluid from any blisters. If infection has occurred, an antibiotic may be prescribed.

For More Information

• American Academy of Dermatology

Swimmer's Ear

Symptoms

- Swelling, pain, and itching in the area of the outer ear.
- Soreness and tenderness in the triangular piece of cartilage in front of the ear opening.
- Discharge from the ear canal.

What Is It?

Otitis externa is the medical name of this painful, itchy condition, which is a bacterial (sometimes fungal) infection brought on when water containing infectious agents gets trapped in the ear and causes inflammation of the outer ear and canal. Just as you needn't be an athlete to get athlete's foot, you needn't be a swimmer to get swimmer's ear.

What Causes It?

Swimming is the most common cause of this problem, but some people may get water in their ears from showering or washing their hair. The longer the water remains in the ear, the more likely it is that any microorganisms will breed.

What If You Do Nothing?

A mild case of swimmer's ear often clears up without treatment. Severe, persistent, or recurring cases require medical attention.

Home Remedies

• **Keep the infected ear dry.** Don't go swimming. When you shower, keep your infected ear turned away from the water while washing your hair, and otherwise wear a shower cap.

• **Use antiseptic eardrops.** You can buy these without a prescription at any drugstore. Or make them yourself: mix equal parts of white vinegar and rubbing alcohol. This solution restores the natural acid balance of the ear canal and helps dry it out; it also kills bacteria. If alcohol irritates your skin, use vinegar diluted with water.

Put one or two drops of this solution in each ear with a dropper. Leave the drops in your ear for two or three minutes, then tilt your head and let them drain out. Repeat three times daily.

• **Don't scratch.** Resist the temptation to scratch inside the ear with an object; you risk rupturing your eardrum.

Prevention

• **Clear your ears.** After swimming, shake your head to remove water trapped in your ears.

• **Keep the ears dry.** Gently dry the external ear with a corner of a towel. Don't insert cotton swabs or anything else into the canal to dry or clean your ears. This could cause injury or infection.

• **If you are prone to ear infection, use antiseptic eardrops (see above).** This is particularly helpful if you've been swimming in a lake.

• **Consider having your ears checked.** People who are prone to itchy ears or ear infections may need to have a doctor check their ears and remove excess wax before swimming season starts. If you have ever had a perforated eardrum or have ever had ear surgery, get medical advice before using eardrops and before swimming.

When To Call Your Doctor

If swelling, pain, and discharge occur, or if mild inflammation persists for more than a few days, contact your doctor.

What Your Doctor Will Do

A thorough examination of the ear will be performed and a culture for bacteria may be taken. Effective treatments include irrigation of the ear and antibiotic eardrops.

Syphilis

Symptoms

- In the initial or primary stage of syphilis, one or more painless sores (chancres) appear on the genitals, mouth, or anus—the sites where the bacteria can enter your body—anywhere from a few days to 12 weeks after the initial infection occurs (but on average 3 to 4 days after infection). Chancres are more obvious in men. Vaginal chancres are rarely noticed and heal without scarring. Lymph nodes near the area of the chancre may become swollen. The infection is highly contagious in this stage.

- If treatment is not received, the secondary stage of syphilis may occur, beginning six weeks to several months after the appearance of the chancre(s). This stage—during which the infection continues to be highly contagious—is characterized by fever, a nonitching rash, and flulike symptoms. Lymph nodes may enlarge. Each of these symptoms may occur, disappear, and then reappear later.

- The untreated bacteria may become latent, and people who reach this stage show no symptoms. Late-stage, or tertiary, syphilis can develop 10 or more years after the initial infection, with symptoms that can mimic many other diseases. This stage can result in damage to internal organs, including the heart and brain, and in death.

- Syphilis can also be transmitted to newborns by infected mothers.

What Is It?

One of the oldest sexually transmitted diseases, syphilis is a highly contagious bacterial infection. Records of the disease go back to the time of Columbus's voyage, and historians argue over whether syphilis originated in the Americas, Europe, Asia, or Africa. After declining in the United States in this century, the number of syphilis cases began to rise in the 1950s, with the height of the most recent epidemic occurring in 1990. At that time the rate of syphilis was near a 30-year high and the number of children born with the disease had also soared. However, the disease has been declining again since then—dramatically so. In 1998, only about 7,000 cases were reported in the United States—an 85-percent decrease from the 50,000 cases reported in 1990.

Syphilis is treatable and curable in its first two stages. If not treated, it becomes latent for a period of years until the outbreak of a final destructive stage.

What Causes It?

Syphilis is caused by the spirochete *Treponema pallidum*, a spiral-shaped bacterium that spreads primarily through sexual intercourse with a person who is in the primary or secondary stages of infection. (Late-stage syphilis is noninfectious.) The bacteria travel quickly and aggressively through the bloodstream and lymphatic system.

What If You Do Nothing?

The initial phase of syphilis will clear up by itself without treatment within a month or so. But the bacteria stay in the body, and within two to eight weeks, second-stage symptoms often appear. These symptoms will also clear up eventually without treatment.

Syphilis may then become chronic and ultimately fatal. The final tertiary, or late, stage of syphilis can begin years after the initial infection. Depending on the course of the disease, late-stage syphilis that has not been treated can cause heart disease, brain damage, destruction of bones or other organs, and, eventually, death.

Untreated syphilis during pregnancy results in infant death in up to 40 percent of cases.

Home Remedies

Syphilis cannot be accurately diagnosed and treated without professional help. There are no home remedies, so see a doctor or another health-care professional if you get infected or think you might be infected.

Prevention

- **Know your partner.** Get to know a potential sex partner before becoming intimate. Avoid anyone whose health status is questionable.
- **Practice safer sex.** Follow the measures described on pages 57-59 for preventing any sexually transmitted disease. Most important, use a latex condom each time you have sexual intercourse.
- **Early detection.** If you or your partner notice any symptoms of syphilis, contact your physician immediately and seek treatment.
- **Get tested regularly if you have multiple sex partners.** Even if you have no symptoms, ask your physician to perform a syphilis test annually.
- **Abstain from sex.** To prevent syphilis from spreading, abstain from sexual intercourse for at least two months after undergoing treatment. Make sure follow-up blood studies show no recurrence of the disease.

- **Inform others.** It's important to notify your local health department. It's also important to tell your sexual partner and make sure he or she also receives appropriate treatment.

When To Call Your Doctor

Contact your physician if you or your sexual partner develops signs of syphilis. Also contact your physician if you have had sexual contact with someone you suspect may have syphilis.

What Your Doctor Will Do

After a careful examination, your doctor will perform blood tests for antibodies to the bacteria and examine the fluid from any lesions under a microscope. Even if no symptoms are present, diagnosis can be made by a blood test—though it usually takes four to six weeks after exposure for a positive result to show up, and in some instances results may be negative for up to 12 weeks.

Penicillin is the primary medication prescribed to treat syphilis; other antibiotics are prescribed for anyone allergic to penicillin.

For More Information

- American Social Health Association
- CDC National Prevention Information Network

Teeth Grinding (Bruxism)

Symptoms

- Grinding or gnashing of the teeth at night; may occur occasionally or so frequently that teeth are worn down or damaged.
- Clicking sound and/or pain in your jaw.
- Jaw pain, earache, headache or facial pain upon awakening.
- Sensitive teeth and/or toothache.

What Is It?

Teeth grinding or clenching of the teeth during sleep, known as bruxism (from the Greek *brychein*, meaning "to gnash the teeth"), can cause facial soreness and pain, headaches, and fractured or abraded teeth, as well as the jawbone pain known as TMD (temporomandibular disorders). Nearly everybody is thought to have occasional episodes of nighttime grinding, but only a small percentage grind so much that they damage their teeth and jaws.

Episodes may occur eight or more times a night and can easily awaken a person in the same room. If your bedmate doesn't tell you, your dentist, at a routine exam, may notice the signs of ground-down teeth and inform you that you're a bruxer.

What Causes It?

Bruxism is a complex phenomenon. There's still argument about probable causes and appropriate treatments.

Emotional stress is a likely cause. People who grind their teeth often report that they are undergoing marital or financial difficulties, taking final exams, fearful of losing their jobs, or otherwise under pressure.

Studies have not agreed on whether one particular personality is associated with bruxism. One small study found that shy, unhappy people tend to grind, but other studies have suggested that hard-driving perfectionists do.

Genetics may play a role, since bruxism seems to run in families. Malocclusion (faulty contact between upper and lower teeth) or restorative dentistry that isn't quite right can cause mouth discomfort that, in turn, makes jaw muscles contract at night. People with sleep disturbances may also be prone to bruxism. Mood-altering substances, including alcohol and amphetamines, can promote the problem.

What If You Do Nothing?

Occasional or light teeth grinding is not considered a serious problem. However, chronic, heavy grinding can result in jaw and ear pain and can contribute to periodontal disease and even the loss of teeth, as well as fractured teeth or broken restorations.

Dealing With A Cracked Tooth

▼

A common side effect of nighttime grinding is a cracked tooth. This is a fracture in the tooth enamel caused by wear and tear; aging; chewing ice, gum, nuts, or hard candies; or biting down hard on a bone, pit, or other hard object. It may be hard for a dentist to diagnose a cracked tooth because the crack may not be visible, even on an x-ray. The first symptom is usually pain in the tooth when you bite down hard or discomfort when inhaling cold air through the mouth.

A crack can get larger and deeper with further wear and may cause serious injury to the tooth or promote infection. In some cases grinding down the chewing surface of the tooth may relieve pressure on the bite and keep the crack from opening when you chew. However, a crack won't heal, and you'll probably need some kind of restorative dentistry.

Home Remedies

• **Reduce stress in your life.** If you suspect that abnormal daily stress is causing the problem, find ways to address the problem. Relaxation techniques may help you to deal with stress or anger. Even something as simple as a warm bath before bedtime may help.

• **Warm your facial muscles.** Place a warm washcloth on your face in the morning. This may help relax your muscles.

• **Chew softly.** Avoid foods like hard candies and crusty bread or bagels, as well as chewing gum. Don't chew on things like pencils or ice.

• **Take pain relievers.** Aspirin, acetaminophen, and other over-the-counter pain relievers can help reduce jaw pain.

• **Reduce or eliminate alcohol intake.** Teeth grinding often gets worse after consuming alcoholic beverages.

Prevention

Follow the tips listed above.

When To Call Your Doctor

Contact your dentist if symptoms of teeth grinding interfere with your normal activities or if you notice that your teeth are being damaged by the grinding.

What Your Doctor Will Do

After a careful examination to rule out other ailments that may cause jaw or ear pain, such as TMD, your dentist may recommend stress reduction counseling to reduce any stress and anxiety. Some simple physical therapy may also be recommended. The dentist should also check for signs of malocclusion and, of course, should repair any damage to your teeth or crowns and bridges.

Occlusal appliance therapy, consisting of an individually fitted mouthguard or splint made of soft or hard acrylic, is a popular item now in preventive dentistry—and frequently suggested for bruxers. Usually worn at night, mouthguards are not designed to prevent clenching or grinding, but they do redistribute the forces exerted while grinding and thus help protect teeth. They can cost several hundred dollars.

You may want to seek a second opinion before investing in a mouthguard. If you do get one, you'll need to go for a checkup every four to six months to make sure it still fits and to get any needed adjustments. You'll also need to keep it clean, brushing it with toothbrush and toothpaste after each use.

A much less expensive solution may be a simple athletic mouthguard, sold at sporting goods stores for about $10. If it fits properly, it should spread the clenching pressure evenly across your mouth. It may not be as comfortable as a custom-made splint and will certainly be bulkier and more visible. You should discuss this measure with your dentist, and should have dental checkups every six months.

For More Information

• American Dental Association

Teething

Symptoms

■ Drooling increases.
■ Fingers are put in the mouth more often.
■ Gums can become red and/or swollen.
■ Irritability may increase.

What Is It?

When a child's new teeth push through the gums, the process is called teething (also known as tooth eruption). It usually begins between the ages of four to eight months and ends around the third birthday. Of the 20 primary teeth, the 8 incisors (sharp front teeth) come in first and are typically all in place at 12 to 14 months. These are followed by molars (back teeth used for chewing) and canines (pointed teeth located between molars and incisors).

As these teeth work their way through the gum tissue, the gums can become swollen and tender, and a teething child may fret, cry, be unwilling to eat, and have trouble sleeping. It is not clear, however, whether these and other symptoms associated with teething are due to tooth eruption. For example, most teething children drool frequently, but the drooling may be caused by the normal development of the salivary glands. Teething has also been blamed for causing infections and high fevers, but these may be separate problems that occur simultaneously with the emergence of new teeth.

What Causes It?

Teething is a normal aspect of development.

What If You Do Nothing?

Any teething-related discomfort, which varies in intensity from child to child, is almost always harmless and temporary.

Home Remedies

Because stimulating the gums helps alleviate any discomfort, a baby who is teething will often chew on fingers and other hard objects. Here are several ways that a parent can help.

• **Give your child an object to teethe on.** Make sure that the object is large enough that your child can't swallow it or choke on it. Usually, a hard rubber pacifier is the best choice. Avoid plastic objects because they can splinter and harm the child. A chilled teething ring or a metal spoon can help numb irritated gums. (But don't use a frozen object; a baby's mouth can get frostbite.)

Do not tie a teething ring around your child's neck; it can become a strangulation hazard.

• **Massage the gums.** Rub the child's gums gently with your little finger for a minute or two. Make sure your finger is clean. Don't rub aspirin on the gums; not only can it cause irritation, but it also may be dangerous if swallowed.

• **Medicate the pain.** If teething pain is especially distressing, acetaminophen or ibuprofen can be used to relieve pain. Follow dosage instructions on the label for your child's age and weight, or consult your pediatrician. Do not apply a teething gel or other topical anesthetic used to numb the gums. Some children have allergic reactions.

• **Skip the bottle at bedtime.** Do not lull a baby to sleep with a bottle of milk, either at nap time or at night. If milk stays in constant contact with the teeth, tooth decay can result. Milk should be used for feeding, not for teething or to quiet your child.

• **Keep your child's face from chapping.** To prevent chapping on the cheeks and around the mouth caused by excessive drooling, rub a thin layer of petroleum jelly on the child's face.

• **Clean gums and new teeth regularly.** Gently clean your child's gums and new teeth twice daily (especially after bedtime feedings) with a clean washcloth, a soft toothbrush, or a piece of gauze. This reduces the amount of bacteria present on the gums, decreasing the risk of infection and irritation.

Prevention
Teething is a natural process.

When To Call Your Doctor
Generally, teething does not warrant calling your pediatrician. But if your child develops a fever, particularly a fever over 101°F, call your doctor, since any fever will probably have a cause other than teething. Likewise, diarrhea, vomiting, or loss of appetite suggest an underlying health problem and can be signs to call your physician.

Occasionally, bluish bruises (blood blisters) will form on the gum opposite the one where a tooth is starting to push through.

What Your Doctor Will Do
Your doctor will determine whether any pain, discomfort, or fever is due to something other than teething.

For More Information
• American Academy of Pediatrics
• American Dental Association

Tendinitis

Symptoms

- Tenderness, pain, dull ache, stiffness, or mild swelling around a tendon or joint.
- Restricted movement.
- Tendon weakness.

What Is It?

Tendons are the fibrous cords that anchor muscle to bone—and they are vulnerable, since the force of all muscle contractions is transmitted through them. Tendinitis is an inflammation of a tendon—the suffix "itis" means inflammation—and is characterized by pain, swelling, warmth, and redness.

Tendinitis is the problem behind many common overuse injuries—and it can be deceptive: the pain can be severe when you start exercising, then diminish as you continue, only to return sharply once you've stopped. Perhaps the most common form of tendinitis is tennis elbow. In sports and activities that involve running and jumping, tendinitis is most likely to develop in the knee, foot, and the Achilles tendon at the back of the ankles. For cyclists, knees are most vulnerable. Shoulder (rotator cuff) tendinitis can develop from pitching a ball, swinging a golf club, or swimming.

What Causes It?

Almost all active people eventually suffer some form of tendinitis. Regular exercisers are especially at risk because of the strong forces produced by their well-conditioned muscles. These increase tension on the tendons, which can then rub against bones, ligaments, and other tendons, causing irritation that leads to tendinitis.

Even if you are sedentary, you can develop tendinitis from repetitive activities like carrying a briefcase or playing a musical instrument for long hours. Posture problems can also lead to tendinitis, as can sudden physical trauma to the tendon resulting from a fall, for example, or a sharp blow or twist to a joint.

What If You Do Nothing?

Tendinitis usually occurs through repetitive physical stress, so altering or eliminating the activity responsible for it should cause the pain to go away. If you continue with the activity that caused the tendinitis and do nothing to eliminate the problem, the ailment may become chronic.

Home Remedies

- **Stop your activity.** At the first signs of tendinitis—pain and swelling—immediately stop the activity that's causing the pain. This will give the tendon a chance to heal. To eliminate the risk of aggravating the injury, don't resume your activity at full tilt until the pain is completely gone.
- **Reduce inflammation.** To quell inflammation and reduce any swelling, ice the injured area 20 minutes a session several times a day for the first 72 hours. After using ice, wrap the area with an elastic bandage. After three days, apply heat—or alternate heat and cold—to increase circulation and speed healing. Hot showers, hot compresses, or a heating pad (at low or medium settings) may be sufficient.
- **Relieve pain.** Use ibuprofen, naproxen, or aspirin according to label directions for relief of pain and inflammation.
- **Begin stretching.** When pain diminishes, start doing stretching exercises to restore flexibility.
- **Begin strengthening.** The stronger your muscles, the less stress placed on your tendons. When pain is gone, use light weights to strengthen the muscle groups around the injured tendon.

465

Prevention

- **Keep muscles flexible.** Stretching and strengthening routines can help prevent tendinitis from developing by keeping the muscles supple and strong.
- **Develop proper technique.** For nearly every sport and recreational activity, certain tendons are vulnerable. But properly executed movements will do a lot to prevent tendinitis problems from developing. Learn the proper movements for any sport you play regularly.
- **Don't overdo it.** Drastically increasing the distance you run or suddenly working out more strenuously or longer than usual can produce muscle fatigue and thus lead to an injury.
- **Compensate for musculoskeletal problems.** If your feet happen to roll inward (overpronate) as you run, you may develop a form of tendinitis in your knee that's commonly called runner's knee (see Knee Injuries, page 364). You may need to consult a physical therapist, orthopedist, or other specialist for treatment.
- **Counter muscle imbalances.** If your calf muscles are very strong from running, but you don't strengthen the opposing shin muscles, you increase the chances of injuring your Achilles tendon. Strengthen the key muscle groups for your activity.

Stress Fractures

These microscopic breaks in bone, usually in the foot, shin, or thigh, are another form of overuse injury. Common among long-distance runners, aerobic dancers, and basketball players, the fractures are caused by the repeated impact of running or jumping. Often the pain is mild at first—a dull ache—occurring during or right after exercise. If you continue the activity, the pain gradually increases, but for the first few weeks such fractures are usually too small to be detected, even by x-ray. Fortunately, the fractures rarely break through the bone, so they don't require splints or casts to heal, only rest.

Prevent stress fractures by increasing the intensity of your workouts gradually, not dramatically. Try to minimize the impact on your legs: run and jump on soft or resilient surfaces—grass, carpet, mats, or suspended wooden gym floors—rather than concrete. Wear well-cushioned exercise shoes.

When To Call Your Doctor

It's usually wise to consult your doctor if you have symptoms of tendinitis, unless it's an injury you've had before and know how to treat. Your doctor may refer you to a physical therapist. Contact your physician immediately if the injured joint appears to be swollen, discolored, or distorted. Also contact your physician if your symptoms don't resolve with the self-care measures described above, or if pain and swelling increase despite the measures.

What Your Doctor Will Do

After taking a careful history, your physician may recommend a course of physical therapy and may prescribe medication to reduce inflammation and pain. In addition, you may be advised to use an elastic support wrap or sling to compress and immobilize the affected body part.

For More Information

- American Academy of Orthopaedic Surgeons

Tennis Elbow

Symptoms

- Tenderness and pain in the muscle connected to the outer side of the elbow.
- Pain in the elbow when hitting a tennis ball.
- Pain in the forearm and elbow when turning the hand and arm, as in using a screwdriver or playing tennis.
- Forearm and elbow pain when lifting a heavy object.

What Is It?

Tennis elbow is a type of tendinitis that at some point sidelines about half of all amateurs who play tennis at least three times weekly. Professional players suffer from it, too.

Tennis players aren't the only ones at risk for epicondylitis—the medical term for tennis elbow. In fact, the pain is not related to tennis in at least 95 percent of patients. Any activity that calls for forceful, repeated contraction of the arm muscles can bring on tennis elbow—for example, working with carpentry tools, shaking hands, gardening, raking leaves, even tightly gripping a briefcase handle. Baseball, golf, bowling, racquet sports, even darts can bring it on. In most cases the dominant side of the body is affected.

What Causes It?

The injury occurs when you flex, extend, twist, or contract your wrist or forearm excessively or improperly, and thus strain the tendons that connect muscles to the elbow joint. In time, the overstressed tendons develop microscopic tears, producing tendinitis (painful inflammation of the tendons) centered around the epicondyle, the point at which the tendons attach to the elbow. The pain can radiate down to the wrist and up to the shoulder. Moving your arm or gripping something aggravates the pain.

The elbow tendons can develop microscopic tears anytime they are exposed to a repeated stress greater than the tissues can withstand. Experts think it's not the vibration that causes the tears but excess torsion—for instance, when the ball hits off center, the racquet twists your arm. Pain on the lateral side of your arm (the side your thumb is on) is 10 times more common than pain on the other (medial) side.

For most recreational tennis players, the backhand may be the main culprit causing the condition. However, the serve or forehand may also promote tennis elbow.

To some extent, whether or not you develop tennis elbow depends on the condition of your muscles and how much they are overused. In tennis, the injury occurs most frequently among recreational players who are 35 to 50 years old—a period during which muscles have begun to lose their resiliency—and who play at least two or

467

Braces May Help

▼

In one study of 2,633 tennis players who suffered from tennis elbow, 84 percent claimed an elbow brace improved the condition. The brace recommended by most health professionals is called a counterforce brace. This is different from the elastic braces you may find in sporting goods stores—elastic doesn't give enough support. The counterforce brace functions as a constraint against muscle contraction and excessive movement of the tendons, thus reducing force and overload on the soft tissues of the elbow. A counterforce brace won't interfere with your game because it does not prevent motion as does a brace with metal supports (such as a knee brace). You can get a counterforce brace through your physician; some sporting goods stores also carry them.

three times a week. In a study of 2,600 amateurs, almost half of those who played daily got tennis elbow.

Occasional players are less vulnerable, as they tend not to play often enough or hard enough to overstress their arms. Pros are generally protected by superior conditioning and stroking technique, though they, too, can develop tennis elbow as they grow older.

What If You Do Nothing?

Tennis elbow will clear up by itself if you are able to rest and stop performing the twisting motions to the wrist and forearm that initially brought on the pain.

Home Remedies

• **Take a break.** If you develop tennis elbow, try to reduce the activity that is causing it—or stop completely—until the pain diminishes. If you must engage in the activity, at least try to warm up your arm for five minutes by stretching it and flexing your wrist. Once you start the activity, take frequent breaks.

• **For pain relief, anti-inflammatories can help.** For mild cases of tennis elbow, nonprescription NSAIDs—aspirin, ibuprofen, or naproxen—will reduce inflammation and pain while you are resting your arm.

• **Apply ice or heat.** For some people, immersing the elbow and forearm in warm water for 15 minutes several times a day may bring some relief. For others, an ice pack placed on the sore area for 15 minutes several times a day can help diminish the soreness.

• **Try an elbow brace.** For players persistently troubled by tennis elbow, some sports physiologists recommend the use of an elbow brace, which supports and protects the muscles and tendons of the forearm; this offers some pain relief without drastically restricting movement.

Protective Conditioning

These two effective forearm strengtheners can help ward off tennis elbow.

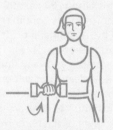

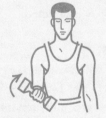

Wrist curls (forearm flexors). Holding a light weight, lay your forearm on a table with your hand over the edge, palm up. Slowly curl up the weight, then lower it as far as possible; repeat. Then reverse the maneuver: turn your palm downward and repeat the curl. Switch arms and repeat.

Arm rotation. Sitting or standing, hold a light weight (one to three pounds) in front of you with your elbow bent at a 90-degree angle and your palm up. Slowly roll your forearm to palm-down position, then return to the starting position. Repeat 20 to 30 times. Switch arms and repeat.

Prevention

If you play tennis regularly, here are the keys to avoiding tennis elbow. To prevent epicondylitis, beginners should remember that technique and conditioning are far more important than the size or type of racquet.

• **Strengthen forearm muscles.** This is the best defense for athlete and nonathlete. According to Dr. Robert Nirschl, director of the Nirschl Sports Medicine Clinic in Arlington, Virginia, half the tennis elbow sufferers he sees have some major strength deficits in the shoulder and upper back. The key therefore is to restore strength, endurance, and flexibility to the arm, shoulder, and back. (If you're under treatment for tennis elbow, you should consult your doctor before embarking on an exercise program.)

One simple forearm strengthener is to squeeze a ball 40 or 50 times with your arm extended horizontally in front of you. (See the box on page 468 for additional exercises.)

• **Work on your form.** Power your serve and backhand with your legs, torso, and shoulder muscles rather than with your forearm and wrist. During a stroke, your elbow should be almost fully extended but not locked, and your grip should be firm but not viselike, so that force is transferred to your shoulder.

• **Try a two-handed backhand.** Some teaching pros recommend this technique to beginners. Players who use two hands seldom develop tennis elbow, since the second hand provides additional support.

• **Choose the right racquet.** Racquets can aggravate tennis elbow. Follow these tips when selecting your equipment.

• **Try a midsize racquet.** This style of racquet has a bigger sweet spot and absorbs vibration better than a small one. It plays softer and gives more power, so you don't need to swing as hard. An oversize racquet, in contrast, can increase the risk of the racquet overtwisting if you hit the ball off center.

• **Choose a flexible racquet, which will dampen shock effectively.** According to Dr. Howard Brody, professor emeritus of physics at the University of Pennsylvania, composite racquets with an increased ratio of nylon matrix, as opposed to epoxy resin, are good models for absorbing shock.

• **An increased grip size can also help.** Too small a grip can lead to arm-muscle fatigue from overtightening. But too large a grip may put you at a strength disadvantage.

• **Lower your string tension to dampen shock.** Higher string tension does give more control, but it also increases the shock to your arm after ball impact.

• **Consider tennis lessons.** A tennis pro can easily help correct any faulty backhand technique and assist you in selecting the tennis racquet that best fits your grip.

When To Call Your Doctor

Contact your physician if, despite self-care efforts, your symptoms don't improve in two weeks.

What Your Doctor Will Do

After taking a medical history and performing a physical examination, your physician may prescribe anti-inflammatory medication and may recommend a course of physical therapy.

For More Information

• American Academy of Orthopaedic Surgeons

Tinnitus

Symptoms

- Ringing, buzzing, humming, or other persistent or intermittent noises in one or both ears.
- Interference with hearing.
- Possible sleep disturbance.

What Is It?

Most of us hear faint ringing sounds occasionally when there's no external noise. Usually such sounds last a few minutes or, at most, several hours. But if ringing or other noises in your head are persistent, you have tinnitus. Though the term is from a Latin word meaning to ring like a bell, people with tinnitus may actually hear many sounds, from buzzing, tinkling, and humming to popping and clanging.

Researchers estimate that about 50 million Americans have occasional or constant tinnitus. About 12 million have such severe symptoms that they have sought medical help. The remainder experience a low level of noise—usually in both ears but sometimes in just one—which can still be a nuisance, interfering with work, social life, and sleep. The onset of tinnitus doesn't signify that you will become seriously or permanently deaf, but tinnitus is often associated with some hearing loss—though it does not cause it. About 80 percent of Americans who have some hearing loss also experience tinnitus.

Tinnitus has been described by one expert as "listening to old age sneaking up on you," since the great majority of tinnitus sufferers are middle-aged or older. It usually comes on slowly, with intermittent episodes that may become chronic with age. But some young people also experience tinnitus.

There is a less common form of tinnitus—objective tinnitus—in which the sounds you hear can also be heard by your doctor listening with a stethoscope. Usually these sounds are produced by either movement of the jaw (the temporomandibular joint) or the flow of blood in major blood vessels of the head and neck.

What Causes It?

While it's true that the sounds of tinnitus are all "in your head," they are nevertheless real. The physiological or neurological cause of such subjective sounds isn't always known, but they are a symptom of something that has gone awry in the auditory system. For example, infections of the middle ear or a perforated eardrum can induce tinnitus, as can a buildup of wax or dirt in the outer ear or damage to the tiny bones of the middle ear that transmit sound.

One of the most common causes is exposure to loud noises such as gunshots, jet engines, jackhammers, chain saws, rock music, or industrial machinery. Tinnitus has also been linked to tumors of certain cranial nerves, head injuries, and excessive use of alcohol and aspirin. More often then not, the specific cause of tinnitus cannot be determined. But whatever factor is responsible, there is usually damage to the microscopic hair cells in the inner ear, particularly those responsible for detecting high-frequency sounds.

What If You Do Nothing?

Tinnitus rarely goes away, and it often intensifies with age. But you can learn to live with it.

Home Remedies

When conductive hearing loss, such as that caused by wax in the ear canal, is involved, treatment is almost always successful. When the cause is unknown—which is generally the case—the chances of medically correcting tinnitus are quite

470

small. No standard drug or medical procedure relieves tinnitus, but the following steps have proved effective.

• **Drown out the noise.** Overcoming the sounds of tinnitus with less bothersome sounds is perhaps the most promising method of dealing with the condition. For people with mild tinnitus, background sound from a radio or television may do the trick. White-noise machines that provide a low, continuous noise can offer the same effect.

For the many tinnitus sufferers with hearing loss, the ambient sounds picked up by a hearing aid can reduce or even eliminate tinnitus of medium or low pitch. A newer device that has been quite successful is the tinnitus masker, which is worn like a hearing aid and emits a steady, monotonous noise like wind in trees or the hum of an electric fan—a sound that quickly becomes familiar and can be easily ignored. One benefit of such a device is psychological: one of the most disturbing aspects of tinnitus is your lack of control over the noise, and a masker gives you back that sense of control.

Masking devices must be approved by the Food and Drug Administration (FDA) because of the potential risk they pose if they are too loud. They are sometimes combined with hearing aids.

• **Cut back on—or avoid—caffeine, alcohol, and nicotine.** These substances can all make tinnitus worse by constricting blood vessels.

• **Reduce stress.** Since stressful situations often seem to aggravate tinnitus—and tinnitus in turn is stressful—almost any type of relaxation technique may help you cope. Some tinnitus sufferers have reported that biofeedback helped them temporarily. Claims have also been made for hypnosis and acupuncture.

• **Join a self-help group.** There are local groups throughout the United States that can offer sup-

port along with information about new techniques and treatments. Check the phone book or contact the American Tinnitus Association (see page 549).

Prevention

• **Avoid loud noise.** This is one of the only preventive steps you can take. Use earplugs when necessary, and make sure that your work environment meets the federal guidelines for noise limits, which employers must follow.

When To Call Your Doctor

If you hear persistent ringing or other noises, you should see your doctor, who will likely refer you to an otologist (ear specialist) or an otolaryngologist (ear, nose, and throat specialist). The specialist can determine if the problem is due primarily to an ear condition or to another medical condition. For instance, if the underlying cause is otosclerosis (a fusing of minute bones in the ear), surgery may help relieve tinnitus. If a middle ear infection is involved, it may be treated with antibiotics.

What Your Doctor Will Do

Your hearing will be evaluated, and the degree of tinnitus will be measured using a technique called loudness matching, in which you compare the noises you hear to external sounds. A complete medical and dental history will also be taken to help determine if the tinnitus is caused by other health problems.

For More Information

• American Academy of Otolaryngology-Head and Neck Surgery
• American Tinnitus Association

TMD

Symptoms

- Sore jaw muscles, difficulty chewing, and pain that spreads to the facial and neck muscles and persists around the clock; in some cases difficulty speaking or singing.
- Painful clicking, popping, or grating sounds in the jaw joint when opening or closing the mouth.
- Headaches, toothaches, and earaches may also be part of the syndrome.

What Is It?

The temporomandibular joint connects the lower jaw—the mandible—to the temporal bone at the side of the head. You can feel the joint move when you place your fingers just in front of your ears and open your mouth. Pain associated with the temporomandibular joint was formerly called temporomandibular joint (TMJ) syndrome and temporomandibular joint dysfunction, but has been renamed temporomandibular disorders (TMD). The new name, it was hoped, would more accurately reflect the complexity of the disorder. All the terms refer to a grinding or clicking sound, plus pain or discomfort, when you open your mouth—a feeling that your jaw has come unhinged.

In most people TMD is not serious, but it can persist painfully. For unknown reasons 90 percent of TMD sufferers are women.

What Causes It?

What causes TMD has been a matter of dispute—emotional stress is often cited—but there is probably no single cause. The bones, ligaments, and muscles of the jaw hinge are a complicated mechanism, and many factors can adversely affect the joint, particularly in combination.

- Teeth grinding (bruxism) and clenching can cause muscle spasm, or be caused by it—and muscle spasm, in turn, produces still more spasm. Many experts think this (and the emotional stress that sometimes leads to teeth clenching and grinding) is at the root of most TMD cases.
- Malocclusion (teeth that don't fit together properly) can throw the jaw out of line.
- Internal derangement of the jaw or other orthopedic problems of the joint (such as arthritis, degeneration of the bone, injury, or developmental disorders) can play a role.
- Postural problems, particularly thrusting the chin forward, can strain the neck muscles and those of the jaw. Beware also of gripping a phone between your shoulder and cheek during a long conversation, or of carrying a heavy shoulder bag for long periods on the same shoulder. Strained neck and shoulder muscles can affect the muscles in your jaw.
- A blow to the jaw can result in TMD, as can whiplash.
- Chewing gum or too many chewy foods (bagels, beef, candies, or dried fruits) can promote or aggravate TMD.

What If You Do Nothing?

For most people, the discomfort from TMD is occasional and temporary; the pain will eventually go away with little or no treatment. However, many people who develop symptoms of TMD consult a physician or dentist to rule out other conditions.

Home Remedies

The first line of treatment for TMD is simple self-care. For nearly everyone, the following measures will cure or control TMD.

- **Try a soft diet.** Going on a soft diet for a few

472

days can help. Good food choices include cereals, soups, and pastas. Also, chew more slowly and eat smaller bites. Avoid steak and other hard-to-chew foods.

• **Use pain relievers.** Aspirin, ibuprofen, or acetaminophen can reduce pain and muscle spasm. Cold or hot compresses to the jaw may also help. Experiment to see which is best for you, or apply ice and then moist heat to the jaw.

• **Rest your jaw as much as you can.** If you chew gum, stop. Excessive chewing will only exacerbate or prolong the problem. Also, squelch cavernous yawns (hold your chin in place with your fingers).

• **Improve your posture.** Correct any poor postural habits that may be contributing to your problem. Try gentle exercises to relax your neck muscles: roll your head in circles, or stretch your chin toward each shoulder in turn and hold for a few seconds. You may need the help of a physical therapist or another practitioner with experience in body mechanics.

• **Relieve stress.** If you believe that emotional problems are contributing to your TMD, try to pinpoint the source of stress or unhappiness and do what you can to alleviate it. Some type of psychological counseling may be worthwhile.

Prevention

No established measures can prevent TMD, but minimizing or avoiding the factors noted under What Causes It? may reduce the risk of getting the condition.

When To Call Your Doctor

Contact your physician or dentist if TMD symptoms interfere with everyday activities. Not all jaw and facial pain is caused by TMD, so other conditions must be ruled out.

What Your Doctor Will Do

Since there are no precise causes and because TMD symptoms are not clear, diagnosing this disorder is often difficult. Currently no standard test is widely accepted for identifying TMD. Your doctor may refer you to a dentist, who will perform a complete oral examination that includes feeling the jaw joints and listening for clicking, popping, and grating sounds.

If the TMD is related to your bite, your dentist may be able to correct your bite simply by grinding down a few tooth surfaces. Before submitting to this or any other procedure, remember that in most cases the discomfort of TMD eventually goes away. Also, be sure to get a reliable second opinion before agreeing to this irreversible treatment. Bite plates or splints, fitted over the biting surface of your teeth, can also help stabilize the bite and eliminate nocturnal tooth grinding.

Another option is to see a physical therapist trained in muscle relaxation techniques for the jaw and neck, which can be very helpful. Ask your doctor for a referral.

Surgical techniques exist for extreme cases, but consider surgery only as a last resort. At least one surgical technique that was touted as "state of the art" some years ago actually caused bone damage. As with any surgery, get a second opinion.

For More Information
• American Dental Association
• American Pain Foundation
• American Psychological Association

Toenail Fungus

Symptoms

- Dry, thickened, or discolored nail that turns white or yellow.
- Scaliness on the skin surrounding the nail.
- Pain while standing, walking, or running, which may be accompanied by blistering or swelling around the nail.
- Nail that has detached from the nail bed (rare).

What Is It?

A nail fungal infection, which is known medically as onychomycosis (on-i-ko-mi-KO-sis), seems to arrive unannounced. At first you may only notice a small white or yellow spot on your nail. Then, months later, your whole nail may be consumed by the fungi. Soon, the nail may turn yellow, gray, black, or brown. As the infection advances, the nail becomes brittle and can crack, sometimes breaking away totally from the nail bed.

Such infections are quite common, affecting between 10 to 12 million Americans of all ages, genders, and races. They primarily affect toenails, but sometimes fingernails, though rarely both at the same time. In most cases the infections are a nuisance that may cause embarrassment over the unsightly nails. In a few cases the infection is severe enough that walking can be difficult.

What Causes It?

Fungal molds called dermatophytes are the cause of fungal nail infections. (Other types of dermatophytes are responsible for athlete's foot and jock itch.) But how nail infections are transmitted isn't well understood. They are more common in people who have infections of the skin adjoining the nail. While warm, moist environments such as gym locker rooms or shower stalls can encourage the spread of skin infections, it isn't evident that these lead to nail infections.

Trauma to the nail appears to be a factor. Regular distance runners who inadvertently bump their toenails against the running shoe toe box on downhill runs—thereby damaging the nail in the process—are prone to the infection. In addition, people who remain on their feet for long periods of time while wearing tight-fitting shoes, such as waiters, policemen, and construction workers, are also more inclined to develop the ailment. And people with compromised immune systems—from HIV infection and chemotherapy—may be more susceptible.

Nail infections also tend to occur more frequently with increasing age.

What If You Do Nothing?

Fungal nail infections are generally harmless, so treatment isn't necessary unless you are bothered by pain or upset by the appearance of the nails. Because prescription medications can be expensive and may have side effects, many people choose to live with the condition.

Home Remedies

Over-the counter antifungal medications do not work (the Food and Drug Administration no longer allows them to claim effectiveness), and topical home remedies—which include tea tree oil, vinegar, Campho-Phenique (containing camphor and phenol), saline solution, and chlorine bleach—haven't been shown to work. Bleach can actually be harmful.

The best way to successfully treat a fungal nail infection is with prescription medications (see When To Call Your Doctor). The preventive suggestions that follow may help keep you from developing the infection in the first place.

Prevention

- **Keep your nails clipped.** Cut the nails straight and make sure they do not extend beyond the tips of your toes (or your fingers). (If you have one or more infected nails, use a separate pair of clippers for infected nails and another for healthy nails. If you have diabetes, consult your physician before cutting your toenails.)
- **Disinfect.** After each use, disinfect any manicure and pedicure tools by wiping them with cotton balls saturated with alcohol. Let them air dry for 60 to 90 minutes before using them again.
- **Be careful at the nail salon.** Make sure the salon has an autoclave (a special heating device for disinfecting instruments) and that it is used after each treatment.
- **Keep clean and dry.** Wash your hands and feet daily with soap and water and dry them well. Be sure to dry between your toes.
- **Use an antifungal foot powder.** Avoid cornstarch because it encourages fungal growth.
- **Make sure your footwear breathes.** Choose leather shoes with plenty of toe room. Have more than one pair and alternate your shoes to make sure they air out at least 24 hours before they are worn again. Also, avoid socks made from nylon or polyester because they don't absorb perspiration as well as cotton or wool. In warm weather, wearing sandals may help prevent infections.

When To Call Your Doctor

Contact your physician if the infection is painful and makes it difficult for you to stand or walk, or if you want to improve the appearance of your nails through treatment.

If you have diabetes, talk to your doctor before trying any kind of foot treatment.

What Your Doctor Will Do

Your doctor will take scrapings from under the nail to discover what type of infection is present. Once the condition is diagnosed, your doctor may prescribe one of the newer oral antifungal medication agents, itraconazole (Sporanox) or terbinafine (Lamisil). Cure rates range from 25 to 80 percent. These drugs occasionally cause skin rash, headache, and gastrointestinal symptoms, but side effects are less likely to occur than they do with earlier oral drugs. The new drugs may interact with other medications, such as some antihistamines and cholesterol-lowering "statin" drugs—so make sure your doctor is aware of any other medications you are taking.

Treatment is not cheap, but it has become less expensive. The usual three- to four-month course costs several hundred dollars, plus the price of blood tests to monitor for liver disease (a very rare complication). But new "pulsed" dosing for itraconazole—you take it daily for one week, then stop for three weeks—reduces the cost by up to 75 percent. (Even with treatment, however, there is a high rate of recurrence—50 percent or more.)

Another option is an FDA-approved topical medication, ciclopirox, sold under the name Penlac Nail Lacquer. You apply it daily to the affected nail and adjacent skin for up to 48 weeks and trim the nail weekly. It may cause skin irritation, but is otherwise safe; it costs less than the oral drugs.

In rare cases, if the infection is extremely painful, your physician may recommend removing the nail (though this alone will not resolve the infection).

For More Information

- American Academy of Dermatology

Traveler's Diarrhea

Symptoms

- Diarrhea, as much as 3 to 10 times a day, often in combination with vomiting, bloating, gas, and abdominal cramps.
- Fever and bloody stools (in severe cases).
- Dehydration (occasionally—and usually not severe).

What Is It?

Traveler's diarrhea, long known as "Montezuma's revenge" among other names, is something of a misnomer. Though it has been defined in the pages of the *New England Journal of Medicine* as diarrhea that occurs when a person living in an industrialized country travels to developing or semitropical regions (Latin America, Africa, Middle East, Asia), some people get traveler's diarrhea when entering the United States or other industrialized nations. Any change of locale and eating habits can make you more vulnerable to it.

Nevertheless, traveler's diarrhea is still more common among travelers from low-risk to high-risk areas—40 to 60 percent of Americans traveling to developing countries are laid low with diarrhea. Wherever you contract it, the illness usually appears within four to six days after arrival, with sudden attacks of loose watery stools often accompanied by abdominal cramps and nausea.

What Causes It?

Up to 80 percent of traveler's diarrhea cases are triggered by bacteria, including the ubiquitous *E. coli* found in fecal matter as well as other bacteria that are transmitted via contaminated food or water. Less common agents are viruses and parasites such as *Giardia lamblia*. Often it's impossible to identify the exact culprit.

What If You Do Nothing?

Traveler's diarrhea is not life-threatening in otherwise healthy people. If you drink plenty of water, you may be uncomfortable, but the condition will clear up on its own—often within two to five days, though in some cases mild symptoms may last for weeks. However, if a parasite such as *Giardia lamblia* is to blame, giardiasis, an infection of the small bowel, may develop (see page 285). Symptoms may persist for four weeks or more if antibiotics are not taken.

Home Remedies

• **Replace lost fluids.** Your goal is to prevent dehydration, which occurs often with diarrhea because the body loses more fluids and salts than it takes in. The most important self-care measure is to rehydrate yourself as soon as you can keep down fluids. Bottled water, flat soft drinks, sports drinks, or tea will help. You can also make your own rehydration drink by adding four teaspoons of sugar and a pinch of salt (a half teaspoon) to a quart of bottled water.

Avoid coffee and alcohol, which can increase dehydration.

For a child who becomes sick, try sweetening water with honey, and add a pinch of salt. Children under age two should drink a commercial rehydration solution, which contains the correct amounts of fluid, salts, and carbohydrates to prevent dehydration.

• **Eat.** If you have no diarrhea after 12 hours, salted crackers are a good way to begin eating again, and the salt helps restore fluid balance. Other foods to consider include dry toast, bread, and clear soup. When the number of stools decreases and your stools have shape, you can add rice, baked potatoes, clear soup, poultry, applesauce, and bananas—or any food, really, that appeals to you, as long as you observe the precautions noted below.

• **Self-treat with medication, if necessary.** If you are otherwise healthy, it's generally best if you give your body a chance to eliminate the diarrhea-causing organism. However, if you are in a situation where diarrhea is inconvenient, you can decrease symptoms with over-the-counter medications.

Loperamide (such as Imodium) is an antimotility drug that works against loose stools, reducing both the passage of stool and the duration of diarrhea by up to 80 percent. Bismuth subsalicylate (Pepto-Bismol, which is also sold in generic forms) reduces the number of loose stools by about 60 percent, but people who are aspirin-sensitive or take aspirin for other reasons, as well as children under the age of 12, should not use bismuth subsalicylate.

Moreover, you should not take any of these drugs if you have high fever and bloody stools; these two symptoms can be signs of a serious infection that requires immediate medical attention, and the medications may make the condition worse.

Prevention

When traveling in developing countries, follow these recommendations.

• **Find out about health precautions.** The Centers for Disease Control and Prevention (CDC) can supply you with information about health risks in different countries. It's also a good idea to get a doctor's advice before you go if you are traveling to developing countries and are pregnant or nursing, are accompanied by infants or small children, or have chronic health problems. Do so as well if you're taking a critically important business trip that would be compromised if you developed traveler's diarrhea.

What To Take Along

Here is a checklist of items for prevention and treatment of traveler's diarrhea:
• An electric immersion coil to boil water if bottled water is unavailable or unsafe. You'll need a conversion plug as well.
• Purifying tablets to add to tap water if you can't boil it and have no alternative.
• Alcohol wipes for hand-washing (when clean water isn't available).
• Antidiarrhea medication—something containing loperamide (Imodium, for example) or diphenoxylate (Lomotil). Pepto Bismal (bismuth salicylate) and its generics are good, too. (Be sure not to dose yourself if you have a high fever or bloody stools—seek medical help.)
• Antibiotics and directions for their use.

• **As a precaution, take diarrhea medications with you.** If you're traveling in out-of-the-way places, beyond the reach of a druggist, it's advisable to take a diarrhea treatment along. If you have any health concerns, consult with your doctor, who can recommend an over-the-counter product or a prescription medication such as Lomotil.

• **Once you've arrived, drink only bottled or canned beverages.** Be sure you're the one who breaks the seal. Or stick to hot drinks like tea or coffee made with boiling water. Bottled wine and beer are safe. In some areas locally bottled water and soft drinks may not be safe. If in doubt, stick to tea and coffee.

• **Never use tap water.** Use bottled or boiled water instead, even for brushing your teeth. Don't swallow water in the shower.

• **Pass up all ice cubes.** The cubes may have been made with contaminated water, and freezing does not kill most microbes.

• **Treat your own water.** If necessary, take along a small electric immersion coil heater and boil your own water. Or add to it a purifying tablet such as Halazone—two and a half tablets per quart for at least 30 minutes.

• **Don't eat anything raw—particularly not salad greens.** Raw fruit is okay only if it can be peeled and if you do the peeling. Be certain not to wash the fruit in tap water. Avoid rare meats, undercooked eggs, and all dairy products, since it's hard to be sure they've been pasteurized.

• **Don't buy food from street vendors.** Even if it's served hot, it still may be contaminated.

• **Wash your hands carefully.** To prevent the spread of diarrhea and eliminate all chances of reinfection, be sure to wash your hands with soap and water after using the bathroom and before eating. Disinfecting alcohol wipes are useful when you have no clean water to wash in.

• **Don't rely on drugs.** It's certainly a good idea to carry antibiotics with you when you travel, along with instructions on how to use them should the need arise. But some travelers take antibiotics before they leave home in order to ward off traveler's diarrhea. Using antibiotics or any other medication prophylactically is generally not recommended. Some medications can produce severe side effects. In addition, taking them can give a false sense of security to travelers who might otherwise be cautious in their choice of food and drink.

People with health problems, however, should check with their doctors before they travel, since some of them will benefit from taking medications prophylactically.

When To Call Your Doctor

The condition is uncomfortable but seldom life-threatening. However, contact a physician if you have diarrhea that lasts more than four days without improvement, a fever of 101°F or higher that lasts more than 24 hours, or if blood is in your stool.

A doctor also should be contacted immediately if severe diarrhea occurs in infants, elderly people, or people with heart disease.

What Your Doctor Will Do

A history will be taken, including how much diarrhea has occurred, whether it is accompanied by blood, mucus, or pus, and if it occurs in combination with nausea, vomiting, or a high fever. The exact cause of the diarrhea may be difficult to determine, but a stool sample can be taken to detect the organism producing the problem.

If diarrhea is frequent and cramps are painful, your doctor may prescribe medications to relieve symptoms, especially if you have serious heart disease or a weakened immune system. Treatment will stop the diarrhea in about a day, compared to two to four days without medication. However, since antidiarrheal medication can delay the elimination of the organism from the digestive tract, it may not be recommended for healthy individuals.

For More Information

• Centers for Disease Control and Prevention
• National Digestive Diseases Information Clearinghouse

Ulcers

Symptoms

- Pain is the distinguishing stomach ulcer characteristic. In most instances there is a burning or gnawing feeling in the upper abdomen, sometimes below the breastbone, which may resemble heartburn. The pain is usually mild to moderate in severity and can last from 30 minutes to several hours.
- Often the pain occurs between meals and may be relieved by eating or by taking antacids, though in some people with gastric ulcer, eating food aggravates the pain. The pain may also awaken you at night or early in the morning. It may come and go for no apparent reason; many people experience multiple-week cycles of pain and freedom from pain.
- Less common symptoms include nausea, vomiting, and loss of appetite and weight.
- 10 to 20 percent of people with ulcers have no symptoms.

What Is It?

A peptic ulcer is a craterlike sore in the stomach or duodenal lining. It's called a gastric ulcer when it occurs in the stomach, and a duodenal ulcer when it occurs in the first 12 inches of the small intestine. Symptoms of the two are similar. (Peptic refers to pepsin, an enzyme in the area of the digestive system where ulcers develop.)

Duodenal ulcers are about three times more common than gastric ulcers and are most likely to affect men. Gastric ulcers are more common in people between the ages of 60 and 70, perhaps because of heavy use of aspirin, ibuprofen, or other nonsteroidal anti-inflammatory drugs (NSAIDs) for managing pain, especially from arthritis. A third type, the esophageal ulcer, is relatively rare and is generally caused by alcohol abuse and/or reflux esophagitis resulting from heartburn.

Up to 10 percent of Americans will have an ulcer at some point in their lives. Although most ulcers occur in people over 30, children may get them as well. Even after pain has subsided and an ulcer has healed, it's common for it to recur. Fortunately, the high rate of ulcer recurrence has been significantly reduced since the introduction of short-term drug regimens that combat the bacterial organism involved in causing most ulcers.

What Causes It?

Many factors contribute to ulcers. For years a stressful lifestyle and a high-fat or spicy diet were blamed for ulcers. Then in 1982 two Australian researchers discovered that a bacterium called *Helicobacter pylori (H. pylori)* was present in more than 90 percent of duodenal ulcers and more than 73 percent of gastric ulcers. Scientists theorize that the *H. pylori* organism weakens the stomach's protective mucous membrane, so that even small amounts of stomach acid can cause new ulcers or delay the healing of existing ones.

Experts are cautious about saying that the bacteria cause ulcers. Other factors, such as heredity and smoking, seem to be involved, and not everybody who is infected with *H. pylori* develops ulcers. Also, some people get ulcers apparently without being infected—as, for example, those who take large doses of NSAIDs over long periods.

It's not known how the bacterial infection spreads, but researchers think it's transmitted orally. Young children and adolescents, when they carry the bacteria, may be more infectious than adults. According to researchers, it's unlikely that one adult can transmit the bacteria to another. But infected children may transmit it to adults and other children.

Once an ulcer develops, several secondary factors may aggravate it. People who often take large doses of NSAIDs are at risk for ulcers, because these drugs may damage the stomach lining, and then digestive acid makes the lesion worse and interferes with healing.

Cigarette smoking is another factor that promotes ulcers, though it's not clear how. Smoking definitely slows an ulcer's healing. Food has also been blamed—coffee, tea, cola beverages, and spicy foods, as well as alcohol. But no food has ever been shown to promote ulcers.

Emotional stress, chronic anxiety, and even an "ulcer-prone personality" have all been blamed, too. But calm, happy people as well as tense unhappy ones get ulcers. There is no "ulcer personality."

What If You Do Nothing?

Ulcers are not contagious, nor do they cause cancer, but they are usually painful. Rarely are ulcers life-threatening, but ulcers that go untreated can sometimes progress and lead to serious complications such as bleeding. In severe cases an ulcer eats a hole in the wall of the stomach or duodenum, and bacteria can spill through this perforation into the abdominal cavity, or peritoneum. This causes peritonitis, an inflammation of the abdominal cavity and wall that usually requires surgery.

Therefore, you should always see a doctor if you suspect you have an ulcer.

Home Remedies

Ulcer symptoms should be evaluated by a doctor. Prescription medications are the most effective form of treatment.

Prevention

The following measures can help you avoid ulcers, or at least reduce the risk of them.

• **Be careful with NSAIDs.** If you must take aspirin, ibuprofen, or other NSAIDs regularly, take the smallest possible dose and always take it with food. If you are prone to ulcers and you must take NSAIDs, your doctor may recommend you take your NSAID with one of several medications that may help prevent the recurrence of NSAID-induced ulcers. Or you may be advised to try one of the newer NSAIDs called COX-2 inhibitors, which carry a lower risk of NSAID-related stomach problems.

• **Eat sensibly.** A diet rich in fiber is recommended because it is thought to reduce the risk of developing a duodenal ulcer by enhancing the development of mucin, which protects the intestinal lining.

• **Quit smoking, if you smoke.** The nicotine in cigarettes may prevent the pancreas from secreting enzymes that protect the intestinal lining. Smoking also slows the healing of existing ulcers and is a cause of ulcer recurrence.

• **Be careful of what you eat.** Though no food is known to cause ulcers, it won't hurt to avoid foods that seem to give you indigestion or cause pain. Spicy foods as well as those that have a high fat content are common problems.

• **Drink in moderation.** If you drink alcohol, drink moderately and never on an empty stomach. Although alcohol consumption and ulcers are not directly linked, ulcers are common in people who have cirrhosis of the liver, an ailment that is associated with excessive alcohol consumption.

• **Reduce stress in your life.** Stress has not been proven to be a cause of ulcers, but it can irritate existing ones.

When To Call Your Doctor

Call your doctor if you develop symptoms of a peptic ulcer.

Contact your physician or a hospital immediately if you vomit blood, if you feel faint or cold, or if you do faint; these are signs of potentially serious blood loss. Also contact your physician if your stools are black, tarry, or bloody, which are signs of internal bleeding.

Call for advice if you develop ulcer symptoms combined with back pain; the ulcer may have perforated into your pancreas. Also contact your physician if you've been diagnosed with an ulcer and now have a pallid complexion and begin to feel fatigued; these are signs of anemia.

What Your Doctor Will Do

A careful history will be taken and other medical conditions will be eliminated as primary causes of your problem. Diagnosing and treating an ulcer can be complex, and your doctor may refer you to a gastrointestinal specialist. The definitive method of determining that someone has an ulcer, and that the cause is *H. pylori,* is to perform an endoscopy, which involves inserting a tube-like instrument down the throat into the stomach and duodenum. This allows the doctor to view tissue and also biopsy samples to test for the presence of *H. pylori* and/or other problems. A barium swallow, visible on an x-ray, is a less precise but noninvasive tool that can detect an ulcer.

Since both tests are expensive, an otherwise healthy person who has an initial bout of pain suggesting an ulcer may first be treated with medication to see if symptoms resolve. If symptoms persist, worsen, or recur, then further evaluation is in order. In addition to endoscopy and barium x-ray, there are less expensive noninvasive tests, including a blood test and an in-office breath test, that can be used in initially detecting *H. pylori* and to monitor the effects of treatment.

For most cases of peptic ulcer, drug therapy will be recommended. If *H. pylori.* is present, your doctor may prescribe a course of antibiotics, usually in combination with acid-suppressing heartburn medications. Treatment with antibiotics greatly reduces the chance of an ulcer recurring. (Never take antibiotics just because you have gastric symptoms, however, unless you're sure you have an ulcer.)

Consult your doctor before using any heartburn medication on your own to treat ulcer symptoms. Some of these medications—which include H2-blockers such as Pepcid, Tagamet, and Zantac—are available in over-the-counter formulations, but the OTC versions are only half the strength of the prescription drugs and may be ineffective for ulcers.

Antacids may also help, but they can interfere with the actions of other drugs if both types are taken in close succession—another reason to see your doctor before taking medication. Antacids and H2-blockers can also help heal ulcers in which *H. pylori* isn't a factor, such as NSAID-induced ulcers.

If you have a severe ulcer that is bleeding or if treatment with medication is unsuccessful, surgery may be recommended.

For More Information
- American Gastroenterological Association
- National Digestive Diseases Information Clearinghouse

481

Urinary Incontinence

Symptoms

- Sudden loss of urine, often triggered by activity that increases abdominal pressure (laughing, sneezing, exercise), or in some cases a change in position.
- Dribbling of urine.
- Strong, imminent urge to urinate.

What Is It?

Urinary incontinence is the involuntary loss of urine. This condition afflicts 15 to 30 percent of older people who live at home, and about half of those in long-term institutional care, such as nursing homes. Younger people, too, can be affected by incontinence, especially women who have had children, because childbirth may weaken pelvic floor muscles that support the bladder. Because of anatomical differences, incontinence is twice as prevalent in women as in men. In all, an estimated 13 million Americans are incontinent.

Despite its prevalence, however, urinary incontinence is not normal at any age, and is not an inevitable consequence of getting older. This condition is very treatable and often curable through behavioral techniques and in some cases surgery.

Some cases of incontinence are temporary, caused by urinary tract infections, constipation, or medications. More commonly, however, incontinence is a persistent, or chronic, condition. There are four main forms of persistent incontinence, and in many patients more than one of these patterns occur simultaneously.

• **Stress incontinence.** More common in women than in men, stress incontinence results from weak pelvic muscles or problems with the urethra. Abdominal contractions that occur when you sneeze, cough, laugh, or lift something increase pressure on the bladder. The muscles of the pelvic floor are not strong enough to override this increase in pressure and so urine escapes, usually a few drops, but sometimes a larger amount. This is the most common type of incontinence.

• **Urge incontinence.** Also called detrusor instability (detrusor is the anatomical term for part of the bladder muscle), urge incontinence is the result of an overactive bladder. The bladder goes into spasm, triggering a sudden strong urge to void and an almost immediate release of a large amount of urine.

• **Overflow incontinence.** In this type of incontinence, the bladder fills until it becomes overdistended, but there is no signal to urinate and the detrusor muscle may not contract. Eventually, however, the bladder gets so full that it overflows.

• **Functional incontinence.** This term is used to describe incontinence that occurs as the result of some degenerative conditions or illnesses, such as severe arthritis, or mental disorders that restrict movement or otherwise make it difficult for a person to reach a bathroom.

What Causes It?

Incontinence that begins suddenly (which is called transient incontinence) usually has very specific causes, including genitourinary infections (such as urinary tract infections and vaginitis) and various medications (especially diuretics, sleeping pills, and tranquilizers).

With persistent incontinence, the cause is typically linked to muscles and nerves involved in urination—a process that we take for granted, yet it is a complex set of actions and reactions coordinated by the central nervous system. Urine produced by the kidneys collects in the bladder, which is able to contract and expand to accommodate the urine. A ring-like muscle called a sphincter prevents urine from leaving the bladder until a sufficient amount accumulates, and muscles of the pelvic floor help support the bladder and urethra (the tube through which urine passes out of the body). Once the bladder reaches a certain level of fullness, it sends a message to the spinal cord, which in turn relaxes the sphincter and signals the muscles in the bladder to contract to force urine through the urethra.

During childhood, we learn to identify and control this reflex by tightening the muscles of the pelvic floor until a toilet is reached. But disruption in the process can cause incontinence.

Stress incontinence often affects women because childbirth weakens the muscles of the pelvic floor. In addition, the drop in estrogen levels that occurs with menopause contributes to the thinning of pelvic muscles and other tissues in the vaginal area and loss of tone of the urethra. In men, prostate or bladder surgery can contribute to stress incontinence.

Overflow incontinence is typically brought about by a physical blockage of urine flow, as can occur in men with prostate problems. It may also be caused by the nerve damage that sometimes results from diabetes, or by certain medications, such as diuretics, antidepressants, sleeping pills, and high blood pressure drugs.

Urge incontinence may be caused by a neurological imbalance—which may be the result of a stroke, for example—but often this condition has no known cause.

What If You Do Nothing?

In most cases, ignoring symptoms of incontinence just makes the problem worse and can also lead to complications. For example, what begins as occasional stress incontinence when sneezing may become more frequent and associated with other activities as the pelvic floor muscles weaken further over time. Being damp all the time, even if absorbable pads are used, can cause skin irritation and lead to sores. There is also an increased risk of developing a urinary tract infection because bacteria breed more effectively in a moist environment. Residual urine that remains in the bladder in the case of overflow incontinence may lead to bladder infections.

There are also psychological consequences of incontinence, including a loss of self-esteem and depression. And people who are incontinent may become socially isolated because they are embarrassed about odor or afraid of not being close to a toilet.

Home Remedies

In many cases, home remedies can eliminate or significantly improve incontinence.

- **Lose weight if overweight.** Excess weight increases intra-abdominal pressure, which can contribute to stress incontinence.
- **Women should wear a tampon while exercising.** Some women experience mild stress incontinence when they exercise. If you have this problem, a tampon inserted into the vagina can compress the urethra and help prevent urine leakage. Remove the tampon after the workout.
- **Strengthen pelvic muscles.** Specialized exercises called Kegel exercises are easy to learn and can be performed anywhere (see page 484). They are helpful for stress and urge incontinence.
- **Cross your legs to prevent accidents.** If you know you leak urine when you sneeze or cough, crossing your legs or squeezing your pelvic muscles may stop it from happening.
- **Practice bladder training.** This strategy helps you regain control of the urinary process. It involves a commitment of time and effort, but is very effective.

• **Start by going to the toilet every two hours.** When you're awake, use the bathroom on this schedule, whether you have to go or not. Maintain the schedule even when you are not at home.

• **Every other day, extend the interval between bathroom visits by 30 minutes.** Aim to achieve four-hour intervals.

• **If you have an urge to urinate in between scheduled bathroom visits, relax.** Do a Kegel contraction to deal with the urge. After the urge has passed, move slowly to a bathroom.

• **Be careful of drinking too much fluid.** Although you need to consume enough water to stay healthy, you may want to cut back on the extra can of soda or fruit juice—especially before bedtime or when you are away from home without ready access to a bathroom.

• **Avoid or minimize caffeine intake.** Caffeine is a natural diuretic—that is, a chemical that clears fluid from the body through increased urine output. Too much coffee, tea, or cola can stimulate frequent urination.

Prevention

• **Get regular exercise.** Physical exercise can help prevent weight gain and also helps keep all of the muscles in the body well-toned.

• **Perform Kegel exercises.** Strengthening the pelvic muscles can help prevent as well as cure incontinence.

• **Get medical attention for any bladder or urinary tract problem.** Untreated bladder or urinary tract infections may lead to incontinence.

• **Consider hormone replacement therapy (HRT).** Treatment with female hormones—either estrogen or a combination of estrogen and progestin—after menopause has a number of benefits, including improving the tone of the pelvic muscles, which in turn can help ease or

---

Strengthening Your Pelvic Muscles

▼

Kegel exercises are highly effective at strengthening the pelvic muscles that support the bladder. They can be used to treat both stress and urge urinary incontinence, and may help prevent stress incontinence. The exercises are easy to do and can be performed anywhere. Most people see improvement in 8 to 12 weeks.

1. The first step is to locate the proper muscles. When you are urinating, tighten up and try to stop the flow. If you cannot do this, try tightening your anal sphincter. Because of its proximity to the bladder sphincter, this helps identify the muscle necessary for maintaining continence.

2. Contract and relax these muscles three times a day, performing 15 to 20 squeezes each time. Your goal should be to hold each contraction for 10 seconds.

3. Practice Kegels during different activities—sitting, lying down, standing, walking.

4. Occasionally monitor your progress by stopping and starting the flow of urine. Do not regularly practice Kegels while urinating or when you bladder is full, however, since this may actually weaken the muscles.

---

eliminate incontinence. (For more information about HRT, see page 382.)

When To Call Your Doctor

If you experience stress incontinence, you may be able to cure the problem by doing Kegel exercises. However, most people who develop signs of incontinence, and especially older people, should see a doctor for an evaluation. Many people are ashamed to tell their doctor that they are incontinent, but there is much your doctor can do to help alleviate the problem.

Note: If you suspect that a medication you are taking is contributing to the problem, don't stop taking it until you consult your doctor.

What Your Doctor Will Do

The doctor will take a detailed medical history, asking questions about the frequency of urination, the approximate volume of urine, and how urgently you feel the need to urinate. (You may be asked to keep a detailed diary recording this information for a few days to provide a better idea of the nature of the problem.) In addition, you should report any medications you take.

A physical exam will check for rectal, genital, and abdominal abnormalities that may contribute to the problem. Laboratory tests, such as urinalysis and culture, are done to check for urinary tract infections or other diseases. The doctor may also order a special test to determine if your bladder is truly emptying after you urinate.

If no underlying cause, such as an enlarged prostate, is found, treatment generally begins with the self-help measures outlined above because they are highly effective and safe. If this regimen does not cure incontinence, the doctor may prescribe medications that can relax an overactive bladder or tighten the urinary sphincter. There are also medications for men who experience overflow incontinence caused by an enlarged prostate. For stress incontinence, doctors sometimes prescribe weighted vaginal cones designed to increase the effectiveness of Kegel exercises.

Several FDA-approved devices may be appropriate for some women with stress incontinence, including women who experience exercise incontinence. So-called barrier devices such as the Reliance Urinary Control Insert and the FemSoft Insert are placed in the urethra to block urine flow; the insert must be removed before urinating and cannot be reused. An intravaginal device, the Introl Bladder Neck Support Prosthesis, is positioned so that it restores the bladder to its normal anatomical position; it can be left in during urination, but must be removed periodically for cleaning. These devices are available only by prescription and require careful fitting by a physician.

Collagen implants and a nerve stimulation implant (which sends impulses to nerves that help control bladder contractions) are other recent nonsurgical options for treating incontinence.

Surgery may be considered to correct anatomical problems causing incontinence. Clinical guidelines from the American Urological Association (AUA) state that surgery may even be considered as an initial treatment for stress incontinence in women. The types of surgery with the best long-term outcomes are retropubic suspension and sling procedures. A third procedure called transvaginal suspension is not as effective over the long term, but it has a lower rate of complications than the other two and the recovery period is shorter, according to the AUA.

You need to discuss with your doctor which treatment—or combination of treatments—is best suited for you.

For More Information
- American Foundation for Urological Disease
- American Urological Association
- National Association for Continence
- Simon Foundation for Incontinence

Urinary Tract Infection

Symptoms

Not everyone with a urinary tract infection will have symptoms, but most people will experience some of the following.

- Frequent urge to urinate.
- A painful burning feeling in the bladder or urethra during urination.
- Despite an urge to urinate, ability to pass only a small amount of strong-smelling, cloudy, sometimes blood-tinged urine.
- Chills, fever, back pain (pyelonephritis).

What Is It?

A urinary tract infection (UTI) occurs when bacteria multiply in the urethra (the tube through which urine flows from the bladder to the outside of the body), in the bladder itself, or in the kidneys, disrupting normal function and causing swelling and infection.

Infection of the bladder or lower urinary tract is called cystitis. Urethritis is an inflammation of the urethra. Cystitis and urethritis usually occur together. In some cases women with painful urination have an infection of the upper urinary tract, which can be difficult to distinguish from a lower urinary tract infection. Upper urinary tract infections can spread into the kidney—a condition called pyelonephritis, which may be accompanied by back pain, chills, fever, nausea, and/or vomiting.

Many women suffer from frequent UTIs, with nearly 20 percent of women who have one UTI also having a second. UTIs are the second most common cause of physician visits each year, after respiratory infections such as pneumonia and bronchitis; approximately eight million women go to their doctors annually with UTI complaints.

Although men can develop UTIs, they are rarer, with infection typically associated with a urinary stone or an enlarged prostate. Women are more susceptible than men to UTIs because the urethral opening in women is close to the anus, where bacteria thrive, and because the female urethra is much shorter than a man's, allowing bacteria quicker access to the bladder.

What Causes It?

Ordinarily, the flow of urine helps wash away bacteria often present in the urethra and bladder. In men, the prostate gland produces secretions that slow bacterial growth. In both sexes, immune defenses also prevent infection. Despite these safeguards, however, infections still occur.

Most UTIs in women are caused by by the *E. coli* bacteria, which live in the colon and can be easily spread from the rectum to the urethra. Often this occurs during sexual intercourse, which can push bacteria from the anal area up toward the vagina and into the opening of the urethra;

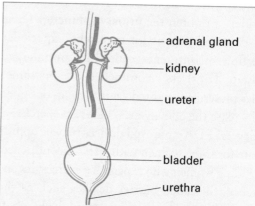

- adrenal gland
- kidney
- ureter
- bladder
- urethra

A woman's urethra is just over an inch long (in contrast to a man's, which is about nine inches). This allows urinary tract infections in women to quickly travel up the urethra into the bladder. If not treated, the infection can move up the ureters into the kidneys, causing more serious problems.

from there they travel into the bladder. Young women who are becoming sexually active for the first time are especially susceptible. Bacteria other than *E. coli* as well as sexually transmitted organisms can also cause infections in both men and women.

Pregnancy also increases the risk of UTIs because as a fetus grows, the bladder becomes compressed and doesn't empty completely, allowing bacteria to reproduce. Diaphragms used for birth control compress the urethra, making infection more likely.

Perimenopausal and postmenopausal women are also susceptible owing to a decrease in estrogen production, which causes tissues in the urinary tract to thin out and become more easily inflamed.

A Home Test That Works

Until recently, testing for a urinary tract infection (UTI) meant a visit to the doctor. But if you're one of the millions prone to recurrent UTIs, there are several home tests that might save you an office visit.

The UTI home testing kit, approved by the FDA and available in drug stores ($6 to $9), consists of six dipsticks and six small plastic urine cups, plus instructions. You test the first morning urine; if results are positive, you can call your nurse practitioner or physician and ask for a prescription. Of course, you may be asked to come in for an exam and further testing, but if you're having a recurrence, the test may save time and money. The test will pick up 80 to 90% of infections.

This is one test where "negative" results are not good news. Painful urination and other common symptoms of UTIs may actually be caused by a sexually transmitted disease. If the test results are negative and your symptoms persist, you should certainly get a medical evaluation.

Some cases of recurring UTIs are due to structural abnormalities that impede the flow of urine, and often correction by surgery is needed to halt the infections.

What If You Do Nothing?

Mild cases of cystitis and urethritis can often clear up without treatment. But if symptoms last longer than two days, you should consult a doctor, since some untreated UTIs may turn into kidney infections, which can be serious and much harder to cure.

Home Remedies

Only women who have had uncomplicated recurring UTIs should consider self-treatment, which will still usually require a supply of antibiotics obtained from a doctor. Before supplying you with antibiotics, your doctor should carry out a thorough evaluation (see What Your Doctor Will Do). The following measures may also help recovery during a bout of cystitis.

- **Use pain relievers.** To alleviate cramps or stomach pain, take over-the-counter pain relievers—NSAIDs (such as aspirin, ibuprofen, and naproxen) or acetaminophen—according to label directions.
- **Try applying heat.** A warm heating pad (on a low setting) or a hot water bottle placed on your lower abdomen may help soothe pain.
- **Drink fluids.** Drink 10 to 14 glasses of water a day to help increase urine flow and flush out the substances causing the problem.
- **Drink cranberry juice.** The juice seems to possess something that keeps bacterial organisms from attaching to the walls of the bladder and urethra, and thereby prevents them from multiplying. Researchers have suggested that cranberry juice might be used as an adjunct to medical treatment—though not as a substitute for it. (Cap-

487

sules containing cranberry extract may help—one small study supports this. However, no one knows what the right dose is, and you can't even be sure the capsules contain what the label indicates.)

Prevention

• **Drink plenty of fluids.** Drink at least eight glasses of liquid a day—enough so that you urinate at least once every four or five hours.

• **Include cranberry juice.** People have been drinking cranberry juice for years to prevent UTIs—and now some research supports this. Studies have shown that it helps keep the bacteria in the urinary tract from settling in. A Harvard study found that women who drank 10 ounces of cranberry juice daily significantly reduced infection rates over a six-month period.

• **Don't delay using the bathroom.** Delayed urination is a major cause of UTIs. Emptying bacteria-laden urine from the bladder helps reduce the bacteria count.

• **Practice bathroom hygiene.** Wipe from front to back to prevent bacteria around the anus from entering the urethra or vagina.

• **Cleanse the genital area before sexual intercourse.** Also, urinate immediately after sexual intercourse.

• **Consider changing your birth control method.** Women who use spermicides containing non-oxynol-9 are often at higher risk for UTIs because it changes the bacterial balance in the vagina, allowing *E. coli* to proliferate. The use of a diaphragm may also promote UTIs. Consider switching to oral contraceptives.

• **Avoid using feminine hygiene sprays and scented douches.** These products can irritate the urinary tract.

• **If you're past menopause, use a water-soluble vaginal lubricant.** Vaginal tissues are drier after menopause, and may be more easily irritated and thus infected during sexual intercourse. A vaginal lubricant will help prevent this.

When To Call Your Doctor

Anyone who is experiencing symptoms for the first time should contact a doctor. Also call your doctor if you are self-treating a recurrent UTI with antibiotics (on your doctor's advice) and symptoms persist for a day or two, or if you develop new symptoms. Call your doctor right away if urinary discomfort is accompanied by fever, chills, or back pain, indicating a possible kidney infection.

What Your Doctor Will Do

After taking your history and reviewing your symptoms, the doctor will do a complete urinalysis and take a urine culture. Specific antibiotics are usually prescribed to fight the infection; often a three- to five-day regimen is sufficient.

If a woman has three or more UTIs in a year, her doctor may recommend low-dose, long-term antibiotic therapy.

If you repeatedly have attacks of cystitis after sexual activity, your doctor may recommend that you take a single dose of antibiotic right after sex. A single dose can be enough to kill bacteria that have just entered the bladder.

For More Information
• American College of Obstetricians and Gynecologists
• American Foundation for Urological Disease
• American Urological Association
• National Kidney and Urologic Diseases Information Clearinghouse

Vaginal Dryness

Symptoms

- Vaginal soreness (may also have itching or burning sensation).
- Painful intercourse.
- Light bleeding after intercourse.

What Is It?

Vaginal dryness, or atrophic vaginitis, is an irritation of the vagina caused by a thinning and shrinking of the vaginal tissues and decreased lubrication of the vaginal walls.

What Causes It?

Decreased estrogen is the most common cause, which is why vaginal dryness most frequently affects postmenopausal women. Removal of the ovaries and radiation treatments also cause decreases in estrogen and thus can cause vaginal dryness. In some cases vaginal dryness is also caused by a lack or loss of estrogen following childbirth (which can occur if the mother is breast-feeding).

Irritation of the vagina caused by tampons, toilet tissue, and contraceptives also can lead to dryness, and in some instances latex condoms can cause an allergic reaction, which can lead to a drying of the vaginal tissue.

For some women, dryness is experienced as decreased vaginal secretions prior to intercourse. However, in this case the cause is more often related to a man's inability to fully arouse the woman sufficiently during foreplay, which normally results in natural self-lubrication of the vagina, or from his unwillingness to wait for his partner's full arousal prior to intercourse.

What If You Do Nothing?

Repeated vaginal dryness is likely to continue until you pinpoint the cause of the problem and resolve it either with the home remedies suggested here or after having it diagnosed and treated by a physician.

Home Remedies

- **Slow down and savor the moment.** If dryness is caused by rushed lovemaking, slow down and spend more time with foreplay, which can help promote vaginal secretions.

Vaginal Moisturizers

▼

A number of over-the-counter moisturizing creams and lotions (including Astroglide, Lubrin, Replens, and K-Y Jelly) are effective in relieving vaginal dryness and accompanying discomfort. These moisturizers work immediately to relieve dryness, unlike replacement therapy (HRT); they also provide a good alternative to women who don't want to take hormones or use hormone creams. Even if you take hormonal pills, vaginal dryness may still be a problem and these nonhormonal creams are helpful remedies.

Some vaginal moisturizers are water-soluble, and at least one (Replens) contains a new type of vaginal lubricant called polycarbophil, which is bioadhesive and binds to the surface of vaginal cells. A controlled study compared Replens (with polycarbophil) and K-Y Jelly (water-soluble) and found that both worked well, but women in the study tended to like Replens better, even though it left a residue. Another small study found that Replens worked as well to counteract dryness as a cream with estrogen. Both Astroglide and Replens are mildly acidic, which helps prevent bacterial vaginal infections.

Ordinary moisturizing lotions can also be used for vaginal dryness. But avoid petroleum-based products, which can break down condoms, foster infections, and interfere with natural lubricants.

• **Lubricate.** If you often have pain during sexual intercourse, even with adequate foreplay, be sure to use a vaginal lubricant prior to sex (see page 489). You can also have your partner use a lubricated condom.

Prevention

• **Avoid douching and using spermicidal foams, creams, or gels.** These can adversely affect the vaginal tissue and lead to drying.

• **Regular sexual activity may help.** This improves blood circulation in the vagina, which helps counter dryness.

When To Call Your Doctor

Contact your physician if the home remedies don't relieve vaginal soreness, burning, itching, or painful intercourse.

490

What Your Doctor Will Do

Your doctor will perform a pelvic exam, specifically checking the health of the vaginal skin. Hormone levels of the blood may also be taken.

Hormone replacement therapy (HRT) or topical estrogen creams may be recommended. Estrogen rings (such as Estring) are a newer option for vaginal dryness. They deliver estrogen continuously in a controlled fashion. Similar to a diaphragm in size, the ring is placed in the vagina and releases estrogen at low doses for 90 days. Two studies have found that women prefer the estrogen rings to the creams, but little is known about any long-term effects. Ask your doctor to advise you about using these products.

For More Information

• American College of Obstetricians and Gynecologists

Vaginitis

Symptoms

- The most common symptom is an abnormal vaginal discharge that varies depending upon the cause of infection.
- **Bacterial vaginosis:** thin, watery discharge, heavier than usual, grayish white or yellow, often with a strong fishy odor ; possible mild burning or irritation of the vulva and vagina, often without redness or itching. (Some women with bacterial vaginosis report no signs or symptoms.)
- **Yeast infection:** white, thick, odorless discharge; possible itching and burning sensations as well.
- **Trichomoniasis:** yellow-gray or green-tinged discharge with intense unpleasant odor; vaginal and vulvar pain and itching, especially upon urination; redness and swelling of the vulva. Symptoms may be more severe just prior to and after menstruation.

What Is It?

The vagina is the part of the female reproductive system that connects the cervix (the entrance to the uterus) with the vulva (the folds of skin around the vaginal and urethral openings). Under normal conditions the vagina, which is self-cleaning, flushes out dead cells and secretions in the form of a discharge. The amount, color, and texture of this discharge varies according to a woman's monthly cycle and her stage of life, but it is usually clear or milky white, and watery or slightly viscous.

Vaginitis is an inflammation of the vaginal lining and vulva that typically includes an abnormal discharge along with itching and burning of the genital area. Most often the problem is caused by an infection, but certain irritants can also trigger it, as can hormonal changes.

At some point in their lives, about one-third of women must deal with this common problem. Though usually not a threat to health, vaginitis is uncomfortable and can be painful. Repeated bouts are common.

What Causes It?

Vaginitis occurs when there is a change in the balance of microorganisms that coexist in the vagina. When the balance is normal, a natural barrier against infection is maintained and organisms that may be harmful are kept in check. Sometimes these harmful organisms suddenly multiply rapidly to cause symptoms. Other times a lowered resistance to infection allows the organisms to thrive.

Three types of infection are the most common causes of vaginitis.

Bacterial (or nonspecific) vaginosis is caused by various types of bacteria that, for reasons not always clear, multiply excessively in the vagina. It's possible that the infection—which is the most common vaginal infection in women of child-bearing age—can be spread by sexual intercourse, though this hasn't been established. But women who have never had sexual intercourse are rarely infected.

Yeast infections, also known as candidiasis, are caused by a fungus normally found in the vagina. Repeated yeast infections are more likely to occur among women who use antibiotics, since these drugs kill off bacteria that keep the yeast in check. Women with weakened immune systems and those with diabetes are also at increased risk. (For more detailed information on yeast infections, see page 501.)

Trichomoniasis is an infection by a tiny protozool organism. The infection, which typically

491

occurs in the vagina in women, is usually passed through sexual contact. (A man can also be infected, but will seldom show symptoms. If not treated, he can infect other sexual partners.) An estimated five million new cases of trichomoniasis occur each year.

In addition to infections, vaginitis can be triggered by allergic reactions to soaps, medications, perfumes, or bath oils. In some women vaginitis is caused by an allergic reaction to the latex in condoms. Douching can also cause symptoms since it disrupts the normal balance of microorganisms in the vagina. Hormonal changes during pregnancy and menopause, which affect the vagina's balance of microorganisms, can also produce symptoms.

What If You Do Nothing?

Many cases of vaginitis will clear up without treatment. But some types of the inflammation are especially stubborn, and the symptoms are often very uncomfortable. In addition, some cases of vaginitis carry more serious risks. Both bacterial vaginosis and trichomoniasis increase a woman's risk of acquiring HIV infection if she is exposed to HIV—and can increase a woman's chance of transmitting HIV infection to a sex partner. Both types of infection can also cause complications in women who are pregnant.

A heavy discharge and burning pain during urination can also be a sign of gonorrhea.

Therefore, it is important to see your doctor if you notice symptoms.

Home Remedies

Self-treatment for vaginitis is advisable only when you have symptoms consistent with a mild to moderate yeast infection, you have had the condition before, and it has been diagnosed previously by a physician. If this is the case, over-the-counter antifungal medications are available in the form of vaginal suppositories and creams (see page 502).

Otherwise, you should consult your doctor and be diagnosed in order to match the treatment with the cause—particularly the first time you have symptoms. It's not wise to treat vaginitis on your own until you know what the problem is. A vaginal discharge can be a symptom of a sexually transmitted disease (for example, chlamydia or gonorrhea), in which case both you and your partner will require diagnosis and treatment.

The preventive measures below will help provide relief during an infection as well as help you avoid recurrent bouts of the problem.

Prevention

You can take a number of steps to decrease your likelihood of getting vaginitis. Prevention is especially important if you have suffered from repeated episodes.

• **Shower or bathe daily.** Use a mild, unscented soap to gently wash the vaginal area, and dry thoroughly.

• **Don't cover up with sprays, douches, or scents.** The vagina cleanses itself naturally, so there is no need to clean it artificially and risk irritation. Also, covering an unpleasant odor with scented sprays or tampons is risky because the odor could signal a problem for which you should see your doctor.

• **Practice careful hygiene.** When you wipe yourself after a bowel movement, wipe from front to back to avoid spreading bacteria from the rectum to the vagina. Also, thoroughly clean diaphragms, cervical caps, and spermicidal applicators after each use.

• **Don't wear tight clothing—and stick to cotton.** Tight pants and underpants made of nylon, silk, or certain synthetics can trap moisture in the genital area. Wear underpants and panty hose with a cotton crotch, which allows excess moisture to escape.

• **Use condoms during sex if you are undergoing treatment for vaginitis.** Also use condoms if you have recurrent infections or more than one sexual partner. This can help prevent infection from vaginitis as well as from gonorrhea and other sexually transmitted diseases.

• **Check on antibiotic medications.** If you are prescribed antibiotics for another infection, check with your doctor about reducing your risk of yeast infection.

• **Complete your treatment.** If you are being treated for vaginitis, it's important that you finish taking the medication and follow any other instructions from your doctor—even if your symptoms disappear. Symptoms can abate, yet the infection can still be present, and stopping treatment may cause it to recur.

• **Make sure your sexual partner sees a doctor.** Both bacterial vaginosis and trichomoniasis can be passed back and forth between partners. If you have been diagnosed with either condition, your partner should be examined to avoid any recurrence.

When To Call Your Doctor

Call your doctor if you experience any of the symptoms of vaginitis for the first time, or if you notice any abnormal vaginal discharge (which could be a sign of some other infection). Also, remember that the most common forms of vaginitis have overlapping symptoms. Therefore, don't assume that symptoms similar to those you've had before signal a recurrence of the same ailment. What appears to be a chronic yeast infection may actually be bacterial vaginosis.

Also call your doctor if you are taking medication for vaginitis and see no improvement after three days; another medication may be more effective or you may have some other type of condition.

What Your Doctor Will Do

Your doctor will perform a pelvic examination and take a sample of vaginal discharge to test vaginal acidity and to inspect secretions under a microscope. This makes it possible to distinguish one form of vaginitis from another. If the diagnosis is unclear, a vaginal culture may be taken. This also allows your doctor to exclude other disorders, including certain cancers, that can cause an abnormal discharge.

Once the doctor has reached a diagnosis, the appropriate medication can be prescribed. Bacterial vaginosis can be treated with the prescription drug metronidazole (Flagyl); metronidazole is used against trichomoniasis as well. Your sexual partner should also be treated if you have trichomoniasis.

For More Information
• American College of Obstetricians and Gynecologists

493

Varicose Veins

Symptoms

- Enlarged, swollen purple or blue veins, usually in the back of the calf and/or along the inner side of the leg.
- Heavy, aching, tired feeling in the legs, accompanied by occasional pain ranging from a dull throb to a burning sensation.
- Brownish gray discoloration, scaling, or itching above the affected veins, particularly around the ankles (advanced cases).

What Is It?

Varicose veins are enlarged, ropelike, or twisted blood vessels near the skin surface of the legs. The veins can be unsightly and uncomfortable, and they can also induce fatigue, aching, and scaling along the legs. In severe cases varicose veins may cause swollen ankles, itching calves, and leg pain.

Less troubling are sunburst patches of finer veins, called spider veins, that can appear on the skin of the legs, ankles, or face. Spider veins don't usually cause pain or interfere with circulation, though sometimes they can ache or burn.

What Causes It?

As part of the circulatory system, leg veins, along with leg muscles, work to send blood back toward the heart, and are equipped with tiny valves to keep the force of gravity from pulling blood back toward the feet. When the valves weaken and malfunction, the blood can't move normally, and varicose veins may result.

No one is sure exactly what causes varicose veins to develop in some people, but hereditary and, apparently, hormonal factors are at work: varicose veins run in families, and of the more than 40 million Americans affected with varicose veins, women outnumber men four to one.

Prolonged standing or inactivity can certainly play a role in people genetically inclined to develop varicose veins. Strain in the abdominal region—from repeated heavy lifting, pregnancy, or constipation—can also be a cause. (During pregnancy, increasing hormone levels may also cause veins in the legs to weaken, contributing to varicose veins.) Age is also a factor. As the skin ages, its connective fibers become less elastic and cannot support veins as firmly.

What If You Do Nothing?

Varicose veins are usually benign and more of a cosmetic than a medical concern. Without treatment, though, the veins may worsen with time (unless they are associated with pregnancy, in which case they may disappear after the birth). If you have a severe case, especially one that involves leg sores, contact your physician.

Spider veins in the legs may fade eventually on their own. If they are too unsightly, you can get medical treatment.

Home Remedies

• **Support your legs.** Special support stockings, available at surgical supply stores, can improve circulation (but won't cure your condition). These stockings, which can be custom fitted, are put on in the morning before your feet touch the floor and taken off before you go to bed.

You can also get special elastic bands that fasten with Velcro and allow you to apply pressure to specific parts of the leg. These also may be easier to put on than compression stockings.

• **Elevate your legs.** When you get a chance, lie down for 15 minutes with your legs on a pillow, elevated above your heart. Or rest your feet on a stool if you're sitting down.

Prevention

If you're prone to developing varicose veins, you may be able to prevent them, minimize their occurrence, or lessen discomfort from them.

• **Walk regularly.** Walking improves overall circulation, without increasing pressure on the legs. However, if you have varicose veins already, you should probably avoid strenuous running, jumping, aerobic dance, or training with heavy weights, since very vigorous or high-impact activity can cause pain and/or swelling in the legs.

• **Avoid prolonged standing or sitting.** This will keep blood from pooling in your legs. Get up periodically and walk around.

• **Perform simple heel rises.** These will get the calf muscle pumping blood back to the heart. Stand flat-footed, then rise up onto the balls of your feet, hold that position momentarily, then go back to the floor. Repeat 10 to 20 times.

• **Don't cross your legs.** Crossing your legs puts pressure on the leg veins.

• **Don't wear tight clothing.** This includes tight shoes, panty hose, girdles, and garter belts—all of which can compress and restrict the veins around the legs.

• **Maintain a healthy weight for your age and height.** Weight gain may cause new varicose veins to appear.

• **Avoid constipation.** Straining at stool can be bad for varicose veins. Drink plenty of fluids and increase the amount of fiber in your diet; start by eating a few prunes every day.

When To Call Your Doctor

Contact your physician if you develop any redness or tenderness, or if you notice a distinct swelling along the length of a varicose vein in your leg. You may have superficial phlebitis, a vein inflammation. Contact your physician if you develop a sore on your leg related to a varicosity. If you are concerned about the appearance of varicose veins, talk to your doctor while they are still in the early stages.

What Your Doctor Will Do

Most people can control varicose veins without surgical treatment, and your doctor may first suggest trying compression stockings or elastic bands. But if varicose veins are causing severe pain, complications, or emotional distress, they can be surgically removed safely and permanently. Blood then reroutes itself through veins that lie deeper in the skin.

One surgical method, whereby distended veins are cut out or tied off, is called stripping. A second option, sclerotherapy, calls for the injection of a solution that hardens the affected veins and blocks the blood flow. The blocked veins form a kind of scar tissue and are eventually absorbed, usually months later. Sclerotherapy is best for treating smaller veins, including spider veins. Laser therapy can also be used to break down smaller veins.

Your doctor will examine you to determine if you are a suitable candidate for surgery, and which procedure would work best for you.

For More Information

• American Academy of Dermatology
• National Heart, Lung, and Blood Institute Information Center

Warts

Symptoms

- A benign, small growth on the skin, typically on the hands.
- May be pale or dark, rough or smooth, raised or flat. Warts seldom bleed or itch.
- Usually painless, although plantar warts, located on the soles of the feet, can be quite painful.

What Is It?

Warts are benign tumors in the outer skin layer caused by the human papilloma virus. They can occur anywhere on the body, but they look different depending on where they grow. Warts typically appear on fingers and tops of hands, where they protrude as dry growths with a horny surface. On pressure areas such as the palms and soles, they grow inward. One of the most painful types is the plantar wart, a light-colored, flat growth on the sole of the foot that extends below the surface of the skin.

Ordinary warts are slightly contagious; they spread most commonly from one location to another—for example, from finger to finger—on an infected person, rather than from person to person. The exceptions are genital warts and warts that appear around the anal area. These are highly contagious and may contribute to the development of penile and cervical cancers. Warts on the larynx can also be dangerous. These three types of warts always require medical attention. (See page 283 for detailed information on genital warts).

Warts, which afflict 7 to 10 percent of the population, never spread from one species to another: that old story about toads causing warts in people is just a myth. (The bumps on toads and frogs, though wartlike in appearance, are unrelated to actual warts, which are found only on humans.) Warts are most common among children and young adults, as well as people with weakened immune systems, such as those infected with HIV. Of the several million people who seek treatment for warts each year, about 70 percent are under 40 years of age.

What Causes It?

Warts are caused by strains of human papilloma virus that can enter the skin through tiny breaks, cuts, or scratches and can be transmitted by direct physical contact with another person. Plantar warts may be spread through swimming pools or showers.

What If You Do Nothing?

Nongenital warts are harmless, and the best treatment for them may be no treatment at all. Up to 80 percent of nongenital warts disappear by themselves in one or two years (typically two years, at least in children). Genital and anal warts, on the other hand, must be treated. And because plantar warts can make walking uncomfortable, they, too, may need medical attention.

Unfortunately, warts that have gone away (a process known as spontaneous remission) can also return just as mysteriously.

Home Remedies

If you think you have a wart, it's a good idea to see a doctor for evaluation, since it might be another condition, such as a skin cancer. If it is a wart, deciding whether to treat it comes down to whether it interferes with your walking or running, or whether it is causing social problems. If not, then it may be best to leave the wart alone. Never cut a wart yourself, as there is a risk of bleeding, infection, and scarring.

The fact that most warts disappear on their own has bred all kinds of legends and given credence to hundreds of home remedies. Huckleberry Finn recommended handling dead cats as a treatment for warts, and Tom Sawyer believed that spunk-water (stagnant water in an old tree stump) could cure warts, at least if you approached the stump backward at midnight and recited the proper spell. Here are some remedies that have proven to be somewhat more effective.

• **Tape it.** This is an inexpensive, noninvasive, and popular remedy. Wrap the area in several layers of waterproof tape and leave it on for one week. Repeat the treatment. Sometimes the wart goes away.

• **Try a wart removal preparation.** Drugstores sell salicylic acid products for the removal of warts. If you decide to try one of these be sure to protect the surrounding skin, since it can get burned. Do not use these remedies on facial, genital, or anal warts.

Paint on the low-strength salicylic acid recommended by your physician or pharmacist. The medication may take weeks to produce favorable results.

Prevention

• **Don't cut or scratch.** Warts can easily spread if cut or scratched.

• **Wear shower shoes.** Plantar warts may be spread through moist environments like swimming pools or showers. Sandals or shower shoes at poolside or in locker rooms can keep you from spreading or exposing yourself to such a wart.

• **Change shaving tools.** An electric razor or depilatory may be used instead of a conventional razor. This will prevent the skin nicks that can easily promote the spread of warts on the legs and face.

When To Call Your Doctor

It's a good idea to have your doctor confirm that a wartlike growth is indeed a wart, especially if you are over 45. New skin growths should be diagnosed to rule out skin cancer.

Also contact your physician if warts develop on the sole of the foot and cause walking difficulties, or if they appear on the face or genitals. Genital warts, transmitted by sexual contact, are associated with the development of cervical cancer and should never be ignored by you or your sexual partner. If you have any type of growth in the genital area, see your doctor right away.

What Your Doctor Will Do

If it is a wart, the safest way to remove it is to have it done by a doctor. There are various methods, including electricity, laser treatment, surgery with a scalpel, and freezing. Cryotherapy (freezing) with liquid nitrogen is generally preferred. There are some prescription medications available for treating external genital warts. Plantar warts, which mainly lie below the skin surface, often require the use of local anesthesia for removal.

For More Information

• American Academy of Dermatology

497

Wrinkles

Symptoms

■ Wrinkles appear as lines, creases, furrows, or folds in the skin, particularly on the face, neck, and hands.

What Is It?

Wrinkles range from fine facial lines around the corners of the eyes and in between the nose and upper lip—the so-called laugh lines—to deep furrows that mark the neck, face, and hands. They are basically depressions in the skin, occurring after the skin has lost its elasticity and becomes thinner and drier. When combined with the effect of gravity, the skin can sag.

What Causes It?

A few mild facial wrinkles are a consequence of aging: the fine hairlike depressions around the eyes and mouth probably occur because elastic fibers that keep the skin taut gradually loosen over time, allowing the skin to sag.

But many wrinkles, including the deepest ones, are caused by overexposure to sunlight. Although the process by which skin damage occurs isn't known, one possibility is that ultraviolet (UV) rays increase the production of certain enzymes that break down proteins in collagen, the connective tissue located underneath the dermis (the layer of skin just beneath the epidermis, or outer layer). You can get a sense of the wrinkling power of ultraviolet rays simply by comparing the skin on your face or hands to skin at a site rarely exposed to the sun, such as the underside of your forearm.

Other factors that contribute to wrinkles include cigarette smoking (which thickens and fragments elastin, the chief constituent of the fibers that give skin its overall resilience) and going on and off crash diets—so-called yo-yo dieting—which causes weight to fluctuate dramatically, thereby stretching and pulling the skin.

What If You Do Nothing?

Wrinkles don't disappear on their own. They also don't pose a health problem—although the presence of severe or premature wrinkles may indicate that your skin has been damaged by too much exposure to the sun, which increases your risk of skin cancer.

Home Remedies

No area is as rich in hype and hokum as the market for "antiaging" and "antiwrinkle" skin-care products. Though the claims made for many of these creams and lotions are without substance, the ingredients in some products described here are being seriously studied by scientists and may hold some promise.

• **Retin-A.** This vitamin A derivative (generic name tretinoin) is a prescription drug that, until recently, was approved by the Food and Drug Administration (FDA) only to treat severe acne. Years ago, however, dermatologists began to notice that in some older patients the drug not only cleared up acne but also smoothed out some wrinkles and reduced blotchiness and blemishes. Subsequent research has found that Retin-A can reduce fine wrinkles and brown spots, and produce rosier skin. A small 1991 study concluded that the drug can help clear stretch marks; a 1992 study found that it can help fade age spots.

In 1996, tretinoin was first marketed in a wrinkle-erasing preparation called Renova. The drug's effect is quite subtle—deep or coarse facial wrinkles are little improved. In addition, the immediate effect of Retin-A is skin inflammation lasting two weeks to several months. In other words, for the sake of eventual minor skin improvements, you may have to walk around with a red, swollen, peeling face for a month or more. No one knows what the long-term consequences may be. Finally, since much isn't known about whether or to what extent Retin-A is absorbed through the skin, and since high doses of vitamin A can cause birth defects, women who are pregnant—or those who may become pregnant—should not use the drug.

• **Retinol, retinyl palmitate, and other vitamin A derivatives.** Because some doctors are reluctant to prescribe Retin-A for people who don't have acne, certain skin-care companies are promoting nonprescription skin creams containing vitamin A relatives as if these ingredients worked against wrinkles like Retin-A, but without the side effects.

Despite the claims, the evidence that these other forms of vitamin A will reduce wrinkles is not conclusive. For instance, some animal studies have found that retinol may improve the skin's connective tissue, which weakens with aging and sun damage. But the amounts of retinol and other compounds actually used in these skin-care products may be too low to have any effect on the skin. And if the concentrations were increased, the risk of side effects would rise as well.

• **Vitamins C and E.** The theory behind using these two antioxidants on the skin is that if they penetrate the outer layer of skin and settle in the dermis, they may scavenge free radicals (created by ultraviolet rays) and retard skin damage. Work by researchers at Duke University suggests that a solution of vitamin C can be absorbed through the skin and seems to protect against sun damage in some people. But other studies, mostly using animals, have had inconsistent results.

The research on the antiaging properties of vitamin E has also been inconsistent. The vitamin

does have a legitimate use on the skin. Because it's an oil, it works as a moisturizer—that is, it coats the skin and keeps the natural moisture from evaporating—whether it's used as a cosmetic ingredient or applied straight from the capsule. But as such, it's no more effective than mineral oil, petroleum jelly, or other moisturizing ingredients. There have been reports of skin irritation caused by vitamin E and vitamin C.

• **Glycolic acid and other alpha-hydroxy acids (AHAs).** Derived originally from fruit, sugar, or milk, these exfoliants have been used for years by dermatologists in facial peels. They are supposed to make the skin smoother by making it shed. The chemical peels done in dermatologist' offices contain high concentrations of these acids, which cause inflammation and so may help the skin regenerate. Over-the-counter products contain lower concentrations and usually have no such effect. In fact, many dermatologists believe that the concentrations are generally too low to have anything more than a very modest effect on fine wrinkles, if that.

Although the cosmetic industry says over-the-counter products are safe, there have been reports of adverse reactions. Products are not required to list their AHA concentrations, but you can call or write the manufacturer. You should not try anything with a concentration higher than 10 percent because it can cause skin inflammation. (If the "acid" ingredient is listed second or third, it's probably less than 5 percent.) AHAs may make your skin more vulnerable to sun damage, so even if you have no adverse reactions—and most people don't—use extra sunscreen when out in the sun.

• **Nayad and liposomes.** These are found in many antiaging cosmetics. Nayad is a yeast derivative that's touted as a restorative for the skin's connective tissue. No published data supports these claims. Liposomes act as fatty envelopes that are supposed to help other ingredients penetrate the skin. Again, the manufacturers supply no data to support any of the claims—it's wishful thinking, at best.

Prevention

• **Protect yourself from the sun.** As much as 70 percent of skin damage comes from the sun. This damage is cumulative, starting in youth, and so much of what is considered an inevitable part of aging is preventable or modifiable. Avoid long periods in the sun; when in the sun, use a sunscreen with a sun protection factor (SPF) of at least 15, preferably 30 or higher.

• **Wear protective clothing.** Dark clothes with a tight weave offer good protection from ultraviolet rays. Special UV-protective garments are also available.

• **Don't smoke.** Premature aging and wrinkling of the face is the logical consequence of smoking. The nicotine in tobacco is a vasoconstrictor that decreases the amount of blood that reaches the capillaries of the facial skin. Since smoking decreases a woman's levels of the hormone estro-

gen—which helps sustain overall skin elasticity—women may be more susceptible to the wrinkling effects of smoking.

When To Call Your Doctor

Wrinkles don't pose any health risk, and cosmetic treatments can minimize mild to moderate lines. If you can't live with your wrinkles, talk to a dermatologist about the pros and cons of Retin-A. If you have deep facial wrinkles that you want to reduce, you need to consult a plastic surgeon to explore possible treatments. Also see your doctor if you experience itching, burning, pain, redness, or stinging from using an over-the-counter cosmetic containing alpha-hydroxy acids (and stop using the product).

What Your Doctor Will Do

A plastic surgeon may offer antiwrinkle procedures such as dermabrasion, chemical peels, or laser resurfacing. Nearly all treatments can be done in an outpatient clinic or physician's office. Results will vary from person to person.

For More Information

• American Academy of Dermatology

Yeast Infections (Vaginal)

Symptoms

- White, thick discharge similar to cottage cheese in appearance and texture, with a sweet or breadlike odor (though it may be odorless). The discharge may not be substantial enough to be noticed.
- In most cases, redness, intense itching, and a burning sensation around the genital area.

What Is It?

Yeast infections are a type of fungal infection that can affect various parts of the body, but those that occur in the vagina are especially common and frustrating. While the condition is not serious, the accompanying itching and burning can be a source of great discomfort. Moreover, yeast infections can recur; for many women they become a chronic problem.

What Causes It?

Fungi that grow normally in the vagina are the cause of yeast infections, and the most common infection—known as candidiasis—results from *Candida albicans,* one of several species of a fungus called candida. A number of factors are associated with sudden and excessive growth of the fungus. Taking antibiotics increases the risk of yeast infections because the medications kill bacteria in the vagina that ordinarily subdue the growth of candida. Infections linked to antibiotics are highly resistant to treatment until you stop taking the medication.

Recurrent attacks are common among pregnant women, since pregnancy disturbs the acidic balance and moisture in the vagina, thereby encouraging the fungus. Birth control pills also disrupt vaginal chemistry and are associated with an increased risk of infection.

Also at greater risk are people with diabetes, possibly because high sugar levels in the vagina promote yeast growth, and those with weakened immune systems, such as people with HIV/AIDS or patients undergoing chemotherapy.

Wearing tight clothing that traps heat and moisture, such as panty hose, has been suspected of promoting yeast infections. It's also possible—but unlikely—for a yeast infection to be transmitted by an infected sexual partner.

What If You Do Nothing?

Some yeast infections clear up spontaneously. Often, however, the symptoms will become so uncomfortable that you will need relief.

Home Remedies

If you have never had a yeast infection before and you develop symptoms, you should see a doctor to be sure that your symptoms are in fact due to a yeast infection and not some other problem. But if you've had the same symptoms previously (and infrequently), and the condition has been diagnosed by a physician, you can try these measures on your own.

- **For mild infections, over-the-counter antifungal medications are often effective.** Available in both cream and suppository form, these products (see page 502) are appropriate and quite effective for treating mild, nonrecurrent yeast infections. Be sure to follow directions and complete the full course of treatment.
- **Yogurt might help.** The use of yogurt is not a completely far-fetched idea, since the same group of bacteria in yogurt—*Lactobacillus*—helps maintain a healthy ecology in the vagina. But studies on the subject are inconclusive and/or have serious problems. Moreover, how bacteria consumed in yogurt would travel from the digestive tract to

OTC Remedies for Yeast Infections

▼

The over-the-counter products for vaginal yeast infections have one of four antifungal agents: butoconazole nitrate (Femstat 3), clotrimazole (Gyne-Lotrimin and others), miconazole (Monistat 7 and others), and tioconazole (Vagistat). These drugs are in the same antifungal family and function in similar ways to break down the cell wall of the candida organism until it dissolves. They generally work well, and you can now buy equally effective generic versions, too, at lower prices.

A number of look-alike "anti-itch" creams are also on the shelves. Some contain benzocaine, which may relieve itching temporarily but can actually make it worse in some people; these products are not meant to be used inside the vagina and can't cure yeast infections.

Some remedies, packaged to look like the others, are homeopathic—they contain tremendously diluted amounts of an herb and the yeast candida. These have never been shown to combat yeast infections. If in doubt about a product, ask the pharmacist.

the vagina isn't at all clear. Douching with yogurt is probably safe (though messy), and it may or may not help with a yeast infection.

Prevention

The measures that help prevent other forms of vaginitis don't guarantee protection against yeast infections, but they may help lower the risk of some occurrences. These include practicing careful personal hygiene, not wearing tight clothing, avoiding vaginal sprays and other irritants, and taking antibiotics only when necessary. If you get recurrent infections, talk to your doctor about using over-the-counter antifungal remedies during any period you must take antibiotics.

When To Call Your Doctor

If you have any symptoms of a yeast infection for the first time, contact your doctor to make sure that the problem is indeed a yeast infection and not another form of vaginitis or a sexually transmitted disease with similar symptoms. Also see your doctor if you are taking over-the-counter medications for a yeast infection and there is no improvement after three or four days.

If you are have had recurrent yeast infections, talk to your doctor about taking preventive doses of medication.

For women who occasionally have yeast infections, an antifungal pill called fluconazole (Diflucan) is available by prescription only. You need to take only a single pill, and symptoms usually clear up in 24 to 48 hours.

Pregnant women should not take fluconazole, and women who are sensitive to other antifungals may react adversely. Fluconazole can interact with a number of medications, so discuss possible interactions with your doctor.

What Your Doctor Will Do

Your gynecologist will perform a pelvic examination and take a sample of the vaginal discharge. This examination allows your doctor to rule out other disorders, including certain cancers, that can cause an abnormal discharge. Once your doctor has reached a diagnosis, the appropriate medication can be prescribed.

For More Information

• American College of Obstetricians and Gynecologists

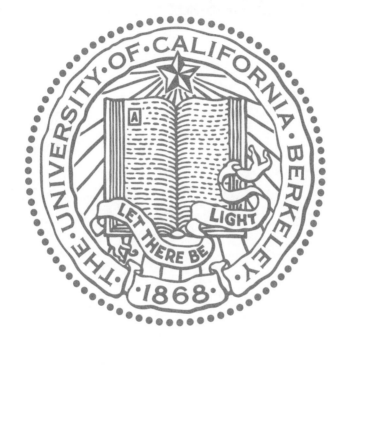

503

Your Health

from childhood to maturity

This section focuses on human growth and development during different stages of life, from infancy and childhood on through adolescence, young adulthood, midlife, and the later years. Along with presenting an overview of the normal physical and emotional changes that occur during each stage, the section highlights common health concerns and problems along with steps you can take to help ensure optimal health.

CHILDREN
(Birth to Puberty)

Watching a child grow physically and intellectually is among the greatest rewards of being a parent. At the same time, parents become easily worried about what is "normal" in terms of their child's growth and development. This section provides a very basic overview of normal developmental milestones, including a chart summarizing the development of some key skills. You will also find measures that parents can take to help ensure a child's health, information on how to recognize and cope with common childhood ailments (pages 516-518), and guidelines for immunizations (pages 519-525).

It is important for every parent to be aware that "normal" really refers to a "normal range" when monitoring a child's progress. Normal rates of development in children vary considerably. Not only do children differ as to when they reach particular milestones, but the same child may develop rapidly in one area and far more slowly in another. It is only when a child falls significantly or persistently outside the normal range that there may be reason for concern—and this applies to a relatively small number of children.

In addition, you as a parent know your child best. If some aspect of your child's growth is troubling you, do not hesitate to consult your pediatrician or family practitioner, who also can take your child's individuality into account. The same advice applies to any health problem your child develops. The information in this book is meant to help and reassure. But if home treatment does not prove effective after a reasonable time, or if a particular symptom seems unusual, by all means talk to your doctor about what action to take.

GROWTH AND DEVELOPMENT: BIRTH TO AGE ONE

Infants seem helpless at first, but within a fairly short time they undergo remarkable changes. In caring for a child's physical health during the first year (as well as thereafter), parents should be sure that the child has regular medical checkups. Your pediatrician or family physician will also monitor the baby's growth and development and advise you about caring for the newborn. At home, you can ensure that your baby is provided good nutrition and good hygiene and also receives the emotional nurturing that is important to a child's well-being. Active engagement between an infant and his or her caregivers helps to establish a secure base from which the child can venture out in the years ahead to explore the world beyond the home.

Birth to three months. During the first week of life, it is not unusual for newborns to actually lose weight, shedding about 10 percent of their birth weight as they expel excess body fluids. By two weeks of age, though, the baby should attain or exceed her birth weight. Thereafter, newborns gain about two pounds a month up to the third month.

A common concern of many new parents is whether a baby is being properly fed. Guidelines on how to best satisfy a baby's nutritional needs are summarized in the box on page 511. Keep in mind that, in addition to providing essential nutrition, feeding is an important component of the baby's emotional development. Holding and cuddling the child during feeding reinforces the child's sense of security and facilitates further development.

SOME EARLY CHILDHOOD SKILL MILESTONES

3 MONTHS

Holds head up when lying on stomach, gazes at hands or feet, clasps hands together, follows objects with eyes through a 180-degree arc, coos and gurgles, reaches out with both arms in response to stimuli, plays with mobiles.

6 MONTHS

Eats solid foods (though milk or formula is the mainstay of the diet), rolls over, holds head up while sitting, plays with feet, passes toy from one hand to the other, moves backward and forward, gets first teeth (6 to 12 months).

9 MONTHS

Sits up without assistance (6 to 9 months), takes bottle without help, pulls himself up to stand with effort (but can't get back down), may stand alone, crawls, feeds self crackers, imitates some adult sounds when playing.

1 YEAR

Says words, responds to "no," plays peek-a-boo, holds spoon, begins to walk (9 to 17 months), stands alone (9 to 16 months), waves bye-bye, helps with dressing by lifting arms or legs, tears and crumples paper, drops toys into container, helps turn book pages.

1-1½ YEARS

Repeats words, puckers and gives kiss, has temper tantrums, identifies body parts, understands simple questions, builds a tower of 2 blocks, throws a ball, walks up stairs (may use wall for help), sits on chair, puts lid on containers.

2 YEARS

Refers to self by name, washes hands, scribbles with crayon, builds a tower of 4 blocks, imitates some adult behavior (housework, talking on the telephone), kicks a ball.

2-2½ YEARS

Refers to the self as "I," helps put things away, speaks sentences of 3 words, counts to 10, walks down stairs, plays hide-and-seek, holds crayon with thumb and fingers, holds book and turns pages.

3 YEARS

Knows full name, rides a tricycle, preference for right or left hand becomes apparent, copies a circle, knows age and sex, unbuttons clothing and puts on shoes, washes hands, has all 20 baby teeth, eats well with spoon, can build a tower of 8 blocks, jumps in place, broad jumps, stands on 1 foot for several seconds.

4 YEARS

Uses scissors to cut out pictures, tells a story, plays with several other children, goes to the bathroom alone, catches a bounced ball, stands on 1 foot for 10 seconds, hops on 1 foot, dresses and undresses with help, knows 3 or more colors.

5 YEARS

Ties shoes, skips, goes up and down stairs carrying something, dresses and undresses with little help, ties shoes, can cut and paste with supervision, knows colors, rides a 2-wheel bike with training wheels, uses eating utensils properly, holds a pencil correctly, understands game rules.

6 YEARS

Waits to take turns, rides bicycle, skates, bounces ball, begins to understand time and directions, answers telephone and takes messages, begins to lose baby teeth (about 4 new teeth grow in each year).

Child and parent also connect through a wide range of gestures. During the first month, a child starts to make eye-to-eye contact with an adult. One of the strongest stimuli for a baby is a parent's smiling face. Babies as young as several weeks can recognize a smile, and they will quiet down when held and gently spoken to. At around two months they will begin to respond by smiling back—one of the most delightful milestones of this age period.

Of course, newborns also cry—and while hunger, a soiled diaper, or some other identifiable source of discomfort may be the cause, babies often cry for no apparent reason, testing parents' patience and accounting for countless frantic calls to the doctor. Crying often peaks at around six weeks of age, when babies may cry for a total of three hours during the course of the day; by three months, crying often decreases to an hour or less. An exception is an infant with a medical condition, such as an earache, that provokes the crying, or an infant with colic. If your child cries for prolonged periods (three hours or longer) for no apparent reason and no amount of cajoling will appease her, see your doctor.

Your baby will also begin to establish predictable sleep patterns. Initially a newborn may sleep and awaken at seemingly random times throughout the day and night, but as the nervous system matures and the infant gradually adjusts to parents' daily patterns, sleep periods gradually lengthen. By two months, infants may wake two or three times during the night. Some will sleep for six hours at a stretch.

Three to six months. During this period, weight gain slows to about 1¼ pounds per month, so that by five months, your baby's weight will have approximately doubled from birth.

Babies this age sleep as much as younger infants—a total of about 16 hours a day—but more sleep occurs during the nighttime. About 75 percent of infants six months old sleep for six to eight hours at a stretch. Sleep cycles are often tied to the baby's feeding schedule.

IS MY BABY GROWING NORMALLY?

Growth charts have been devised by the National Center for Health Statistics, compiled from a sample of more than 20,000 healthy children in the United States. The charts provide detailed percentiles for height and weight for children from birth to age 18. Your doctor will likely tell you during checkups where your child falls—for example, in the 55th percentile for height and the 40th percentile for weight.

These charts are useful for purposes of general comparison and for following trends, since growth problems may become apparent when a child's progress is followed over time. However, it is important not to read too much into one or two numbers. Prematurity, medical conditions, ethnicity, genes, parents' height, and many other factors all play a role in what is "normal" for your child. Size at birth, for example, largely reflects the newborn's environment in the womb. By two years of age, on the other hand, a child's percentiles more closely reflect the growth patterns of the parents, indicating the strong contribution of genetic factors.

During feeding, a child this age will look around more and become distracted by his surroundings, rather than focus solely on the person feeding him. The baby will also become more aware of his own body. He will touch his ears, cheeks, and genitals, blow bubbles, and wiggle his fingers.

His legs will also start to gain strength. When you pull him to a standing position, he will extend his legs and put weight on them. Likewise, he will progress from being able to hold an object for only a few seconds to holding it for minutes at a time and then voluntarily letting it go.

You can also expect to see him express a wider range of emotions—joy, anger, fear, and surprise, as well as coos and other vocalizations in response to a parent's verbal and facial expressions. If these expressions aren't beginning to show themselves, or if your baby exhibits any persistent lethargy or unwillingness to engage in interactions, you should talk to your doctor.

6 to 12 months. At a year old, your child's weight will be about triple her birth weight and she will be about 50 percent taller. Her strength and agility will increase. At six to eight months, her first teeth will appear—a process that may be heralded by increased crankiness (see Teething on page 463). If no teeth emerge by about the thirteenth month, a problem may exist that needs medical attention.

Your baby will begin to understand simple commands like "no" and "give me," though it will be several more months before she speaks her first words. She is also naturally curious about her environment and will use her newly developed motor skills to explore. By eight months, many infants can drag themselves along the floor on their elbows, and they may get up on all fours and begin to crawl, often backward at first. A baby's urge to move and explore may seem limitless. Babies this age will tear the pages out of books, open cabinets, pick up objects, move them from hand to hand, and put just about anything into their mouths. It's important that you keep a close eye on your child so that she doesn't swallow anything dangerous or get into trouble. Now is the time to take steps to childproof your home to prevent accidents—as explained in the section on Children and Safety (page 525).

Emotionally, children in this age range make their preferences increasingly well known. They may refuse food or insist on feeding themselves (facilitated by their new ability to grasp with the thumb and forefinger—a skill that develops at around nine months). Their willfulness may culminate in another, less welcome milestone by the end of the year: the first temper tantrum.

Anxiety around strangers is another normal stage that occurs toward the end of a child's first year. A child who previously babbled and smiled when meeting new adults may, at nine months or so, suddenly become guarded and cautious at the stare or approach of a stranger.

Regular sleep patterns may also become disrupted, as your child wakes during the night and cries because you aren't in the room. If nighttime awakening is a problem, try putting your child to bed while she is drowsy but still awake, and encourage her to go to sleep on her own. This may help ease her anxiety if she awakens in the middle of the night.

GROWTH AND DEVELOPMENT: AGE ONE TO TWO

During the second year, infants show more and more independence as they learn to communicate their needs more effectively.

12 to 18 months. This is an exciting time for

509

parents, as language begins to take shape. At 12 months, babbling will be interspersed with your baby's first words. By 18 months, he may be stringing several words together, though he won't be talking in true sentences. Your baby will know the names of a few body parts, like nose or eyes, and be able to point to them. He will also continue to assert himself by showing strong preferences, such as for specific foods or mealtimes.

Youngsters this age exhibit a healthy degree of guardedness, particularly in unfamiliar situations. A child may readily explore the pediatrician's office, for example, but cling to a parent when the examination begins. The parent becomes a secure base from which the child can explore.

Your child will move about and explore a room by grabbing onto furniture for support before taking his first steps. Many parents get needlessly upset if other children of the same age are already beginning to walk and their own child is not; as with all stages of development, there are normal variations. Highly active and fearless babies tend to walk earlier—at 12 or 13 months. More timid children may be temporarily scared off by a fall, and others are content to sit and concentrate on toys for several months before taking their first steps.

Your child may be frustrated by early, unsuccessful efforts at walking, but once he has mastered those first few steps, his mood dramatically lifts. Most babies are truly delighted by their newly achieved freedom to explore. By 15 months, your child may even be climbing up and down stairs (usually backward).

All that activity helps to burn off "baby fat." Weight gain slows to about a pound every two months. Your child's appetite will also decrease, but as long as he is still alert, active, and growing, he is getting enough to eat.

18 to 24 months. By 18 months a child is walking well and may even begin to run. During the next 6 months, development is rapid, so that by her second birthday she may be able to walk up and down stairs. Fine motor skills also mature, allowing her to stack several blocks, dismantle toys, feed herself with a spoon, open doors, help undress, or drink from a cup with few spills. A favorite activity for many children this age is climbing. Keep an eye on your child to avoid accidents like falling out of a crib.

Many parents notice that their children become increasingly "clingy" at around 18 months. Toddlers this age may also be particularly fussy at bedtime and may throw tantrums when put to bed. A favorite blanket or stuffed animal often provides comfort.

An improvement in language ability may be the most prominent milestone of this period. A child of 18 months knows about 10 words. As a child approaches her second birthday, she knows 100 or more words and begins creating simple sentences of two or three words. She may also begin to relate immediate experiences and will understand more complex commands.

Pay close attention to your child's requests. If a child asks what something is, teach her the word. Speak in clear, simple sentences. Ask questions. Respond to even incomplete requests or gestures from your child. At this stage of development, language is becoming an important part of parent-child communication.

Failure to thrive. A child under age two who weighs less than 80 percent of the average for children with the same birth weight may be diagnosed with *failure to thrive*—a term that refers to abnormally slow development in infants and young children. Other signs of failure to thrive include being withdrawn, apathy, and slow devel-

NUTRITIONAL GUIDELINES: BIRTH TO AGE TWO

High metabolism and a rapid growth rate make it especially important to meet calorie, nutrient, and fluid requirements for children younger than two. (Fluid intake is critical because water makes up a greater percentage of an infant's body weight than an adult's or an older child's.)

• A newborn needs about 50 calories per pound of body weight daily—a requirement that drops to about 45 calories per pound by the first birthday. You probably won't have to calculate how much to feed your baby, since infants will signal when they are hungry and simply stop eating when they are full.

• Breast milk is the best food for infants. It is the only food or fluid needed for the first six months of life. It provides not only nutrients and calories but other components that contribute to the baby's immune system and may also help offer protection against future allergies. If a mother cannot breast-feed, infant formula is satisfactory.

(Mothers who wish to breast-feed benefit from taking a breast-feeding class. The La Leche League and the Nursing Mother's Breast-feeding Council are also good sources of information. Your pediatrician or health clinic can direct you to a local group. You can also contact La Leche by telephone at 1-800-525-3243.)

• Nutritional deficiencies in infants must be diagnosed by a physician. Iron deficiency, for example, is common in infants, and a pediatrician may prescribe an iron supplement. Other nutrients that may require supplementation in infants are Vitamin D and fluoride.

• The American Academy of Pediatrics recommends introducing solid foods between four and six months of age. For a baby, solid foods include anything served with a spoon: mashed vegetables, fruit, cereals, or meat. Introduce foods one at a time over consecutive weeks, so that you can test for any adverse reactions or food allergies. If a food causes vomiting, diarrhea, or blood in the stools, withdraw it. (Call your doctor if you find blood in the stools.) Your child may be better able to tolerate a particular food a few months later.

Check with your doctor if you have concerns about food allergies or specific foods.

• Don't restrict fat intake in children younger than two. Fats, especially cholesterol, are essential for the developing nervous system.

• Check with your doctor about when to switch from breast milk or formula to cow's milk. Many experts recommend this be done at one year of age. Babies should be fed whole milk until they are two years old. Reduced-fat and fat-free (skim) milk contain a high proportion of protein relative to total calories, and an infant may have trouble digesting them.

511

opment in speech and motor control.

Malnutrition is one cause of failure to thrive, and that in turn may be the result of poor parenting skills, depression or some other psychological problem affecting the mother, or a lack of time or money to adequately care for a child. Children who are on a nutritious diet can also be afflicted, in which case the cause is likely to be a congenital defect or an underlying disorder that interferes with eating and metabolizing food.

If an infant is failing to grow at any point, a doctor should be consulted to determine the cause. The doctor will take the baby's history, including patterns of weight loss and previous illnesses, and ask about the baby's feeding habits. If the cause is organic, the underlying medical problem will be treated. If psychological factors are identified, individual counseling and family therapy may be recommended. In addition, nutritional counseling may be necessary to make sure that the baby receives a proper diet. Often, social workers or nutritionists can provide low-income families with information on how to provide a well-balanced diet at below-average cost. Families can also obtain help from federal or state programs.

GROWTH AND DEVELOPMENT: AGES TWO TO FIVE

The preschool years are a time when the child's unique personality begins to emerge more dramatically—which can include willful and contradictory behavior. A youngster may vacillate from clinging demands for attention to rebellious independence, testing a caregiver's limits and patience. Children are learning new rules of behavior and modes of self-expression and widening their social universe. So many changes are occurring that it may be very difficult to know whether your toddler is progressing normally or encountering stumbling blocks in his development. Talk about any concerns openly during regular visits with your doctor.

The rate of physical growth slows during these years. On average, a child gains about five pounds and grows about three inches each year. Your child's appetite may decrease, which should not be a source of alarm. Children normally regulate their nutritional intake. They may eat a lot one day and little the next, but from one week to the next their intake should remain relatively stable. Forcing or withholding food is discouraged; not only is it unlikely to produce healthier eating habits, but it can also lead to eating disorders in adolescence (see page 531).

The need for sleep also decreases somewhat. Two-year-olds who were sleeping 13 or 14 hours a day (including a nap) may sleep only 11 hours a day without a nap by age five.

Toilet training is another milestone at this age. It's generally best to wait until a child is able to stay dry for several hours at a time and remain dry after a nap before teaching him to use a potty. Training may take until age three and a half or later, and once a child has learned to use a toilet during the day, he may still wet the bed at night for another six months or so. Remember that bed-wetting accidents are normal in young children (see page 169). If bed-wetting remains a persistent problem beyond age five, however, you should consult your pediatrician.

Interest in the genitals and masturbation, which is universal among children, will often become increasingly apparent during this stage of development. Although in the past children were often routinely punished or humiliated for genital activity, it is completely safe and natural. Unless the practice becomes obsessive, parents shouldn't be concerned by it. Most children begin to acquire a degree of modesty with respect to their genitals between the ages of four and six, depending on family practices and cultural traditions.

These years are marked by dramatic strides in communication skills. From the ages of two to three, youngsters progress from knowing roughly 100 words to up to 1,000, and they pepper their conversations with endless questions about their surroundings. Language acquisition emerges as an important gauge of intellectual and emotional progress. Delayed speech in a two-year-old, for example, may be the first indication of a learning disability or a medical problem like mental retardation. Language can also be an important emotional outlet for children. Encourage your child to express his feelings, rather than acting them out, by teaching him the meaning of words like "afraid" or "angry."

Despite your best efforts, children will have times when they lose emotional control. Temper tantrums, which may begin toward the end of a child's first year, tend to peak between the ages of two and four. Children use tantrums in part to maintain a sense of control and to test their parents' limits. Tantrums can also occur when children are overly tired or fearful, or if an ailment is causing discomfort. They may become entrenched if parents give in to them. (One popular strategy for dealing with tantrums is the "time out"—explained in the tips for disciplining a child on page 514.) Tantrums that last more than 15 minutes or that occur more than three times a

---

NUTRITIONAL GUIDELINES: AGE TWO AND OLDER

Children over two need to consume enough calories to sustain periods of rapid growth. Pay special attention to ensuring proper intake of calcium (for growing bones) and iron (to prevent anemia). Whereas children under two should not restrict their fat intake, older children can be started on a diet low in fat and high in complex carbohydrates, the same as for a healthy adult (see page 17). Keep these points in mind:

• Fat intake should be no more than 30 percent of the total calories, with less than 10 percent of daily calories coming from saturated fat.

• Cholesterol intake should not exceed 300 milligrams a day.

• The average daily diet for a child under 12 should include low-fat dairy products, few meats, and should offer plenty of fruits, vegetables, and whole grains.

• The total calorie count should be adjusted to your child's growth rate so as to maintain a desirable body weight.

Cardiologists generally agree that limiting a child's fat intake from age two onward will help reduce the odds of eventually developing coronary heart disease. Although symptoms of heart disease seldom become manifest before middle age, damage to the coronary arteries begins to appear in early childhood. It is estimated that 5 percent of all children 5 to 14 years old in the United States have blood cholesterol levels above 200 mg/dl. (All children at high risk—those with a parent who develops any form of cardiovascular disease before age 55 or a parent who has high blood cholesterol that is not controllable by diet—should have a cholesterol test. See page 201.)

Try to limit sugary snacks, and teach children to stop eating when they are full. But avoid disputes over food. If a child doesn't want to eat the meal provided, don't force the issue. You can help ensure proper nutritional intake by offering a variety of healthy food choices, not by urging—or forcing—a child to eat something.

day may be a sign of a medical or an emotional problem.

Children's thinking is sometimes described as "magical" during these early years. Reasoning tends to center around the self, and there is a lot of fantasy play. This is normal and healthy. Irrational fears of the dark or of monsters may also arise. You can best deal with these by talking

DISCIPLINING A CHILD

Physical punishment may not only endanger the welfare of a child but is likely to be counterproductive. According to the National Committee for Prevention of Child Abuse, kids don't need to be hit in order to learn proper behavior. This is not to say that parents can't occasionally swat the small hand that's reaching for a hot stove or a forbidden treat. But using physical force as a routine form of discipline can have disastrous results. Here are some positive steps:

• **Show respect for the child** and expect respect in return. Aim to teach self-esteem, which motivates youngsters to discipline themselves.

• **Set an example** of self-control and good manners. If you lose your temper, try to get away for a few minutes if you can, or at least turn on the radio or find some other way to distract and calm yourself. Anybody who looks after children gets angry sometimes. But what you do sets an example for the child. If you get so angry that you scream or lose control, apologize when you've calmed down.

• **Set rules for behavior** and for the daily routine when caring for children. Small kids, especially, feel more secure if they know when to expect a bath, meals, play, or sleep.

• **Remember that babies and most toddlers** are not yet capable of following rules. Children under the age of three or four may endanger themselves, break objects, and do the exact opposite of what you tell them. If you fight with

them, you're sure to lose, and hitting them accomplishes nothing. (An infant, of course, should never be hit, and no child should ever be shaken.) If a toddler heads into danger, it's the adult's job to rescue her. Offer an explanation: "You'll get hurt out in the street; I don't want you to get hurt." But if she doesn't understand you or repeats her action anyway, remove her from temptation.

• **When you say no,** be sure the child understands your reason. Be sure you understand it, too.

• **Always praise good behavior.**

• **Give the child some voice** in decisions that affect him. Allow him to say how he feels and what he thinks. When setting limits, offer choices when possible: "You can play in the sandbox or on the swing, but you can't throw sand."

• **Call "time out."** If the child loses his temper or disobeys repeatedly, try isolating him for a while and offering some quiet but constructive activity. Later, give him a chance to make amends or apologize. Don't hold his anger against him. Make him feel worthwhile.

• **If a child has broken a rule** (for example, "you can't hit your brother") and you feel punishment is in order, take away privileges for a limited time, or if she is hitting and fighting, isolate the child from playmates. If a child has broken something or written on the wall with crayon, get her to clean it up or at least help you clean it up. Always be clear about what the punishment is for, how long it is to last, and what you expect it to accomplish.

them through with your child. Not until age five or so will a child truly begin to distinguish fantasy from reality.

Concurrently, your child will be developing a moral sense that helps in adapting to an expanding social world. A three-year-old may have a hard time understanding what it means to share, but by age four or five she will be taking turns at the playground. Children this age will also begin to comprehend concepts like honesty as they interact more with other youngsters. Solitary play, so common in a child of one or two, gives way to true group play in a favorite pastime such as playing house, in which each child assumes a different role.

The child's entrance into kindergarten at age five marks a major milestone for parents and child alike. Seeing a child board a school bus for the first time can bring tearful joy to a parent. Children are also often simultaneously anxious and eager to begin a new social and intellectual adventure. And by this age, they have indeed grown up considerably. They have a greater command of their emotions and are able to focus on immediate tasks without being unduly distracted by diversions. These skills all help to set the stage for success in the upcoming school years.

GROWTH AND DEVELOPMENT: AGE SIX TO PUBERTY

During these years, children become more aware of being part of a larger world. Consequently, they grow more independent from their parents and seek approval from peers, teachers, and others they come in contact with. External factors like good grades, establishing a circle of friends, physical attributes, or prowess in competitive sports take on increasing importance as children branch out socially from home. By age seven or

eight, most children develop a sense of continuity with friends, usually of the same sex. Social milestones may include the first "sleep-over" at a friend's house or going away to camp. A good general strategy for parents during these years is to expose a child to a wide range of activities, so that he or she can learn to develop new areas of interest, discover hidden talents, and build up confidence.

Physical growth rate continues to slow. Boys and girls grow, on average, about two inches each year and gain about five to seven pounds, though there are wide individual variations. Physical features may become an important source of pride or shame. Though most children in this age range remain sexually immature, there is still interest in gender differences and sexual issues.

Because children are developing increased muscle strength, coordination, and stamina, this is a good time to encourage them to make exercise a lifelong habit. Even at this age, being sedentary is associated with an increased lifetime risk of obesity and heart disease. On average, schools are offering fewer physical education classes—and gym programs tend to stress competitive sports rather than cardiovascular fitness. Yet all youngsters can participate in aerobic activities, since they require minimal hand-eye coordination and athletic talent. Running, for example, can be a good aerobic activity for children. Long-distance running poses an increased risk of injury for prepubescents, but if a running program is gradual and well supervised, the risks should be minimal. Swimming, cycling, brisk walking, and hiking are other good aerobic options that can easily be shared as family activities—and are likely to become lifelong habits.

Behavioral problems or learning disabilities may become more apparent during these years and may affect school and social performance. If your child finds schoolwork or reading unusually difficult, talk to a teacher or to your doctor about having the child tested for developmental problems such as attention deficit hyperactivity disorder (ADHD) or a specific learning disability, such as dyslexia. Such problems demand attention and usually can be successfully treated with medications, special classes, and various forms of psychotherapy. (Usually the family should be involved in the therapy.) Depression has also been recognized increasingly in children. It may be marked by withdrawal and a loss of interest in activities. Studies indicate that antidepressant medications may be helpful, especially as adjuncts to therapy, in treating depressed children.

Once children are in school, they are more likely to be exposed to contagious ailments ranging from lice to colds. Some of these can't be avoided, but it is important to continue getting regular medical checkups and recommended immunizations. Regular dental exams are also important, since during this period a child's baby teeth fall out and all the permanent teeth, except for wisdom teeth, come in.

HEALTH PROBLEMS AFFECTING CHILDREN

All children—even the healthiest—get sick from time to time. Infants and young children can get sick frequently; colds and other viral illness typically occur at least six times a year in children in kindergarten. Fortunately, most ailments are self-limiting and resolve in a few days with rest or other home measures.

Many of the health problems included in the "Ailments and Disorders" section of this book can affect children, and there are a number of complaints that are specific to children (see the index on page 141). In each of the entries, you will find measures for home treatment along with advice on when to call your doctor.

Three symptoms that appear repeatedly in children and that can be especially worrisome to parents are rashes, fever, and diarrhea.

Rashes. The vast majority of rashes in children are not serious. Common causes include heat (see page 415), irritation caused by dampness (see page 238), contagious infectious diseases like chicken pox (see page 194), and allergic reactions to drugs, other ingested substances, or environmental toxins.

Many newborns develop red splotches on their skin within the first five days, but these disappear within a day or two. Older babies also commonly develop a rash similar to acne on the face and neck at one to three months of age. The rash may come and go and worsen with crying or heat. It may be related to hormonal changes in the infant and is nothing to worry about. It, too, will disappear on its own. Another common skin complaint in infants is cradle cap (page 224), which typically appears on the scalp but which may spread to other areas.

Call your doctor in the following situations: if a rash does not clear up with home treatment; if it involves extensive areas of skin or unusual areas like the eyes or genitals; if itching is severe or persistent; if it appears to be infected (red, swollen, sensitive to touch); if it occurs after a bee sting or insect bite or appears to be the result of a particular medication; or if other symptoms occur, such as wheezing, difficulty breathing, or fever.

Fever. Fever is the body's natural response to infection. An elevated body temperature can help the immune system kill off harmful germs. But fevers can be uncomfortable, and high fevers, particularly in children younger than age two, can cause dangerous complications, such as seizures.

What constitutes a high fever? Children's body temperatures are generally higher and more variable than those of adults; also, a child's age is taken into account in assessing a fever.

• For a child up to a month old, a high fever is 100°F.

• Up to three months: 101°F.

• Up to two years: 103°F.

• For older children: above 104°F.

Call your doctor promptly if your child has a high fever. Also call the doctor if any fever is accompanied by other symptoms like sore throat or listlessness, or if it persists for more than five days despite home treatment.

Children with fever should never be given aspirin (or other salicylates) because of the risk of Reye's syndrome, a potentially fatal brain and liver disorder. Acetaminophen should be used instead, unless your doctor directs otherwise.

Diarrhea. Diarrhea is common in children of all ages. In infants, stools are commonly soft, and young infants may have up to a dozen bowel movements a day. If the consistency is runny and liquid, it may be a sign of diarrhea. In older children, two or three soft or runny stools a day may indicate diarrhea. Diarrhea in children is commonly caused by viral or bacterial infections, though it may also be a response to particular drugs (such as antibiotics) or food allergies. In chronic cases it may reflect a bowel disorder.

For information on treating diarrhea in children, see page 241. Most instances of diarrhea are not serious, though it's important that infants get enough fluids to avoid dehydration. Call your doctor if blood appears in the stools (it may be either bright red or black in color), if your child is experiencing severe abdominal pain, if mild diarrhea persists for more than five days, or if diarrhea seems to be causing dehydration.

When to seek medical assistance. While fever, rashes, or stomach or ear pain are readily apparent, it is not always obvious when a child is sick. Look for any changes in your child's appearance

517

Taking a Temperature

There are several ways to take a child's temperature. An **oral thermometer** should generally not be used with children younger than age five, because they have trouble holding the thermometer properly under the tongue. Instead, use a **rectal thermometer,** which has a rounded bulb. The thermometer has to be inserted only about an inch into the rectum (you can use a lubricant on the tip) but should be kept in place for about two minutes to obtain a good reading.

Axillary thermometers that read the temperature under the armpit or **temperature strips** applied to the forehead are the least reliable gauges of body temperature. **Ear thermometers,** which measure infrared energy from the eardrum, are fast (a few seconds) and accurate, though they are expensive (costing $60 or more) and generally are used by health professionals. (The tip of the device must be inserted precisely into the ear canal—otherwise you will get a lower temperature.) Some studies question their accuracy in children under three because kids that age squirm so much.

or behavior, such as unusual fussiness in an infant, poor appetite, or loss of energy. As you get more familiar with your child's behavior and personality, you'll grow more confident about assessing his state of health. Older children will often let you know if they're not feeling well.

Although most minor ailments can be safely treated at home, call your doctor if you're unsure about any situation. Also call if your child exhibits any of the following:

• A high fever.

• Blood in the stools; blood may appear bright red or black in color.

• Blood in vomit (red or brown vomit), persistent vomiting, or projectile vomiting (forceful vomiting in an infant younger than three months).

• Severe stomach or abdominal pain lasting more than 30 minutes.

• An unusual rash or inflammation.

WHEN IT'S AN EMERGENCY

You should contact the nearest medical facility for the following:

• **Dehydration.** Signs include no urination for eight hours, little or no tears, dry lips, thirst, irritability, sunken eyes, dry and pale skin, or (in an infant) a sunken fontanel (the soft spot on top of the head). Dehydration is particularly serious in infants.

• **Breathing difficulty** such as wheezing or blueness in the lips.

• **Seizures.**

• **Obvious trauma, serious bleeding, or unconsciousness.**

EARLY PREVENTION: TEETH, VISION, HEARING

Here are preventive measures you can take in three crucial areas of your child's health to prevent problems or to detect them early so that corrective measures can be taken.

Tooth care. Tooth cleaning should begin as soon as the first teeth come in, around one-and-a-half to two years of age. Children love to imitate their parents, so encourage your child to brush along with you as soon as she is able to hold a toothbrush. You can help out with the toothbrushing until your child becomes proficient, usually around age five or six. Any toothpaste you use should contain fluoride to help prevent tooth decay. Be sure to supervise small children so they don't swallow too much of the toothpaste. Also talk to your dentist about fluoride treatments for your child, which can be very effective in preventing decay.

The American Dental Association (ADA) recommends that parents also floss their children's teeth from age 1½ until the children are able to do it themselves (about age eight). Children should be supervised during flossing so that they do not injure their gums.

Take your child along with you to the dentist and show that this is a positive experience. Most dental squeamishness in adults can be traced to an unpleasant childhood experience. Making a youngster comfortable with dental treatment can do much to eliminate lifelong anxiety.

Dental sealants are also recommended for all children by the American Dental Association and the federal government. Fluoride and brushing are effective against cavities on the smooth surfaces of the teeth, but they have little effect in preventing cavities on the biting surfaces, where 80 percent of cavities in children occur. The dentist applies dental sealants on the pits and fissures of the teeth to form a tight protective seal against decay. In combination with fluoride, sealants virtually guarantee a cavity-free mouth.

Vision. Scientists now generally believe that even newborns can see, although vision is not sharp in infants. Vision generally improves to about 20/30 by age three and 20/20 by age four.

The U.S. Preventive Services Task Force recommends that all children should have their eyes examined at age three or four, before starting school. Eye-care professionals can often detect and treat common problems such as amblyopia (lazy eye) or cross-eyes in children this age. During the school years a child should see an eye doctor if visual problems develop, such as difficulty reading small print (farsightedness) or a blackboard (nearsightedness). Many schools conduct regular vision checks for all students. A routine professional vision check at age 13 is also a good idea.

Hearing. Newborns usually react to loud sounds by startling. Older infants will turn their heads toward the sound. Parents are usually the first to suspect a hearing problem. Impacted earwax can sometimes muffle hearing, particularly if children stick things in their ears and wedge the wax in further. A cotton swab should be used to clean the outside of the ears only; it should never be inserted into the ear canal.

If you are concerned about your child's hearing ability, arrange to have a hearing test done. Hearing tests are generally more precise after the first year, when children are better able to understand and communicate.

CHILDHOOD VACCINATIONS

Mass vaccination programs in the United States and other developed countries have been highly effective in curbing a number of once common and devastating diseases such as polio, diphtheria, whooping cough, and tetanus. The scourge of smallpox has been effectively eliminated thanks to a vaccine. American children are supposed to be routinely immunized against the leading contagious diseases—and for the most part they are. According to recent estimates, 79 percent of preschoolers have now received the complete vaccination series.

Yet as long as even a few cases of disease occur within a population, people who are not immunized are at risk of contracting it. Moreover, when immunization coverage drops, diseases can return with a vengeance, as has happened with whooping cough and measles. Therefore, the success of vaccination efforts should not lull parents and guardians into a false sense of security. Continued vaccination efforts are essential to ward off a host of common contagious bacterial and viral childhood illnesses that in many cases cannot be effectively treated with drugs or other therapies.

How immunization works. Vaccines create immunity by boosting the body's natural immune response. Most vaccines contain components of infective microorganisms or toxins that have been markedly weakened so that they are no longer capable of causing disease. When these vaccines are injected (or taken orally in the case of some types of polio vaccine), the immune system's cells recognize the invading pathogen and mount an immune response against it. If a vaccinated person is later naturally exposed to these infectious agents, the body has been primed to mount an immune response that effectively prevents disease.

Some vaccines afford lifelong immunity. Others require regular booster doses, often at 10-year intervals. While no vaccine is 100 percent effective, most provide protection for the vast majority of those vaccinated. Even in children who do

519

later develop a clinical illness, symptoms are usually mild and the duration of illness short.

The argument for immunization. Concerns linger about vaccinations, and some people are reluctant to have their children (and themselves) immunized. The concern has in part been fueled by media reports of dangerous reactions to particular vaccines, such as the swine flu scare of 1976-77, which might have caused rare cases of Guillain-Barre syndrome, or older pertussis vaccines that might have been associated with convulsions. Some people believe that vaccination is unnecessary, since once-common childhood contagious illnesses are now so rare. But as experience continues to show, when vaccination levels in a community drop (to below 70 percent or so), outbreaks of disease are likely to occur. In children who have not been immunized, disease may be severe and sometimes fatal.

Today's vaccines are safe and effective. Such groups as the American Academy of Pediatrics, the American College of Physicians, and the Centers for Disease Control and Prevention (CDC) concur that the enormous benefits of vaccination greatly outweigh the small potential risks. This does not mean that the adverse effects from vaccines have been eliminated; rather, the chances of a severe reaction occurring are extremely slim. For most individuals as well as for the society at large, the benefits of immunization far outweigh the risks.

The key recommendations and guidelines for childhood vaccinations are given below.

Diphtheria. A disease that typically produces a severe sore throat, diphtheria is spread by airborne bacteria that release toxins that in turn can attack the heart and other internal organs. Because of widespread immunization with a toxoid vaccine, diphtheria has almost disappeared in the United States, but recent outbreaks among unvaccinated individuals in the United States and elsewhere (especially Russia) have renewed fears that diphtheria may reemerge as a public health threat.

Vaccination with inactivated diphtheria toxin is very effective in preventing or limiting the severity of the disease. Initially, five doses are typically given in conjunction with tetanus toxoid and pertussis vaccine. A booster dose of diphtheria and tetanus toxoids should be given at age 11 to 12, and then every 10 years.

Tetanus. Also known as lockjaw, tetanus is now rare in the United States because of effective immunization programs with tetanus toxoid. Still, despite the dramatic increase in vaccinations, about 50 cases are diagnosed each year in the United States, most of them in older people. In developing countries where vaccination is uncommon, tetanus accounts for a million deaths annually, half of those in newborns and young children.

The bacterium that causes tetanus usually enters the body through a contaminated wound and can cause painful muscular contractions, often starting with a stiff neck and difficulty opening the mouth (lockjaw), which may prove fatal. Infants should receive diphtheria-tetanus-pertussis (DTP) vaccine at two, four, and six months of age, with a fourth dose at 12 to 18 months and a fifth at four to six years of age. A booster of tetanus and diphtheria toxoids is recommended at 11 to 12 years of age if five years or more have elapsed since the last dose of DTP. Booster doses should be continued every 10 years.

Pertussis (whooping cough). Pertussis, or whooping cough, is now fairly uncommon in the United States, although outbreaks occur from time to time in communities where vaccination levels are low. Vaccination is important, because infection with the whooping cough bacterium causes severe coughing fits and can be fatal, particularly in infants younger than six months.

As noted above, the pertussis vaccine is typically combined with the diphtheria and tetanus toxoids (DTP) and given as a five-shot series at two, four, and six months of age, 12 to 18 months, and four to six years. It prevents whooping cough in most of those who receive it, and the remaining recipients have a milder and shorter course of the disease.

There was concern about the safety of older pertussis vaccines, which caused many side effects, including seizures in susceptible people. But serious reactions were rare, and many health experts argued for continued vaccination.

The most convincing evidence for continued widespread use of the vaccine showed up in the late 1970s, when routine vaccination declined in Great Britain and Japan as a result of vaccine scares. Within two years, 100,000 cases of pertussis (with 28 deaths) appeared in Great Britain and 13,000 cases (with 41 deaths) in Japan.

Moreover, newer generations of pertussis vaccine have been developed and are safer. The vaccine may cause soreness at the injection site or mild fever, but these effects subside quickly.

Some public health experts have argued that additional booster doses of pertussis vaccine should be given to adolescents and young adults as well to assure continuing immunity, since mild whooping cough in older adults is often the cause of severe infection in infants. This issue is under study.

Polio. Prior to the introduction of Jonas Salk's inactivated polio vaccine (IPV) in 1955, followed by the Sabin oral polio vaccine (OPV) in 1961, tens of thousands of cases of paralytic polio occurred each year in the United States. Mass vaccination programs against the polio virus have proven spectacularly effective. The last natural case of polio occurred in the United States in 1979, and the last case in the Western Hemisphere in 1991. Efforts are under way to eliminate the disease globally in the near future.

Vaccination can be accomplished with either OPV or IPV, which uses a killed virus and needs to be injected subcutaneously (under the skin). Until recently, a vaccination schedule utilizing two shots of IPV followed by two doses of OPV was generally recommended. In 2000, however, the government's Advisory Committee on Immunization Practices recommended that routine vaccination be done entirely with IPV because OPV can, very rarely, cause polio (a condition referred to as vaccine-associated paralytic polio, or VAPP). Individuals receiving OPV are at risk, as are people with whom the recipients come into close contact (because live virus is sometimes shed by vaccinees). Since the risk of getting polio in the United States is extremely low, experts believe that using oral vaccine is no longer worth even the slight risk of VAPP.

All children, therefore, should receive four shots of IPV at ages two months, four months, six to eighteen months, and four to six years. OPV, if available, should be used only in special circumstances, such as outbreaks of paralytic polio or with children of parents who don't accept the recommended number of IPV injections (and who should be made aware of the risk for VAPP).

Hemophilus influenzae type B. Routine vaccination of children with *Hemophilus influenzae* type B (HiB) vaccine is important to avoid infection with this harmful bacterium, which can cause potentially fatal brain infections (meningitis), throat swelling (epiglottitis), pneumonia, and other complications. Doses are given at two, four, and

521

ROUTINE CHILDHOOD VACCINATION SCHEDULE

The chart below outlines recommended vaccinations for infants and children. *Age guidelines are approximate* (see pages 519-525 for more detail). Children can safely be vaccinated with most vaccines at a later age than indicated; consult your doctor. Also let your doctor know if your child has any of the following:

• Fever or infection.

• A medical condition that requires your child to take steroids or impairs your child's immune system.

• A bad reaction to a vaccine in the past.

• A history of seizures or other nervous system disorders.

Your doctor may decide to delay or modify the vaccination schedule until a particular condition clears up or changes.

Be sure to keep a record of current and future vaccinations.

Possible side effects. It is not unusual for vaccines to cause mild and fleeting side effects, most commonly low fever, redness or soreness at the injection site, or muscle or joint aches. Most clear up within a day or so. But more serious adverse reactions do occasionally occur. Call your doctor if your child exhibits any of the following signs or symptoms after vaccination:

• A fever of 104°F or higher, with or without convulsions.

• Crying that persists more than a few hours.

• Persistent sleepiness, lethargy, limpness, or paleness.

	DTP (diphtheria, tetanus, pertussis)	Polio (IPV)	HiB (*Hemophilus influenzae* type B)	MMR (measles, mumps, rubella)	Chicken Pox (varicella zoster)	Hepatitis B	Pneumococcal Conjugate
Birth						X	
1 month						X	
2 months	X	X	X				X
4 months	X	X	X				X
6 months	X		X			X	X
12 to 18 months	X	X*	X**	X**	X		X**
4 to 6 years	X	X		X			
11 to 12 years	X			X***		X****	

*6 to 18 mos **12 to 15 mos ***if second dose was not given previously ****if vaccination was not given during infancy six months of age, with a fourth dose given at 12 to 15 months. Side effects are minor and include redness at the injection site and/or mild fever.

Measles. Once a common childhood illness with potentially devastating consequences, measles is now fairly uncommon. The introduction of the measles vaccine in the 1960s and its subsequent widespread use has prevented millions of cases of the disease as well as thousands of deaths and cases of mental retardation due to such complications as infection of the brain with the measles virus.

In the late 1980s, measles cases began to increase in the United States, with a number of outbreaks among college students. Apparently, the single dose of vaccine given to these young adults as children was not providing adequate and lasting immunity. As a result, the U. S. Public Health Service (USPHS) now recommends that young adults born after 1957 be revaccinated, and that two doses of measles vaccine now be given routinely to children. The first dose is given at 12 to 15 months of age, and the second is routinely recommended for 4 to 6 years of age (when children are entering kindergarten or first grade). But the second dose can be administered earlier, provided at least four weeks have elapsed since receiving the first dose. Children who have not received the second dose should do so by age 10 or 11. The vaccine is usually given as the MMR vaccine, offering protection against measles, mumps, and rubella.

Because measles can be very severe in infants, vaccination is recommended for those as young as six months if there is a high risk that they might contract the disease; for example, during a community outbreak or travel to exotic locales. Children vaccinated before their first birthday should be revaccinated at 15 months and again when they enter school.

The vaccine is effective and safe.

Mumps. Mumps is a viral infection of the salivary glands causing swelling ("chipmunk cheeks") and fever. Like measles, it was once a common disease of childhood. Its symptoms include headache and a variable fever, followed by swelling of one or both salivary glands. Only a couple of thousand cases now occur each year in the United States, thanks to the effectiveness of the MMR vaccine. Most cases occur in school-age children, though about a third occur in adolescents and adults. In older persons the disease may be more severe, with a greater likelihood of serious complications such as inflammation of the testes (which rarely can cause sterility), deafness, or infection of the brain.

Mumps vaccine should be given routinely to children (as MMR vaccine) at 12 to 15 months, with a second dose at school entry (though it can be given earlier). The vaccine is safe and effective. Occasionally, a child will have a mild allergic reaction marked by soreness or redness at the inoculation site.

Rubella (German measles). Initially, rubella, or German measles, causes only a few days of fever and rash, but it can cause devastating congenital defects or miscarriage if it occurs in a pregnant woman, particularly during the early stages of pregnancy. In 1964, during the last rubella epidemic in the United States, tens of thousands of newborns suffered from heart defects, blindness, and deafness as a result of the disease. Since then, congenital rubella infection has been virtually eliminated in the United States, due to the effectiveness of the MMR vaccine. Children should be vaccinated at 12 to 15 months of age and again at school entry.

Chicken pox. Although a chicken pox vaccine

523

has been available in the United States since 1995, many parents and doctors opt to forgo vaccination. Some believe that natural chicken pox infection offers better and longer-lasting immunity than the vaccine does, and that youngsters who are vaccinated are at risk for more serious complications if the effects of the vaccine wear off and they subsequently contract chicken pox as adults. But the vaccine has been in use for many years in Japan, and studies continue to show that concerns about its safety and effectiveness are unfounded. The vaccine can also help to prevent rare but serious complications like Group A streptococcal infection.

Similar reluctance was seen with the introduction of the mumps vaccine in 1968, but that vaccine is now widely used. Public health officials remain concerned that some—but not enough—children are being immunized, raising the likelihood that outbreaks of chicken pox will increasingly occur in older age groups, in whom complications may be more serious. The current recommendation is that all babies be vaccinated between the ages of 12 and 18 months, and that older children who haven't had chicken pox be vaccinated by age 13. (Children that age who may be susceptible because they weren't previously immunized and/or haven't had chickenpox should receive two doses at least four weeks apart.)

Hepatitis. Hepatitis B is caused by a virus that often lingers in the body for decades before causing actual illness, including potentially fatal liver disease (hepatitis or cirrhosis) and liver cancer. The virus is not easily transmitted. A person must have contact with infected blood or bodily secretions (such as during sexual relations) to become infected, and only sometimes will a chronic infection occur. It is estimated that more than 200 million people worldwide carry the hepatitis B virus, and that as many as 300,000 Americans each year acquire the disease (see page 324).

Hepatitis B vaccination is recommended for all newborns in order to give children lifelong protection against the virus. (Vaccination is also recommended for certain adults who are considered at high risk for hepatitis B. These include health-care workers, injection drug users, and sexually active people who are not monogamous.)

Three doses of vaccine are given. In infants, the first injection is given within 12 hours of birth, the second at one month of age, and the third at six months of age. Some studies suggest that better protection may be provided by giving the third dose at 12 months of age instead. Children who did not receive three doses of hepatitis B vaccine as infants should be vaccinated when they are 11 to 12 years old.

A vaccine is also available for hepatitis A, a less serious form of infection from which most people recover completely. The vaccine is recommended only for certain people at high risk, including children over age two who will be traveling to areas where hepatitis A is common, and children living in communities with a high rate of hepatitis A. (Information on rates of hepatitis A can be obtained from your local public health authority.)

Pneumococcal disease. Pneumococcal disease causes many health problems in young children, including meningitis, blood infections, and, most commonly, ear infections (about five million each year). The bacterium that causes it—*Streptococcus pneumoniae* (also known as the pneumococcus)—is spread from person to person through close contact, and the resulting infections can be difficult to treat because the organism has become resistant to some of the drugs used to treat it. Fortunately, a pneumococcal vaccine is now available that can prevent the disease in young children. (A vaccine for adults has been available for some time—see page 407.) The vaccine for children—called pneumococcal conjugate vaccine—offers protection for at least three years, and so will protect children during their first two years of life, when they are at greatest risk for serious illness.

All healthy infants and toddlers should get four doses of the vaccine: one dose at two months of age, then repeated at four months, six months, and twelve to fifteen months. The vaccine is also recommended for children between ages two and five who have diseases that affect the immune system, such as HIV, diabetes, or cancer.

CHILDREN AND SAFETY

Injury experts do not like to use the word *accident,* since it suggests that the event just happens out of the blue or is an act of fate. To them, most injuries are preventable and occur in predictable patterns—and thus are no accident.

Children, in particular, are at great risk from injuries, and when they are injured, their wounds can be devastating. They are also at risk for poisoning. Often they playfully emulate adults, which sometimes leads to serious or even fatal results when medications are accessible.

For children as for adults, a disproportionate number of injuries are associated with stressful life events, such as the arrival of a new baby, divorce, death of a family member, or marriage of a parent. The effect of stress is cumulative, so during a period of multiple stressful events, it's especially important to be on guard against childhood injuries.

Learning to foresee "accidents" is the best way to prevent them. If you have children in your household, or if children visit you often, there are many steps you should take to childproof your home.

• *Remove all hazardous substances from the kitchen and dining areas;* do not keep them in old food containers. Almost 75 percent of poisonings involve kids under five, who mistake household cleaners for beverages, for instance, or medicine for candy. Store paints, lacquers, and other toxic substances in locked cabinets. Keep all medicine, including aspirin and other over-the-counter drugs, in containers with safety caps. Better yet, keep drugs out of sight and/or locked up. That advice also applies to dietary supplements: vitamin and mineral pills, especially iron pills and children's vitamins shaped like cartoon characters, are a leading cause of poisoning.

Flush all old medications down the toilet instead of throwing them away in the garbage where children or pets may find them.

• *When bathing a small child,* test water temperature by putting your whole hand in the water and moving it around for several seconds; if it feels even slightly hot, it's too hot for your child. Don't leave a small child alone in the water for even a few seconds, since she can turn on the hot water. A child can also drown in a tub, even in shallow water.

• *Keep electrical appliances away from a filled tub or sink.* Unplug bathroom appliances after using them: they can cause electrocution if they are plugged in and fall into water, even if they are turned off. *To prevent severe or lethal shocks, install ground-fault circuit interrupters in outlets in the bathroom and kitchen.*

• *Install slip-proof padded carpets* at the foot of all staircases.

• *Be aware of hazards* to a child left alone in a playpen, high chair, or crib. For instance, a string of toys across the top of a playpen can strangle a child, and fingers can get stuck in hinges. A baby can slip out of a high chair in a minute, or topple over if it's unstable.

In a crib, if there's too much room between the mattress and side of the crib, an infant's head can get caught in between and he could suffocate. Get a mattress that fits the crib; otherwise, place bumper pads or rolled-up bath towels in the space. Don't place cribs or playpens near windows.

Remember, hand-me-down cribs may not meet current safety standards. *Use only cribs approved by the U. S. Consumer Product Safety Commission,* an independent federal regulatory agency that develops and enforces safety standards for thousands of consumer products.

• ***Don't use a walker.*** Walkers for babies cause more injuries than any other baby product. In a walker, the baby can scoot down a flight of stairs, into a table edge, or into a glass door. And an unstable walker can tip over.

• ***Surround swimming pools*** with high fences and locking gates. This is the law in many localities.

• ***Replace an automatic garage door*** that does not reverse if it lowers onto a person or object.

• ***Keep portable heaters*** away from play areas—and away from curtains and furniture.

TRANSPORTATION SAFETY

• **Children in cars should ride in the back seat,** in proper safety seats or restraints, until they are old enough and big enough to use seat belts, usually after the age of 12. This protects them from being struck by an air bag, which can deploy at 150 to 200 miles per hour—fast enough to seriously injure or even kill a child (or a small adult). Younger children should also be in a safety seat that has them facing backwards.

A child riding in the front seat should be at least 4 feet 11 inches tall, able to put his or her feet on the car floor, and able to wear a seat belt so that it fits across the shoulder and chest. (All states require the use of safety seats or restraints for children.)

• **Infants and small children should ride in proper safety seats.** Older kids—40 to 65 pounds—can use a booster seat and a seat belt. Never place a child safety seat in the front seat, especially if you have a passenger-side air bag. (Some new cars may offer the option of disengaging the air bag—but a child is still safer in the back seat.)

• **Any seat belt is better than no belt.** If your rear seat has shoulder straps, you can buy the kind of booster seat that raises your child so that the shoulder strap crosses the chest. If the rear seat has only lap belts, choose a booster seat that has a harness or shield.

• **Make sure children wear helmets.** The fact that fewer than 10 percent of children wear helmets when bicycling is one reason why three out of four child-bicyclist deaths involve head injuries. Children should wear helmets not only when cycling but also when riding scooters, on horseback, in-line skating, rock climbing, and playing sports such as football, baseball, and hockey. Helmets may be certified by various testing organizations. For instance, look for a bike helmet with a sticker from ANSI (American National Standards Institute) or the Snell Memorial Foundation. Set a good example by wearing a helmet yourself.

• *Use care when cooking.* Put pans on rear burners. Turn pot handles toward the back of the stove. Keep hot foods away from the edge of tables and counters and not on a tablecloth that a small child can grab.

• *Don't smoke.* Adults' cigarettes are a leading cause of childhood burns.

• *Keep disposable lighters out of the reach* of young children. These lighters are easy to use, and kids may be attracted by their bright colors. About 140 youngsters under the age of five die each year as a result of playing with such lighters.

• *Keep toothpicks out of the reach* of children under age five, because of the risk of injury to an eye or ear.

• *If you keep a gun in your home,* keep it locked up and unloaded, and store the bullets in a separate location. Buy a trigger lock or other device to prevent accidental shootings. Every year about 3,000 American children and teenagers die as a result of gunfire—intentionally (homicides and suicides) or unintentionally. Most of these shootings involve handguns. Kids may play with guns because they resemble toys; few children have been taught how to handle guns safely.

• *Don't let children use a microwave oven* without supervision, and be careful with microwaved baby formula. Microwaved foods get very hot quickly and may feel only warm on the outside, but be scalding inside. Microwaved coffee can be boiling while the mug is cool. Most important, your baby's formula can be scalding, though the bottle is merely warm to your touch. Use the old arm test before giving an infant microwaved formula—the baby can't react to hot liquid until it's too late.

• *Maintain swings, slides, and other outdoor play equipment* and make sure they are in safe condition. Install matting or other soft material on the ground.

• *Install window guards.* Don't depend on screens to prevent kids from falling out of windows—screens aren't strong enough. Make sure the bars are not fixed in place, but rather can be easily removed from a window in case of fire.

• *Don't let kids play with plastic bags of any kind.*

• *Keep your eye on toy balloons.* During a 15-year period, 121 American children suffocated after inhaling balloons. Don't let young kids blow them up on their own; don't let kids chew or suck on balloons.

• *Choose safe toys.* For small children, avoid toys with sharp edges or points, brittle materials, small removable parts, projectiles, poorly constructed electrical components, or cords or strings. Look for age recommendations.

• *Don't let kids play with discarded refrigerators and deep freezers,* since they can get trapped inside. Remove the doors immediately.

LEAD POISONING

Though lead in exterior and interior house paints was banned in 1978, more than 24 million homes in the United States are at risk of lead paint hazards, which are by far the most common source of lead poisoning for children. Much progress has been made in reducing exposure to lead, but nearly one million American children have lead levels in their blood high enough to risk impairing their mental abilities as well as their physical growth and stature.

Older oil-based paints were particularly heavily leaded and may flake or peel off and be swallowed by children. Paints that are in good condition or that have been painted over with lead-free paints are not a problem, unless painted surfaces rub together and create dust (as on window frames). Remodeling that involves removing leaded paint, particularly by chipping or

527

sanding the paint, can be extremely hazardous and should be done by experts.

Because any kind of dust, especially paint dust, may contain lead, it's important to keep a child's environment as dust-free as possible. Clean windowsills and floors frequently with detergent and water. Make sure children wash their hands before eating. Keep kids from chewing on painted objects. If you're not sure the paint on an old toy is lead-free, dispose of it.

The American Academy of Pediatrics recommends screening all children for blood lead levels. If a child is at high risk (for example, lives in old housing), the first screening should be done at the age of six months. The interval for rescreening will depend on the results of the first test. Children at low risk should be screened at 12 months and retested at age two. Children with low blood levels need not be tested again.

If your child's test shows lead levels of 10 micrograms per deciliter or higher, you will need help from your physician and the health department to track down the lead sources and correct the problem.

For more information on handling lead hazards, including advice on removing old paint, you can call the Department of Housing and Urban Development (HUD) at 202-708-0685 or go to their Web site, which has an area devoted to lead hazards (at www.hud.gov/offices/lead/index.cfm). Another source is the National Lead Information Clearinghouse hotline (800-424-LEAD).

ADOLESCENTS
(Puberty to 19)

Teenage bodies undergo dramatic changes, though the rate at which adolescents mature varies markedly from person to person. Many boys grow three to four inches in a year, for example, while some grow twice that amount. It is both realistic and reassuring to think of a range when assessing what is a "normal" indicator of a teenager's development—from the onset of adult sexual characteristics to the sudden appearance of skin blemishes (see Acne, page 142). The following milestones are based on averages and general recommendations; they should be viewed as a guide rather than a rigid standard.

CHANGES IN GIRLS

The onset of sexual maturation in girls usually begins about two years earlier than it does in boys. The process of puberty can take anywhere from two to six years and can begin anytime between ages 8 and 14. (If a girl begins developing before age 8, puberty is considered to be premature, and a doctor should be consulted.)

• *An increase in height* usually begins at age 10 to 11 and continues to age 15 to 16. If a noticeable increase in height has not started by age 15, consult a physician.

• *Breast development* usually begins at age 10 to 11, but it may start as early as 8 or may not occur until age 14 or 15. One breast may start to develop before the other. If noticeable breast development doesn't begin by age 16, consult a physician.

• *The emergence of body hair* usually begins in

the pubic area about the same time as breast development, usually starting at age 10 or 11 but sometimes not occurring until age 13 or 14. Underarm and leg hair appears a year to two later. In general the color, thickness, and pattern of body hair is quite variable.

• *Menstrual periods* usually begin between ages 11 and 14, about one year after breasts begin to develop, although periods may not occur until ages 15 to 17. If menstruation begins before age 10, or has not begun by age 17, or if periods are irregular, a physician should be consulted.

On average, a menstrual period occurs every 28 days and lasts 4 days, although periods occurring 23 to 35 days apart and lasting 2 to 7 days are still considered normal. Painful menstrual cramps, or dysmenorrhea, are unusual during the first year or two of menstruation but may occur in later adolescence.

During the first year or two after menarche (the first menstrual period), an adolescent girl may experience irregular periods, skipping one or many months between periods. It can take a while for the hypothalamus, the part of the brain that regulates reproduction, to coordinate the release of the various hormones that control the menstrual cycle. This is quite common and is not cause for concern. However, it is possible for pregnancy to occur any time after menarche, so sexually active teenage girls need birth control, and a missed period in a sexually active girl should not be ignored.

A certain amount of body fat appears to be necessary for menstruation to occur, and some young female athletes, such as gymnasts or ballet dancers, have so little body fat that menstruation is delayed. This is not harmful as long as menstruation begins by age 16. After that, a failure to menstruate can indicate a lower-than-nor-

STRONG BONES: NOW IS THE TIME

The more bone you build early in life, the better you will be able to withstand the bone loss that starts to occur by about age 35. Years later, the loss of bone mass can result in the debilitating disease called osteoporosis. To develop bone mass, you need to make weight-bearing exercise part of your daily life—with activities like walking, running, and weight lifting.

The mineral calcium also plays a crucial role in building strong bones and maintaining bone density. Older children and adolescents (ages 9 to 18) should consume at least 1,300 milligrams of calcium a day. Low-fat or nonfat dairy products are the best source, but many other foods can supply calcium (see pages 23-24).

529

mal level of estrogen, which can contribute to thinning and weakening of bones.

• *An increase in weight and body fat* begins at ages 10 to 11, when female hormones trigger an increase in fat in the breasts, hips, thighs, and buttocks. Fat makes up about 25 percent of total body weight in girls, compared to 15 to 20 percent in boys.

If body weight does not increase, or if it increases and then drops, consult your physician, since this may be an indication of an eating disorder or another medical problem.

• *The development of sweat glands,* which are responsible for increased perspiration, usually begins at age 12 to 13. These glands can cause underarm odor (which is not present in young children).

CHANGES IN BOYS

Growth in teenage boys occurs in spurts, generally over four to five years. The first growth spurt may start anytime between ages 10 and 14. Outside that age range, puberty is either delayed or premature. The following changes occur in a boy's physical development.

• *An increase in height* usually begins at age 12 or 13 and continues until age 17 or 18. (If some visible growth has not occurred by age 15, consult your doctor.)

• *Body hair appears,* usually beginning in the pubic area at ages 11 to 12. Hair is first visible on skin around the base of the penis, then thickens and extends to the scrotum. Underarm hair subsequently develops at age 13 to 15, along with the first appearance of facial hair (which generally develops more slowly than other body hair). The color, pattern, and thickness of body hair varies considerably from person to person.

• *The testicles, penis, and scrotum enlarge,* starting at about age 12 to 13. The skin of the scrotum and penis also darkens, and about a year after the penis begins to lengthen, most boys are able to ejaculate semen for the first time. Genital growth is usually completed by age 17.

• *The larynx, or voice box,* begins to grow at age 13 or 14; approximately a year later the voice begins to deepen. (If the voice has not deepened by age 16, consult a physician).

• *The development of sweat glands,* which are responsible for increased perspiration, usually begins at ages 13 to 15. These glands can cause underarm odor (which is not present in younger children).

LIFESTYLE HABITS
AFFECTING ADOLESCENTS

Teenagers are intent on experimenting, and sometimes this entails adopting lifestyle habits that seem attractive to them—either because adults who are role models embrace the habit, or because a teenager wants to be included in a particular group of peers. Also, some habits can produce pleasurable sensations without any apparent ill effects. But several lifestyle habits that appeal widely to adolescents are also bad for their health.

Tobacco. At least 3,000 young Americans (age 11 to 20) become established smokers every day. Cigarette smoking among high school students is more prevalent today —by about 27 percent— than it was at the beginning of the 1990s, according to a nationwide survey on adolescent health by the Centers for Disease Control and Prevention (CDC). People who start smoking when they are teenagers (which is when most smokers take up the habit) and continue to smoke are five times more likely to have a heart attack in their 30s or 40s than nonsmokers. Smoking will also make your teeth yellow and your breath smell bad, and it will prematurely wrinkle your skin. It's certainly best not to start—but if you have started, the sooner you quit, the easier quitting will be. (For tips on quitting, see page 39.)

Substance abuse. The use of alcohol is widespread among teenagers: in the CDC survey cited above, half of those surveyed reported consuming alcohol in the previous 30 days. Nearly a third of the students—including 28 percent of the women—said that, during the same period, they had engaged in binge drinking (consuming more than five drinks on one occasion). A third of them also reported that they had first consumed alcohol (more than a few sips) before age 13.

The use of illicit drugs, after a temporary drop in the early 1990s, may be on the increase, according to the survey. About 47 percent of high school students reported that they had used marijuana— and more than 25 percent had used it recently one or more times. (In a 1990 survey, by contrast, only 31 percent reported ever having used marijuana.) About 4 percent of the respondents in the 1999 study reported using some form of cocaine; less than 2 percent reported cocaine use in 1991.

Of course, not all teenagers who experiment with alcohol or marijuana use these substances regularly or go on to experiment with harder drugs. But for those who do, drinking excessive amounts of alcohol and using illicit drugs can harm the cardiovascular and respiratory systems. These substances can also interfere with proper growth and development in adolescents, whose bodies are not completely mature.

In addition, even occasionally using alcohol or drugs can cause a teen to participate in activities that he or she might normally avoid, because these substances alter a person's perception and judgment. Fights, accidents, and unplanned or unprotected sexual intercourse are more common among teenagers who drink alcohol or use drugs than those who don't.

Sun abuse. A suntan may look healthy—but sun exposure is the leading cause of wrinkles. It also increases the risk of skin cancer. Teenagers should take the same precautions that adults do: don't sunbathe for extended periods, and take steps—including the use of a sunscreen—to protect skin when in the sun (see page 55).

Unhealthful eating patterns. As with adults, the key to healthy eating for adolescents is variety—of the sort suggested by the U.S. Department of Agriculture food pyramid illustrated on page 19. However, growing teens often need more calories than adults, especially if they are active in sports. As a result, it is common for teenagers to snack, and indeed parents should encourage snacking. The problem is that adolescents, studies have shown, tend to eat a good deal of junk food—sweets or meals from fast-food restaurants that are high in fat and low in fiber, vitamins, and minerals. Parents can help by serving well-balanced meals at home and by stocking the kitchen with healthy snacks that include fruit, yogurt, low-fat chips, and unbuttered popcorn. It's also important not to skip meals, since this can easily lead to snacking on junk foods.

Physical inactivity and obesity. Nearly half of all American youths between 12 and 21 years old get no vigorous exercise on a regular basis. Engaging in physical activity drops dramatically with age—73 percent of ninth graders get some form of regular exercise, compared to only 61 percent of twelfth graders, according to data from the Centers for Disease Control and Prevention (CDC). One result of declining physical activity among young Americans, coupled with the consumption of high-fat fast foods, is that the percentage of adolescents who are overweight has nearly doubled during the past twenty years. Like adults, young people can benefit from a moderate amount of physical activity. And increasingly, it falls to families and friends to encourage this: many overweight children do not have access to comprehensive weight-loss programs, and participation in school physical education programs has dropped significantly during the past decade.

Eating disorders. Some young women become focused on being as thin as fashion models—even though few adult women develop a model's figure naturally. Watching your weight so as not to become overweight is fine. But be aware of how much you should realistically weigh (see page 36). Half of all white adolescent girls think they are overweight when, in fact, their weight is normal, according to a National Health and Nutrition

531

PREVENTIVE SERVICES RECOMMENDATIONS

The following table highlights the major screening tests (that is, routine tests for people without symptoms) and immunizations for healthy adolescents. This advice is based in part on the recommendations of the U.S. Preventive Services Task Force. (*Pregnant women need other kinds of professional preventive care that are not covered here.*)

PREVENTIVE SCREENINGS AND CHECKUPS

FOR WOMEN

Pelvic exam: Every adolescent girl should have a pelvic examination at age 18 or when she becomes sexually active, whichever comes first. After that, pelvic exams should be performed annually. In between regular visits, young women should see a doctor if any of the following occur:

- Missing a menstrual period for the first time.
- Unusually heavy or painful periods.
- Vaginal spotting (intermittent bleeding between periods) or heavy bleeding.
- Pain in the lower back, abdomen, or vagina that worsens while menstruating.

Pap smear (for detecting cervical cancer): The Pap smear is a simple test to detect cervical cancer—which, because it develops far more slowly than most other cancers, is almost 100 percent curable if detected early. A woman should have a Pap smear when she turns 18 or becomes sexually active. Thereafter, she should have a Pap smear at least every three years and possibly more often, depending on risk factors for cervical cancer, such as smoking and/or multiple sex partners. (Not all authorities agree on how often to have a Pap smear—see page 74.)

IMMUNIZATION

Tetanus-diphtheria booster: This should be given between the ages of 11 and 14, and every 10 years thereafter.

Hepatitis B vaccine: If not already vaccinated, adolescents should receive three doses of hepatitis B vaccine. (For a description of hepatitis B, see page 325.)

Varicella chicken pox vaccine: If an adolescent has not had chicken pox by age 13, getting vaccinated is important, since the illness is more serious in adolescents and adults than in young children. For those who aren't sure if they have had the disease, a blood test is available.

532

Examination Survey. (African-American children of both sexes and white boys were much less likely to have such misperceptions.)

In some cases, being thin becomes an obsession and leads to the eating disorders anorexia and bulimia. Combined, these conditions affect about 4 percent of adolescent and young women. Anorexia is self-starvation to the point that a woman's weight is at least 15 percent below average for her height. People with anorexia often simply stop eating, sometimes consuming as few as 100 calories a day. They tend to be obsessed with food composition and calorie counting and may consider only low-calorie foods, such as raw vegetables, acceptable to eat. They often deny feelings of hunger and fatigue and have an unrealistic image of their bodies, thinking they are fat when they are actually quite thin, even emaciated.

Bulimia is often called the "binge and purge" disease. People with this condition eat large amounts of food at one sitting, often very quickly and in secret, and then vomit or use laxatives to get rid of the extra calories. Others exercise obsessively to stay thin. The bingeing and purging is often accompanied by feelings of guilt and depression. This condition is more prevalent than anorexia among young women. (Bulimia also occurs more in men than anorexia does—though both are far less common in men than in women.)

In some cases these disorders develop because a young woman participates in an activity that values extreme thinness—gymnastics, ballet, or ice skating, for example. In other cases the eating disorder is a manifestation of underlying psychological issues, including low self-esteem, poor self-image, family problems, stress, or feelings of not being in control.

Signs of eating disorders include unusual weight loss; preoccupation with food; peculiar eating habits; and menstruation that ceases for three or more consecutive months. It is more difficult to spot someone with bulimia, compared to anorexia, since people with bulimia typically maintain a normal weight and tend to do their bingeing and purging in secret.

Both anorexia and bulimia have serious consequences and in extreme cases cause death. About 20 percent of people with anorexia die because of complications related to the disorder. The vomiting that occurs with bulimia can erode tooth enamel; cause electrolyte imbalances that can lead to kidney or heart abnormalities; or rupture the stomach or esophagus. The disorders are also difficult to treat, often because the person denies that anything is wrong and hides the behavior from friends and family. Nutritional and psychological counseling are required. The earlier treatment is begun, the better the chances for recovery.

STDs and birth control. Contrary to what many adults may believe, the majority of adolescents who are sexually experienced use some method of contraception to protect themselves and their partners from unintended pregnancy and sexually transmitted diseases (STDs). But for adolescents who do not use contraceptives, or don't use them effectively or consistently, the consequences can be serious, especially for teenage girls.

Every year an estimated three million teenagers are infected with an STD, and between 900,000 and one million teenagers become pregnant—nearly all of them unintentionally. Older teenagers, African-Americans, and teenagers who are poor are more likely to get pregnant than those who are younger, white, and better off economically. Yet the rates of certain STDs—especially genital herpes—has increased dramatically among white teenagers in recent years.

533

Teenagers who are in a sexual relationship or intend to become sexually active should be aware of the different birth control options available (see the following section). They should also take steps to protect themselves against STDs (see page 57)—first and foremost by using latex condoms. (Nonlatex condoms do not provide protection against STDs.) Adolescent girls may be more likely to contract a sexually-related cervical infection than older women, since their cervixes have not undergone age-related developmental changes.

(If you have symptoms of an STD or you suspect that an infection has occurred, contact a doctor. The index on page 141 in "Ailments and Disorders" can guide you to information about specific STDs.)

YOUNG ADULTS
(20 to 39)

For most Americans, these are years of relatively good health. With the exception of pregnancy, men's and women's bodies don't change much physiologically, and health concerns are often focused on sexuality, reproduction, and accident prevention. Today, many Americans postpone marriage and often have more than one sex partner before they do get married. Once married, they often postpone having children. Consequently, choosing a method of birth control is a major concern, as is preventing sexually transmitted diseases (STDs).

Once a couple has decided to have a child, the concern shifts to wanting to ensure a healthy pregnancy. Each of these issues is outlined below, with the latest recommendations and guidelines. Other health concerns that tend to arise during this stage of life are also noted. (The section on pregnancy is intended to convey some key points about having a healthy pregnancy; anyone who is pregnant or planning to become pregnant should consult additional sources.)

During these years it can be tempting to ignore general health practices, since the consequences of doing so—of being sedentary, for example, or of eating a diet full of fatty foods—may not be immediate. You are unlikely to die in your 20s or 30s from a lack of exercise. But sooner or later unhealthy habits will have an impact on most people's health, often starting with excess weight gain. This stage of life is an ideal time to begin taking an active approach to improving and maintaining your health—and to integrating the healthy practices covered in the section "Wellness Strategies" into your daily life (starting on page 14). Doing so will offer immediate rewards and will also prepare the way for your later years to be vital and healthy.

WOMEN: BIRTH CONTROL CHOICES

In the area of contraception, women have wider choices than men—and far more often than not, women are responsible for choosing and using contraceptives. Yet American women have more unplanned pregnancies and more abortions than women in most industrialized countries. Part of the reluctance to use contraceptives stems from a belief that those available to women pose medical risks. Also, American women have fewer choices than do women in many European countries. Because not every type of contraceptive is appropriate for every woman, nor for every stage of a woman's reproductive life, the more choices available, the more likely she is to find one she can comfortably use regularly—the only way birth control devices can be effective.

Women who are reluctant to use a medical method of birth control can, of course, use such "natural" methods as coitus interruptus (withdrawal) or periodic abstinence—known as natural family planning—based on monitoring ovulation patterns and abstaining from sex at times of fertility. These methods have a high failure rate.

In recent years a woman's choice of contraceptives has significantly widened with the introduction of two long-term and very effective hormonal methods. Norplant consists of tiny capsules that are implanted under the skin of the upper arm; they release a constant low flow of a hormone that prevents ovulation. Norplant provides protection for five years. Depo-Provera is an injection lasting about three months. Besides these new forms, improvements have been made in other methods—and users have also come to realize that some contraceptives have advantages in addition to preventing unwanted pregnancies (such as more-regular periods in the case of the birth control pill).

Aside from abstinence and coitus interruptus, there are four types of contraception:

Barrier methods. Used during intercourse, and applied prior to it, these methods prevent sperm from reaching the egg. Barrier methods include condoms, the diaphragm, and the cervical cap. (Another barrier method, the sponge, was taken off the U. S. market by the manufacturer in 1995, but a new manufacturer announced plans to resume production in 2001.) Diaphragms and cervical caps should be used in combination with spermicides. Spermicides should not be used alone because they provide limited protection against pregnancy. (The only method that effectively protects against STDs is the latex condom, used correctly and consistently—see page 58.)

Hormonal contraception. This involves modifying sex hormones to imitate the natural suppression of fertility that occurs during pregnancy and breast-feeding. Birth control pills—also called oral contraceptives, OCs, or simply the Pill—contain estrogen and a form of progesterone; they prevent ovulation. Others (the minipill) contain progesterone only and cause the cervical mucus to thicken so that the sperm cannot reach the egg. Progestin or other forms of progesterone can be delivered via implant (Norplant) or long-lasting injection (Depo-Provera).

The Pill cannot be surpassed for safety and reliability (when correctly used), and it can also make irregular periods more regular, reduce the amount of menstrual bleeding, and relieve menstrual cramps. Yet many women have had fears that the Pill increases the risk of breast cancer later in life. However, an exhaustive analysis of virtually all studies on the subject concluded that the Pill does not increase the long-term risk of breast cancer. Moreover, the Pill reduces the risk of ovarian cancer, as well as endometrial cancer. It also helps protect against ovarian cysts, pelvic inflammatory disease, and benign breast disease.

Evidence also shows that the oral contraceptives do not put healthy women at risk for heart disease or blood clots, unless they smoke. One study in *Circulation* found that low-dose pills do not increase the risk of a heart attack even in women who smoke or have another major risk factor for cardiovascular disease, such as high blood pressure. Still, the Pill is not recommended for women over 35 who smoke.

535

EMERGENCY CONTRACEPTION

Several types of oral contraceptives (OCs) can prevent pregnancy after unprotected intercourse if they are taken in sufficient doses within 72 hours. Depending on where a woman is in her menstrual cycle, the pills can prevent ovulation, disrupt fertilization by sperm, or prevent a fertilized egg from implanting itself in the uterine wall. While emergency contraception should not be considered a substitute for ongoing contraceptive methods, it can be useful in the case of contraception failure (a broken condom or displaced diaphragm), lack of access to contraception, or in the event of sexual coercion or rape.

If you need emergency OCs, you will have to contact a physician or contraceptive clinic to get the pills in the correct dose, which varies from brand to brand. Ovral, Nordette, Levlen, Lo/Ovral, Triphasil, and Ti-Levlen are OCs commonly used for this purpose. The Food and Drug Administration (FDA) has also approved two prescription kits—Preven and Plan B—especially for emergencies. The pills are safe and inexpensive (about $20 for a kit).

These pills must be taken within three days: usually one set of pills is followed by another set 12 hours later. The second dose must not be skipped. Therapy is more effective the sooner it is begun within the 72-hour time frame. (A possible side effect of high-dose OCs is nausea and vomiting, so an antinausea drug such as Dramamine is usually recommended.)

Even a woman who might not be able to use OCs regularly can take them once. If for any reason a woman cannot take estrogen, she can try another OC, or her physician can provide her with a copper IUD, another form of emergency contraception that can be utilized up to five days after intercourse. In addition, hormones similar to those in OCs can be taken by injection to achieve the same effect.

Taking emergency OCs reduces the risk of pregnancy by about 75 percent, but this does not mean that 25 out of 100 women using this method will become pregnant. If 100 women have unprotected intercourse during the middle of their menstrual cycles, about 8 will become pregnant. If those same 100 women used emergency OCs, only 2 would become pregnant (a 75 percent reduction).

For some women emergency contraceptive methods do not work. If your period does not start in two to three weeks after taking the pills, you should have a pregnancy test.

Intrauterine devices (IUDs). These small plastic devices are inserted into the uterus; how they prevent conception is not well understood. They may alter the uterine environment or inhibit the transport of sperm. Of three IUDs on the market in the United States, ParaGard is covered with copper, which seems to give it its contraceptive properties, and another, Progestasert, delivers progestin. ParaGard can remain in place for about eight years; Progestasert must be replaced annually. Recently, the Food and Drug Administration (FDA) approved a new IUD that has been used in Europe for years. Called Mirena, it's a small flexible device that releases tiny amounts of a progestin hormone and is effective for up to five years.

Surgical sterilization. For women this means tubal ligation, which involves sealing the fallopian tubes to prevent transport of the egg. (For men this means a vasectomy—see below.)

For further details on the advantages and disadvantages of each method, see the chart on pages 538-539. Except for condoms and spermicides, obtaining a contraceptive requires contacting your doctor. Be sure to talk to your doctor about the various options, and choose your contraceptive method according to your health, personal preferences, plans (if any) for future pregnancies, your sexual history, and your partner's sexual history.

MEN: BIRTH CONTROL CHOICES

Three modes of contraception are available for men, aside from abstinence. Withdrawal before ejaculation is probably the most common worldwide, but it is so ineffective that it can't be recommended. Two very different methods, condoms and vasectomies, are far more effective.

Condoms. A common argument made by those afraid of encouraging the use of condoms is that they are not foolproof, either for birth control or preventing STDs. But in addition to being an extremely effective contraceptive, condoms offer the only known effective protection against transmission of HIV (the virus that causes AIDS). Also, most of the time, condom ineffectiveness is due to human failure, not product defects. As a contraceptive, condoms are 85 to 95 percent percent effective—offering substantial, but not surefire, protection.

Failure rates vary not only from brand to brand but also from batch to batch; the user's age and experience also play a part. But you can take steps to enhance condom effectiveness. Researchers estimate that when condoms are used properly (see page 58), failure rates can be as low as 1 to 2 percent.

Vasectomy. This contraceptive method entails the severing of the tube (the vas deferens) through which sperm travel from the testicles to the penis. Vasectomy is probably the safest and most effective means of contraception—its success rate is more than 99 percent. In recent years approximately 500,000 men have been getting vasectomies annually. Fears about a possible risk of prostate cancer have convinced some men not to undergo a vasectomy. But the most rigorous studies conducted over the past decade have shown no link between vasectomy and prostate cancer. In some studies the men who had a vasectomy actually had a lower overall death rate than men without vasectomies. Vasectomy still appears to be one of the safest means of contraception.

The procedure is also fairly simple and inexpensive (and has no effect on sexual desire or sexual performance). In a new technique called no-scalpel surgery, the physician makes an incision so small it requires no stitches. Any soreness is gone in a week or two. Because some sperm remain stored in the reproductive tract, a couple should continue to use some other form of birth control until at least two sperm counts show no sperm in the semen—which usually requires 20 or more ejaculations.

Reversing a vasectomy is not nearly so simple. It usually requires general anesthesia and can cost upwards of $10,000. Moreover, it is successful less than half the time. Therefore, a man should have a vasectomy only if he is certain that he won't want children in the future.

A HEALTHY PREGNANCY

Every aspect of a woman's health takes on new meaning when she becomes pregnant, since taking care of her body will directly affect the health of the unborn child. While pregnancy has a self-

COMPARING CONTRACEPTIVES

TYPE AND ESTIMATED EFFECTIVENESS	ADVANTAGES	DISADVANTAGES	COMMENTS
Male condom (rubber, prophylactic, sheath) 85-95%	Latex condom protects against STDs, including HIV and herpes. May also offer protection against cervical cancer.	Must be applied immediately before intercourse. May break, may blunt sensation. There are rare cases of allergy to rubber.	New one must be used for each act of intercourse. No prescription.
Female condom (with spermicide) 74%	Some effectiveness against STDs, including HIV. Offers women a choice if partner refuses to use male condom. (However, no clinical studies. Not known to be as effective as male condom.)	Must be handled carefully and used correctly to avoid breakage.	New one must be used for each act of intercourse. Nonprescription.
Vaginal spermicide (used alone) 70-80%	Available over the counter as jellies, foams, creams, and suppositories. Active agent usually nonoxynol-9.	Messiness. Must be applied no more than 1 hour before intercourse. May cause rash. No protection against STDs.	Most effective against pregnancy when used with a diaphragm or cervical cap. Nonprescription.
Diaphragm (with spermicide) 82-94%	No side effects. Can be inserted up to two hours before intercourse (rather than immediately before). May protect against pelvic infections and human papilloma virus, but not HIV.	Increased risk of urinary tract infection. Rare cases of allergy to rubber. No protection against STDs.	Must be used with spermicide. Prescription.
Cervical cap (with spermicide) 82-90%	Less fragile than diaphragm; can be left in place for up to 48 hours; spermicide needn't be replaced for subsequent intercourse.	Can be hard to insert or remove; may cause unpleasant odor. Pap test required before fitting of cap. No protection against STDs.	Approved only for women with a normal Pap smear prior to use and after 3 months of use. Prescription.

538

TYPE AND ESTIMATED EFFECTIVENESS	ADVANTAGES	DISADVANTAGES	COMMENTS
Birth-control pill (oral contraceptive) 99% (combination) 97% (mini)	Most effective reversible contraceptive. Results in lighter, more regular periods. Protects against cancer of the ovaries and uterine lining. Decreases risk of pelvic inflammatory disease, fibrocystic breast disease, and benign ovarian cysts. Does not affect future fertility.	Minor side effects similar to early pregnancy (nausea, breast tenderness, fluid retention) during first 3 months of use. Major complications (blood clots, hypertension) may occur in smokers and those over 35. Must be taken on a regular daily schedule. No STD protection.	Combination types contain both synthetic estrogen and progesterone (female hormones). Mini-pill contains only progesterone and may produce irregular bleeding. Prescription cost: $25 to $35 monthly.
Implant (Norplant) 99%	Effective for 5 years with no further effort. Can be removed anytime. Does not affect future fertility.	Menstrual cycle irregularity. In some women, weight gain, headaches. Removal of the device may be uncomfortable. No STD protection.	Hormones, progestin only. Released from 6 silicone rubber tubes implanted under the skin. Prescription cost: about $550 or more for implant, $200 or more for removal.
Injection (Depo-Provera) 99%	Good choice for women who have trouble remembering OCs and who don't like Norplant.	Menstrual cycle irregularity. In some women, weight gain, headaches. No protection against STDs.	Progesterone given by injection once every 3 months. Prescription cost: $50 or more per injection.
Intrauterine device (IUD) 99%	Once inserted, usually stays in place. One type, Progestasert, requires annual replacement. Other types last longer: ParaGard for up to 8 years and Mirena for up to 5 years.	May cause cramping and other side effects as well as increased risk of pelvic inflammatory disease. If pregnancy occurs, increased risk that it may be ectopic (tubal).	Should be used by women who are over 25, have had a child, and have no history of pelvic inflammatory disease or tubal pregnancy. Prescription.

539

care component, it is emphatically a time in a woman's life when consulting a physician or a licensed nurse midwife is essential—not only for the prospective mother's health but for the baby's as well. While general issues of health, safety, and nutrition apply to all pregnancies, each case differs, and it is of paramount importance that a woman's condition be evaluated and monitored by a health-care professional who specializes in childbirth and pregnancy. During your pregnancy, any particular concerns you have should be addressed to your doctor or midwife.

You should expect to see your doctor every four to six weeks during the first seven to eight months, then weekly during the ninth month.

Before pregnancy. If you are planning to have a child, you should see your doctor for a thorough physical examination before you attempt to become pregnant. One reason for this is that you may have a condition that can complicate your pregnancy, but that initially has no obvious symptoms (such as diabetes, high blood pressure, or genital herpes). Your doctor can advise you about how to deal with any health problems before you try to become pregnant. You can also find out whether any medication you are taking could be harmful and if a safer substitute is available. If you are overweight, your doctor may advise you to slim down to prepare for the weight gain that will occur during pregnancy.

If you plan to become pregnant (or already are an expectant mother), a doctor or another health-care professional can also counsel you (and your partner) about prenatal care and help you evaluate your diet, physical activity, and lifestyle as it will affect your baby. During the time you are trying to become pregnant, you should avoid smoking and drinking alcohol, and either avoid caffeine or minimize it (no more than one cup of coffee a day), since these substances increase the risk of miscarriage and other complications. (Smoking also affects your chances of conceiving: according to a study from the School of Public Health at the University of California, Berkeley, a woman reduces her chances of becoming pregnant by 50 percent if she smokes even less than half a pack a day.)

All women capable of becoming pregnant are also advised to consume 400 micrograms of folacin daily, from foods or supplements, in order to ward off birth defects such as spina bifida (see opposite page). Because spina bifida and similar birth defects occur in the first two weeks of pregnancy—long before most women know they have conceived—women must start building up folacin stores at least 28 days before becoming pregnant. Since half of all pregnancies are estimated to be unplanned, it's recommended that intake should be kept high at all times.

Pregnancy after 35. Women over 35 now account for about 13 percent of births, or about 1 in 8. In 1999, the birth rate for women ages 40 to 44 was the highest reported since 1970. Some studies have shown that as women grow older, they run a greater risk of miscarriage, premature birth, birth defects, having a low-birth-weight baby, and experiencing complications. Yet other research suggests that the risks of delaying pregnancy until late in the reproductive years (after 35) are not related only to age but to preexisting disorders such as high blood pressure or diabetes that may worsen with age. Studies do continue to show that women older than 35 are at higher risk for miscarriage and having babies with birth defects, as well as for cesarean delivery—although the latter may reflect physician-patient anxiety rather than an absolute need for cesareans. In addition, fertility in women declines with the years.

FOLACIN FACTS

Folacin is a B vitamin known to reduce the risk of certain birth defects by at least 50 percent when consumed before conception and during early pregnancy. These birth defects include spina bifida (in which the spinal cord is improperly encased in bone) and anencephaly (a fatal defect in which a major part of the brain never develops). The latest research shows that folacin can also help prevent oral and facial birth defects such as cleft palate.

In addition, folacin (also called folate or, when used in a supplement or to fortify foods, folic acid) may help protect against cervical cancer, particularly in women at high risk for the disease (such as those infected with certain forms of human papilloma virus). It also helps protect against heart disease (along with other B vitamins such as B_{12} and B_6).

Fortification of grain products with folic acid has been in effect since 1998. This has helped raise blood levels of the vitamin among Americans, but not enough to prevent birth defects. The Centers for Disease Control (CDC) and the March of Dimes recommend that all women who can possibly become pregnant consume 400 micrograms of folic acid daily from vitamin supplements and/or fortified foods, in addition to eating naturally-occurring folate (see page 27 for food sources). If you don't eat at least five fruits and vegetables a day, as well as fortified cereals and small servings of lean meat, poultry, and fish, consider taking a daily multivitamin supplement providing 400 micrograms.

To obtain the benefit of preventing birth defects, it's important to start building up folic acid stores at least four weeks before becoming pregnant. Many pregnancies (as many as 50 percent) are unplanned, so it's important for any woman who is capable of becoming pregnant—even if she is not planning on pregnancy—to be sure she is consuming the recommended amount of folic acid.

541

None of this means, however, that it's inadvisable to have a baby when you're over 35 or even in your 40s. A woman attempting a first pregnancy at 35 or older should take the following precautions (in addition to those already noted):

• If pregnancy does not occur readily, seek professional advice early. If either partner needs treatment for infertility, the sooner it is begun, the better.

• Women over 35 should consider amniocentesis to determine whether there are genetic abnormalities in the fetus. Genetic counseling for couples is a good idea.

• Try to embark on pregnancy before age 40, since fertility declines quickly after that, and the chances of genetic abnormalities in the fetus increase. Nevertheless, women in their early 40s can still conceive and bear healthy babies.

Signs of pregnancy. The absence of a menstrual period is one of the first indications you are pregnant. Other early signs are enlarged and tender breasts, needing to urinate frequently, feeling tired, minor weight gain, and possibly nausea or vomiting.

If you suspect you are pregnant, it's fine to use a home pregnancy test (which detects a fetal hormone in the urine). These tests are not always reliable, so if the result is negative and you still think you are pregnant, you should see your doctor or go to a clinic or health-care center for more accurate testing. One reason to do so is to make sure you don't have an ectopic pregnancy—a circumstance in which the pregnancy develops outside the uterus, usually in the fallopian tube. Ectopic pregnancies are often missed by home pregnancy tests because the fetal growth hormone is present in much lower amounts than when the pregnancy is uterine. Though relatively rare—ectopic pregnancies occur in about 1 in every 100 pregnancies—the condition can become life-threatening and needs to be dealt with surgically.

About one in six pregnancies ends in miscarriage. But most miscarriages occur early, often before a woman is aware of being pregnant, so the true incidence of miscarriage is unknown. Usually there are no lasting consequences.

Prenatal care should start as soon as you know you are pregnant—at which point (if you haven't already heard it) your doctor will caution you about the potential hazards of using tobacco, alcohol, and drugs. All three can impair fetal development in different ways, and you should avoid them entirely, except for drugs that you take at your doctor's direction.

PREGNANCY AND NUTRITION

Nutrition can have a profound effect on your health and your baby's. Poor eating habits not only can interfere with your baby's growth but can also aggravate some of the common discomforts of pregnancy.

The 38 weeks of a normal pregnancy is one period in your life when you are encouraged to gain weight. Recommendations about healthy weight gain vary somewhat among experts, but according to current guidelines from the Institute of Medicine at the National Academy of Sciences, most women should gain 25 to 35 pounds:

three to five pounds during the first trimester, and one to two pounds per week after that. A large percentage of this weight gain is from the baby, the placenta, and the increased volume of fluid in a woman's body. Failing to gain sufficient weight can be harmful to the baby's health. At the same time, pregnancy is not an excuse to become excessively heavy. Too much weight can complicate delivery, impede postpartum weight loss, and result in other complications such as hypertension. It is also harder to lose excess weight after pregnancy.

Your doctor or other caregiver will assess how much weight is best for you to gain. Women who are overweight at conception may need to add weight at only half the rate of an average-weight woman, but it is important that they gain at least 15 to 25 pounds, since lower increases are associated with retarded growth of the fetus. Similarly, underweight women and some very young women may need to gain more weight than the average woman—up to 40 pounds, depending upon their stature and weight at conception.

The demands of pregnancy will require, on average, an additional 300 calories daily. In addition to extra calories, pregnant women should eat a nutritious diet based on the food groups and portions shown in the food guide pyramid devised by the U.S. Department of Agriculture (see page 19), which provides specific amounts of food to be eaten daily. If you're having trouble gaining weight, eat more breads and other grains, rather than consuming foods high in fat. If you're gaining too much weight, reduce your consumption of high-fat foods like butter and margarine, packaged snack foods, salad dressings, and rich desserts. (See page 37 for additional advice.)

The National Research Council, which sets recommended daily amounts of nutrients, advises

PREGNANCY: COMMON COMPLAINTS

The great majority of pregnancies are medically uneventful; only a small percentage of women experience medical complications, and those can usually be dealt with successfully. What most women have to contend with are discomforts that aren't major problems but are nevertheless vexing.

One of the most common problems is the nausea and vomiting referred to as morning sickness—which actually can occur at any time, though it usually strikes in the morning, often immediately after awakening. Morning sickness typically begins in the first month of pregnancy and continues through the fourth or fifth month. Eating a few crackers before getting out of bed in the morning can help. Eating frequent light meals and sweet foods, avoiding spicy and high-fat foods, and drinking plenty of fluids may also ease the problem.

Other problems include backache, constipation, heartburn, hemorrhoids, and varicose veins—all of which are covered elsewhere in this book. You can treat most of these complaints yourself, but you should discuss the problems and any treatments or remedies with your doctor, including any over-the-counter medications, which can be dangerous to unborn babies and pregnant women. (Also, always check warning labels of any products.) These problems generally subside soon after the baby is born.

543

that pregnant women who eat a well-balanced diet don't need vitamin and mineral supplements. Many women, however, may have trouble meeting the recommended amounts of iron, calcium, and folacin, and, depending on their diet, other nutrients as well. Women following a vegetarian diet, for example, may need additional zinc and possibly some B vitamins. Many doctors, therefore, will prescribe a supplement especially formulated for pregnant women to provide various essential nutrients. These supplements are not a substitute for a balanced diet; your health and that of your child depend on getting the bulk of your nutrients from foods.

PREGNANCY AND EXERCISE

Proper exercise during pregnancy can have many benefits. For a woman who enjoys working out, it can be important psychologically to continue with a regular exercise program after she becomes pregnant. If you do not already exercise, pregnancy can help you feel more in control as your body changes. Moderate exercise during pregnancy can also help prevent pregnancy-related complaints such as excessive weight gain, back strain, and constipation. Another potential benefit: Exercise may help ease or shorten labor and delivery, and help speed recovery after birth.

Medical experts say that your exercise program must be geared to your level of fitness, your medical history (particularly any problems during past pregnancies), the stage of development of the fetus, and maternal complicating factors. Therefore, it is important to consult your physician.

Remember that being pregnant puts extra demands on your heart and lungs, so cut back on the intensity of any exercise routine. As pregnancy advances, breathing becomes harder work because each breath must displace the enlarging uterus downward.

For exercise to be effective, it should be regular. Try to exercise at least three times a week in half-hour sessions. The best exercise is an activity you enjoy. Walking and swimming are particularly good for pregnant women who have been relatively sedentary. Muscle-strengthening and joint flexibility exercises are also excellent for helping you support the extra weight you'll carry and improving your balance.

Be sure to warm up and cool down—but stretch carefully because muscles and joints are looser than usual. Cool down with leisurely walking, which helps return blood to your heart from your lower extremities.

If you feel comfortable and your doctor allows it, you can continue most forms of exercise into your ninth month, although you may have to make some modifications to meet your body's changing demands.

What to avoid. Avoid bouncing, jarring, twisting, and any activity that could lead to a fall or a blow to the abdomen. Contact sports are too risky, as is any activity that requires rapid stops and starts, since your center of gravity has changed and it is easier to lose your balance. In addition, take the following precautions:

• Avoid exercising to exhaustion. If you feel very tired or experience discomfort, stop and rest. You should not exercise so intensely that you are unable to talk. You should recover your preexercise heart rate within 15 minutes after your exercise session.

• After 20 weeks into your pregnancy, don't exercise for more than a few minutes while lying on your back This can block the blood supply to the uterus and depress the fetal heart rate.

• If you need to rest during an exercise session, lie down on your side, not on your back.

• Don't exercise vigorously in hot, humid weather; always drink plenty of water before and after exercising. This avoids the dehydration and elevated body temperature that could injure the fetus.

• Remember that your muscles and connective tissues are gradually undergoing hormonal changes that will relax them. This will facilitate the baby's birth, but it also makes you more susceptible to strains and sprains. Wear properly fitting shoes that support your feet in whichever activity you choose.

AFTER PREGNANCY

All women should seriously consider breast-feeding their babies, as breast milk is an ideal source of nutrients and can supply the newborn with antibodies to various infections. Breastfeeding also helps a woman's uterus return to normal size after delivery. And the contact between mother and child provides a nurturing psychological bond.

Nevertheless, some women dislike the idea of breast-feeding or have a job that would make it very inconvenient to breast-feed. Also, some women should not breast-feed, including those taking certain medications that pass into breast milk or women with certain infections, such as HIV, chicken pox, or active tuberculosis. A woman who cannot or chooses not to breast-feed should not feel guilty, since babies do fine on formula.

If you decide to breast-feed, talk to your doctor about the care and preparation of your breasts. Even though breast-feeding is a natural process, many women can benefit from learning how to do it properly. Your doctor can instruct you or may refer you to a "lactation coach." Some women develop sore, swollen breasts and/or cracked nipples; if this happens, see your doctor.

Also, talk to your doctor about when you can resume having sexual intercourse (generally about three weeks after birth) and about any steps you want to take to avoid another pregnancy right away. (Breast-feeding does not prevent pregnancy.) You should also have a pelvic exam four to six weeks after the birth.

Postpartum depression. After a child is born, it is normal for the mother to experience a range of feelings. Joy and a sense of relief are part of this emotional spectrum, but it is common for new mothers to feel inexplicably "blue" at times, which may stem from fatigue, hormonal changes, and shifting emotions. Such intermittent feelings often develop a few days after the baby is home and may persist for several weeks. The support of family members in taking care of the baby usually helps diminish the blue feelings, and so does talking to other new mothers. It's also important to avoid becoming too tired. If you feel overwhelmed, you should talk to your doctor, who may be able to help you work through your feelings or can recommend a counselor or support group to provide assistance.

Severe depression is rare, but a few women do become so depressed after childbirth that they cannot take care of themselves or their babies. Depression of this nature is usually evident within a month of the birth. If it develops, the mother and/or father or other family members should seek professional help right away.

INFERTILITY

If you are unable to become pregnant after one year of having sexual intercourse without using any contraception, you and your partner need to consider that one or both of you are infertile. Age is certainly a factor: in both men and women alike, fertility peaks sometime in the 20s. But while a man can produce sperm most of his life, a woman's fertility begins to decline markedly in her 30s and ends at menopause.

In younger adults capable of conception, infertility has other causes. Sometimes the cause is simple—such as not having intercourse at the optimal time. More commonly, causes include a blockage or other abnormality in a woman's fallopian tubes; the inability of her ovaries to release an egg; a low sperm count or low sperm motility in men; or a number of conditions that interfere with ovulation and fertilization.

Numerous treatments are now available for infertility, and many of the causes are correctable—about half of the couples who seek help are eventually able to have a child. However, the treatments are often expensive, and they may involve emotional and ethical issues that should be discussed before you and your partner make a decision about pursuing a particular course of action. Often physicians who specialize in fertility problems can offer guidance, as can support groups.

SEXUAL DYSFUNCTION

Nearly everyone experiences a diminished sexual response from time to time, because of such routine difficulties as fatigue, stress, or acute illness. This is normal and nothing to worry about. But some people of both sexes find themselves experiencing a chronic loss of sexual desire, and some men struggle with frequent bouts of impotence, or erectile dysfunction—the inability to achieve and maintain an erection. Most men who are chronically impotent are over 50, but younger men can suffer, too.

Although impotence in older men is often linked to a physical or medical problem (see page 347), most cases of impotence, particularly in younger men, have a psychological component—anxiety, depression, or relationship problems are common causes. When a man who experiences impotence wakes up at night or in the morning with a full, firm erection, the cause of the impotence is most likely psychological. But for any case of chronic impotence, a doctor should first be consulted to eliminate a possible physiological cause.

The physiology of the female sexual climax, or orgasm, has been studied extensively. The ability to have orgasms, and indeed multiple orgasms, can last throughout life for a woman. But women, too, may experience a variety of problems, including reduced desire.

Once known as frigidity, sexual disinclination in women may arise from many factors: an unskilled partner or an unsatisfactory relationship with a partner; anxiety and depression; lack of knowledge; feelings of shame about sex; unsatisfactory prior sexual experiences; or underlying disease. Surveys indicate that many women do not have orgasms through intercourse alone and need direct stimulation of the clitoris to have an orgasm either during foreplay or intercourse.

Lifestyle habits such as excessive alcohol consumption, drug abuse, and smoking can also be at the root of sexual problems. Alcohol in particular is associated with impotence. When a substance or habit is the cause, the remedy is fairly straightforward. If the problem persists, talk to your doctor, who can assess your physical condition and, if necessary, help you (and your partner) find a qualified sex therapist.

OTHER HEALTH CONCERNS FROM 20 TO 39

Although most young adults are healthy, it pays to be aware of certain health risks at this stage of life.

Weight gain. Americans have been gaining weight, as a number of recent studies have indicated. As doctors have observed for many years, being overweight is associated with disease, including heart disease, hypertension, and diabetes. Furthermore, it isn't only older Americans who are gaining weight. A 1999 study published in the *Journal of the American Medical Association* comparing the prevalence of obesity among different age groups found a dramatic increase in 18- to 29-year olds: between 1991 and 1998, the proportion of obese Americans in that age group grew from 7 percent to 12 percent—an increase of 70 percent. (Subjects were considered obese if they had a body mass index of 30 or higher.)

Part of the reason for this national weight gain is that, while Americans are eating less fat, they are consuming more calories—and calories do count. Even a low-fat diet can be high in calories if you depend too much on some of the new low-fat or nonfat cakes, cookies, ice creams, and other products that contain lots of sugar and calories but few nutrients and little fiber.

The other part of the equation is the continuing epidemic of physical inactivity among Americans. The key to successful weight control is not simply the calories you consume but also the ones you expend in physical activity.

It's important at any age to maintain a healthy weight. For strategies to achieve this goal, see pages 37-39. And remember that, although low-fat foods can help promote weight loss, if you don't cut down on calories (and/or add exercise) over the course of the day, you won't lose weight.

Breast cancer. The risk of breast cancer increases with age, and the disease is far more common in older women. But young women can also get breast cancer. Those who do often have a mother or sister with the disease, and the cancer is pre-

PREVENTIVE SERVICES RECOMMENDATIONS

The following table highlights the major screening tests (that is, routine tests for people without symptoms) and immunizations for healthy adults ages 20 to 39. This advice is based in part on the recommendations of the U.S. Preventive Services Task Force (see page 70). (*Pregnant women need other kinds of professional preventive care that are not covered here.*)

PREVENTIVE SCREENINGS AND CHECKUPS

FOR MEN AND WOMEN

Blood pressure measurement (to detect hypertension). Once every 2 years for those with normal blood pressure.

Cholesterol measurement. At least once every 5 years; more often if the total cholesterol number is elevated (above 200 mg/dl) or the HDL cholesterol is low (below 35 mg/dl), and/or you have cardiac risk factors such as hypertension, diabetes, or cigarette smoking.

Dental checkup: Every 6 months or on professional advice; should include cleaning.

FOR WOMEN

Pap smear (for early detection of cervical cancer): Every 3 years for all women with a cervix. Possibly more often, depending on risk factors such as smoking or multiple sex partners (see page 74).

Rubella (German measles): All women should be tested for immunity to rubella before getting pregnant. A blood test can determine whether a vaccination (which confers lifetime protection) is necessary. Serious birth defects can occur in the fetus of a woman who develops a rubella infection during pregnancy.

IMMUNIZATION

Tetanus-diphtheria booster: Every 10 years. Relatively few cases of tetanus occur in the United States, but it can strike adults who aren't immunized. Tetanus, which is often fatal, can develop after even a minor wound or scratch.

Hepatitis B vaccine: Recommended for any adult at high risk. This includes health-care workers who are exposed to blood or blood products, injection drug users, people not in a long-term monogamous relationship who have a history of sex with multiple partners, and people with other sexually transmitted diseases (see page 326).

sumably caused by inherited genetic factors. Because the cause of breast cancer is not fully understood, there are no firm guidelines for women to follow to reduce their risk. Eating a healthy diet, not smoking, and drinking little or no alcohol may help cut the risk. Exercise may also have some protective effect against the disease.

Every woman should also examine her breasts monthly (see page 61). Most palpable lumps are found by women themselves during self-exams.

Usually, there is no reason for women in their 30s to have a mammogram. But if breast cancer runs in your family, you should discuss your risk factors, and your wishes, with your doctor.

Ovarian cancer. This cancer is most commonly diagnosed in women in their 50s and older. Because the disease is hard to detect, it is seldom curable. Fortunately accumulating evidence shows that oral contraceptives greatly reduce the risk of ovarian cancer (as does tubal ligation). No one understands why this is so. Risk factors for ovarian cancer include a family history of the disease, as well as never having had children. Women at high risk of ovarian cancer can now help themselves by using birth control pills. The longer you use them, the lower the risk of cancer. Even women who use the Pill for as little as six months lower their risk. The protection lasts for many years.

Skin cancer. If you have fair skin that burns easily, or you had severe sunburns as a child or teenager, or you spend a good deal of time in the sun, you are at increased risk of skin cancer. Most skin cancers are detected by people examining their own skin, which you should do regularly (see page 60). If you notice any unusual change, see your doctor. You should also take precautions to protect yourself from sun exposure (see page 56).

Testicular cancer. Testicular cancer is rare, accounting for just 1 percent of all cancers, but it comprises 23 percent of all cancers in males ages 20 to 34—making it the most common form of cancer among men in this age range. Although testicular cancer can strike at any age, the prime years are between 15 and 40, with white males at highest risk. The rate among African-American men is about one-sixth that of whites.

Each year close to 7,000 cases are diagnosed and about 300 deaths are caused by the disease. This form of cancer is on the increase in the United States for no apparent reason. According to the National Cancer Institute, from 1976 to 1997 the incidence increased 50 percent among Americans, jumping from 3.2 to 4.8 per 100,000 men. The incidence has more than doubled among white Americans during the past 40 years.

The main known risk factor is an undescended or partially undescended testicle (normally, the testes descend soon after birth). Men with this condition are 3 to 17 times more likely to develop testicular cancer—but they account for just 10 percent of all cases. An undescended testicle is easily corrected, but this doesn't reduce the risk of cancer. Children or men who have this condition should be checked by a physician.

Although testicular cancer cannot be prevented, a regular monthly three-minute self-exam, like a monthly breast self-exam for women, is the best way to detect it in its earliest stages. The cure rate is more than 95 percent if the cancer is detected early. Otherwise, the survival rate drops considerably. (See page 63 for how to perform a self-exam.)

Symptoms of testicular cancer include a slight enlargement of one of the testes, a lump in the testes, or a change in its consistency. There may be no localized pain, but often a dull ache is experienced in the groin area and lower abdomen.

Despite the increase in the incidence of testicular cancer in the United States, the mortality rate has dropped 60 percent, thanks to advances in treatment. The preferred treatment is surgical removal of the affected testicle, usually followed by chemotherapy. This surgery doesn't affect sexual response or fertility, since one testicle is sufficient, but chemotherapy may reduce fertility, at least temporarily.

MIDLIFE ADULTS
(40 to 65)

Because life expectancy in the United States has increased so dramatically in this century, the definitions of middle age (as well as old age) are undergoing significant change. In 1890, life expectancy was only 42 years for men and 45 for women, so that 65 seemed—and indeed was—a venerable age. Average life expectancy did not rise to 65 until 1940. Today, as the first baby boomers have entered their 50s, there are people who regard themselves as young at 40 or 45 and may not feel "middle-aged" even by their late 50s and early 60s. This perception of age has to do with not only increased life expectancy but also the quality of life—the sense of vitality and well-being (or lack thereof) that one feels at any age.

Still, our bodies noticeably change as we grow older—that is universal—and healthy adults in this age range tend to display certain physical signposts and often share particular health concerns, which are discussed below. As we all know from personal observation, however, not all of us age in the same way or at the same rate. Biological aging among humans is amazingly varied, and so the point at which these changes occur differs from person to person, sometimes dramatically.

This variability is in part programmed by our genes—for example, the onset and rate of hair loss in men is almost entirely genetically determined and is nearly impossible to prevent. But it is also clear that some aspects of aging are a matter of lifestyle—and that as people enter their 50s and 60s, the consequences of diet and other health-related habits become increasingly evident. Poor nutrition, obesity, smoking, and excessive use of alcohol and drugs tend to accelerate aging and illness, while eating nutritiously and exercising regularly tend to offset or prevent a number of the changes associated with aging. Access to adequate health care is also a key factor in how successfully someone ages—because it allows medical problems to be dealt with as they arise and because it makes preventive services available.

CHANGES IN MEN AND WOMEN

Aside from changes in eyesight, hearing, and hair loss, which for the most part can't be prevented or delayed (but can be partially to completely corrected), the other changes noted here can be prevented to varying degrees or, in some cases, reversed.

Eyesight. The lens of the eye hardens with age, usually starting when people are in their 40s. This hardening makes it more difficult to change focus, especially to see near objects sharply. Reading glasses are usually needed for correction.

549

Hearing. Loss of hearing is a gradual process that starts with a decline in the ability to hear high frequencies. Most people don't notice any hearing loss until their 60s, a decade or two after it actually begins, when voices can become harder to perceive as low-frequency hearing also starts to fade. Heredity affects hearing loss, but so does exposure to loud noises (see page 312).

Hair. About half the people of European descent will develop some gray hair by age 50. In African-Americans, onset of graying occurs about a decade later. Roughly half of all men show some hair loss by age 50. In women, hair loss (when it occurs) usually begins at about age 30, becomes noticeable around age 40, and may be more noticeable after menopause.

Skin. At age 40 you may have no wrinkles, but most people by age 50 show some wrinkling and sagging, which occur as collagen—a connective tissue—declines, causing a loss of elasticity in the skin. But most wrinkling is caused by exposure to sunlight. Painless and harmless age spots, which may be yellow, tan, or brown and variously shaped, tend to appear after age 40, usually on the back of your hands or on your face (see page 62). Reddened, itchy skin and other forms of dermatitis are also associated with aging.

Muscle mass and body fat. In sedentary adults, muscle tissue tends to shrink with age, and the rate of loss speeds up after age 45. Adults can lose 30 to 40 percent of their muscle strength over the course of a lifetime. This loss of muscle leads to a decline in resting metabolic rate—the amount of energy your body uses in a given period of time—since muscle demands more energy use by your body than does fat. As a result, older people tend to have a higher percentage of body fat than they did when they were younger. Body fat is also redistributed: in men, it tends to settle around the abdomen; in women, around the breasts and hips. Exercising regularly to gain muscle mass and maintaining a healthy weight (see page 33) can slow these changes.

Aerobic capacity. The ability of your body to deliver oxygen to working muscles—and of the muscles to utilize oxygen—constitutes aerobic capacity. Normally, this declines by about 1 percent a year after age 30. But the decline is not inevitable: people in their 50s and 60s who exercise regularly can display the aerobic capacity of sedentary people in their 20s. Even people who have been sedentary can improve aerobic capacity significantly (though the maximum gains a person can expect from training are different at age 50 or 60 than they are at 20).

Heart and blood vessels. Some narrowing and hardening of the arteries occurs in almost all people as they grow older, and by midlife this process may be forcing the heart muscle to enlarge and work harder to pump blood through the arteries. Large and medium-size arteries can become affected by atherosclerosis—characterized by deposits of cholesterol, fatty substances, and cellular waste products (plaque) in the inner lining of an artery. As plaque builds up inside coronary arteries, the arteries can narrow to the point where they block the flow of blood to the heart muscle, and the result is coronary heart disease, or CHD. This process of plaque formation can be slowed or halted in many people through diet, exercise, and other lifestyle measures.

Blood pressure. In the United States and other Western countries, aging is accompanied by a mild rise in blood pressure—though whether this is normal is not clear, since in many other countries, blood pressure does not rise with age. As a rule, women have slightly lower blood pressure than men; high blood pressure, or hypertension, is more common before age 55 in men than in women. (After age 65, blood pressure numbers are also affected by activity level, weight, and other factors—see page 332.) Systolic blood pressure (the top number in the blood pressure measurement) increases by about 15 percent between ages 35 and 70. For the general population, a systolic pressure of 120 or less over a diastolic pressure of 80 or less is optimal; a blood pressure of 140/90 or higher is classified as hypertension. Exercising regularly, not smoking, limiting alcohol and sodium consumption, and maintaining a healthy weight are the best strategies for preventing high blood pressure.

Cholesterol levels. Blood cholesterol levels are not directly linked to age, but they do tend to rise as people get older—in part because of eating and exercise habits, which can lead to high cholesterol levels that increase the risk of developing heart disease (see page 199). At menopause, low levels of estrogen lead to an increase in a woman's LDL ("bad") cholesterol and a drop in HDL ("good") cholesterol—though this is by no means uniform or universal. Low-dose estrogen therapy (ERT) and hormone replacement therapy (HRT) can have a positive effect on blood cholesterol, but to varying degrees, and there is controversy about using hormone replacement to prevent heart disease in postmenopausal women (see page 382).

Bone density. Bone loss begins to exceed bone growth around age 35, and this loss accelerates in women after menopause, when production of the female sex hormone estrogen (which is a major influence on calcium uptake by bone tissue) begins to decline. Bone loss does not mean that the bone is diseased or abnormal—just that there is less of it, and any new bone that forms is less dense. Bone loss also affects men, but at a much slower rate, so that the consequences—especially osteoporosis (see page 397)—usually don't appear in men until their 70s or 80s.

Memory. Anyone over the age of 45 or so is familiar with a slowdown of memory: names, arbitrary facts, and sequences of words or numbers may become harder to retrieve. These types of memory lapses can be ameliorated with some simple training techniques (see page 562). Long-ago memories typically remain intact. Knowledge and good judgment are cumulative; they can and do increase with experience. Studies have found that many mental capacities—including verbal abilities, sense of spatial orientation, judgment, and reasoning—are stable across the years.

MENOPAUSE

At some point, usually about age 50, ovulation and menstrual periods in women will stop. Menopause—which specifically refers to the cessation of menstruation—is part of a biological process (unless it is the result of surgery) that begins about five years before menopause, when the ovaries begin to produce decreasing amounts of progesterone and then estrogen, the two principal female hormones. About half of all women stop menstruating by age 48; by age 52, 85 percent will have reached menopause (which is complete when a year has passed since the last menstrual period). Some women, however, enter menopause in their early 40s, while a few continue to have menstrual periods into their late 50s.

In itself, menopause is a normal, healthy transition in life, not a disease. It may bring certain worries to the fore, for example, fear of aging, or of being defeminized or desexualized. Yet most women find the passage relatively smooth. Some of the changes are for the better: no more menstrual cramps, no need for contraceptives, and no more worry about pregnancy. A woman's interest in sex may actually increase after menopause. However, the reduction of estrogen can have wide-ranging effects, some of which are noted below.

Irregular periods. Irregularity in the menstrual cycle as well as changes in the amount of blood flow are usually the first obvious signs of impending menopause. You should see your doctor if you have bleeding between periods, if you experience excessive or prolonged bleeding, or if you go more than eight weeks without a period.

Weight gain. Many women, as they pass through menopause, experience a gain in weight and a redistribution of body fat concentrated around the abdomen. The shifts in hormone levels may contribute to weight gain, and being sedentary can compound it. Because even a gain of 10 pounds can increase your risk of high blood pressure, heart disease, type 2 diabetes, and some cancers, you should try to keep your weight at recommended levels for your height and build (see page 36).

Bone loss. The decline in estrogen production that accompanies menopause also produces a loss of bone mass, causing bones to become thinner and more brittle—the condition known as osteoporosis, which can lead to debilitating fractures later in life. To help prevent or delay the onset of bone loss, it's important to consume adequate amounts of calcium and to perform regular weight-bearing exercise.

Mood swings. Some women experience mood swings during menopause, which may include bouts of depression. The causes of mood swings are not understood: they may result from hormonal fluctuations and may also be triggered by menopausal symptoms (such as hot flashes that disrupt sleep). In addition, shifts in mood may be brought on by new roles that women take on at this stage of life—and of old roles that are dropped, as when children leave home. The departure of grown-up children from home—once thought to result in severe depression for mothers—may actually improve their lives. One study of women with "empty nests" found that they often emphasize their opportunities to take on new roles, to function assertively and independently, and to enjoy their freedom once the daily responsibilities of parenthood are behind them.

If depressive feelings or other emotional upsets are severe or persistent, you should consult your doctor or a qualified therapist. (For a more detailed description of menopause and problems associated with it, see page 379).

SEXUAL FUNCTION

Sexuality is no longer seen as coming to an end in middle age. As many studies have shown, interest in sex can and does endure, change, renew itself, and develop throughout the life span.

Sexual desire varies from one person to another and over a lifetime. Reduced sexual desire is a common concern. Depression, anxiety, workplace stress, and underlying health problems, including drug reactions or hormonal abnormalities, can all play a role in the diminution of desire. Also, a lack of sexual desire and loss of physical intimacy between partners often reflects unresolved conflicts about nonsexual problems, rather than some underlying psychiatric or physical condition. Another difficult situation may arise after a divorce or death of a spouse or life partner: many people feel guilty or anxious over embarking on a new relationship after so many years with one person. Longstanding feelings of shame about sex can also dilute sexual desire in middle age (just as they can in younger people).

Many factors can keep desire alive: adequate self-esteem, previous good sexual experiences, the availability of a partner interested in sex. Perhaps as important as any other factor is a good relationship with this partner in nonsexual areas. Love is always a big help.

Even in a long-term relationship, partners often have different ideas about what constitutes normal sex, along with different ideas about arousing sexual desire. According to scores of studies and a string of best-selling books, women tend to value the emotional side of sex more than men do, while men place greater emphasis on the physical aspect of the sex act itself. Like most generalizations about gender differences, these lines break down quickly when you look at individual cases. For women as well as men, physical satisfaction is as important as romance, and for both sexes emotional involvement is highly correlated with physical satisfaction.

Changes in men. Many men experience a gradual lessening of desire. It also takes middle-aged men increasingly longer to get an erection, and to regain an erection after climax. This is neither a reflection of decreased sexuality nor a symptom of impending impotence. Rather, it is the result of the male body secreting less testosterone (the hormone that regulates sexual performance and desire) and conducting nerve impulses more slowly. In addition, the arteries in the penis are less able to maintain the blood pressure necessary for a full erection.

These changes needn't be alarming; indeed, they can be turned to advantage since they allow a man to prolong foreplay, sustain intercourse longer, and delay orgasm until the moment when both partners will be satisfied.

At the same time, the rate of impotence (the inability to have and maintain an erection suffi-cient for sexual intercourse) increases after age 40. All men experience occasional brief episodes of impotence, which are normal. But an estimated 5 percent of men at age 40 have chronic erectile problems, and the percentage increases with age (it is most common among men over 65). The causes are complex, combining physical and psychological factors. If you are having erectile problems, it is a good idea to seek a medical evaluation to determine if your problem can be treated medically or through counseling or other means (see page 347 for more information).

Changes in women. Menopause signals the end of a woman's fertility, but not necessarily the end of her sexuality. Indeed, some women, freed of worries about birth control, pregnancy, and the bother of having a monthly period, report that their sex lives are better than ever. But after menopause, women may have physical problems that interfere with sexual satisfaction, including a drying of the vaginal tissues and a failure to lubricate during intercourse, which can make it painful or impossible. Most of these problems are treatable, and you should not hesitate to seek help for them. If you have an underlying disease, diagnosing and treating it may restore sexual desire. Drying of vaginal tissue can be corrected either with hormone therapy or with a simple nonhormonal vaginal moisturizer.

Pregnancy and birth control. While rare, pregnancy can occur during perimenopause (the three- to five-year period preceding a woman's final menstrual period), when a woman still occasionally ovulates. It is possible for a woman in her early or mid-40s to safely bear a healthy baby—though both mother and child are at greater risk for certain health problems than is the case with women under 35, particularly if it is a first pregnancy (see page 540). A woman who wants to be sure of

553

ADULTS 40 TO 65

PREVENTIVE SERVICES RECOMMENDATIONS

The following table highlights the major screening tests (that is, routine tests for people without symptoms) and immunizations for healthy adults ages 40 to 65. This advice is based in part on the recommendations of the U.S. Preventive Services Task Force (see page 70). (*Pregnant women need other kinds of professional preventive care that are not covered here.*)

PREVENTIVE SCREENINGS AND CHECKUPS

FOR MEN AND WOMEN

Blood pressure measurement (to detect hypertension): Once every 2 years for those with normal blood pressure.

Cholesterol measurement: At least once every 5 years, more often if the total cholesterol number is elevated (above 200 mg/dl) or the HDL cholesterol is low (below 35 mg/dl), and/or you have cardiac risk factors. These include age (men over 45; women over 55), family history of heart disease, diabetes, hypertension, or cigarette smoking.

Colorectal cancer screening (fecal occult blood test and/or sigmoidoscopy): At age 50 and then annually for the occult blood test; at age 50 for sigmoidoscopy and then every 5 years thereafter (or for colonoscopy every 10 years). A digital rectal exam (DRE) should also be done annually.

Diabetes mellitus screening: The American Diabetes Association recommends that everyone age 45 and older should be tested for non-insulin-dependent (type 2) diabetes.

Glaucoma screening: The American Academy of Ophthalmology recommends eye exams, including glaucoma testing, every three to five years, beginning at age 39. People at high risk, which include the very nearsighted, people with diabetes, African-Americans over the age of 40, and those with a family history of the disease, may need more frequent screenings. How often depends on professional advice (see page 289).

Thyroid disease screening: For people over 50, especially women, who have experienced possible symptoms of hypothyroidism or who have high cholesterol levels; they should discuss this test with their doctors (see page 84).

Dental checkup. Every 6 months or on professional advice; should include cleaning.

FOR WOMEN

Pap smear (for early detection of cervical cancer): After 4 consecutive normal pap smears, every 3 years for all women with a cervix. Possibly more often, depending on risk factors such as smoking, multiple sex partners, or a history of genital warts (see page 74).

554

Breast cancer screening (mammogram and clinical breast exam): Every year for all women age 50 and over; those 40 to 49 should discuss their risk factors with their doctors, since there is still debate about screening women in their 40s (see page 76).

FOR MEN

Prostate cancer screening (prostate specific antigen, or PSA, test and digital rectal exam): All men 50 and older should have a digital rectal exam (DRE) annually. The usefulness of the PSA for screening all men remains controversial. Routine screening with the PSA is not recommended, but men 50 or older who are African-American or who have a family history of the disease should begin screening. (Some doctors advise that men in this category should begin at age 40.) Consult your doctor as to how often. If you are 50 to 75 with no family history or other risk factors, you may choose not to be screened. (See page 80 for more information.)

IMMUNIZATIONS

Tetanus-diphtheria booster: Every 10 years. Relatively few cases of tetanus occur in this country now, but most cases occur in people over 50, who are least likely to be adequately immunized because they have not kept up with their shots.

Influenza vaccine: Recommended for all adults 50 and over; research indicates that even healthy younger adults can benefit and should consider getting a flu shot annually in the autumn.

avoiding pregnancy should continue using some form of contraception until menopause is complete (one year after the final period).

STDs. Even though you may not need birth control, you still need to protect yourself against sexually transmitted diseases (see page 57).

HEALTH CONCERNS: MEN AND WOMEN

Heart disease. The risk of coronary heart disease—which is caused by restricted blood flow to the heart and can result in heart attacks—starts to increase significantly in men older than 45 and women over 55. Based on the Framingham Heart Study (an ongoing long-term study of risk factors for heart disease), about 45 percent of all heart attacks occur in people under the age of 65.

Before menopause, few women suffer from heart disease. But after age 50, women begin to develop the disorder at an increasing rate, such that by age 65 the risk of heart attack is as great in women as in men. Coronary heart disease is by far the major cause of death among women after menopause. A number of lifestyle measures, summarized on pages 64-65 and explained in detail elsewhere in this book, can reduce your risk of a heart attack.

Hormone replacement therapy (HRT), which can alleviate or prevent symptoms (such as hot flashes) associated with menopause, may also help reduce a woman's risk of heart disease. It also offers some protection against osteoporosis. But HRT has its downside, including monthly bleeding in some cases and, possibly, a slight risk of breast cancer. Therefore, every woman should decide about HRT in consultation with her physician, who can help her weigh the benefits of HRT against personal risk factors (see page 382.)

Diabetes. Each year more than 700,000 Americans are diagnosed with type 2 diabetes—a dis-ease that typically affects middle-aged to older people, and thus was formerly called *adult-onset* diabetes, as compared with type 1 diabetes, which is usually diagnosed in young people. Diabetes is a breakdown in the body's ability to efficiently utilize glucose (blood sugar), which can be used by cells only in the presence of the hormone insulin (see page 233). In type 2 diabetes, the body produces insulin, often in increased amounts, but the cells are resistant to the effects of insulin, and thus blood levels of glucose rise. (This type of diabetes has been called *non-insulin-dependent*, since injections of insulin are often not required for treatment, as they almost always are for type 1, formerly called *insulin-dependent* diabetes.)

Diabetes that is not well controlled greatly increases the risk of hypertension, stroke, and diseases of the heart, eyes, nerves, and kidneys. There is as yet no foolproof way to prevent diabetes, but you can improve your chances of avoiding it by staying within a healthy weight range, eating a low-fat semivegetarian diet, and exercising regularly (which lowers blood sugar). Regular testing for diabetes is recommended for everyone beginning at age 45 (see page 82). The earlier the disease is detected, the earlier treatment can be started, which will help prevent the complications of the disease .

Colon cancer. Colon cancer is the third most common cause of cancer deaths, after lung cancer (which is difficult to detect early) and—in women—breast cancer and—in men—prostate cancer. If you are 50 or older, you should be regularly screened for colon cancer (see page 78). Getting plenty of fiber in your diet (from plant foods) may help protect you from the disease.

Skin cancer. Your risk of developing this disorder increases as the years of sun exposure accumulate. Take steps to protect yourself from the sun (see page 56) and check your skin regularly for any changes in moles or other growths (see page 60).

Cataracts and glaucoma. The risk for both of these eye problems increases with age. Many eye specialists advise screening for glaucoma—which may have no symptoms—starting at age 40 or 50 (see page 289).

HEALTH CONCERNS: WOMEN

Breast cancer. Asked what they fear most, many women say breast cancer—even though the risk of getting breast cancer is much lower than the risk of stroke, heart disease, osteoporosis, or type 2 diabetes. Breast cancer is undeniably the most common cancer among women in the United States and Canada, but it is very much a disease associated with aging. It is rare among women under age 40. For a 40-year-old woman, the risk of breast cancer is 1 in 233 (compared with 1 in 2,000 for a 30-year-old woman); by age 60 the risk is about 1 in 22.

Survival rates for breast cancer have improved dramatically in recent years, no doubt because of better treatments but also because of early detection. If you are a woman over 40, it is important that you perform monthly breast self-exams (page 61), see your doctor regularly, and and get regular mammograms (page 76).

Ovarian cancer. In women over 50, persistent digestive upsets such as gas or stomach discomfort that can't be explained by any other cause may indicate the need for a thorough evaluation for ovarian cancer, which causes more deaths than any other cancer of the female reproductive system.

Although it can occur at any age, this cancer is most common in women ages 50 to 75. Women who have never had children are at greater risk than those who have, as are women who have never taken oral contraceptives. Having an annual pelvic exam is still the main way of detecting ovarian cancer.

Osteoporosis. The chief risk factor for osteoporosis is age: the condition usually doesn't show up in eventual sufferers—most of whom are women—until they are in their 60s, 70s, or beyond. But the bone loss that causes osteoporosis accelerates sharply after menopause. Even though young adulthood or even adolescence is the right time to form the health habits that prevent osteoporosis, it's never too late to begin. For postmenopausal women, hormone replacement therapy, or HRT, can help prevent or reverse osteoporosis, as can weight-bearing exercise. To maintain bone mass, it's also important that postmenopausal women consume sufficient amounts of calcium—at least 1,200 to 1,500 milligrams per day. (See pages 23-24 for more information on calcium intake, including good dietary sources and the use of supplements.)

HEALTH CONCERNS: MEN

BPH. The enlargement of the prostate known as benign prostatic hyperplasia (BPH) is common in men over 40. Many people fear that an enlarged prostate is a prelude to cancer, or *is* cancer, but this is not the case; hence the term *benign*. If you have any urinary difficulties, it's wise to discuss them with your doctor. They may be caused by something more serious that needs immediate treatment. If you have BPH, your doctor will be able to diagnose it. (For more information on how to manage BPH, see page 178.)

Prostate cancer. For men over 50, cancer of the prostate is the most common cancer and the second leading cause of cancer deaths after lung cancer. Nobody knows the underlying cause of

557

prostate cancer, and there is still no known way to prevent it. Often no symptoms appear in the earliest stages of the disease.

Therefore, it is important for men at risk to be screened for the disease by seeing their doctor and getting a digital rectal exam and prostate specific antigen (PSA) test (see page 80). Risk factors for prostate cancer include advancing age and a family history of the disorder. African-American men are also at significantly higher risk than white men.

The outlook for men with early prostate cancer is good, and many cases can be cured.

OLDER ADULTS
(65 and over)

A great many of us can look forward to long lives. Today in the United States about one person in eight—or about 35 million people—is 65 years of age or older, and the numbers will continue to increase: experts project that by 2030, one in five people will be over 65.

Moreover, once people move into this age group, the longer they are likely to continue living. At age 65, the average life expectancy for women is 84, and for men, 80; 75-year-olds can expect to live, on average, to 87 and 85, respectively. As the average American lifespan has lengthened and the possibility of living eight or nine decades has become a realistic prospect for many of us, scientists have begun to examine the capabilities and special needs of older people. What they have found is that the way people age is largely a matter of how they live—which is why there is no hard and fast boundary between middle age and old age.

It is true that physical changes that began in midlife continue to make their mark. For example, in many older people, the senses—eyesight, hearing, and taste—decline by varying degrees with advancing age. Skin continues to lose the resilience of youth. The lungs can't take in as much oxygen as they once did, and the myocardium—the heart muscle—contracts less forcefully during exercise. It is also true that serious health problems can occur in the last decades of life. But as in midlife, each body system ages according to its own timetable, and these schedules vary dramatically from person to person. More emphatically, many things we associate with aging, from "middle-age spread" and brittle bones to forgetfulness and loss of muscle strength, are not the inevitable results of growing old but are brought on, in part, by factors extrinsic to aging—notably inactivity, both physical and mental.

That is why the benefits of preventive health during this stage of life can't be overstated. It is never too late to improve habits affecting your health. While a person's maximum ability may be slowly decreasing, most people haven't been working at anywhere close to their maximum. And if a health concern does arise, do not presume that you have to be resigned to it: seek early diagnosis and treatment, because relief is often available.

PHYSICAL CHANGES

The changes discussed on pages 549-553 that mark midlife for most people continue to develop gradually into old age. What follows are changes and health concerns that, for many people, become most evident after age 65.

Height. One of the most common signs of aging is a gradual diminution in height. After years of use, the fibrocartilage that acts as the cushion and connection between the bones can naturally lose some of its capacity to withstand repetitive impact. It loses water and also shrinks, which is partly what accounts for the height reduction.

A decrease in height is also caused by osteoporosis, the thinning of bone that often doesn't become detectable in people until after 65. Osteoporosis can cause a decrease in height because of the compression and remodeling of the vertebrae in the spine, and it can also cause the stooped posture known as dowager's hump. Though it is mostly elderly women who are diagnosed with osteoporosis (about 90 percent of American women over 75 are affected), older men can suffer from it as well (see page 399).

Of course, poor posture may be caused by many factors, including disease, years of poor muscle tone, and previous injuries. At any age, good posture is worth achieving and maintaining (see page 409). However, if standing up straight is painful, or if you have chronic neck or back pain caused by poor posture and your own efforts to correct the problem are not successful, you should consult your physician or an orthopedic specialist.

Eyesight and hearing. The condition known as presbyopia (an inability to focus sharply on near objects), which usually begins in the 40s and eventually affects nearly everyone, starts to stabilize around the age of 65, so that the need for new glasses tapers off. But a number of conditions that affect eyesight, including glaucoma and cataracts, are more prevalent in older adults. Therefore, it is crucial that older adults have their eyes examined regularly.

By 65, most people have also suffered some degree of hearing loss and related symptoms (see page 312). Most hearing problems can be alleviated by a hearing aid (yet only about one-third of the individuals who need hearing aids actually have them).

Skin and hair. Aging takes a toll on the skin. The most noticeable creases and furrows, which are often labeled as age lines, are actually caused by ultraviolet radiation from sun exposure. But even skin protected from the sun continues to lose the resilience it once had, taking on a lightly wrinkled appearance. Wrinkles or folds can also appear as body fat is redistributed—typically, from the face and upper body to the abdomen and, in women, to the thighs and buttocks as well. It is important to continue to monitor the skin for any changes that may signal skin cancer (see page 60).

Hair shafts often grow thinner with age—though as hair turns gray, the shafts may thicken. Men who started to lose hair in middle age may continue to lose hair on their heads, while hair may emerge on the ears—and be all the more noticeable since the ears, along with the nose, tend to enlarge in one's 60s or 70s.

Mobility. The cartilage that cushions and lubricates our joints undergoes some wear and tear over the years, but for most of us remains resilient enough so that we don't feel our mobility is significantly hampered. There may be less flexibility, and reflexes may be slower. But we start to feel truly old when we experience painful movement or a loss of mobility—which are among the symptoms of osteoarthritis, one of the most widespread ailments after 65. Fortunately, a number of measures, including exercise and medication, can make the effects of arthritis bearable, and many people can minimize or avoid pain and maintain good joint flexibility (see page 392).

Osteoporosis can hamper mobility by contributing to falls and fractures. About 1.5 million older people in the United States suffer fractures each year because of osteoporosis. Not only do osteoporotic bones break easily, they also heal more slowly, which is why the disease is a major cause of disability among older women. The best time to begin prevention of osteoporosis is early in life, but you will still benefit even if you've waited until you're in your 60s (see page 397).

Also affecting mobility are a host of overuse injuries (including tendinitis, tennis elbow, knee injuries, and carpal tunnel syndrome) that can strike at any age, but often take longer to recover from in your 60s and beyond—which is why it pays to take measures to prevent them.

Physical conditioning. Even by age 70, there is nothing "normal," much less inevitable, about experiencing a sharp decline in aerobic capacity (how well the heart and lungs bring oxygen to the muscles, and then how efficiently the muscles use the oxygen to generate energy during sustained exercise). Experts have estimated that much of the functional loss in aerobic capacity that sets in between the ages of 30 and 70 (about 1 percent per year) is in fact attributable to a lack of regular exercise. Likewise, while aging continues to cause a decrease in muscle mass, it is possible to stem this loss at virtually any age with strength training.

Cholesterol levels. Studies show that the adverse effects of high cholesterol levels persist well into old age, and that for people over 65, lowering cholesterol offers much the same benefit derived by people under 65. This is particularly important for women, whose risk of heart disease rises significantly after menopause. Twenty percent of women over 65 have symptoms of coronary heart disease—double the percentage for women under 65. Aggressive

BUILDING MUSCLE: NEVER TOO LATE

Women in their 60s and beyond have been shown to benefit from strength training. In a study published in the *Journal of the American Geriatric Society*, 36 women over the age of 60 who were already engaging in some form of regular aerobic exercise were given training sessions on heavy-resistance weight-training machines. After six months, the women experienced significant decreases in body fat and increases in lean muscle mass. Their muscle strength also improved, and no injuries were suffered.

Even more surprising results came from a study conducted at Tufts University in which 10 very frail 90-year-olds, already institutionalized, participated in a 9-week program of high-intensity weight training. They began slowly, lifting only 50 percent of the maximum they were capable of (8 repetitions 3 times a week), then moving up to 80 percent of their maximum capacity and increasing their exercises in number and intensity each week. They were able to build muscle mass and become more mobile and self-sufficient.

cholesterol reduction may not, however, make sense for people who are over 75 years of age. More moderate measures, such as daily walking and a healthy diet, make more sense.

Sleeping patterns. About 80 percent of people over 65 find that they are waking up more often during the night and earlier in the morning. Though the amount of time spent in bed may remain fairly constant, actual sleep time lessens: while eight hours of sleep is typical at age 20, six hours is closer to the norm at 60. According to sleep researchers, these changes in sleep patterns are a natural part of the aging process and nothing to worry about. You can take steps to compensate for changing sleep patterns (see page 352). Sleeping less than five hours or more than ten hours a night may be a sign of clinical depression; if this is the case for you, you should check with your physician.

Sexuality. Experts in this field indicate that, in the absence of disease, sexual expression may endure throughout life. While the *intensity* of sexual interest may generally decline with age, an active sex life, contrary to myth, is by no means unusual in old age. Research indicates that the great majority of men in their late 60s continue to be interested in sex. At 80 or older, one out of every four men is sexually active. Decreased sexual activity in older women usually arises from lack of a partner, rather than lack of interest. Indeed, sex may be freer and more satisfying, since it is now separated from reproductive worries.

It's true that sexual capacity in men (the ability to achieve and sustain an erection) can be altered by age. Among 65-year-olds, about 30 percent report that they are impotent, and that figure rises to 55 percent by the age of 75. Most older women experience a decline in vaginal lubrication. But these problems can be treated medically, if necessary—they need not limit sexuality. Also, coital performance is not the only expression of sexual love. A sexual bond can endure, change, and be renewed and developed throughout the lifespan.

MEMORY AND AGING

It is normal for a certain amount of forgetfulness to occur with age—and for older people to worry about it. Yet even as you search for someone's name or for your car keys, remember that many people can and do retain a very high level of mental ability as they grow older. Studies repeatedly show, in fact, that older people whose performance is inferior to college students on timed tests actually do as well or better than the students when they are allowed to pace themselves. It's not so surprising, given their far larger stores of experience.

Research suggests a number of causes behind memory lapses (known clinically as age-associated memory impairment, or AAMI). An aging brain produces smaller amounts of the chemicals called neurotransmitters, which facilitate the passage of electrical impulses that are involved in short-term memory. The brain's cells, or neurons, shrink over time, which could also account for some of the general slowing of mental functioning that occurs in old age. There is also evidence that blood flow to the brain decreases gradually over the years, which may be a contributing factor. And some researchers suspect that cultural attitudes and stereotypes toward older people play a role, causing them to lose confidence in their mental abilities.

Of course, memory loss is also the primary symptom of Alzheimer's disease and other forms of serious dementia—the majority of which are irreversible. Only a small percentage of the population over 65 come down with true Alzheimer's.

561

ASSISTING YOUR MEMORY

Even late in life, it's possible to train our memories to retain or improve overall ability. Here are some of the steps you can take to keep the mind supple with age.

Know your health status. Untreated high blood pressure, for example, can mildly impair memory and lengthen recall time. If you have high blood pressure, this is one of many reasons to treat it and keep it under control.

Be patient with yourself. Don't worry if your short-term recall slows down, or if it takes you longer to rummage through your memory to come up with the fact you want. The process of retrieval may slow down, but age usually enhances "intelligence" and may even result in "wisdom," in part because our store of information has grown so much.

Stay active mentally. Pursue old interests and cultivate new ones. Play Scrabble or bridge; work on puzzles. Read the newspaper. Take a course in some subject that interests you, or learn a craft or skill. All these are good exercises for improving memory and maintaining intellectual function.

Use mnemonic devices. These are methods that depend on strong visual images and meaningful associations to improve short-term recall and ferret out stored facts. For example: Helen's three-number telephone exchange, 744, is easy to remember, but you won't forget the rest of the number either, 4591, when you reflect that she looks to be about 45, almost halfway to 91. Or form mental images with people's names (picture someone named Appleton sitting in an apple tree). Books are available describing dozens of mnemonic strategies.

Write things down. Jotting down notes and making lists will help fix things in your mind. You may find you don't even have to refer to the notes and lists.

Structure your life. The hook for the house keys by the back door is a mnemonic device: you'll always look there first. For example, keep your checkbook in the third drawer of your desk, or park your reading glasses on the night table.

Be physically active. While there's no proof that physical fitness goes along with intellectual fitness, regular exercise confers a sense of well-being and may help control or ward off health problems.

Still, because early symptoms of the disease can appear trivial, "normally" forgetful people sometimes feel anxious over memory lapses. The difference between age-related memory lapses and serious dementia can be summed up in an old adage: "You need not worry if you forget where you put your car keys; you only need worry if you forget what they're used for." In fact, worrying about a memory lapse is considered a good sign that no other serious problems are the cause of it:

people with serious impairment tend not to worry or be aware of memory lapses.

Fortunately, we can do a number of things to improve our memory (see above). Research has shown that people in their 70s and 80s are quite capable of learning and can even reverse mental declines—which, when they do occur, happen gradually over many years.

Signs of a problem. If memory lapses in an older person seem to interfere with daily functioning, or if relatives and friends think lapses are serious, then the cause may be more complex than age-related memory impairment. A person who exhibits one or more of the following traits should be evaluated by a physician, who will perform a thorough physical exam and test the patient for any basic cognitive impairment:

• **Trouble retaining recent information.** The person misses appointments, forgets recent events or conversations, or regularly loses things.

• **Becoming disoriented.** The person gets lost while strolling or driving through familiar neighborhoods, or has trouble recognizing familiar landmarks.

• **Difficulty with previously easy tasks.** Examples include trouble balancing a checkbook, playing a card game, coordinating a social occasion, cooking a meal, or doing a similar task requiring a fair degree of intellectual function.

• **Personality changes.** Traits emerge that weren't previously apparent: a person becomes more passive than usual, a trusting person acts suspicious, an easygoing person is irritable or quickly provoked.

Keep in mind that a number of reversible conditions can mimic symptoms of Alzheimer's. Memory problems can be triggered by minor head injuries, high fever, poor nutrition, alcohol consumption, tranquilizers, adverse reactions to medication, or the emotional problems common to old age—depression, loneliness, and boredom. In such instances the problems are often eminently treatable.

OTHER HEALTH CONCERNS

The following health problems are not restricted to older people, but they are more common after 65 and can pose special risks.

Chronic diseases. The risks for the chronic diseases noted on pages 556-557—heart disease, certain cancers, and diabetes—continue to increase as people age. The risk of breast cancer, for example, is far higher in women over 60, and the risk of prostate cancer in men jumps dramatically. The estimated prevalence of coronary heart disease in both men and women climbs steadily with increasing age, as does the death rate from heart disease. About 60 percent of whites over age 60, and 71 percent of African-Americans, have high blood pressure (hypertension), a risk factor for heart disease. About 9 percent of whites ages 64 to 75 and 17 percent of African-Americans in the same age bracket are diagnosed with type 2 diabetes—as compared with 6 percent of whites and 11 percent of African-Americans ages 45 to 64.

These figures underscore the importance of preventive measures to reduce the risk of these diseases, and of regular tests and screenings to improve the chances of early detection.

Falls. Each year about one-third of adults over age 65 sustain a fall. Falls are the leading cause of nonfatal injuries among older adults, and deaths from falls, or from complications directly related to falls, are responsible for more than half of all accidental deaths of older people. Up to 25 percent of those who have fallen find themselves limiting their activities because they fear another accident.

Among the causes of falls are physical changes such as gait and mobility problems or diminished vision; unsafe elements in the environment (such as poor lighting, loose rugs, slippery surfaces, and objects on the floor); and the use of multiple medications, which can cause dizziness as a common side effect. Sedatives and alcohol also increase the risk of falls. Adopting some relatively simple measures can help prevent falls (see page 564).

563

PREVENTING FALLS

Older adults can take a number of simple precautions to reduce the risk of falling—starting with fixing household conditions that pose a hazard. Among the precautions: remove throw rugs; make sure stairways and hallways are well lighted and that handrails are installed along stairways; have grip bars and nonskid mats installed in bathrooms, along with shower chairs and bath benches; use nightlights in bedrooms, hallways, and bathrooms; finish wax floors with nonskid wax.

In addition, take these commonsense preventive health measures:

- Have your eyes and ears checked regularly.
- Stay active—with regular exercise and, as much as possible, during your daily routine (by taking stairs, for example, instead of an elevator).
- Wear well-fitting rubber-soled shoes—and never walk in your stocking feet, because you can slip. Use a cane or walker if you feel unsteady.
- Get up slowly—if you stand up quickly, you may get dizzy because of a momentary drop in blood pressure.
- Be careful drinking alcohol—even a small amount can impair balance and coordination.
- Review all your medications with your doctor, including their side effects, and see if it is possible to eliminate any of them.

Flu and pneumonia. Older people, as well as those with medical problems that may affect their immune systems, are at increased risk of serious illness from both influenza and pneumococcal infections. All adults 50 years of age and older should receive a vaccine annually that protects against the most recent flu viruses. Adults over 65 should also get a vaccine for protection from pneumococcal disease One shot provides protection for at least five years, at which time a booster shot may be needed.

Gastrointestinal ailments. The gastrointestinal tract remains highly functional throughout life, but aging gives rise to certain complaints. Older people are five times more likely than younger people to report problems with constipation. Poor diet, lack of exercise, an insufficient amount of fluids, and medications can all be causes of constipation in older people. But many complaints, according to experts, may stem from a preoccupation with having a daily bowel movement, rather than from being truly constipated. A concern with bowel movements can lead older people to depend on laxatives, and over time this reliance causes the natural mechanism of the digestive tract to falter. Most cases of constipation can be remedied with dietary changes and exercise (see page 217).

Diverticulosis is another gastrointestinal condition that is common in people over 60. For most people it does not develop into a health problem, but sometimes the diverticula—small pouches that form in the walls of the intestines—become inflamed, and the resulting condition, called diverticulitis, is more serious and requires medical treatment (see page 244).

Older people are also more prone to hiatal hernia—a condition that can produce symptoms that mimic heartburn (see page 328).

Heat and cold. A sharp rise in air temperature

can put older adults at risk because normal aging reduces the body's ability to cool off—in effect by raising the temperature threshold for sweating, thirst, and heat-related discomfort. Medical conditions such as heart disease or diabetes can worsen the problem. When air temperatures start to climb, older people should take protective measures against heat exhaustion (see page 119).

As we age, we also become less sensitive to drops in temperature—and so an older person's reaction to cold is slower and less acute. Older people therefore may not realize they are in a chilly environment that makes them susceptible to hypothermia—in which core body temperature falls below what is safe. Older people (and/or their friends and relatives) need to be sure that their homes are adequately heated and that they are well clothed against any chill. If you find an older person who appears to be suffering from hypothermia, you need to take emergency measures (see pages 121-122).

Incontinence. Experts estimate that 13 million older Americans must contend with urinary incontinence, or the involuntary loss of urine. Manufacturers of adult diapers often imply in their advertising that incontinence is an inevitable consequence of normal aging. In fact, incontinence is a symptom of some underlying disorder—and while it requires evaluation by a doctor, several of the most effective methods of treating it can be done at home (see page 482).

Thyroid problems. If the thyroid gland in your neck fails to produce enough thyroid hormone, you can gain weight, experience memory problems, undergo hair loss, feel tired all the time, and have trouble sleeping—all symptoms of hypothyroidism (insufficient levels of thyroid hormone). It may be hard for a doctor to spot thyroid problems: the symptoms may be mild or nonexistent, and many symptoms are not unique to thyroid disease. Therefore, people over 50, especially women, should be alert to the possibility of hypothyroidism. According to the American Association of Clinical Endocrinologists, disorders of the thyroid are underdiagnosed in Americans, and all older women—because they are at the greatest risk for thyroid disease—should talk to their doctors about a blood test (the TSH assay) for thyroid function as part of their regular physical checkup. If you do need thyroid hormones, you must be carefully monitored to make sure your dosage is correct. You will also need to take steps to reduce your risk of bone loss.

PREVENTIVE SERVICES RECOMMENDATIONS

This table highlights the major screening tests (that is, routine tests for people without symptoms) and immunizations for healthy adults ages 65 and older. This advice is based in part on the latest recommendations of the U.S. Preventive Services Task Force (see page 70).

PREVENTIVE SCREENINGS AND CHECKUPS

FOR MEN AND WOMEN

Blood pressure measurement (to detect hypertension): Once every 2 years for those with normal blood pressure.

Cholesterol measurement: At least once every 5 years, more often if the total cholesterol number is elevated (above 200 mg/dl) or the HDL cholesterol is low (below 35 mg/dl), and/or you have cardiac risk factors such as a family history of heart disease, diabetes, or hypertension.

Colorectal cancer screening (fecal occult blood test and/or sigmoidoscopy): Every year for the occult blood test; sigmoidoscopy every 5 years (or colonoscopy every 10 years). A digital rectal exam (DRE) should also be performed annually.

Diabetes mellitus screening. The American Diabetes Association recommends that everyone in this age group should be tested for non-insulin-dependent (type 2) diabetes.

Glaucoma screening: Many eye specialists advise screening all adults in this age group. People at high risk, which include the very nearsighted, people with diabetes, African-Americans over the age of 40, and those with a family history of the disease, may need more frequent screenings. How often depends on professional advice (see page 289).

Thyroid disease screening. For people in this age group, especially women, who have experienced possible symptoms of hypothyroidism or who have high cholesterol levels; they should discuss this test with their doctors (see page 84).

Dental checkup: Every 6 months or on professional advice; should include cleaning.

FOR WOMEN

Pap smear (for early detection of cervical cancer): Every 3 years for all women with a cervix. Possibly more often, depending on risk factors such as smoking or multiple sex partners, or a history of genital warts. Some experts advise that women who have never had an abnormal result can stop being screened after age 65 (see page 74).

Breast cancer screening (mammogram and clinical breast exam): Every year for all women in this age group.

FOR MEN

Prostate cancer screening (prostate specific antigen, or PSA, test and digital rectal exam): All men in this age group should have a digital rectal exam (DRE) annually. The usefulness of the PSA for screening all men remains controversial. Routine screening with the PSA is not recommended, but older men who are African-American or who have a family history of the disease should consider testing. Consult your doctor as to how often. If you are 65 to 75 with no family history or other risk factors, you may choose not to be screened; this also applies if you are over 75 and symptom-free. (See page 80 for more information.)

IMMUNIZATION

Tetanus-diphtheria booster: Every 10 years. Relatively few cases of tetanus occur in this country now, but most cases occur in older adults, who are least likely to be adequately immunized because they have not kept up with their shots.

Influenza vaccine: Everyone in this age group.

Pneumococcal vaccine: Everyone in this age group. One shot is effective against most strains of the bacterium *Streptococcus pneumoniae*, the most common bacterial cause of pneumonia in people over 40. Protection lasts at least 5 years.

The point of stocking medical supplies is to have essential items on hand in case of emergencies. But medicine chests tend to become an elephant's graveyard: out-of-date drugs pile up, making you think you're better stocked than you really are. Outdated drugs are generally not harmful, but may not be as effective.

Check expiration dates every few months. If a drug doesn't have an expiration date, write the purchase date on the label. Then check with your pharmacist before using a drug that is more than a year old. Discard old drugs by flushing them down the toilet; children could find them in a wastebasket.

A bathroom is actually a poor place to store drugs because the high heat and humidity from the bath or shower causes pills and powders to deteriorate. Choose a cool, dry spot instead, like a closet shelf. If a drug needs to be kept in a refrigerator, it will be indicated on the label.

What to Consider Discarding

• Prescription drugs you didn't use up. Medications prescribed for a specific condition that has since cleared up should be thrown away, not kept around "just in case." Get rid of outdated medications, too.

• Hexylresorcinol, Merthiolate, Mercurochrome, and similar products. These are not effective disinfectants and can burn the skin under a tight bandage. Be wary, generally, of products that claim to promote healing.

• Hydrogen peroxide. This old standby for "cleansing" can actually damage skin and retard healing. Water is better.

• Stimulant laxatives (such as Ex-Lax, Feen-A-Mint, and Cascara). A diet high in fruits, vegetables, and whole grains, plus two quarts of fluid daily, should keep you from needing a laxative. (See page 589 for more information on laxatives.)

If you have any questions about the condition or potency of a drug, call your doctor or pharmacist. Since medicines don't last forever, it may be a waste of money to buy large, family-size bottles of drugs. They may go bad before you use them.

If there are children in the house or coming to visit, be sure that potentially toxic medicines are in childproof containers or in a locked box. Don't rely on keeping them out of reach.

What To Keep

• A pair of thin-tipped tweezers for removing splinters, dirt particles from a wound, or ticks.

• Bandages (assorted sizes), gauze, and adhesive tape.

• An over-the-counter pain reliever. Because no single pain reliever is right for every situation or every person, you might keep more than one type on hand.

• A simple antacid, especially one with calcium, such as Tums or Rolaids.

• A remedy for mild diarrhea, such as Pepto-Bismol or Imodium, which can be bought in generic form.

• Calamine lotion for soothing insect bites or poison ivy.

• OTC hydrocortisone cream (1 percent) for skin rashes, insect bites, and contact dermatitis. It should not be used on any eruption caused by fungi, viruses, or bacteria (such as athlete's foot, ringworm, or cold sores).

• A fever thermometer.

The Drugstore Guide

Over-the-counter (OTC) drugs can play an important role in managing your own health care, and drugstores now also carry a wealth of dietary supplements that consumers are turning to as remedies. This section explains safety and effectiveness issues concerning drugs and supplements, provides guidelines for choosing and using key OTC products, and offers profiles and recommendations on the most popular supplements.

Guide to Over-the-Counter Medications

The modern Food and Drug Administration (FDA) was created in 1938 in the aftermath of a tragedy. An adulterated sulfa drug killed 107 people in 1937, most of them children. The new legislation covered not only drugs, but also cosmetics and therapeutic devices, and the agency was given broad powers of enforcement.

DRUGS AND THE FDA

For the first time, the burden of proof for a fraudulent or harmful drug or device lay with the manufacturer, not the government. Before companies could market new drugs, they had to offer proof of safety and efficacy. Only in 1951, however, were rules laid down as to which drugs must be sold by prescription: basically any drug deemed unsafe for use without medical supervision.

Getting a drug approved by the FDA has been a painstaking, time-consuming, expensive process—the toughest approval process for drugs in the world. Manufacturers must pay for and conduct animal and human trials to demonstrate safety and efficacy. The FDA also does "postmarketing surveillance," because even after all this testing, drugs sometimes prove unsafe in the marketplace. In 1938, when the FDA was formed, many existing drugs were "grandfathered" as approved, though some had never been rigorously tested; these have gradually come under review. Labeling is also under constant review.

Clinical trials are relatively brief, small, and include only certain groups of people. The FDA keeps track of adverse side effects and can take a

drug off the market or restrict its use. For instance, the diet drug Redux was withdrawn in 1997 because it caused heart damage. And in 2000, dozens of over-the-counter cold remedies, along with OTC appetite suppressants marketed as aids in weight control, were ordered off the market because a six-year study concluded that an ingredient in these products—phenylpropanolamine, or PPA—was linked to a small but significant risk of hemorrhagic stroke in young women.

OVER-THE-COUNTER DRUGS

OTC drugs, which include many pain relievers, laxatives, cold remedies, and antihistamines, are under the surveillance of the FDA, just like prescription drugs. It's a myth that OTC drugs are essentially harmless. OTC drugs, according to the American Pharmaceutical Association, are "powerful chemical entities" that should be viewed just like prescription drugs. Many, in fact, were once prescription drugs. Of course, self-medication with OTC drugs is a reasonable way to manage minor, self-limiting problems. But not everything that has been on the shelf really works (see the listing on page 571). And things that do work can have side effects or adverse effects that may turn out to pose a health risk, as was the case with products containing PPA.

OTC drugs are much cheaper and easier to get than prescription drugs. For one thing, you can skip the medical consultation—thus consumers, drug companies, and health insurers are usually

---

OTC Drugs That Don't Work

The FDA's review of OTC drugs is a massive and continuing project. Some drugs have been sold for decades and have never really been reviewed under the newer laws. Some ingredients once thought safe and effective have proven otherwise. Recalling a product is a complicated, time-consuming business, and some products may remain on the shelves after a recall, but they are gradually being removed from circulation.

According to the FDA, *none* of the following OTC products, for example, have been proven safe or effective:

- Antifungal diaper rash products.
- Nail fungus remedies (there are effective prescription drugs).
- Aphrodisiacs (sexual stimulants).
- Boil remedies.
- Digestive aids (such as cellulase, garlic, ox bile extract).
- Products for pancreatic insufficiency.
- Ingrown toenail relief.
- Nail-biting or thumb-sucking deterrents.
- Remedies for eye infections.
- Oral treatments for fever blisters and cold sores.
- Oral agents for wound healing.
- Insect repellents to be taken orally.
- Products to relieve urinary urgency and benign prostatic hypertrophy.
- Daytime sedatives for nervous tension.
- Nocturnal leg cramp remedies.
- Preventives for swimmer's ear.
- Smoking deterrents such as ginger, silver acetate, and lobelia (however, nicotine-delivery products such as patches and gums, now sold OTC, may help some people).
- Stomach acidifiers.
- Asthma remedies containing theophylline.
- Topical hormone products claiming to remove wrinkles.

---

happy to see a drug reclassified. Certain heartburn drugs (such as cimetidine, brand name Tagamet), pain relievers (naproxen, brand name Aleve), and antiyeast products for vaginal infections are examples of products formerly available only by prescription. Hundreds of other drugs have also made the switch. In reclassifying a drug, the FDA considers the safety record of the drug, its toxicity, its potential for misuse, the difficulty of labeling it adequately, and other factors. Opinions are solicited from many scientific advisors. For consumers, this process has benefits, but also dangers, since it's up to the individual to be aware of warnings and to monitor effects and side effects. (See page 573 for pointers on using OTC drugs.)

SORTING OUT THE CHOICES

There are over 100,000 nonprescription drugs available in the United States. This gives consumers plenty of choice, but sorting out these products can be bewildering. Rather than clearly tell you what a product contains, manufacturers want you to rely on choosing a product by its brand name—which is not the way you might shop for, say, a pain reliever ("Brand X Pain Reliever" vs. "aspirin"). And even brand names that are familiar can confuse: for example, there are now a dozen different Tylenol formulations with multiple—and different—ingredients.

So if you decide to use an over-the-counter remedy, it's important that you inspect a particular product to establish precisely what active

Brand Names Vs. Generics

Generic drugs—which are sold under the chemical name of the principal active ingredient rather than a brand name—are on the rise. Most over-the-counter medications are available in generic formulations, and half of all drug prescriptions filled today are generics. Generics are cheaper than brand-name drugs, which is why insurers, as well as Medicare and Medicaid, favor them for filling prescriptions. Yet many people worry that generics aren't the same as the brand-name drugs, and doctors sometimes refuse to switch a patient from a brand name to a generic.

In most cases, there's absolutely no reason to shy away from generics. For the generic to be regarded as interchangeable with the original, the active ingredients must be identical. In addition, the generic must be the bio-equivalent of the original: this means that the active ingredients must be absorbed by the body at the same rate and with the same effects. The medication may contain a different inert ingredient, however, and it's possible that someone might have a minor side effect from that, but it's rare.

Over-the-counter generics are safe and often much less expensive than brand names. An aspirin is an aspirin, no matter what it costs or what the ads tell you about the supposed advantages of sticking to the brand your mother used to buy. And increasingly, the same big drug companies are manufacturing both the brand name and the generics. Almost all HMOs, hospitals, and government agencies use generics whenever possible.

Of course, the choice of a prescription drug is up to a physician's best judgment, and your doctor is the person to consult if you are worried about any drug you are taking. If you do plan to discuss your medication with your doctor, keep taking it in the meantime. It can be dangerous to make changes on your own.

Your pharmacist should also be able to answer questions you have about any differences between a brand name and a generic.

ingredients it contains—and to choose a product that contains only what has a good chance of really helping you. Because of a labeling regulation passed in 1999 (to be phased in over several years), OTC products will start to carry a new easy-to-understand "Drug Facts" label that clearly list a product's active ingredients first, along with the purpose for each, followed by uses, warnings (including interactions with other drugs and side effects), directions, and inactive ingredients.

Medicines that can be obtained over the counter, by law, must be safe for use without the supervision of a physician. They are not addictive if used correctly, and they must have clear warnings and instructions for consumers printed on the labels. Yet there's a difference between "safe" and "harmless." Over-the-counter drugs can do damage if they are used incorrectly, and some can lead to physical dependence if overused. Some nonprescription drugs should not be taken by children, pregnant or lactating women, or the elderly. Some OTC drugs are also not meant to be taken in combination with other drugs.

OTC drugs are also supposed to be effective as well as safe. But the degree of effectiveness varies greatly: some drugs don't actually do very much, and you may be just as well off either doing nothing or using the nondrug remedies discussed in other sections of this book.

This section provides information on widely

used over-the-counter medications that can cause confusion for consumers. You will also find information on medications in entries on specific ailments. Different treatments for skin problems, for example, are discussed under *athlete's foot, dermatitis, dry skin, diaper rash, warts, wrinkles,* and other skin-related disorders. You can also check the index for a particular product or ingredient.

USING OTC DRUGS SAFELY

Remember these pointers when using any OTC drugs:

• Read the label before buying and taking medication. Heed warnings about possible side effects and interactions with other drugs (including alcohol) or food.

• Be certain that your self-diagnosis is correct. What seems like heartburn, for example, may actually be heart disease.

• Pregnant and nursing women and children under 12 should generally not take any OTC drug except on medical advice and under medical supervision. People with serious disorders, and especially those with chronic liver, heart, or lung disease, should also check with their physicians before using an OTC medication.

• Follow dosage instructions. If the drug isn't working, get medical advice from your pharmacist or doctor—don't simply increase the dosage on your own.

• If you are 65 or older, check with your doctor about the doses of any over-the-counter medications you take regularly. Many older people do not need—and should not take—full adult doses. Age-related changes in the liver may increase the amount of medication in the bloodstream, resulting in greater therapeutic effects and the possibility of more-pronounced side effects.

• Buy drugs with only the ingredients you need.

Multi-ingredient products (such as cold remedies with antihistamines) may give you drugs you don't need.

• Don't take the drug for longer than recommended.

• If you are taking any other drug, prescription or OTC, ask your pharmacist or doctor about possible interactions.

• Keep all drugs out of the reach of children.

Rule of thumb: OTC drugs are only for temporary use, and in the dosage prescribed, unless you have other advice from a physician. If you are in chronic need of OTC drugs (antacids, for example, or pain relievers), that's a signal to seek medical advice. You may have misdiagnosed yourself, or you may need some other medication.

Antihistamines

573

When pollen or some other airborne allergen strikes, your body reacts by producing a chemical called a histamine, which helps trigger symptoms of a hay fever attack. The drugs known as antihistamines, which have been on the market for years, are effective against three primary symptoms of hay fever: itching, sneezing, and a runny nose (as well as postnasal drip).

Antihistamines are also used in many brand-name products labeled as cold remedies. But many health experts, including those responsible for the FDA's recommendations concerning cold and allergy medications, do not advise using antihistamines for alleviating cold symptoms, even when cold symptoms mimic symptoms associated with hay fever. Histamine plays no part in viral infections such as colds or flu, and in fact, antihistamines may make cold congestion worse:

although they can dry up secretions, they may make mucus too thick, and thus difficult to expel by coughing. They can also induce drowsiness in many people, and have other possible side effects, including dry mouth, blurred vision, and urinary retention. (A number of cold and allergy products with antihistamines also contained phenylpropanolamine, or PPA—a decongestant ingredient that acted as a stimulant to counteract the sedative effect of the antihistamine. Because of an FDA warning about PPA, products containing it must either be removed from the market or reformulated without PPA.)

A new class of antihistamines, known as "second-generation" antihistamines, are nonsedating. These newer drugs—which include loratidine (Claritin) and fexofenadine (Allegra)—can be bought only by prescription. Most work with just one dose a day, and they also don't cause dry mouth. However, they are not recommended for treating cold symptoms.

Over-the-counter antihistamines come in many chemical classes, and are sold under scores of over-the-counter brand names and as generic "allergy pills." Since they have no effect on nasal congestion, antihistamines are often combined with a decongestant. Decongestants, which are also used in many cold remedies (see page 576), can produce a stimulating effect that may help to counter the drowsiness caused by antihistamines. (Antihistamines are also used in other types of over-the-counter products, including those for pain relief and for treating insect bites and stings.)

Here are the leading over-the-counter antihistamine ingredients used for the treatment of hay fever, and some single-ingredient brand products in which they're found. (There are also generic equivalents available for each of these brands; the label will show the ingredient, or

generic, name, indicated here in italics.)

Brompheniramine maleate (Dimetapp Allergy)

Chlorpheniramine maleate (Chlor-Trimeton 12-Hour Allergy)

Clemastine fumarate (Tavist-1)

Diphenhydramine hydrochloride (Benadryl Allergy)

• *Doxylamine succinate* and *phenyltoloxamine citrate* are antihistamine ingredients used in a number of "night-time" cold formulas because they induce drowsiness. Another ingredient, triprolidine hydrochloride, is used in combination with a decongestant (for example, Actifed).

• The antihistamine ingredient *pheniramine maleate*, in combination with *naphazoline*, a decongestant, is approved for over-the-counter use in eyedrops (Opcon A) to relieve eye redness and itchiness caused by airborne irritants and allergens.

Choosing a product: All of the over-the-counter ingredients cause drowsiness, but the effect can be minimized by starting at low dosages and gradually increasing them. Still, don't ignore the warnings about drowsiness and impaired performance: one study found that drugs with diphenhydramine, one of the most popular antihistamine ingredients, may impair driving ability nearly as much as alcohol.

• Chlorpheniramine and brompheniramine are considered the least sedating, and so are preferred for daytime use.

• Diphenhydramine is quick-acting, but also may be the most sedating; it is used in a number of night-time formulas, and some people even use it occasionally as a sleeping pill. It is also approved for use as a cough suppressant.

• Clemastine fumarate is in the same class as diphenhydramine, but is longer-acting and less sedating.

• Pay attention to side effects. Each ingredient

has side effects in addition to drowsiness, including urinary retention, constipation, and blurred vision. Special warnings apply to individuals taking other medications or who have other medical problems. Antihistamines are usually not recommended for pregnant or nursing women.

You may be one of the lucky people who don't become drowsy when taking over-the-counter antihistamines, or you may at least be able to find one brand that doesn't affect you that way. But an antihistamine can still slow motor reactions, even if you feel alert. Over-the-counter allergy pills that claim to be nonsedating (usually labeled "for daytime use" or "non-drowsy formula") do not contain an antihistamine, and are not as effective as products that do contain an antihistamine.

You may need to experiment to see which antihistamine provides the best relief while causing the least drowsiness. Also, some people find that the effect of an antihistamine diminishes when it is used regularly over weeks or months; in that case, switching to another ingredient may boost relief.

Another option is a nasal spray specifically approved for preventing and treating nasal allergy symptoms. Called Nasalcrom (cromolyn sodium), the spray is available without a prescription and can be used regularly by adults and children age 6 and older (see page 305 for more information).

Cold and Cough Medications

There are no cures for the common cold. (Contrary to what many people think, antibiotic medications cannot kill cold viruses or any other type of virus; they are effective only against bacterial infections.) But in response to the millions of people who seek relief from the discomfort brought on by colds, drug manufacturers have concocted an enormous variety of products that promise to alleviate symptoms. More than 800 over-the-counter cold and cough products are available in the United States, making up the largest segment of nonprescription medications. (A recent FDA warning about phenylpropanolamine, or PPA—an ingredient commonly used in cold remedies—affected dozens of products that had to be removed from pharmacy shelves.)

In contrast to products like pain relievers, which are readily available in single-ingredient formulations, the majority of over-the-counter cold and cough remedies contain multiple ingredients. In effect, they are "shotgun" formulas that attack several symptoms at once with as many as six ingredients. Some of these ingredients will be of no value to you if you don't have the symptoms they address, yet you will have to put up with any side effects they cause. In addition, all the ingredients in a combination product must be taken in fixed amounts; you can't vary the dosage independently as your symptoms change. Combination products are also usually more expensive than single-ingredient formulations.

The effectiveness of cold products is another issue. Not only won't these products prevent or cure colds, but often the symptomatic relief they provide is limited. Some approved over-the-counter ingredients aren't all that effective, and many of them have noticeable side effects, even at recommended dosages. So they won't necessarily make you feel better. (In fact, rather than rush out to buy a cold remedy, consider first trying the self-care measures that are listed on page 210.)

If you decide to use an over-the-counter remedy, it's important that you inspect a particular

575

product to establish precisely what it contains—and to choose a product that contains only what has a good chance of really helping you.

The different types of active ingredients that can be included in cold and cough formulations are discussed here, along with the symptoms they address and which ingredients are worth trying.

FOR A STUFFY NOSE: DECONGESTANTS

Of all the over-the-counter products marketed for cold symptoms, decongestants may provide the most noticeable relief for many people. Swollen or dilated blood vessels are a major cause of congestion, which occurs in membranes lining the nose and can also affect the sinuses, throat, and lungs. Decongestants relieve congestion by constricting blood vessels and opening nasal passages temporarily, and they may also dry up mucus. (They are also used in "allergy" products aimed at relieving congestion that is caused by hay fever.)

Topical decongestants, which are applied directly to membranes by means of sprays, drops, or inhalers, act quickly, but the relief they provide is temporary—your nose clears for a few hours, then you want to repeat the dose. Yet after only a few repeated doses, these drugs can have a rebound effect—an increase in swelling and more congestion than ever. Many people take this rebound effect as a sign that they need more medication, but taking more only makes the problem worse.

Because the rebound problem is so prevalent, topical decongestants should be used only rarely, if at all. If you do choose one of these products, *it's important not to use it for more than one to two days*—used longer, it will almost surely cause rebound congestion.

Most topical decongestants rely on one or more of four active ingredients.

• Because it is long-acting and has relatively few side effects, *oxymetazoline* (Afrin 12-Hour, Neo-Synephrine 12-Hour) is the ingredient used most often.

• *Xylometazoline* (Otrivin) lasts eight to ten hours per dose, *naphazoline* (Privine) four to six hours.

• *Phenylephrine* (Dristan) has less strength than the other ingredients but fewer adverse effects.

• Recently, a drug called l-desoxyephedrine (also called levmetamfetamine) was approved by the FDA for over-the-counter use in decongestant inhalers (Vicks Vapor Inhaler).

Oral decongestants (in pill form) take longer to act than topical decongestants (nose drops, sprays, and inhalers), but their effect may last longer. Because they act systemically, however, oral decongestants can increase heart rate, induce insomnia, cause headaches, cause palpitations, and elevate blood pressure in some people.

By far the most common active ingredient is *pseudoephedrine*, which is used as a single ingredient in Sudafed and many other brand-name and generic products as well as in dozens of multiple-ingredient products. It has the fewest side effects of any oral decongestant, and is the ingredient most often used in children's products.

Another decongestant ingredient, *phenylpropanolamine* (PPA), was used for decades in cold and allergy remedies (such as Comtrex, Contac, Dimetapp, Naldecon, Triaminic, and others). But in 2000 the FDA asked drug manufacturers to stop marketing products containing PPA after a study linked it to an increased risk of stroke in young women. Brand-name products containing PPA must be reformulated to remain on the market. If you have a product containing PPA in your medicine cabinet, you should discard it. You can ask your pharmacist about replacing it with a new and comparable product.

Choosing a product: Nasal sprays or drops are fast-acting, but should only be used for a day or two at most. Because drops allow doses to be more precisely controlled, they are good for using with small children. Sprays are better suited for older children and adults.

For congestion that lasts longer (which is more often the case with hay fever than with a cold), try one of the oral decongestants. Start with a product containing pseudoephedrine, which is the ingredient least likely to cause adverse effects. In regular tablet form, the decongestant effect lasts only about four hours, but pseudoephedrine is now available in sustained-action formulations, which may be preferred by people whose sleep is

interrupted by congestion or who need to take a decongestant for long periods.

However, don't use an oral decongestant for more than ten days without consulting your doctor.

Avoid decongestant products that contain acetaminophen: the acetaminophen may increase nasal congestion, thereby fighting the effect of the decongestant.

FOR COUGHS: SUPPRESSANTS (ANTITUSSIVES) AND EXPECTORANTS

In the first stages of a cold, a cough is probably dry. Coughing seems to further irritate the throat and make you cough more. Thus you may want a cough suppressant, which acts on the cough center in the brain. Some suppressants contain the narcotic *codeine*, which is approved for over-the-counter sales in several states. It works, but can cause stomach upset and promotes constipation. A better choice is a suppressant with *dextromethorphan*, a synthetic relative of codeine that works on the same nerve center to suppress coughing but with much less of codeine's side effects. A third type is one containing *diphenhydramine*, the only antihistamine recommended for treating coughs. Like codeine, it may make you drowsy.

Camphor and *menthol* are two ingredients approved for use by the FDA as topical antitussives. Each is available as an ointment (such as Vapo-Rub), which you spread on the throat and chest, and solutions containing menthol or camphor can be added to a vaporizer; the medicated vapor can then be inhaled. (Be careful not to accidentally ingest ointments or solutions containing either of these ingredients. It's also important not to use them near an open flame or to heat them in a microwave oven, since they can ignite.)

Using Nose Drops and Sprays Properly

▼

Before using either drops or a spray, clear your nose by blowing it gently.

For drops: It's best for the person receiving the drops to lie down on a bed and tilt his or her head over the side. Release the drops into each nostril, then move the head gently from side to side so the medicine will bathe all the nasal membranes. Rinse the dropper with hot water and let it dry.

For sprays: Insert the tip of the open bottle into a nostril. Be sure to keep the head upright. Squeeze the bottle quickly and firmly, and take a deep sniff as the spray is released. Rinse the spray tip with hot water (but don't let water get into the bottle). Dry with a clean tissue and replace the cap.

Remember to limit use of drops or sprays to one to two days.

577

Cold and Cough Formulas for Children

▼

Drug manufacturers are marketing more cold products than ever aimed at the parents of young children, since children are especially prone to colds. Many of these products are combination formulas. But the American Academy of Pediatrics advises against the use of combination cold and cough medications, and recommends that if parents choose to use a medication, they use single-ingredient products targeted at the leading symptoms. Also, don't give cold medications made for adults to children; many adult products contain ingredients and/or dosage levels that are harmful when taken by children. Decongestants and antihistamines in particular should not be given to young children without consulting a physician.

578

Later you may have a "productive cough"—that is, you bring up phlegm when you cough. That's usually a good sign, meaning that your infection is on the way out. It's best not to suppress this kind of cough, since it serves a useful purpose by clearing secretions from your throat and lungs. But if the cough is keeping you awake, you may need to take a suppressant at bedtime.

If you're congested but your cough is *not* productive, you may wish you had something to loosen up the mucus. Plenty of products, known as expectorants, claim to do just that. All contain *guaifenesin,* the only expectorant ingredient classified as "safe and effective" by the FDA. However, guaifenesin has never been proven effective in clinical trials.

Choosing a product: Choose either a suppressant (preferably one containing dextromethorphan) or an expectorant, depending on what kind

of cough you have. Avoid using cough formulas that contain both a cough suppressant along with guaifenesin. These products encourage you to cough up phlegm while also suppressing the urge to cough—a combination that makes no sense. Cough drops will do little to relieve a cough, but they may soothe a throat that is raw from coughing (see below).

FOR A SORE THROAT: ANESTHETICS & ALTERNATIVES

Lozenges, cough drops, sprays, and gargles are widely marketed as a treatment for sore throat. Despite the medicinal taste and smell of some of these medications, there's no clinical evidence that they're better than simply sucking on a piece of hard candy. Topical anesthetics, mentholated cough drops, and other ingredients may not help you any more than a plain lemon drop. Sucking on a hard candy (or any cough drop) probably works by promoting saliva flow, which is soothing; the sugar can also soothe the throat.

Here's what throat products may contain:

• Topical anesthetics such as benzocaine or dyclonine.

• Hexylresorcinol, an antibacterial completely ineffective against cold viruses.

• Sugar in the forms of sucrose, corn syrup, or honey; artificial sweeteners such as saccharin, sorbitol, or aspartame.

Choosing a product: Topical anesthetics may provide some relief for three to four hours (though in some people these compounds can trigger an allergic skin reaction). A warm saline gargle (see page 451) may be just as soothing. Like hard candies, cough drops with sugar can contribute to tooth decay, so use them sparingly or avoid them.

Taking acetaminophen, aspirin, or another pain reliever may also help ease sore throat pain. However, don't treat a sore throat with aspirin-containing chewing gum or aspirin gargles. Aspirin applied directly to the mucous membranes won't reduce the pain and can act as an irritant.

FOR ACHES AND FEVER: NSAIDS AND ACETAMINOPHEN

Over-the-counter non-steroidal anti-inflammatory drugs, or NSAIDs—which include aspirin, naproxen, ibuprofen, and ketoprofen—can relieve muscle aches and fever associated with colds and flu. Acetaminophen, which is not an NSAID, is also effective for cold- or flu-related aches and fever.

Choosing a product: If your cold is accompanied by aching, consider taking a pain reliever. Pregnant women, especially in the last trimester, should avoid NSAIDs. Children 19 years of age or younger should not take aspirin, which may cause Reye's syndrome, a potentially fatal disorder in children who have flu or chicken pox and use aspirin. Heavy drinkers or people with liver or kidney disease should avoid acetaminophen. (See pages 594-605 for more information on pain relievers.)

ADDITIONAL GUIDELINES FOR COLD MEDICATIONS

In addition to the advice for selecting each type of product, here are general recommendations to consider when shopping for a cold medication.

• *Skip the antihistamines if you have a cold.* Many products labeled as cold remedies contain antihistamines, even though antihistamines—which are effective against symptoms of allergic rhinitis, or hay fever—do nothing to alleviate similar symptoms caused by cold viruses. Persistent, repeated sneezing is one indication you have hay fever rather than a cold. While the sinus drainage

from a cold is usually murky, that from a hay fever attack is clear and thin. Hay fever is also often accompanied by itching around the eyes and mouth.

• *Read labels carefully—don't rely on brand names and marketing claims.* These can often be misleading. A "cold relief" product may contain an antihistamine, which won't help your cold symptoms. A term like "maximum strength" in a brand name could mean that the product contains maximum recommended levels of one ingredient, or of all the ingredients, or it may simply refer to the fact that the product contains many ingredients. Likewise, terms such as "fast-acting" and "slow-release" have no specific meaning when used on these products.

You need to read what is actually in the product, and try to choose a product that clearly states the ingredients and their functions.

• *Single-ingredient products are usually the best choice.* If you find a combination drug that works well for you, you needn't avoid it. But don't assume that because combination products are the norm, they are preferable. Single-ingredient products have several advantages.

You can match ingredients to your symptoms, which may change during the course of a cold. Your cold may start off with just a stuffy nose, so if you have no cough or muscle aches, take a simple decongestant (if you wish) instead of one of the many decongestant products that also contain a cough formula and a pain reliever. Take a cough medicine once you actually develop a cough, if the cough is bothersome enough that you want to do something about it. Add a pain reliever if you develop muscle aches.

You can better control the timing and dosage of an ingredient. For example, in the evening you could take a cough suppressant but lower the dose of a

579

decongestant (which can be stimulating). A combination product may not even have a sufficient dose of the ingredient that provides you with the greatest benefit.

Combination products also multiply side effects and may compound them. Single-ingredient products confront you with only one set of side effects.

If you have multiple symptoms and want to try a multiple-symptom medication, at least try to select a product with ingredients for your specific symptoms.

• *Be wary of "night-time" formulas.* Generally, products that promise to help you sleep carry a full arsenal of ingredients, including an antihistamine that may induce drowsiness (but won't necessarily alleviate cold symptoms). There is no more reason to consume all of these ingredients at night than there is during the day. If a cough is keeping you awake, take a cough suppressant before you go to bed. Take a decongestant and/or a pain reliever in addition only if a stuffy nose and a headache have also been interfering with your sleep.

• *Check warning labels.* If you choose a cold remedy that contains an antihistamine, it can cause drowsiness, which can be more than an inconvenience if you will be driving or performing work that requires alertness. Other ingredients interact with various medications or aggravate certain health problems. The more ingredients a product contains, the greater the number of warnings to keep track of.

• *Generics are as effective as the comparable brand-name product.* Many active ingredients for colds and hay fever are packaged generically. Not only are they far less expensive—half the price or less of comparable brand-name products—but their labels are often more straightforward.

• *Talk to your pharmacist.* Many people are con-

fused by these medications. If you have questions about a particular product, or want advice on what is appropriate for you, a pharmacist should be able to help.

Diarrhea Medications (Antidiarrheals)

Simple diarrhea is usually self-limiting—it gets better without treatment in a day or two. Although there a number of over-the-counter products sold to combat diarrhea, many are not effective, and even those that are effective in relieving symptoms may not be warranted. If you have an attack of mild to moderate diarrhea, it's important to drink plenty of fluids and follow the other measures spelled out on pages 240-243. See pages 476-478 for information on treatment and prevention of traveler's diarrhea.

It's also important to be sure that you don't have inflammatory diarrhea, signaled by a small volume of stool, blood and/or pus in the stool, fever, and abdominal pain. These symptoms are indicative of a more serious bowel disease and should not be self-treated with an antidiarrheal remedy or any other over-the-counter product. Anyone with these symptoms needs to be diagnosed by a physician before beginning treatment.

GUIDELINES FOR DIARRHEA MEDICATIONS

Some over-the-counter medications to alleviate diarrhea can be useful in certain cases. But wait a few hours after the onset of diarrhea before using one of these medications. Diarrhea is a purging of the intestines, so you want to give your system a chance to get rid of or decrease whatever irritant is causing the problem. Once that occurs, some of the medications designed to alleviate diarrhea can be useful in certain cases.

There are a number of products sold in drugstores for easing symptoms of run-of-the mill noninflammatory diarrhea, but only three have been shown to be safe and effective.

Consider loperamide first. Loperamide (Imodium A-D), which is available generically, is the preferred nonprescription medication for treating diarrhea. Known as an antiperistaltic or antimotility agent, it slows the peristaltic contractions of the intestines and therefore the passage of intestinal contents, reducing the frequency of stool by up to 80 percent. It also helps relieve cramping.

Bismuth subsalicylate and polycarbophil can also help relieve symptoms. More commonly known by a brand name, Pepto-Bismol, bismuth subsalicylate (which is also sold in generic forms) works by inhibiting the secretion of fluid into the intestine and by binding diarrhea-causing bacterial toxins. It reduces the number of loose stool by about 60 percent.

However, anyone taking aspirin should not use bismuth subsalicylate. It contains varying amounts of salicylate, the pain-relieving ingredient in aspirin, and levels of salicylate from both sources could reach toxic levels in some people. Bismuth subsalicylate is also not suitable for aspirin-sensitive individuals or for children 19 or younger, who are at risk of the rare but serious illness called Reye's syndrome, which is induced by aspirin and can strike children and teenagers who have or are recovering from chicken pox or influenza.

Polycarbophil is a synthetic fiber-like compound, available in chewable tablets (such as Mitrolan), that absorbs up to 60 times its original weight in water. Also used in the treatment of constipation, it can help form firmer stools and slow the loss of intestinal fluid. It may take up to a day to work effectively.

Products containing attapulgite or kaolin and pectin are generally not effective. These agents, known as adsorbents, bind (or adsorb) with irritants in the bowel and also absorb water, theoretically resulting in larger, firmer, and less frequent bowel movements. However, there is little evidence that attapulgite preparations (such as Donnagel or Kaopectate) or those containing kaolin and pectin (Kapectolin or Kao-Paverin) actually diminish intestinal fluid loss. In addition, they may bind with—and so hamper the absorption of—needed nutrients, digestive enzymes, and other medications.

Be alert to signs of dehydration. Contact your doctor if you suspect dehydration has occurred in someone with diarrhea. Children are most susceptible, but elderly adults can also become dehydrated. Signs include cool, dry, pale skin; dry tongue; thirst; listlessness; rapid pulse; sunken eyes; changes in posture; in small children and infants, no tears when crying and a sunken fontanelle (the soft spot on top of an infant's head). See page 241 for more information about treating diarrhea in children.

Be sure to contact your doctor if your diarrhea lasts more than 48 hours or is accompanied by severe cramping, blood in your stool, or fever (see page 243).

EYEDROPS AND OTHER EYE-CARE PRODUCTS

Eye-care products sold in drugstores tend to fall into two categories: those that provide relief from minor eye discomfort, and products used for cleaning, soaking, and wetting contact lenses. Although contact lens products are sold without a prescription, they should be purchased on the recommendation of a competent eye-care professional, either the one who fitted you for the lenses or someone else knowledgeable about the products best suited for your type of lens.

Therefore, the information below focuses on products intended to help treat irritation, redness, and other temporary vexations of the eye. But it begins with this caveat: *Most nonprescription eye-care medications, which by and large are eyedrops of one type or another, are rarely necessary.* Your eyes do an excellent job of protecting themselves from irritants and infectious agents. Eyelids and eyelashes help keep foreign particles, such as dust, out of the eye, while tears help cleanse the eye of particles, allergens, surface infections, and other sources of irritation that come in contact with the cornea, the clear protective tissue covering the front of the eyeball.

Hence, normal eyes don't need "soothing" or "refreshing" or "redness relief"—the benefits promoted on many eyedrop products. Yet many consumers not only use eyedrops unnecessarily, but choose a "redness reliever" (such as Murine or Visine) containing a decongestant for any type of eye irritation. The use of these products, as noted below, can produce a rebound effect, and may also mask symptoms of serious eye infection and disease.

If you think you can benefit from using eyedrops, keep these recommendations in mind:

For minor irritation, try artificial tears. These lubricating drops, which are intended to help alleviate the condition known as dry eyes, are the preferred choice for relief of any minor eye irritation. (See below for more detail.)

Avoid using decongestant eyedrops. Bloodshot eyes will usually clear up on their own, and any persistent redness indicates that something else

is wrong with your eyes. It's especially important not to use "redness relievers" if you have glaucoma, except under a physician's advice.

Don't use any over-the-counter eyedrops on your own for more than three days. Otherwise, you may be masking—and possibly worsening—a problem that needs medical attention.

Know when to see your doctor. Aside from the few minor conditions described in this section, eye problems should be diagnosed by a physician—for which your regular doctor may refer you to an ophthalmologist, a medical doctor who specializes in diagnosing and treating all sorts of eye disorders. Symptoms indicating medical evaluation include any kind of change in your vision, signs of infection (such as a discharge of mucus), objects embedded in the eye, burns, injuries from exposure to chemicals, and redness or irritation that persists for more than a day or two.

Children with eye redness should be seen by a doctor before they use any eye-care product, since red, inflamed, or irritated eyes in children can accompany illnesses requiring medical attention, such as colds and measles.

As part of caring for your eyes, you should also have your vision checked regularly by an eye-care professional.

LUBRICANTS: ARTIFICIAL TEARS AND BLAND OINTMENTS

Our eyes should stay moist. Artificial tear solutions, also called demulcents, can temporarily moisten and cleanse eyes. Examples of brand-name products are Hypo Tears, Moisture Eyes, Refresh, and Murine Tears Lubricant; most drugstores also carry generic or store-brand equivalents that are usually less expensive.

Artificial tears are intended to help treat dry eyes, but can also provide temporary relief to eyes

Administering Eyedrops

Any liquid you put in your eye should be sterile, which is why it's important to purchase eyedrops from a drugstore. (There is one exception: emergencies. If you get dirt or a toxic chemical in your eye, there probably won't be time to find a sterile solution—just wash your eye with plenty of tap water.)

To keep eyedrops from becoming contaminated, observe the following steps when using them:

1. Whenever you are using an eye medication, be careful not to let the tip of the eyedropper or container touch any surface, including your fingers, eyes, or eyelids.

2. Wash your hands before using a medication.

3. Tilt your head back, then use one hand to pull the lower eyelid out to form a pouch.

4. Hold the dropper or container above the eye and look directly at it, then look upward and release one drop of solution. Look downward for several seconds to distribute the solution around the eye, then release the eyelid.

5. With a finger, press gently against the inner corner of the eye, which keeps medication from draining too soon and also prevents any systemic absorption of the medication. Keep the eye closed for a minute or two.

6. Wipe away any excess fluid secreted from the eye with a tissue.

7. If directions call for applying more than one drop, wait a few minutes between drops to let each drop work its way around the eye.

8. Note the expiration date on any label, and don't use a product after that date. Once you've broken the seal on a medication, use it within 30 days.

9. Be sure to discard any eye medication that has turned cloudy.

irritated by air pollution, chlorinated pool water, or fatigue. The agents in them, which include polyvinyl alcohol, methyl cellulose, and povidone, work to slow down the evaporation of your eye's actual tear film, supplement tear production, and increase tear viscosity, so that tears stick to the surface of the eye.

Many artificial tear solutions contain preservatives that help keep them sterile, but the preservatives can also cause allergic reactions. In recent years, manufacturers have introduced preservative-free preparations (such as Bion Tears and Tears Naturale Free) that don't trigger reactions. These must be administered carefully, however, since they can become easily contaminated while you are using them (see "Administering Eyedrops," above). As noted on the label, these products must be refrigerated after opening.

There are also ointments that perform the same lubricating function as artificial tears, but stay in contact with the eye longer. (Artificial tears can start to lose their effectiveness within an hour after application). The ointments (such as Acu-Tears and Lacri-Lube) contain white petrolatum (petroleum jelly) and mineral oil, usually without preservatives. Because the ointments can blur vision, people using them for treating dry eye often prefer administering them at bedtime.

Don't use any eye lubricant while you are wearing contact lenses.

DECONGESTANT EYEDROPS

Eyedrops that promise to "relieve redness" or "get the red out" contain decongestants (naphazoline, oxymetazoline, phenylephrine, or tetrahydrozoline) that act as vasoconstrictors, contracting the blood vessels in the eye so that the eyeball appears to whiten. Brand-name products include All Clear, Murine Tears Plus, Relief, Vaso Clear, and Visine.

Some formulations (such as OcuHist and Opcon-A) also contain antihistamines to help relieve eye irritation due to hay fever, and a number of products include an artificial tears lubricant to relieve irritation and dryness.

The effect of decongestants is completely cosmetic—no healing is taking place. And like decongestant nasal sprays, decongestant eyedrops can have a rebound effect—that is, they can produce acute and chronic forms of redness, known as noninfectious conjunctivitis, a form of "pinkeye." Unfortunately, some people deal with the rebound effect by applying more eyedrops to lessen the redness, which simply aggravates the problem. The cure is to stop using the eyedrops, though you may need medical advice to clear up the problem, which can take several weeks to resolve.

It's best not to use decongestant eyedrops (which can also cause dryness of the eyes as a side effect). If the cause of redness is external and temporary, give the redness a chance to clear. Applying cold compresses can help, and you can take steps to help avoid redness in the first place (see page 175).

If you insist on trying one of these products, drops containing naphazoline or tetrahydrozoline are probably the best choice, since these ingredients appear to have less rebound effect than the others. Don't use the drops more than four times a day or for more than three days. Decongestant ingredients may also cause your pupils to dilate, though this side effect is not clinically significant.

People with high blood pressure, heart irregularities, or glaucoma should check with a doctor before using decongestant eyedrops. Never use these products when wearing contact lenses. If the redness doesn't clear up in a day or two, or you think you have conjunctivitis or some other eye infection, contact your doctor.

EYEWASHES

Eyewashes can be used to irrigate the eye. But while they may feel refreshing, they have no medicinal effect and are no more effective than cold tap water. Though eyewashes are generally harmless, there is no reason to use them except in cases of chemical injury to the eye. (If that occurs, you should immediately begin washing the eye with cold running water for at least 10 to 15 minutes and then seek medical attention right away.)

Some eyewashes contain boric acid, an antibacterial agent that is so mild and in such a small concentration that it won't help you if you have an eye infection. Other eyewashes are preparations of saline (sodium chloride and water) that can cleanse the eye, and may include ingredients to help maintain the acid (pH) balance of the tear film.

Even though eyewash solutions are sterile, products administered with an eyecup carry a risk of contamination that could lead to an eye infection. Use disposable eyecups or select an eyewash available as eyedrops, which is safer.

EYELID SCRUBS

Eyelid "scrubs" can help remove scales, oil, or other debris that accumulate on eyelids, usually as a symptom of the condition known as blepharitis. A scrub is applied after softening the material on the lid with a hot compress. Baby shampoo can accomplish the same effect, though it may sting more than a scrub. You can also clean the eyelid quite effectively with a cotton-tip applicator (see page 172). Scrubs can also be used for cleaning deposits from eyelids that occur because of wearing contact lenses.

Heartburn Medications

Dozens of preparations aim to alleviate the conditions we call heartburn, acid indigestion, and sour stomach. All of these problems are often loosely attributed to overindulging in food and alcohol, and certainly overindulgence can cause stomach discomfort. But heartburn—which is usually first signaled by a burning sensation in the upper abdomen or lower chest—is a specific ailment that is often accompanied by sensations of sourness or acidity in the stomach, throat, or mouth. The cause is stomach acid backing up and irritating the lining of the esophagus, the tube that runs from the throat to the stomach. This typically occurs after meals, when the stomach is secreting gastric juices and when pressure in the stomach is more likely to push stomach contents, including acid, up through the lower esophageal sphincter, a muscle that should close to keep stomach acid from splashing into the esophagus. Heartburn—technically called gastroesophageal reflux—occurs because the muscle is malfunctioning, which allows a backwash, or reflux, of stomach acid.

Both conventional antacids such as Alka-Seltzer, Tums, and Maalox and the newer heartburn drugs called H2-blockers can, when used judiciously, offer short-term relief from mild heartburn symptoms. Some H2-blockers also claim to prevent heartburn symptoms when taken before meals. (Neither antacids nor over-the-counter formulations of H2-blockers are effective for treating chronic or severe heartburn symptoms).

All antacids are generally safe, rarely causing serious side effects, when used occasionally—once or twice a month—by healthy people. But more frequent use of either conventional antacids or H2-blockers, especially daily use, can mask a serious problem, such as a peptic ulcer. Taken regularly without a doctor's supervision, antacids may cause bowel irregularities (constipation or diarrhea), aggravate kidney disorders, and cause other problems. And prolonged use can actually cause an increase in the production of stomach acid if you suddenly stop taking antacids—an effect called acid rebound.

Of course, it's better not to have heartburn in the first place. Lifestyle habits are often the cause of heartburn, and most people can avoid the problem with some straightforward preventive measures (see page 316).

CONVENTIONAL ANTACIDS
Antacids work by neutralizing stomach acid and inhibiting the conversion of pepsinogen to pepsin, a digestive enzyme that, in the presence of stomach acid, breaks down protein. In excess amounts, acid and/or pepsin can irritate the lining of the esophagus and stomach. Antacids don't reduce the amount of acid or slow its production, nor do they coat the stomach lining; they only neutralize acid already present in the stomach.

Most antacids—which come in chewable

tablets, liquids, and foams, and in regular and extra-strength formulations—are effective and easy to use, which accounts for their popularity. They also work quickly, providing relief within 15 minutes. The relief typically lasts from one to three hours.

Active ingredients. Four principal agents are used to formulate most antacids: sodium bicarbonate (the active ingredient in Alka Seltzer); calcium carbonate (Amitone, Tums); aluminum compounds (ALternaGEL, Amphojel); and magnesium compounds (Phillips' Milk of Magnesia). Products are also available that combine aluminum and magnesium, sometimes in a chemical form called magaldrate (Maalox, Riopan). And there are antacids containing three or more ingredients (Gaviscon Extra Strength).

An antidiarrheal drug, bismuth subsalicylate, which is found in Pepto-Bismol and its generic forms, has no measurable neutralizing effect on stomach acids, and is not considered an antacid. But it is often used to combat "sour stomach" and the effects of overeating.

Some brands of antacid also add other types of ingredients, such as simethicone, an antifoaming agent that is supposed to reduce gas (or at least reduce the size of gas bubbles). Simethicone has never been proven to provide relief. Aspirin and acetaminophen are other combination ingredients, though they contribute nothing to neutralizing stomach acid (and in fact, aspirin can aggravate heartburn).

Special concerns. Antacids are safe for most people—to such an extent that the FDA has not set maximum daily dosages based on effectiveness. However, some ingredients can cause special problems for certain people. For example, high amounts of sodium may aggravate hypertension (high blood pressure), especially in older

586

people, and antacid labels must now indicate sodium content. Similarly, antacid products containing aluminum or magnesium carry a warning for people whose kidney function is impaired, since these ingredients pose a risk of serious side effects. And taking frequent doses of calcium-based antacids can increase the risk of kidney stones in some people. Therefore, it is important to read the warnings on antacid labels.

POTENCY AND EFFECTIVENESS

Every antacid is tested by its manufacturer to establish how much acid can be neutralized by a single dose of the product. This measure of potency is known as *acid-neutralizing capacity,* or ANC, and it varies considerably among antacid products. One advantage of antacids with a relatively high ANC is that they can neutralize stomach acid with lower doses than products that are less potent. In fact, many manufacturers of antacids recommend similar doses, and products with a very low ANC may have an almost negligible effect at those dosage levels. Higher doses may be necessary to obtain relief; consequently, less potent products may end up costing more to provide an effective dose.

The chart opposite, which shows ANC figures for a sampling of different antacid tablets, indicates how widely doses can vary to obtain the same effect. Antacid manufacturers, however, cannot include ANC information on their labels. This is because the FDA doesn't want consumers focusing solely on potency in choosing a product—because a more potent product isn't necessarily better. Since the amount of stomach acid being secreted varies greatly from person to person, as well as within the same person at different times, a product with a mid-range ANC may be more than sufficient for providing relief.

Comparing Potency in Antacids

▼

This chart indicates the acid-neutralizing capacity, or ANC, of some common brands of antacid tablets. Four tablets of Extra-Strength Maalox, for example, have the same acid-neutralizing effect as nine tablets of regular Maalox.

PRODUCT (TABLETS)	NUMBER OF TABLETS*
Extra Strength Maalox	4
Gelusil-II	4
Amphojel (600 mg)	5
Riopan Plus	6
Mylanta	7
Tums	8
Maalox	9
Gaviscon	160

* Number of tablets required from each brand to provide an equivalent ANC.

There are also other factors to consider: for example, aluminum compounds tend to have the lowest potency and are slower-acting than other types, but they also have the longest duration of neutralizing action. Side effects and taste are other considerations.

H2-BLOCKERS

Four drugs, formerly sold only by prescription, were approved in 1995 and 1996 for over-the-counter sale in lower-dose versions. They are Pepcid AC (meaning "acid control"; the active ingredient is famotidine) and Tagamet HB (for "heartburn"; active ingredient, cimetidine), as well as the anti-ulcer drug Zantac (ranitidine), one of the world's largest-selling drugs. The fourth drug is Axid AR (for "acid reducer"; active ingredient, nizatidine). As prescription drugs, these medica-

tions are used for helping to heal peptic *ulcers*. But the lower-dose OTC versions are approved by the FDA only for the relief of heartburn, sour stomach, and acid indigestion.

Are these new heartburn remedies any better than plain antacids? Certainly they are different. The drugs they contain, known as H2-blockers or H2 "antagonists," suppress the production of stomach acid, rather than just neutralizing it the way conventional antacids do. Pepcid AC can, and does, claim to prevent heartburn as well as relieve it, if you can predict when heartburn is about to strike and take the medication about half an hour in advance. Tagamet simply claims to "reduce the production of stomach acid." Axid AR is approved only for the prevention of heartburn, not as a means of relieving symptoms.

Individual reactions to H2-blockers are quite variable. What works fast for one person may not work for another. Expect these drugs to keep working for about three to five hours—though this, too, can vary from person to person. Side effects are rare, as are interactions with other drugs. (One exception is Tagamet, which does interact with a number of drugs, including warfarin, a widely used blood-thinning medication.)

Remember also that these OTC drugs contain only 50 percent of the minimum dosages in the prescription versions. According to testimony submitted to the FDA, dosages at these levels are only about as effective as conventional antacids.

GUIDELINES FOR CHOOSING HEARTBURN MEDICATIONS

• *If you already have heartburn,* you will get faster relief from a conventional antacid.

• *If you think you are going to get heartburn,* H2-blockers may be worth a try. They are similar in their effects and side effects, though cimetidine (Tagamet) is more likely to cause interactions with other drugs. Be aware of these if you are taking other medications.

• **If you tend to become easily constipated,** consider a magnesium antacid, since aluminum-based antacids can cause constipation. Conversely, if you have a history of diarrhea (for example, from irritable bowel syndrome), it's best to avoid magnesium antacids and start with aluminum products. Aluminum-magnesium combinations generally have the least potential for these side effects.

• **Sodium bicarbonate is the least-preferred type of antacid.** Antacids containing sodium bicarbonate, which include Alka Seltzer, Gaviscon Extra Strength, and plain baking soda, are short-acting and they also carry a number of potential risks for certain people—in part because normal doses of sodium bicarbonate deliver large amounts of sodium into the bloodstream. Alka Seltzer Extra Strength, for example, contains 588 milligrams of sodium per dose, which is nearly one-fourth of the 2,500 milligrams recommended as the daily maximum for people trying to reduce their sodium intake.

Hence, these antacids are not suitable for anyone on a salt-restricted diet, and they can also cause serious adverse effects in pregnant women, post-menopausal women taking calcium supplements, and others. An excess intake of sodium bicarbonate can also lead to alkalosis, an abnormal shift in the acid-base balance of body fluids that, among other effects, can increase the risk of kidney stones.

• **Check the inactive ingredients.** For most people, these won't make much difference. But if you are lactose intolerant, you may want to avoid antacids containing lactose. (Any antacid containing more than 5 grams of lactose per day in a maximum daily dosage must carry a label warning that cautions individuals "allergic to milk or milk products" to consult a physician before using the product.) People with diabetes should be aware of any sugar content.

• **Don't choose a liquid antacid assuming that it will work better**—it depends on where your burning sensation is. Liquid antacids have long been considered more effective than tablets at neutralizing stomach acid. But a study from the University of Oklahoma found that tablets are better at reducing acid in the lower esophagus, where reflux of stomach acids causes heartburn. The researchers suggest that the tablets become gummy when chewed and thus stick to the wall of the esophagus longer and better than liquids. Also, chewing the tablets stimulates the production of saliva, which contains a natural antacid.

• **Choose a form of antacid you will stick with.** One reason for the popularity of H2-blockers is that they come in pill form. You need not chew a chalky tablet or swallow a liquid. With conventional antacids, many people find tablets more convenient than liquids, particularly at work.

• **Taste is also a consideration.** The more palatable an antacid is, the more likely you are to use it properly.

• **If one brand doesn't work well, try another.** If one brand isn't providing sufficient or long-lasting relief, try a "high-potency" version. One advantage of high-potency antacids is that smaller amounts can neutralize a large amount of gastric acid—which means that you can take less medication than you would with a less potent product to obtain the same effect.

If you experience bothersome side effects, try a different type of active ingredient.

GUIDELINES FOR USING HEARTBURN MEDICATIONS

• *Take an H2-blocker well before trouble starts*— as, for example, before you eat a spicy meal or cut a big piece of chocolate cake late in the evening or do anything else that you know brings on heartburn. Whatever brand you choose, expect it to take at least 30 minutes to have any effect.

• *Take antacids about 20 to 30 minutes after meals.* An antacid taken on empty stomach will be effective for about 20 to 40 minutes; taken after a meal, when food slows the emptying of the stomach's contents, the same antacid may neutralize acid up to three hours.

• *Don't take an antacid with milk.* Contrary to popular belief, milk is not a recommended remedy for heartburn. Milk may initially provide some relief, but eventually triggers the production of even more stomach acid, so that you may develop heartburn that is more severe than the case you're treating.

• *Calcium-based antacids can be used to supplement your calcium intake.* But if you are using antacids only to increase your calcium consumption, take doses yielding no more than 1,000 to 1,500 milligrams of calcium a day. To determine how much elemental calcium your antacid or other calcium supplement contains, see product labels. And avoid aluminum-based antacids, which can actually deplete calcium. (See page 24 for more information on calcium supplements.)

• *Children under 6* should not take antacids unless prescribed by a physician. And children 19 or younger should not take bismuth subsalicylate (Pepto-Bismol) because, like aspirin, it can cause Reye's syndrome, a potentially fatal illness.

• *Never use one of these drugs for more than two weeks for heartburn relief.* If symptoms persist, or if side effects from any medication are persistent, contact your doctor. Also check with your doctor if you develop more serious symptoms, such as wheezing, difficulty swallowing, or vomiting blood (see page 317).

Laxatives

Probably no drugstore products are as overused and abused as laxatives, nor as misunderstood. Worry about "irregularity" leads many people to rely routinely on over-the-counter products that promise quick relief for constipation, the number-one gastrointestinal complaint in the United States. Americans now spend more than $650 million annually on laxative products. Yet this is a mostly useless expenditure that fails to promote normal bowel movements or accomplish any health objective.

Products marketed as "laxatives" actually fall into several distinct groups that have different chemical properties and are meant to be used for different purposes, as explained below. Not all laxative products are intended for the self-treatment of constipation. Moreover, in the great majority of cases, the use of laxatives for relieving constipation is unnecessary; people turn to them in large part because of common misconceptions about constipation and how best to prevent or alleviate it.

Unfortunately, many people, particularly older adults concerned about how often they should have a bowel movement, begin taking laxatives as a quick fix, and then become dependent on them for prolonged periods—a habit that can produce adverse effects ranging from the depletion of essential vitamins and minerals to a weakening or even impairment of bowel function (see

589

"Avoiding Laxative Abuse," page 594). Recognizing that the ingredients in laxatives are, after all, drugs, the FDA has issued, over the past decade, label warnings for laxative products and banned more than 20 active ingredients because manufacturers failed to demonstrate their safety or effectiveness.

In some instances, discussed below, certain types of laxative products may be appropriate for relieving occasional constipation and for specific medical uses recommended by your doctor. But it's rare when someone truly needs a laxative. Despite claims of being "gentle and safe" or "natural," laxatives are one over-the-counter remedy that most of us can do without.

Alleviating constipation depends on the specific cause and severity of the problem. If constipation is due to a medical condition or a drug you are taking, you need to consult your doctor. But in most cases when you have no other symptoms, you can get quick relief with the straightforward measures provided on page 218 (which should also prevent constipation from recurring).

WHEN A LAXATIVE MAY BE APPROPRIATE

Some people experience temporary constipation from changes in eating, fluid intake, or exercise habits that have been altered by travel, work, or some other circumstance. When this happens, the use of a laxative may be warranted, though only if you have no other symptoms and preferably only for a day or two. (The labels on all laxatives now caution that they shouldn't be used for more than one week without consulting a physician.) As soon as possible, you should follow the dietary and other lifestyle measures described on page 218 to remedy your constipation.

For constipation associated with medical dis-orders, pregnancy, or with the use of certain medications, consult your doctor before using a laxative. In these circumstances, a laxative may not be appropriate or, if it is, your doctor will want to base the type of product and the dosage on your specific situation.

Over-the-counter laxatives are also used in preparing for diagnostic tests of the gastrointestinal tract and before or after abdominal surgery. Here, too, the choice and use of a laxative should be undertaken in consultation with a physician.

PREFERRED LAXATIVES FOR CONSTIPATION

When you look for products under "Laxatives" in the drugstore aisle, you'll find such common brand names as Cascara, Citroma, Dulcolax, Metamucil, and Senokot—all of which have generic equivalents—along with mineral oil and castor oil, and products in suppository and enema form as well as oral laxatives. What these products have in common is that they all promote a bowel movement. But they do so in different ways, with ingredients that have distinctly different effects.

Two types of products, based on their active ingredients, are most appropriate for temporary relief of occasional constipation.

Bulk-forming laxatives. If treating constipation through dietary measures isn't feasible or fails to be effective, bulk-forming laxatives are the best choice for an over-the-counter remedy. Generally considered the safest type of laxative, bulk-forming agents—which include methylcellulose (the active ingredient in Citrucel), calcium polycarbophil (FiberCon), psyllium (Metamucil), and bran supplements—are made up of fiber or fiber-like compounds derived from seeds and plants or created synthetically. These compounds help the body to eliminate waste products much like the dietary fiber in food you eat. When taken with plenty of fluid, a bulk-forming agent can absorb up to 25 times its weight in water as its passes through the intestinal tract. This added water increases the bulk of stool and, along with other compounds in these agents, also softens stool—effects that make the stool pass more readily and easily.

Bulk-forming products, which come in powders, granules, or compressed wafers, can relieve constipation within a day, but may take up to three days to work effectively. When taken properly, these products have fewer side effects than other laxatives. Indeed, they are generally safe to use on a long-term basis, and may be recommended for increasing fiber intake (especially for people who can't get sufficient fiber through their diet) or for preventing or managing other health problems (see "Psyllium" on page 592).

Docusate stool softeners. Also called emollients, these products (Colace, Correctol Stool Softener) make use of docusate, an ingredient that doesn't stimulate a bowel movement, but provides moisture to stool to promote smoother passage. Stool softeners are useful when hard stool will cause pain during a bowel movement, and are often recommended by doctors to prevent hard stool from forming after childbirth or following abdominal surgery or treatment for hemorrhoids. Products using docusate are usually effective in one to two days, but for some people it may take three to five days to act.

MINERAL OIL

Also known as liquid petrolatum, mineral oil coats the stool so that it slips through the intestine more easily and also helps it retain water to maintain softness. The effect of mineral oil products (Haleys M-O, Fleet Mineral Oil) is similar to that of a docusate stool softener, but docusate is usually a better choice because small amounts of mineral oil can be absorbed by the body and may interfere with the body's ability to absorb certain nutrients, especially fat-soluble vitamins. Also, in rare cases, mineral oil may be aspirated (inhaled into the lungs), especially in the very old or very young, so docusate or another type of laxative is recommended for these two age groups.

STIMULANT LAXATIVES

These are the products that people often reach for first to relieve constipation—but they shouldn't. Stimulant laxatives contain such active ingredients as bisacodyl (used in Correctol, Dulcolax, Ex-Lax tablets, Feen-A-Mint), cascara sagrada (Cascara), and senna and sennosides (Perdiem, Senokot). These chemicals agitate the wall of the intestine, causing muscular contractions that speed passage of the stool. Many stimulants also contain docusate to soften stool.

Stimulant laxatives act forcefully and quickly, usually within 12 hours. However, taking too large a dose of these laxatives, or using them habitually, can cause diarrhea, fluid loss, cramping, inflamed hemorrhoids, and, most seriously, a poorly functioning colon with impaired peristalsis (the muscular action that moves food through the intestinal tract).

Because of the risk of adverse effects, the FDA has banned a number of ingredients used in stimulants. Phenolphthalein, used in several common brands, is no longer on the market in the United States (though it is in other countries). Other ingredients, including those mentioned above, are currently under review by the FDA.

For these reasons, stimulant laxatives should play a very small role in treating constipation. They are suitable only for occasional use and

591

when other treatments have failed, or when a rapid onset of action is required. Because the effective dosage can vary from person to person, and because stimulant laxatives can have adverse side effects that include dehydration, cramping, and diarrhea, it's best to use them under a doctor's direction.

SPECIAL-PURPOSE LAXATIVES

Several types of laxative products sold over-the-

Psyllium: More Than A Laxative

Psyllium, one of the primary agents used in bulk-forming laxative products, is derived from the seeds of the plantago plant. A tablespoon of psyllium powder contains about 4 grams of dietary fiber—not as much, by weight, as the amount of fiber in a serving of some whole-bran cereals or certain legumes, but still substantial. Like many other forms of fiber, psyllium is surprisingly complex and has a number of varied effects in the body.

For simplicity, fiber can be divided into two broad categories: compounds that are insoluble in water and those that are soluble. Most plant foods contain both types in varying amounts. About 20 percent of the fiber in psyllium is insoluble fiber, which draws in water to add bulk to stool. The larger proportion of soluble fiber helps produce a softer stool, and also enhances regularity by forming emollient gels that facilitate the passage of intestinal contents.

In addition, soluble fiber works chemically to prevent or reduce the absorption of certain substances into the bloodstream, including cholesterol. Hence, some products that contain psyllium are also recommended for helping lower blood cholesterol levels, especially LDL ("bad") cholesterol. The FDA now allows foods containing significant amounts of psyllium (at least 1.7 grams per serving) to claim on their labels that they may reduce the risk of heart disease, when the foods are part of a diet low in fat and cholesterol.

Like other sources of soluble fiber, psyllium may also help control blood sugar and insulin in some people with diabetes. And psyllium and other bulk-forming laxative products may help in the prevention or management of other disorders, including diverticulosis and irritable bowel syndrome.

Psyllium products are safe to use on a daily basis for an extended period. But you should consult your doctor before using any bulk-forming agent on a long-term basis to treat or prevent a health problem. As the labels warn, psyllium may interfere with prescription medication, so talk to your doctor or pharmacist if you take psyllium and a drug at the same time.

While bulk-forming agents are safe and effective for relieving occasional constipation, no one has recommended that they be used as a substitute for increasing daily fiber intake. It's much better to get your fiber from food sources, rather than from bulk laxatives or other type of fiber supplement. These products lack the variety of fiber compounds found in fiber-rich foods, not to mention the vitamins, minerals, and other nutrients they contain. Fiber supplements contain no nutrients.

Fiber also binds some minerals in the foods you eat, so it may interfere with their absorption by your body—though research suggests that any such effect from consuming moderate amounts of fiber is small and not a worry. Still, foods high in fiber contain minerals, so you more than make up for any losses.

counter are intended to be used primarily for evacuating the bowel prior to surgery or in preparation for a diagnostic evaluation of the gastrointestinal tract, such as a sigmoidoscopy or colonoscopy. Therefore, use these products only on your doctor's recommendation. (Prescription laxatives are also available for these purposes, and your doctor may recommend one of these.)

Osmotic laxatives—which contain magnesium salts (Citroma) and sodium biphosphate (Fleet Phospho-Soda)—trigger a complex series of reactions that bring on a bowel movement quickly, usually within 30 minutes to three hours. These laxatives can also be used to treat constipation that doesn't respond to bulk-forming laxatives or stool softeners.

Castor oil is another over-the-counter agent used for colonic preparation. It is a powerful stimulant laxative that empties the entire gastrointestinal tract, and should not be used to treat constipation without a doctor's approval.

Enemas and suppositories are forms of laxatives that can be self-administered rectally, and are used to prepare patients for diagnostic exams and surgery. They may also be prescribed for helping to manage constipation in severely constipated children or elderly patients. Sodium phosphate is an effective enema ingredient (for example, Fleet), while bisacodyl, a stimulant agent, is commonly used in suppositories.

LAXATIVE GUIDELINES

Try to use dietary and lifestyle measures to relieve an occasional bout of constipation. But if you decide to use a laxative temporarily, take the following into account when selecting a product.

Try a bulk-forming laxative first. These products are the safest and come closest to duplicating the normal process of elimination. Choosing among the different types of bulk laxatives is a matter of personal preference. A more important consideration is to take each dose with plenty of water—at least eight ounces. Otherwise fiber compounds in bulk laxatives can swell in the intestine or the esophagus to form an obstruction.

If hard stool is a problem, consider a laxative containing docusate or mineral oil. Both help soften stool. Docusate products are more convenient to use, and are also considered safe in almost every situation. However, this type of laxative should not be used if you are taking any prescription drug. Also, do not use docusate in conjunction with mineral oil.

Mineral oil should not be given to young children or used by older or debilitated adults because of the risk of side effects.

Consider stimulant laxatives only after you've tried other strategies. Not only is there a higher likelihood of adverse effects, but laxatives containing bisacodyl, senna, and similar stimulant chemicals are more likely to become habituating than milder-acting laxatives. If you decide to try a stimulant, the less strong it is, the better. For example, a combination product that mixes senna (one of the weaker stimulants) with psyllium has a lower amount of senna per dose than a pure stimulant product. Always take the minimum dose needed to produce an effect, and only for a day or two.

Don't reach for osmotic laxatives, suppositories, or enemas. Even though you can buy these products in a drugstore, you shouldn't rely on them as a remedy for simple occasional constipation. Only use them under a doctor's direction.

Consult your doctor or pharmacist if you are taking a prescription medication. Laxatives can interfere with the absorption of certain drugs, including aspirin, antibiotics, and anticoagulants.

593

Don't use any laxative if you have other gastrointestinal symptoms. Severe abdominal pain, vomiting, nausea, diarrhea, cramping, and/or a loss of appetite are signs of some other disorder that could be aggravated by taking a laxative.

AVOIDING LAXATIVE ABUSE

A routine and chronic use of laxatives occurs for a variety of reasons. People who abuse laxatives frequently believe that they must have a daily bowel movement, and turn to laxatives to ensure this—often strong stimulant laxatives that produce a bowel movement overnight. Although many laxative abusers are elderly, a child may be given laxatives by a parent intent on the child having a daily bowel movement. Some adolescents and young adults also use laxatives routinely to help control weight. The laxative abuse may be part of a pattern of bulimia nervosa, an eating disorder characterized by purging food after meals with self-induced vomiting.

The way many laxatives are packaged may foster laxative abuse. It can be easy to forget that products in the form of chewing gum, wafers, chocolate tablets, and effervescent granules are drugs, not food or candy. The fact that some laxatives are "pleasant-testing" can make it that much easier to use them on a daily basis and/or in excessive doses.

One problem with stimulant laxatives, which work by irritating the walls of the intestine, is that they can cause the entire colon to empty, rather than just the lower portion of the bowel (which is the area emptied during a normal bowel movement or when a bulk-forming laxative is used). Because of this effect, not enough stool forms to produce a normal bowel movement the next day—and so the laxative user may take another laxative to force a bowel movement.

Over time, the colon fails to function properly, and a bowel movement without the stimulus of laxatives becomes more and more difficult. The prolonged use of laxatives ends up causing chronic constipation, rather than alleviating it. Excessive laxative use can also cause severe diarrhea and/or vomiting, which in turn leads to fluid loss, the risk of dehydration, and a loss of essential vitamins and minerals.

Someone who has been using stimulant laxatives for many years can incur permanent bowel damage. Before that occurs, it is possible for an abuser to withdraw from a laxative by eating a high-fiber diet, possibly supplemented with a bulk-forming laxative as needed. Gradually, normal bowel function will begin to return—a process that can take several months.

Pain and Fever Medications

A splitting headache, a sore arm after a weekend baseball game, achiness and fever from flu, menstrual cramps—these are just a few of the many reasons people reach for nonprescription pain relievers each day. According to a survey by the American Pharmaceutical Association, two thirds of adults in the United States use nonprescription pain relievers at least once a month, and one-third use them at least once a week. In total, more than 50 billion of these pain pills—medically known as analgesics (from the Greek for "no sense of pain")—are consumed each year.

Pain relief, in fact, is the most common reason people take nonprescription medications. In answer to that need, drugstores stock a multitude of brand-name products that come in a variety of strengths and forms, and are aimed at alleviating practically every sort of pain. But this seemingly vast choice is misleading; in fact, there are only two basic types of these over-the-counter medications, acetaminophen and NSAIDs (nonsteroidal anti-inflammatory drugs). Acetaminophen was introduced in an over-the-counter formulation more than 30 years ago. Aspirin, an NSAID, has been around the longest, just over one hundred years. The other pain-relief formulations are more recent: ibuprofen was approved for nonprescription use in 1984, followed by naproxen sodium in 1994 and ketoprofen in 1995.

BASIC BENEFITS

As pain relievers, these over-the-counter medications are effective for alleviating mild to moderate pain associated with a variety of conditions, from muscle soreness to headache pain to arthritis. For some more severe types of pain, over-the-counter pain relievers are usually not strong enough to control the discomfort, but they may still be used in combination with prescription analgesics so that the dosage levels of the stronger drugs can be lower, minimizing their side effects.

In addition to relieving pain, the NSAIDs and acetaminophen have an *antipyretic* (antifever) effect. Fever is the body's natural response to infection and other illnesses, and it can help the immune system kill off harmful bacteria and fight infections. But fevers can be uncomfortable, and a high fever, particularly in children younger than age two, can cause dangerous complications like seizures. Nonprescription antipyretic/analgesics can not only reduce a fever, but also alleviate aching, soreness, and other discomforting symptoms associated with the condition causing the fever. (Using these drugs to treat a fever won't help speed recovery from the underlying ailment, however.)

As their name suggests, NSAIDs (but *not* acetaminophen) also help reduce inflammation, stiffness, and swelling. These symptoms (along with pain) can accompany conditions such as muscle strains, sprains, bursitis, tendinitis, tennis elbow, plantar fasciitis, and other localized pain syndromes involving tissues around the joints. (The non-steroidal part of the NSAID name distinguishes these drugs from corticosteroids, which also control inflammation.)

A key advantage of NSAIDs is that they are nonaddicting, in contrast to narcotic analgesics such as codeine, Percodan, and Demerol, all of which act like morphine by inhibiting pain impulses in certain centers of the brain. Available only by prescription, narcotic analgesics (also called opiates, though not all are opium derivatives) are useful as short-term treatments, but are usually not suitable (except as a temporary measure) for chronic pain because the body may develop a tolerance to them—that is, experience a diminished effect with prolonged use. Addiction, a component of which is physical dependence, is another danger. Narcotic analgesics can also impair physical and mental function.

While there is no risk of addiction when using nonnarcotic analgesics, using them improperly may cause adverse side effects, which are discussed on the following pages.

NONSTEROIDAL ANTI-INFLAMMATORIES (NSAIDS)

NSAIDs act to quell, or interfere with, the production of hormone-like chemicals called prostaglandins. There are many types of prostaglandins, and they perform a number of different functions. Some of them raise body temperature, others cause inflammation or pain when cells are injured or infected. They also control

Over-the-Counter Pain Relievers

PRODUCT	USE/EFFECTIVENESS	CAUTIONS	COMMENTS
Acetaminophen (Tylenol, Panadol, Anacin-3)	Aches, pain, fever. Useful for children under 19 with chicken pox or flu or those allergic to aspirin. Does not cause gastrointestinal bleeding. Does not prevent blood clotting. Safe after oral surgery.	Rare reactions include skin rashes and painful urination. High doses over long periods may damage the liver and kidneys. Should not be used by alcoholics nor people with liver or kidney diseases. Pregnant and breast-feeding women should check with their doctors. Do not take acetaminophen when you have been drinking alcohol.	Will not reduce inflammation. Do not combine with aspirin.
Aspirin	Aches, pain, fever, inflammation. On medical advice, daily low dosages (like an 81-mg baby aspirin) can help prevent heart attack, because aspirin inhibits blood clots. Some evidence indicates a preventive effect against colon cancer and non-hemorrhagic strokes, but more research is needed.	Not recommended for pregnant women (can cause bleeding); breast-feeding mothers; those with known aspirin allergies or people with ulcers, gout, or stomach bleeding; children age 19 or younger with chicken pox or flu, because of risk of Reye's syndrome; people taking anticoagulants; people undergoing surgery. Frequent use can lead to ulcers. Excessive doses may produce stomach upset, ringing in the ears.	A highly effective, inexpensive drug. At least 40 percent of people have some stomach bleeding (usually inconsequential) after taking aspirin. Those who experience stomach upset may be helped by taking aspirin with food.

PRODUCT	USE/EFFECTIVENESS	CAUTIONS	COMMENTS
Ibuprofen (Advil, Nuprin, Mediprin)	Pain, fever, inflammation.	Less gastrointestinal distress than with aspirin. Those who are allergic to aspirin may experience similar side effects with ibuprofen. In some people, may cause stomach bleeding, like aspirin. May interfere with diuretic and antihypertensive drugs. Children and pregnant or breast-feeding women should take it only on medical advice.	Better for menstrual cramps than the other NSAIDs.
Naproxen sodium (Aleve)	Pain, fever, inflammation.	May cause stomach upsets and stomach bleeding in some people, but less likely to than aspirin or ibuprofen. Not recommended for those with ulcers, asthma, or kidney disease, or heavy drinkers. Children under 12 and pregnant or breast-feeding women should take it only on medical advice.	Longer lasting relief than aspirin or ibuprofen; thus good for taking at bedtime. Good for menstrual cramps, postpartum pain. Worth trying if other OTC pain relievers haven't worked. Sold in tablets of 200 mg. For those over 12, maximum daily dose is three tablets with 8 to 12 hours between doses.
Ketoprofen (Actron, Orudis)	Pain, fever, inflammation.	May cause gastrointestinal, kidney, and other problems. Should not be given to children age 19 or younger with flu symptoms or chicken pox.	No significant advantages over other OTC pain relievers. Actron comes as a very small pill, which may help make it easier to swallow (though people with arthritis may find it harder to handle).

597

muscle contractions and the dilation of blood vessels, and they affect blood clotting. When you take NSAIDs, the resulting decease in prostaglandins lowers the sensitivity of pain receptors at the sites where injury or inflammation has occurred. (Narcotic pain relievers, by contrast, work centrally on the brain, rather than by a localized action at the site of injury.)

NSAIDs work quickly and effectively, providing initial relief for acute pain and fever within an hour. (Relief for chronic or progressive pain or inflammation, such as that from arthritis, takes more time.) When used for the temporary relief of pain, and in the proper dosages, these medications are also safe for most adults—though some individuals and children should check with their doctors before using a pain.

However, all the NSAIDs can cause adverse effects that range from nausea, upset stomach, and mild gastrointestinal bleeding to more serious symptoms when the drugs are taken daily on a long-term basis. In fact, the use of NSAIDs is the most common cause of gastrointestinal bleeding in the United States. Ibuprofen, naproxen sodium, and ketoprofen generally cause less gastrointestinal bleeding than aspirin, but can still be very harsh on your stomach, especially when used for weeks or months.

NSAIDs hurt the stomach and duodenum (the first portion of the small intestine) in two ways—through a direct "irritative" effect on the stomach lining, and, more significantly, by interfering with prostaglandins that help protect the stomach wall from the irritating effects of digestive acids. This systemic effect can produce damage to the stomach in people even when they take steps to minimize local irritation, such as by using enteric-coated aspirin. It is also the principal cause of more serious problems—which include anemia, gastritis, ulcers, and kidney damage—associated with long-term use of NSAIDs. For people who take NSAIDs on a long-term regular basis, new prescription drugs called COX-2 inhibitors can help to minimize gastrointestinal side effects (see page 603).

ASPIRIN

Although technically an NSAID, aspirin belongs to a group of drugs called salicylates. Other salicylates include choline salicylate, sodium salicylate, and magnesium salicylate, all of which are available in nonprescription formulations and may be less irritating to the stomach in some people than aspirin, though they are also usually less effective. As a practical matter, people who can't tolerate aspirin's side effects can first try acetaminophen or another NSAID.

As a pain reliever, aspirin acts much like the other NSAIDs, but it also has effects distinct from ibuprofen, naproxen sodium, and ketoprofen—most notably the unique ability to keep platelets in the bloodstream from sticking together and blocking blood flow, an effect that can help to prevent heart attack and some types of strokes. Aspirin has other health benefits as well, but this doesn't mean that it should be taken casually. In some people, aspirin's anticlotting effect may increase the chance of severe bleeding, including hemorrhagic stroke (a stroke caused by bleeding in the brain). Using aspirin too often, or taking inappropriate doses, is also a leading cause of gastrointestinal complaints. Because of its potential for good and harm, it's important to know when and how to take aspirin safely, as explained on page 600.

ACETAMINOPHEN

Acetaminophen was first synthesized in the 19th

century. Exactly how it controls pain is not known. Many experts believe that, unlike NSAIDs, which work on peripheral pain receptors, acetaminophen works directly on the brain to raise the threshold at which pain is perceived. Researchers aren't certain if or how acetaminophen affects prostaglandin production. It may inhibit prostaglandins responsible for causing fever. But acetaminophen has no significant effect on prostaglandins that promote inflammation, so it is less effective than NSAIDs at relieving soft tissue injuries, such as muscle strains and tendinitis.

It also does not block the production of prostaglandins that maintain the stomach lining, and so doesn't cause stomach distress or damage, making it a good choice for people who cannot tolerate NSAIDs. Acetaminophen can also be taken by people who should avoid NSAIDs because of potential interactions with other drugs they are taking, especially oral anticoagulants (blood-thinning agents)—though there is some evidence that acetaminophen interferes with one such drug, warfarin.

Because it is relatively free of adverse effects when taken in recommended doses, acetaminophen is the pain/fever remedy of choice for pregnant women and children. But although it is generally considered the safest analgesic for short-term use, acetaminophen can pose health risks—notably liver toxicity (especially when taken with alcohol) and decreased kidney function—when used for long periods and/or in high doses. Therefore, long-term use of acetaminophen should only be undertaken in consultation with your doctor.

COMBINATION PRODUCTS AND ADDED INGREDIENTS

Many products contain more than simply a single pain reliever. Here are the most common examples:

- ***Aspirin or another salicylate and acetaminophen.*** These two pain relievers can be combined in one product, though there is no evidence that they are consistently more effective in combination than taken singly, except possibly in treating some migraine headaches (see page 310). At present, this is the only combination of two over-the-counter pain relief agents approved by the FDA.

- ***Buffering agents and aspirin.*** Buffering compounds such as calcium carbonate are intended to protect or "buffer" the stomach against aspirin's acidity. Buffered products typically cost more than plain aspirin, but their benefit is dubious. The gastric irritation and damage from aspirin are primarily due to its systemic action, not from its local impact on the stomach lining, and comparisons of the amount of gastric damage from buffered and non-buffered products have shown there is no difference in the two products.

- ***Enteric-coated aspirin.*** Enteric-coated aspirin—which is coated in cellulose, silicon, or some other inactive ingredient—can benefit some people. The coating keeps the aspirin from being absorbed until it reaches the small intestine, and so the release of salicylate is delayed, which helps reduce direct irritation of the stomach lining (though it doesn't protect against systemic effects that are damaging to the stomach). The pain-relieving benefit of enteric-coated aspirin is also delayed, however, so it may not be suitable for someone who wants rapid pain relief. Its preferred use is in long-term aspirin therapy, such as the management of arthritis, when it may produce less damage than either plain or buffered aspirin.

- ***Caffeine.*** Though not recognized as a pain reliever, caffeine has been reported to increase the

599

Aspirin, the Wonder Drug

Aspirin is not only the most popular drug in the world, it is also one of the most useful. Not only does it alleviate pain and fever, but studies show that even in small doses, aspirin can prevent heart attack and stroke. In addition, preliminary evidence suggests it may help protect against colon cancer, Alzheimer's disease, and possibly breast cancer.

The power to protect the cardiovascular system is unique to aspirin. The majority of heart attacks and strokes are caused by blood clots, which are formed by blood platelets sticking together. Aspirin inhibits the type of prostaglandins that promote the stickiness of platelets. It also appears to stimulate the production of two other substances—gamma-interferon and interleukin-2—that seem to discourage the proliferation of cancer cells.

Guidelines and Precautions

Taking low-dose aspirin daily to ward off heart attack is such a common practice that many people do it on their own. But dosing yourself without medical advice to prevent a heart attack or for any other reason is not a good idea. Even low-dose aspirin poses a risk of gastrointestinal bleeding, so if you want to take it, or already do, you need to discuss this risk with your doctor.

Here are other reasons not to start preventive therapy with aspirin on your own.

• **If your risk factors are low, you may not need to take aspirin.** To evaluate your risk factors for heart attack, you need to have your blood cholesterol and blood pressure measured and discuss other risk factors, such as family history, with a health-care professional. If you have one or more risk factors for heart disease, your doctor may recommend aspirin therapy.

• **There is a slight risk of stroke.** Though aspirin therapy is very safe, studies have consistently shown that that it does slightly increase the risk of one kind of stroke (hemorrhagic). For the great majority of people, this small increase in risk does not outweigh the heart-protective benefits. But your physician should help you evaluate your risk for hemorrhagic stroke.

• **If your blood pressure is high, it's essential to get it under control before you begin taking aspirin.** Studies of aspirin and heart attack have found that people who take aspirin might be at a slightly increased risk for stroke, especially those whose systolic blood pressure (the top number) was high. Hypertension (systolic pressure greater than 145) itself increases your risk of stroke. In a study published recently in the *British Medical Journal*, researchers concluded that bringing systolic blood pressure down to 130 or below means that you can have the benefits of aspirin without significantly increasing stroke risk.

• **You need to know how much aspirin to take.** A very low dose works as well as a high dose to reduce the risk of heart attack. You can take half (160 milligrams) a regular tablet every other day, or a "baby" aspirin (one-quarter aspirin, or 80 milligrams) every day. Once every 15 days (on the first and fifteenth of the month), we recommend that you take a whole aspirin instead of your regular dose. This "booster dose" further reduces the risk of clots.

• **Aspirin can interact with other drugs you take.** Be sure your doctor is aware of any other medications you take regularly.

• **Don't rely on aspirin alone for preventing a heart attack.** See the other steps that can help lower your risk on pages 64-65.

pain-relieving effects of both aspirin and aceta-minophen. How it works is unclear: It may help relieve pain by elevating mood. Also, since caffeine is a mild diuretic, the relief it provides may also come from reducing water retention, a factor in menstrual discomfort. Aspirin or aceta-minophen pills with caffeine may be more potent than pills that contain the active ingredient alone, increasing effectiveness of a particular dose by about 40 percent.

Actually, you don't have to buy special caffeinated pain relievers to get caffeine's effect. Studies have shown that taking aspirin with a caffeinated beverage such as coffee or tea increases the aspirin's effect.

If you choose to use a pill containing caffeine, keep in mind that these products may contain up to 65 milligrams of caffeine per dose, as much as a cup of coffee. If you're sensitive to caffeine, you may want to avoid these products, or at least not use them within two or three hours of bedtime.

• **Effervescent solutions.** A product like Alka-Seltzer promises to deliver fast pain relief because the aspirin in it is dissolved in water, and so doesn't have to be broken down in the stomach. But there is no evidence that such products deliver pain relief more quickly or effectively than solid dosage forms of aspirin. Moreover, they may contain large amounts of sodium that should be avoided by individuals whose sodium intake should be restricted, such as people with hypertension or heart disease.

• **Antacids and cold remedies.** Acetaminophen and aspirin may be combined with antacids for treating headache or other pain that accompanies acid indigestion or heartburn. Pain relievers are also combined with some nonprescription cold remedies to relieve headache and muscle aches associated with cold and flu.

WHICH TYPE OF PAIN RELIEVER?

No single pain reliever or fever reducer has been shown to be consistently more effective than the others. But pain is an individual matter, involving complex physical and psychological variables. Your backache or tendinitis may be relieved by aspirin, while someone else's may not. No one medication or treatment will work for all people, all types of pain, or even for all people with the same complaint or apparent underlying condition. People also vary considerably in how they experience side effects: You may get an upset stomach from one dose of an NSAID, while someone else can take the same medicine for a week with no adverse reactions.

Choosing a specific pain reliever entails balancing the beneficial effect it has for your particular problem with the side effects and potential risks. Many people will find that it takes some trial and error to find the agent that works best for them.

Be sure to check all warnings or precautions, indicated in the entries that follow as well as on product labels, since a particular product might be inadvisable, depending on other medical conditions you might have as well as any medications you are taking.

Here are a few common conditions that aren't chronic for which one type of OTC pain reliever may be preferable. (For arthritis pain relief, see pages 393-395.)

Exercise-related injuries. Whether it is general muscle soreness brought on by overdoing an activity, or a sports-related injury such as tendinitis, ankle sprain, or a rotator cuff strain in the shoulder, inflammation is usually a symptom. In that case, an NSAID, rather than acetaminophen, is the preferred choice.

601

Colds. All pain relievers are effective at reducing muscle aches accompanying a cold. But some studies indicate that ibuprofen may be preferable because it does not seem to promote nasal congestion, unlike aspirin and acetaminophen.

Headache. Headaches vary greatly in severity, duration, and cause. For most people a headache is a passing discomfort that results from a lack of sleep, an argument at work, polluted air, a hangover, or some other temporary situation. For these occasional headaches, no one pain reliever has been proven more effective than another.

For *migraine* headaches, which can be accompanied by incapacitating pain that may last from a few minutes to a few days, a panel of headache experts, convened by Chicago's Diamond Headache Clinic Research and Educational Foundation, recommended a combination of acetaminophen, aspirin, and caffeine to treat mild to moderate migraines.

If you suffer from persistent migraines or any severe headache pain, you should see your doctor for diagnosis and treatment. Often in these cases, prescription drugs offer the best pain control.

Menstrual cramps. Most women find that NSAIDs, especially ibuprofen or naproxen sodium, offer the best control of painful menstrual cramps, which are caused by uterine contractions. This is probably because they inhibit prostaglandins released during a woman's period that cause the contractions. NSAIDs are most effective when started two days before a period and continued through the second day of menstrual flow, when prostaglandin production is at its peak. Take the medication on a regular schedule for these four days, whether you feel the need or not, to best control prostaglandin formation. For women who cannot tolerate NSAIDs or who are breastfeeding, acetaminophen may provide pain relief.

Pain Relievers and Children

A number of pain-relief products are "specially formulated" for children. These products are typically in lower doses, and come in liquid preparations or chewable tablets (usually flavored) to make them easier to take. A distinguishing feature of these products is that they don't contain aspirin, which can cause a rare but potentially fatal brain and liver disorder called Reye's syndrome in children and teenagers when they have influenza or chickenpox. The symptoms of Reye's syndrome include tiredness, severe headache, disorientation, and vomiting; symptoms usually occur near the end of the original illness. While no one knows the cause of Reye's syndrome, it is associated with the use of aspirin during a viral illness.

Acetaminophen and ibuprofen are the preferred medications for children age 19 or younger. If the medications are for children age 12 or older, there is no reason to pay extra for specially packaged formulas. Children that age can take adult doses of generic acetaminophen or ibuprofen as well as naproxen sodium (which is not recommended for children younger than 12).

Toothache. Any of the pain relievers can be used to control the pain of tooth decay or the soreness that may develop after you've had some dental work, such as a filling or root canal. However, aspirin should not be used after any form of dental surgery or tooth extraction because it inhibits blood clotting. Even one aspirin tablet can double the bleeding time after dental surgery.

Fever. Fever is defined as a body temperature higher than 98.6°F, the normal core temperature.

But because "normal" temperature can vary slightly, an adult's temperature usually isn't considered abnormal unless it exceeds 100° F. Eliminating a fever is controversial, since fever reduction could mask infection and delay treatment. (Reducing the fever, of course, doesn't treat the infection or other problem causing the fever.) Most fevers run their course if left untreated. So the principal reason to treat most fevers is because of the discomfort they cause.

If an adult or a child age 12 or older isn't uncomfortable with a temperature below 102°F, then you don't need to lower it. But you should take steps to lower a fever if a fever is uncomfortable or when it exceeds 102°F in adults and older children. When infants develop fever, it's best to contact your doctor.

Acetaminophen is the preferred agent for reducing fever in children, but ibuprofen is also approved as a children's fever reducer. All nonprescription pain relievers take about the same amount of time to achieve maximum reduction of temperature (two to three hours) and last for approximately the same length of time (four to six hours), though ibuprofen may last longer, especially in children.

Children 19 or younger should not be given aspirin to reduce fever because of the risk of Reye's syndrome, a potentially fatal illness (see the box, opposite).

If you have a chronic condition (such as heart disease, arthritis, or chronic pain) that might be helped by regular long-term doses of a pain reliever, you should talk to your physician. Among the questions to ask: Would I be better off with acetaminophen than aspirin or another NSAID? What is the lowest dose of a medication I can take? Am I at high risk for stomach bleeding? What are the warning symptoms?

Depending on the answers to these questions, you might be a candidate for the new form of aspirin known as a COX-2 inhibitor, available only by prescription. COX-2 inhibitors "inhibit" a pain-producing enzyme, but do so without blocking an enzyme that protects the stomach lining. Hence, they relieve pain and inflammation with a lower incidence of gastrointestinal side effects than older NSAIDs. Two such drugs—celecoxib (Celebrex) and rofecoxib (Vioxx)—are approved for managing both osteoarthritis and rheumatoid arthritis. Follow your doctor's advice: if you have arthritis and are doing well on acetaminophen, aspirin, or another over-the-counter NSAID, you probably don't need to switch to one of these newer drugs, which are much more expensive.

PAIN RELIEVER GUIDELINES

• *Look beyond brand names and claims.* Certain brand-name products, such as Bayer and Anacin, used to be synonymous with aspirin. However, these companies are now marketing a variety of pain relievers under their brand names. For example, Anacin is aspirin and caffeine, but Anacin 3 is acetaminophen. Manufacturers are also "targeting" products to specific conditions, such as headaches, arthritis, or menstrual cramps. But there is nothing truly new about these products: for example, a brand-name "menstrual cramp formula" may simply contain ibuprofen and caffeine, but at twice the price of a generic product.

• *For longer-lasting pain relief, consider naproxen sodium.* This drug works for 8 to 12 hours (compared to 4 to 6 hours for the other drugs). It's also good for overnight use.

• *People allergic to aspirin should use acetaminophen.* Although the other NSAIDs contain no aspirin, they may still produce a reaction in

603

someone with an aspirin allergy. And pain relievers other than aspirin that contain salicylates (such as magnesium salicylate and Pepto-Bismol) may also cause an allergic reaction. (True aspirin allergy is relatively rare, affecting less than one percent of the population. Some people who experience heartburn or intense stomach upset assume they are allergic to aspirin, but these are side effects. Allergy or hypersensitivity is signaled by symptoms such as hives, itching, facial swelling, and difficulty breathing.)

• *Start with the lowest dose.* This minimizes side effects. Taking the lowest dose is especially advisable for people over 65, since older people are more likely to experience side effects. Moreover, large doses of a pain reliever are not necessarily more effective. There is a "ceiling effect," such that increasing the dose beyond a certain point doesn't result in greater benefit.

• *Avoid alcohol when taking any pain reliever.* Consuming alcohol with pain relievers increases the risk of certain side effects. Acetaminophen and alcohol may promote liver damage, while combining alcohol with aspirin or other NSAIDs can cause gastrointestinal bleeding. If you habitually have more than three or more alcoholic drinks per day, consult your doctor before using any pain reliever. (The FDA now requires a warning to this effect for all over-the-counter drug products labeled for adult use that contain internal analgesic/antipyretic active ingredients.)

• *Avoid mixing pain relievers.* Unless your doctor has specifically told you to do so, it's best to avoid combining pain relievers, especially NSAIDs. Products containing aspirin and acetaminophen are the only combination deemed safe for short-term use. Taking other pain-relief ingredients in combination can increase the risk of potentially serious side effects. Combining

---

Don't Always Rely on Medication

▼

Many aches and pains are amenable to other forms of self-treatment and prevention that can complement medication and/or reduce the need for it. Relaxation training, for example, can help prevent or reduce the severity of some headaches, while backaches and other types of muscle strains and sports injuries can often be prevented by appropriate conditioning exercises, by warming up carefully, and by easing into new sports and fitness activities. Ice and heat, properly applied, are also effective at relieving pain and swelling from injuries to muscles and joints.

---

ibuprofen or ketoprofen with acetaminophen, for example, increases the risk of kidney damage.

If you take low-dose aspirin regularly to reduce your risk of heart disease, and you need an additional pain reliever for up to several days, you probably won't need to alter your aspirin schedule. But talk to your doctor first.

• *Use caution when buying combination products.* Cold, flu, sinus, and sleep remedies usually combine aspirin, acetaminophen, or ibuprofen with one or more of the following: a decongestant, an antihistamine, and a cough suppressant. Read labels carefully to make sure you really can benefit from all the active ingredients, and remember that the additives can produce undesirable effects. (For example, antihistamines sometimes cause drowsiness.) Also check the label to make sure that you don't exceed daily recommended dosages of pain relievers by taking these combination products in addition to a separate pain reliever.

• *Limit your use.* Don't take any product for

more than ten days for pain, more than three days for fever, or more than 48 hours for a migraine headache unless directed by your doctor. If you are using any pain reliever daily, you need medical supervision.

• **Contact your physician if any pain or ache is severe.** This is especially important for a severe head pain or pain in the stomach or abdomen. If you are self-treating mild to moderate pain related to a headache, muscle injury, or cold or flu, call your doctor if the pain doesn't improve after several days of self-treatment, if it gets worse, or if new symptoms appear (such as a rash, a severe sore throat, or severe redness or swelling in a painful area).

Fever. Call your doctor promptly if you or a child has a high fever. For older children and adults, a high fever is more than 104°F; for children up to two years, above 103°F; for children up to three months, above 101°F; and for month-old infants or younger, above 100°F.

Call your doctor if any fever is accompanied by other symptoms, such as a sore throat, persistent vomiting, or an unusual rash. If you are taking a pain reliever according to directions, and the fever remains above 102°F for more than a few hours, call your doctor. Also contact your doctor if the fever lasts for more than three days, if it returns after diminishing, or if the fever worsens or new symptoms occur.

Side effects. If, despite taking pain relievers with food and water, you develop gastric distress or other minor side effects that persist or become annoying, call your doctor. Also notify your doctor of any serious side effects associated with taking a pain reliever.

Once your problem has been diagnosed, your doctor may recommend another medication and/or provide special dosage instructions for your particular situation. Ibuprofen, naproxen sodium, ketoprofen, and acetaminophen all come in prescription-strength formulations, and your doctor may prescribe one of these. There are also other NSAIDs and other types of salicylates available only by prescription that may be more appropriate for relieving your discomfort.

Sunscreens

Sunscreens can be confusing. Their labels contain numbers and acronyms (UVA, UVB, SPF) that often aren't clearly explained, and ingredients with long technical names. There are more than 150 brands to choose from—perhaps double that if you include private store brands along with national brands—and brand names and ingredients change with surprising frequency. Also confusing is the fact that some researchers have questioned whether sunscreens actually offer protection against skin cancer, specifically against malignant melanoma, the most serious form of skin cancer.

Don't let any of this persuade you that choosing a sunscreen is too much trouble or that you might just as well skip the sunscreen and work on your tan. In fact, sunscreen use has a number of benefits, and, once you know which ingredients to look for, choosing a product isn't complicated. At the same time, too many people seem to believe that wearing a sunscreen practically reduces their risk of skin cancer to zero. It doesn't. A sunscreen should always be thought of as back-up protection, to be used in conjunction with other measures —above all limiting your sun exposure—that can substantially reduce your risk of skin cancer (see page 443).

Protection from UV radiation. There are two types of UV radiation. UVA, or ultraviolet A, is long-wave radiation that's part of the ultraviolet spectrum. It penetrates more deeply than UVB, or ultraviolet B, and causes wrinkling and leathering, damages connective tissue, and promotes tanning, although it is less likely to cause an immediate burn. It may be crucial in the development of melanoma. (Tanning lamps emit mostly UVA rays.) UVB is short-wave radiation. It reddens and burns the skin and causes tanning. It also promotes basal cell and squamous cell carcinoma, the two most prevalent forms of skin cancer, and may worsen the effects of UVA.

Even brief exposure to UV radiation can, in addition to causing sunburn, cause allergic reactions such as hives, trigger reactions to certain commonly used medications that increase skin sensitivity, or worsen certain medical conditions, including cold sores, systemic lupus, and many others (see page 55).

SUNSCREEN PROTECTION

Sunscreen preparations—in the form of oils, lotions, creams, or gels—contain compounds that minimize the damage inflicted on the skin by filtering out some or most of the sun's UV rays, which cause both suntan and sunburn.

Chemical agents in sunscreens. A chemical agent known as PABA was once the most common active ingredient used in sunscreens, but it often causes itching or rashes and is only effective against UVB radiation. Newer active ingredients, which include salicylates, cinnamates, and benzophenones, are far less likely to cause skin irritation, even at high concentrations, and offer protection against UVB. And other ingredients, such as anthranilates and certain benzophenones, protect against part of the UVA spectrum.

Most products contain two or more ingredients to provide protection against both UVB and UVA radiation; hence, nearly all sunscreens today offer "broad spectrum" protection. Most are also water-resistant.

One ingredient—avobenzone (originally called Parsol 1789)—protects against the widest spectrum of UVA rays (which are an important cause of skin aging). Though once hard to find, more and more products containing avobenzone are coming on the market.

Physical sunscreens. Some sunscreens use physical sunblocks—compounds such as titanium oxide and zinc oxide that actually block or reflect light, thus protecting from both UVA and UVB. Sunblocks used to be available only as opaque creams or pastes intended for protecting the nose or lips, but were messy to use and unattractive. But now these ingredients can be manufactured as ultra-fine powders, and new products formulated with them are less visible and less messy.

UNDERSTANDING SPF

Every sunscreen product is labeled with a number indicating the SPF, or Sun Protection Factor, for that product. This number tells you the length of time you can stay in the sun before you burn from exposure to UVB, compared to using no sunscreen. For example, if you start to turn pink in 20 minutes on a hot day, an SPF 15 would, in theory, allow you to stay out for 300 minutes (15 multiplied by 20 minutes), or five hours, before burning. (These numbers can produce more confusion than clarity, and the FDA is planning to replace the numbers with a simple rating system, such as high, medium, low.)

In real life many variables, such as skin color, the season, and your location, come into play to determine the effectiveness of sunscreens. The

606

amount of protection also depends on how much sunscreen you apply. Studies have shown that people tend to apply only about half the amount of sunscreen that the FDA used to determine SPF. So it's very likely that you would have to reapply the sunscreen to be protected for five hours.

Also, SPF 30 does not offer twice the protection of SPF 15, which blocks 93 percent of UVB. SPF 30 actually blocks only 4 percent more, or 97 percent. For this reason, although there have been sunscreen products with an SPF of 50 or higher, the FDA has indicated that there is no incremental benefit from an SPF of more than 30. Also, to achieve this benefit could require up to 25 percent more sunscreen chemicals, increasing the likelihood of skin irritation and toxicity.

What SPF doesn't tell you. Not all sunscreens with the same SPF offer the same protection. Although it is a fairly reliable indicator, the SPF pertains only to UVB rays—those mainly responsible for sunburn and skin cancer. Most of the active ingredients in chemical sunscreens effectively absorb UVB rays, but let through varying amounts of longer-length UVA rays, which can

damage the skin's connective tissue, leading to premature aging, as well as playing a role in causing skin cancer. There is, however, no rating system to indicate the degree of UVA protection. Instead, you need to check the list of active ingredients to see if any that protect against UVA are present (see below).

SUNSCREEN GUIDELINES

Your skin type and the amount of time you spend in the sun are the two most important factors to consider when choosing a sunscreen. Some sample brand names are mentioned in these guidelines. But remember that the ingredients of products frequently change, so you need to check labels to see which active ingredients are actually used in a product. Remember, too, that the best step you can take to save your skin is to avoid long sun exposure, even if you are wearing a sunscreen.

607

Look for a broad-spectrum sunscreen rated SPF 15 or higher. The slightly greater protection offered by SPF 30 may be needed for children, for very long exposure, in climates where sunlight can be very intense (high altitudes or southern latitudes), or for people who are very fair-skinned or who have had skin cancer or lupus (an autoimmune disorder with symptoms that often include sensitive skin which burns easily in sunlight).

For extra protection against UVA rays, consider a product with avobenzone ((Parsol 1789), which is now used, along with UVB-screening ingredients, in a dozen or so leading brands. There are also more widely used sunscreen ingredients that offer some UVA protection; these include oxybenzone, octocrylene, and menthyl anthranilate. Check for these ingredients on labels and for the degree of UVA protection they offer.

If you are in the sun often or are very fair or have had skin cancer, get a sunscreen with titanium oxide or zinc oxide. These physical sun-blocking agents offer maximum protection against all UV radiation. Some products combine sunblockers with chemical sunscreen agents. Also check with your pharmacist, since new products with sun-blocking ingredients are coming on the market.

If you have sensitive skin, especially sensitivity to certain medications, avoid sunscreens with a PABA derivative, such as Padimate-O. These derivatives are less irritating than PABA, but they are still more likely than non-PABA products to cause a skin reaction or rash.

If you're taking medication, ask your doctor or pharmacist about possible reactions to sunlight and interactions with sunscreens.

For infants, use sunscreen only when a baby is at least six months old. The chemicals in sunscreen may have an adverse effect on children younger than this. Special-formula sunscreens for babies may be less irritating, though there is little evidence for this. Choose a product with an SPF of 15 or greater. (Infants six months old and younger should never be exposed to the sun for extended periods because the melanin in their skin will not yet protect them significantly. When you go outside, cover a baby in a tightly woven long-sleeved shirt, long-legged pants, and a wide-brimmed sunbonnet.)

Don't confuse sunscreens and "sunless" self-tanning products. The latter are cosmetic creams and lotions for coloring the skin without the damaging effects of sun exposure. A pigmenting agent called dihydroxyacetone (DHA) is a major ingredient, and the FDA has determined that while it is safe to use, it provides no protection against UV radiation. Several self-tanning products combine DHA with sunscreen agents for people who don't want to be completely sunless. But if you are spending any time outdoors, you will be bet-

ter protected by applying a separate strong sunscreen beforehand.

Put sunscreen on half an hour before you go outside. Studies show that this allows it to penetrate the skin for optimal effectiveness.

Use a generous amount, and reapply it often. One ounce is about right to cover all exposed skin for an average-size adult in a swim suit (of average size). If you're perspiring or swimming, apply sunscreen frequently and generously while you're outdoors, even if the product is labeled "very water resistant," "waterproof," or "all day."

Apply extra sunscreen if you're also using an insect repellent. A concentration of 33 percent DEET (the most common active ingredient in insect repellents) spread on top of a sunscreen with SPF 15 decreases the effectiveness of the screen by about 40 percent, according to one study, probably because DEET is a solvent. The alternative is to apply the repellent only to your clothes.

Combination products, containing both DEET and a sunscreen, are available, but the separate products are better because you can keep reapplying sunscreen without having to reapply DEET.

Apply a lip balm. The lip area is one of the most common locations for oral cancer. Choose a balm rated SPF 15 or higher.

Be sure to follow the other steps listed on page 56 to protect your skin from the sun.

Guide to Dietary and Herbal Supplements

In the United States, "dietary supplements" encompass an array of different products that include vitamins, minerals, herbs, botanicals, and other plant-derived substances, as well as enzymes, amino acids, and even some human hormones. At first glance, you might think that supplements, like over-the-counter medications, have passed some sort of scrutiny: their labels typically carry dosages and make various claims related to health matters. But there is a huge difference between the two types of products.

CONFUSIONS AND DILEMMAS

In 1994, federal legislation, passed after intensive lobbying by the supplements industry, essentially removed "products that supplement the diet"—which included herbal products as well as vitamins and minerals—from control of the Food and Drug Administration (FDA) and dramatically relaxed restrictions on their manufacture and marketing. The Dietary Supplement Health and Education Act, or DSHEA, has allowed supplement manufacturers to make claims about a product's health benefits without any real scientific evidence of the product's actual effects. Before a drug can be marketed, its safety and efficacy must be demonstrated. Supplement manufacturers, by contrast, don't have to submit data in advance of making a claim; the law merely stipulates that they need to have the evidence of safety on hand. But since the FDA cannot possibly inspect the claims of the thousands of products that flood the marketplace, manufacturers have little to fear

as far as being challenged to produce the evidence behind their claims. No one can be sure about the degree of compliance.

What are the consequences for the consumer?

• ***Dubious and deceptive health claims.*** For years now the FDA has attempted to make a distinction between "disease claims" (also called "medical claims"), which it strictly limits, and "structure or function claims" or "health maintenance claims," which are essentially unregulated. Unfortunately, it's still often impossible for consumers to tell the reasonable sorts of claims from the overblown ones.

Disease claims say something about preventing, treating, or curing a disease or one of its symptoms—for example, "reduces the pain of arthritis" or "alleviates constipation." Such claims require prior FDA review for efficacy. Among the few explicit disease claims on supplements are the claim that calcium can prevent osteoporosis and that folic acid can help prevent birth defects.

Even claims that imply disease prevention or treatment—such as "prevents bone frailty" or "promotes urinary tract health"—require FDA approval. But supplement manufacturers, denying that such statements are medical/disease claims, often push to see how far they can go with so-called implied claims

Claims relating to the "structure or function" of the body are permitted on supplement labels. But this is where language becomes murky, since such claims may imply that a product can also help prevent or treat health problems. For example, the label on a bottle St. John's wort cannot claim to treat depression. But it can state that the product "helps improve mood"—begging the question as to whether it will actually reduce depression. Likewise, people with high cholesterol may be eager to try a supplement that claims to "promote healthy cholesterol"—even though there may be little or no evidence that the product can lower high cholesterol levels. None of these claims require FDA approval.

Products that make any kind of structure of function claims must also carry the following disclaimer: "This statement has not been evaluated by the Food and Drug Administration. This product is not intended to diagnose, treat, cure, or prevent any disease." But the disclaimer can appear in tiny type, and many people only see "Food and Drug Administration," which can lead them to think this indicates approval.

Overall, the new regulations, rather than limit unsubstantiated pseudo-health claims, have allowed manufacturers to make broader and bolder claims than before. Moreover, manufacturers and marketers can now suggest almost anything in ads, on the Internet, in stores, and on TV and radio. They don't need any proof of safety or efficacy. Flawed studies are vigorously cited in support of dubious or even dangerous products. Studies that show a negative effect are never mentioned, and indeed may never be published. Yet some supplements are highly beneficial: Under certain circumstances, they can truly supplement your diet and help prevent or treat a health problem. No wonder people are confused.

• *No standardization or quality control.* The deregulation of supplements basically leaves the purity and content of products up to manufacturers. The result is that consumers can't be sure that any supplement contains exactly what the label says it does. Odds are good that straightforward vitamin and mineral supplements accurately reflect their labels: the chemistry of vitamins and minerals is well understood, and standardizing them is simple compared to herbal products or supplements like glucosamine or melatonin, which are more complex. Even so, in one lab test of 26 vitamin C pills, three had less C than the label claimed.

Herbals and other types of supplements are more problematic. Little is known about which constituents of each plant are the important ones. And even when that information is available, the amount of active ingredients can vary from plant to plant, making it difficult to produce standardized products with consistent amounts of active ingredients. Both consumer magazines and professional journals have published test results in recent years showing that different brands of herbal remedies such as St. John's wort or saw palmetto contain widely varying amounts of the herb in question. There are no tests for bioavailability—that is, whether the active ingredient will be absorbed and actually utilized by the body. And in the case of chemicals like SAM-e or glucosamine, to name two popular supplements, the active ingredient is known, but there is no "standardized" method for measuring it or its effect.

• *No guarantee of effectiveness or safety.* Even if a product contains exactly what it claims, will it have any benefit? There is no assurance it will. This is not to say that some herbs aren't helpful or that some manufacturers aren't conscientious in trying to manufacture products with consistent levels of active ingredients. But in many cases, reliable information on health benefits or the dosages needed to produce results is hard to come by. Nobody knows because the necessary research hasn't been done.

Then there is the safety issue. Because herbs come from a natural source or have been traditionally used for centuries, many people consider them safe. In fact, herbs have side effects ranging from inconsequential to life-threatening, just like drugs—many of which originally came from plants. (Aspirin, for example, was discovered in the bark of the white willow.) Herbs can also interact with conventional medications. Unfortunately, if an herb does have serious side effects, it is now up to the FDA to prove this, not the manufacturer.

MAKING SUPPLEMENTS MEASURE UP

Ideally, all supplements would meet standards of identity that would ensure quality and purity. But because most supplements can be derived directly from plants and other natural sources, they can't be patented. Therefore, drug and supplement manufacturers have little financial incentive to devote the kind of money that is spent researching and getting approval for drugs, since any company would be able to make the same product.

Eventually, American regulations and/or practices may approach those in a number of European countries, where herbal remedies are examined with some scientific rigor and products must conform to manufacturing standards. In this regard, Germany stands out for maintaining a special board—Commission E—that has evaluated the safety and efficacy of some 300 herbs by making use of information obtained from clinical trials, field studies, scientific literature, and the opinions of medical organizations.

To that end, here is what consumers need and can legitimately demand from the FDA and from supplement manufacturers:

• Standards of identity that ensure quality and purity; assurance that products don't vary from batch to batch.

• Herbs sold under their official Latin name, as well as their common name, with lists of scientifically established uses for each herb.

• Proof of "equivalence"—that is, a given dose of a product must contain a certain amount of key ingredients in order to produce a known effect.

• Proof that products actually will be absorbed and utilized by the body.

• Assurance that the substance is nontoxic, along with lists of any potential side effects and interactions with drugs.

This is a big and expensive order, but it's the least we can ask for.

IF YOU WANT TO TRY SUPPLEMENTS

The entries on the following pages sort through the claims made about best-selling herbal remedies and other types of supplements—from coenzyme Q-10 to SAM-e—being marketed in the United States. (For general recommendations on vitamin and mineral supplements, including vitamins C and E, see pages 21-27.)

Recent regulations from the FDA require that all supplements must start to carry a "Supplements Facts" panel on product labels that clearly identifies a list of all ingredients and gives the name and address of the manufacturer or distributor. The new ruling also specifies the meaning of terms such as "high potency" and "antioxidants," and in the case of herbs, the part of the plant used in the product must be identified. But you have no way of knowing whether a bottle's contents conform to what is on the label.

If you decide to try a supplement, remember that herbs especially can have potent effects and side

611

effects. Keep the points below in mind, along with specific precautions in the entries that follow.

• *Don't self-treat a serious or chronic health problem with supplements.* See your doctor.

• *Always tell your doctor about any supplements you are taking*—or supplements you want to try. *This is especially important if you are taking any medication,* so your doctor can tell you about any interactions that might occur. More and more evidence is accumulating that herbs and other supplements can interact dangerously with prescription medication. A wide range of supplements, for example, including garlic, gingko, and feverfew can boost the effect of the widely-used blood-thinning drug warfarin, thus increasing the risk of bleeding. Other supplements, such as coenzyme Q-10 and ginseng, reduce its effect. It's also essential that you tell your doctor about any supplement you take if you are scheduled for surgery.

• *If you are pregnant or potentially pregnant, or breastfeeding, avoid medicinal herbs.* Don't dose children with herbs without checking first with a physician.

• *Be careful of overdosing.* With many supplements, no one knows what the proper dose is. But as with conventional drugs, too much of a medicinal herb can have serious consequences. As a precaution, when a dosage range is given, start with the lowest dose.

• *Herbal remedies should be short-term.* There are no established guidelines as to how long you should take a supplement for it to have an effect. But generally, if you are taking an herbal remedy to treat a specific health problem, stop if the herb doesn't seem to be working after one or two weeks at most.

• *If you experience any adverse effects,* stop taking the supplement.

Alpha-Lipoic Acid

▶ **What It Is**

Alpha-lipoic acid is an antioxidant that is now sold as a dietary supplement. Scientists first discovered the importance of this substance in the 1950s, and recognized it as an antioxidant in 1988, but only recently has it made its way into American health-food stores. Very potent, alpha-lipoic acid is apparently a special antioxidant. It has been the subject of a substantial amount of basic research around the world.

▶ **How It Works**

The human body needs alpha-lipoic acid to produce energy. The body actually makes enough alpha-lipoic acid for these basic metabolic functions. This compound acts as an antioxidant, however, only when there is an excess of it and it is in the "free" state in the cells.

However, there is no free alpha-lipoic acid circulating in your body, unless you consume supplements or get it injected. Except for yeast and liver, foods contain only tiny amounts of it.

What makes alpha-lipoic acid so special as an antioxidant is that it helps deactivate a wide array of fat- and water-soluble free radicals in many bodily systems. In particular, it may help protect the genetic material, DNA. It is also important because it works closely with vitamins C and E and some other antioxidants, "recycling" them and thus making them much more effective.

▶ **Health Claims**

Alpha-lipoic acid is being studied—and already marketed—as a preventive and/or treatment for many age-related diseases, from heart disease and stroke to diabetes and cataracts. In Germany, in particular, it is often prescribed to treat long-term complications of diabetes, such as nerve damage, thought to result in part from free-radical damage.

What we know. Some studies—mostly in animals, a few in humans, often using intravenous doses—do show that supplemental alpha-lipoic acid can help keep nerves healthy and play other beneficial roles in the body.

What we don't know. Research on alpha-lipoic acid is still in its infancy. The studies have been small, and the results sometimes inconsistent. There has been little good research in humans. Large, long-term, well-controlled studies need to be done. No one knows what dose should be used for what ailment. Studies in humans have used much larger doses than are found in most supplements. If alpha-lipoic acid is as powerful as it seems, there may be a danger in too much of a good thing.

In addition, while in Germany it is sold only by prescription and is monitored by the government, in the United States you have no way of knowing what's in the bottles.

▶ Possible Side Effects

Though alpha-lipoic acid so far appears to be safe (except for a few reports of allergic skin reactions), no one knows what the long-term side effects of large supplemental doses may be.

▶ Wellness Recommendation

In a few years, alpha-lipoic acid may be seen as important an antioxidant supplement as vitamin E. Meanwhile, don't be a guinea pig. Not enough is known now to recommend it.

If you have diabetes or heart disease, in particular, you may be unwilling to wait until more research is done. In that case, it is crucial that you talk to your doctor before taking it. The supplement may, for instance, affect the dosage of your diabetes medication.

Black Cohosh

▶ What It Is

A member of the buttercup family, black cohosh (*Cimicifuga racemosa*) is a native American plant, also known as black snake root or rattleweed, long used to treat "female complaints" when these symptoms could not be mentioned in polite society. It was the chief ingredient in Lydia E. Pinkham's Vegetable Compound—a famous patent medicine of yore that claimed to cure menstrual cramps and menopausal symptoms, as well as nervous tension and other conditions. The vegetable compound was a tincture—that is, the herbs were dissolved in alcohol. At 36-proof, it was more alcoholic than wine. Some people thought this was Lydia's true secret.

You can still buy Lydia Pinkham's, now reformulated with vitamins E and C and other substances, and not quite as alcoholic. It no longer contains black cohosh. Black cohosh itself, used in various products (such as Remifemin or Black Cohosh Power), is one of the best-selling herbs for menopausal symptoms.

▶ How It Works

Some researchers think black cohosh contains plant estrogens and thus has hormonal effects, but the latest reports have found no estrogens or hormonal effects.

▶ Health Claims

Black cohosh is being promoted as a "natural" alternative to hormone replacement therapy for treating symptoms related to menopause.

What we know. Although the herb has been much studied, evidence is still pretty thin. Some studies have found that it relieves hot flashes, sweating, headache, dizziness, and other

613

menopausal symptoms—but few of these studies have been well designed.

What we don't know. It's unknown whether black cohosh has any effect, positive or negative, on breast cancer risk. And it is also not clear whether women taking birth control pills or hormone replacement therapy can safely take black cohosh.

Other claims: Black cohosh was used at one time to treat joint pain, and it does contain salicylates, which are similar to the compounds in aspirin—but in amounts too small to have a therapeutic effect.

▶ Possible Side Effects

These include stomach upset, headache, dizziness, and weight gain.

▶ Precautions

• Women who are pregnant or breast feeding should steer clear of black cohosh. It seems to increase the risk of miscarriage.

• Because black cohosh may work as a mild sedative, avoid taking the herb if you are taking tranquilizers.

• Black cohosh may interfere with hypertension medication.

▶ Wellness Recommendation

Even its advocates (one of them is the herb expert Varro Tyler) say that women who decide to try black cohosh for menopausal symptoms should not take it for more than six months; others say three months. Since so little is known about it, and there's no guarantee how much of it is in any given product, it's difficult to say how these experts arrived at such a conclusion.

Perhaps good studies will one day be done, so that you could be more certain of its benefits and

side effects. Thus far its traditional uses and benefits have no solid support from scientific research.

In the meantime, if you try black cohosh, be sure your physician knows. Ask whether it might interact with other medications you are taking.

Coenzyme Q-10

▶ What It Is

Coenzyme Q-10 (CoQ-10) is one of the most popular dietary supplements—not just in this country, but around the world, especially in Japan. It's claimed that CoQ-10 prevents and/or combats many disorders, including heart disease, cancer, AIDS, lung disease, hypertension, gum disease, obesity, impaired immunity, chronic fatigue syndrome, asthma, Alzheimer's, allergies, and aging itself. In recent years much research on CoQ-10 has confirmed that it is indeed a very important substance. But even so, the clinical research is still in its infancy, and thus the marketing claims remain overblown.

▶ How It Works

CoQ-10 is necessary for generating energy in all human cells, as well as in all living organisms. The substance is manufactured by the liver; it is also found in many foods, but is most concentrated in meat and fish.

First isolated in 1957, it was named ubiquinone because it belongs to a class of compounds called quinones, and because it's ubiquitous. It also acts as a powerful antioxidant, meaning that it helps prevent the cellular damage caused by free radicals in the body.

▶ Health Claims

CoQ-10 is one of many substances (including

DHEA and melatonin) in the body that tend to decline as people age and/or develop certain diseases (such as various cardiac conditions and Parkinson's Disease). Supplemental CoQ-10 is reputed to combat or reverse the effects of aging or disease, even though lower levels of CoQ-10 don't necessarily *cause* aging or disease.

What we know. Interest in CoQ-10 began after early research in Texas showed that CoQ-10 supplements can help treat otherwise unresponsive congestive heart failure and certain other heart problems. Studies since then have had inconsistent results. Further clinical trials are underway.

An international conference on CoQ-10, held in 1998 in Boston, but only recently published, included three dozen studies and reports. Among the findings: CoQ-10 may work even better than vitamin E against two kinds of free radicals. But, unfortunately, it can also "auto-oxidize"—that is, it can become a free radical itself under some circumstances. Vitamin E can prevent this, however. Indeed, studies suggested that these two substances work synergistically, as do many other antioxidants, such as vitamins C and E, beta carotene, and alpha-lipoic acid.

Another study found that the more CoQ-10 there is in LDL ("bad") cholesterol, the less susceptible it is to oxidation. It's theorized that the oxidation of LDL increases plaque development in artery walls. Vitamin E also helps reduce the oxidation of LDL, thus reducing the risk of heart attack.

Other researchers at the conference reported that the cholesterol-lowering drugs known as "statins" (which include lovastatin and the dietary supplement Cholestin) reduce the body's synthesis of CoQ-10, but the health effects of this are unknown.

What we don't know. Most of these studies and presentations were highly theoretical and/or preliminary, merely suggesting potential benefits of CoQ-10 supplements. There is still no solid clinical evidence that CoQ-10 supplements are actually beneficial.

▶ **Possible Side Effects**

Side effects with CoQ-10 have rarely been reported, but no one knows what the long-term effects are.

▶ **Wellness Recommendation**

This interesting antioxidant may be helpful in treating heart failure, but it has not been adequately tested, and does not appear to be nearly a effective as medications currently being used. Its benefits for healthy people remain unproven.

Is there any reason not to take CoQ-10, just to be safe? There doesn't seem to be any danger, but no one knows what the long-term effects are. Talk to your cardiologist about it if you have heart disease. If you're taking it on your own, make sure your doctor knows.

Make sure you also take vitamins E and C, and don't think that CoQ-10 can take the place of proven, reliable treatments and preventive strategies for heart disease.

DHEA

▶ **What It Is**

Discovered in the 1930s, DHEA (dehydroepiandrosterone) is a hormone manufactured in the human adrenal gland; other primates also produce it. DHEA-sulfate, or DHEAS, is a related form of the hormone. There's more DHEAS circulating in the body than any other hormone. It's a "precursor" hormone—that is, it

615

is a basic chemical that the body uses for different purposes. It can be converted to androstenedione, and then to testosterone or estrogen. Production begins in the fetus, stops at birth, resumes around age 7, peaks at about age 25, and then begins to decline. By age 70 production falls to one-fifth or as low as one-twentieth of what it was at age 25.

These days, DHEA is promoted as a "clinically proven fountain of youth" and a panacea in ads and catalogues and on the Internet. At the same time, many of the scientists who consider DHEA "promising" look upon the sale of DHEA pills as alarming.

▶ Health Claims

If a hormone increases along with youth and vigor and then almost disappears, it's logical to wonder whether it might prevent or slow aging as well as the chronic diseases of aging—which are some of the leading claims made for DHEA.

What we know. We don't know much. Most of the studies so far on DHEA have been with lab animals, chiefly rodents. This is a drawback because rodents produce negligible amounts of DHEA, and the results in rodents probably don't apply to humans. In any case the results have been unclear: sometimes DHEA seems to improve rodent immunity or confer other benefits, while in other studies DHEA appears to cause cancer.

Studies of humans have also yielded confusing results. At least 21 studies of DHEA have been done in people, using widely varying doses and administered either by injection or orally. Researchers are interested in its possible effects on the cardiovascular, immune, digestive, and nervous systems, and in whether it promotes or protects against tumor growth, as well as obesity. But no answers have been forthcoming. Studies of

DHEA and immunity in older people have had disappointing results. An early study found that high blood levels of DHEA are associated with a lower risk of heart disease—in men but not women—but this is far from definite.

Other studies suggest that high natural levels of DHEA are linked to a lower risk of breast cancer in premenopausal women, but to a higher risk in postmenopausal women. As reported in the *Journal of the National Cancer Institute*, a research study found that postmenopausal women with the highest blood levels of DHEA (occurring naturally, not administered experimentally or as a dietary supplement) had the *highest* risk of breast cancer.

What we don't know. It's much too early, most scientists think, to launch big clinical trials, since so little is known about the basic biology of DHEA. No one even understands what it does in adults, except that it affects many bodily systems.

But studies continue, here and in other countries. DHEA might prove useful against such immune-system disorders as lupus or AIDS. It might slow aging. On the other hand, it may prove to promote cancer. Little is known about lesser side effects, which in women may include the growth of unwanted facial hair, male-pattern baldness, deepening voice, and acne.

It's not possible to say of DHEA, as is often said of various herbal remedies, "It's widely used in other countries." No country with a regulatory system for drugs allows DHEA to be sold over the counter. In Canada it is not available even by prescription.

▶ Wellness Recommendation

DHEA is a substance so poorly understood and so potent that you may wonder how it can be sold as an unregulated product. Because of the U.S. Dietary Supplement Health and Education Act of 1994, which relaxed the rules for "dietary supplements," DHEA can be sold without testing, so long as the label makes no specific medical claims. DHEA doesn't even exist in foods, except in the adrenal glands of monkeys and other primates, which are not sold for human consumption.

To add to the confusion—and perhaps it's a lucky break for the public—what's sold as DHEA may not be DHEA. Our bodies synthesize DHEA from cholesterol, but what's sold over the counter is synthesized from plants (which don't contain any cholesterol). Wild yam extracts and soy do contain substances that can be converted into human hormones such as DHEA and cortisone, but only by a long, complex manufacturing process. Scientific investigators require (and get) a product that's pure and consistent—the real thing. However, the wild yam extracts billed as DHEA in stores are plant products that the body can't convert to DHEA or any other hormone. Even if the product you buy does contain real DHEA, there's no guarantee it has the amount claimed on the label.

DHEA is not a "natural medicine" and not a dietary supplement—and how the FDA could allow it to be classified as such remains a mystery. What's currently on the market is probably a complete waste of money. If this supplement really works like a hormone, then it's risky business. We think you should avoid DHEA.

Echinacea

▶ What It Is

Echinacea is part of the sunflower/daisy family, and its extracts have been used medicinally for centuries. Nine kinds of echinacea grow in the Unites States, the most common being *Echinacea purpurea,* which is known as purple coneflower. The active ingredients in echinacea are thought to strengthen the immune system, and it has become extremely popular in recent years as an herbal medicine for fighting colds, flu, and other infections. It comes in tinctures (dissolved in alcohol), capsules, pills, and teas. An ounce and a half of liquid can cost up to $15. Even the teas come at a premium price.

▶ How It Works

Like all plants, echinacea is a complicated mix of chemicals. No single constituent has been identified as the "active ingredient" in echinacea. But some of the herb's constituents, working in combination, might actually stimulate the immune system or promote healing (though none of these has been substantiated).

▶ Health Claims

Echinacea has been promoted as a cold remedy, an aid to healing wounds, and for treating various kinds of infections. Some supporters have suggested it may even be helpful against cancer. None of these claims, however, has been substantiated.

What we know. Echinacea has been extensively studied, but with conflicting results. One study recently found that a commercially made supplement did seem to stimulate immune cells, but in a test tube. In some studies involving humans, echinacea seems to have no effect on colds or immunity; in others, it seems to help.

In most studies that find echinacea to be an immune booster, however, the herbal extract was injected, which is not possible with the products on the market here. Studies of echinacea taken

617

by mouth have had inconsistent results. The commercial preparations you can currently buy in this country have not been tested at all.

What we don't know. Like all herbal products, echinacea is completely unregulated. What you're buying may not contain much, if any, echinacea. And nobody knows what a proper dosage might be. No one even knows what the active ingredient is, though 15 different compounds have been identified. No clinical trials have been done with any of these compounds. Little is known about toxicity.

▶ Possible Side Effects

Adverse effects with echinacea have rarely been reported, but that doesn't mean that it is safe. Some researchers think it could have an adverse effect on T-4 cells, an important component of immunity.

▶ Precautions

According to Commission E, the German board that rigorously assesses the efficacy and safety of herbal medicines, the following individuals should not try echinacea:

• People who know they're allergic to daisies.

• People with diseases such as lupus, rheumatoid arthritis, tuberculosis, and multiple sclerosis.

• Anyone who is HIV-positive, including anyone with AIDS.

• Pregnant or nursing women and small children.

▶ Wellness Recommendation

Though the supplements are prescribed in Germany for colds and flu, studies on them have yielded conflicting results. Because echinacea is not regulated by the FDA, active ingredients may vary among brands, and you may not be taking the same preparation that has been used in research studies or, for that matter, by someone who recommended it to you. Similarly, the doses you'll find on echinacea products will often vary according to the form of the herb. Until the government sets labeling standards and requires herbal manufacturers to meet them, consumers will continue to be part of what amounts to a haphazard marketplace experiment.

Evening Primrose Oil

▶ What It Is

Native to North America, the evening primrose is a tiny and short-lived wildflower and not a true primrose. When Europeans found it and took it to Europe, its purported healing properties for skin diseases and flesh wounds quickly earned it the name "King's cure-all." Evening primrose is now grown in 30 or more countries, and the oil pressed from its seed is marketed as a nutritional supplement and indeed as a miracle drug.

▶ How It Works

Like other nuts, seeds, and fruits (including olives, rapeseed, corn, and so forth), evening primrose seeds contain some vitamin E, and in addition what are known as essential fatty acids (EFAs)- so called because the body needs them in order to function properly, but does not produce them. We have to consume them. The chief EFAs are linoleic acid and linolenic acid, both of which are plentiful in foods. It's almost impossible to imagine a diet deficient in EFAs.

Evening primrose oil, however, is a source not only of linoleic acid but also of another kind of fatty acid called gamo-lenic acid (also known as gamma linolenic acid, or GLA). This fatty acid, normally manufactured by the body from linoleic acid, is important in many ways. It is transformed by the body eventually into eicosanoids, hormone-like chemicals that include the prostaglandins. The latter control such processes as inflammation, blood clotting, and cholesterol synthesis.

▶ **Health Claims**

Since the body produces its own GLA, why consume it in evening primrose oil? According to the label on one bottle of evening primrose gel capsules, "modern diets and lifestyles" may block conversion of linoleic acid into GLA. That's an interesting claim, but it has never been shown to be true. It is true that in several diseases, such as cancer, eczema, multiple sclerosis, and diabetes, the body seems to have a decreased ability to convert linoleic acid into GLA. But this is a long way from saying that swallowing GLA will cure or prevent these diseases.

What we know. There have been a large number of scientific studies of evening primrose oil. In England it is an approved medical treatment for breast pain and eczema, and is widely used for premenstrual syndrome, psoriasis, high cholesterol levels, rheumatoid arthritis, asthma, and nerve damage in people with diabetes.

What we don't know. There is actually little good clinical evidence that the oil has any benefits. An article in the *British Medical Journal* in 1994 concluded that although the oil was in wide use, there was hardly any justification for such use because the studies were flawed. However, the author called evening primrose oil "an interesting substance," and thought it might prove promising for such conditions as diabetic neuropathy, rheumatoid arthritis, and other ailments. Further research was called for.

That's pretty much the situation today—studies since 1994 have had conflicting results, but most have been negative.

Dr. Varro Tyler, an expert on plant medicines who is generally favorable toward them, is not convinced that evening primrose oil is efficacious. He also points out, in his book *The Honest Herbal*, that there are no data to support the safety of long-term consumption.

▶ **Possible Side Effects**

There is no evidence that evening primrose oil is toxic or produces any side effects except occasional headaches and nausea.

▶ **Wellness Recommendation**

You can buy some brands of evening primrose with standardized doses, but nobody knows what the right dose might be, or whether a healthy person would need any at all.

Capsules cost anywhere from 10 to 30 cents apiece. And manufacturers typically advise you to take three to six daily. If you took the larger dose, that could run from $18 to $54 a month—a lot of money for the EFAs you can get easily and cheaply from food. Also, some products on the market may be adulterated with other vegetable oils or may have decomposed

Because evening primrose oil is so expensive, some people have turned to borage seed oil or blackcurrant oil (also called beebread or starflower oil), another rich source of GLA. However, borage may contain liver toxins and should probably be avoided until more is known about it.

Feverfew

▶ **What It Is**

A common garden flower *(Tanacetum parthenium)* sometimes called a "summer daisy," feverfew has been used as a medicinal plant for centuries, and is one of the most interesting and potentially valuable of herbs. It's been used to treat headaches, menstrual irregularity, and fever.

How It Works
Experiments with animals have shown that feverfew may reduce inflammation as well as the hormonelike substances known as prostaglandins; among other effects, prostaglandins play a role in producing pain sensations and migraine. Feverfew's actions might resemble those of aspirin, and it might therefore prove useful in treating arthritis. But no one is sure which chemical in the plant may have medicinal effects.

Health Claims
Studies of feverfew as a migraine preventive have had confusing results.

What we know. One or two studies have shown that the leaf of the plant can prevent (not relieve) migraines, meaning that you'd have to take it all the time.

What we don't know. In an issue of *Cephalalgia*, researchers in the Department of Complementary Medicine at the University of Exeter in England reviewed the clinical work on feverfew and concluded that the jury was still out. As quoted in a later interview in *The Lancet*, one of these researchers, Dr. Edzard Ernst, doubted that feverfew's active compound had been identified.

Possible Side Effects
Side effects may include mouth ulcers, stomach irritation, and nausea.

Precautions
• Feverfew may interact with aspirin, so if you take aspirin or any anti-inflammatory drug regularly, consult your doctor before trying feverfew.

• If you are allergic to chamomile, ragweed, and yarrow—or if feverfew gives you a rash—you should steer clear of swallowing it. There's some evidence that if you take it and then discontinue its use, you can get rebound headaches.

• Children and pregnant or nursing women should not take this herb.

Wellness Recommendation
People suffering from migraines might try feverfew: it's not expensive, it's not risky, and it has helped in some studies. However, you may be wasting your money on what you find in the drugstore or health-food store. Dr. Varro Tyler, an American herb expert interested in the potential of feverfew, says that commercially available preparations usually have very little plant material in them.

If you have feverfew in your garden—and are certain that's what it is—you could try the fresh leaves: two to three leaves daily taken with food is the dose recommended by herb experts. An infusion (that is, tea) is another way to take feverfew.

Canada's Health Protection Branch recognizes feverfew as a nonprescription drug for preventing migraines and reducing the nausea and vomiting that sometimes accompanies them. In Canada, standardized doses of dried leaves are sold over the counter.

5-HTP

What It Is
5-HTP is among the growing array of do-it-yourself attempts to enhance brain chemistry. This "nutritional neuroscience," as it's been dubbed, includes supplements as well as a variety of dietary strategies that affect the brain

chemicals known as neurotransmitters. Depression, obesity, pain, aggression, insomnia, irritability, addictions, PMS, food cravings, panic disorder, and headaches are some of the problems now linked—with varying degrees of scientific certainty—to abnormalities in serotonin or other chemicals in the brain. Research into this vast subject has yielded drugs such as antidepressants (notably Prozac) and diet drugs (such as Redux, now banned because it caused heart damage).

The brain makes its supplies of neurotransmitters mostly from amino acids, the building blocks of protein, and these enter the brain from the bloodstream. The proteins in foods we eat are broken down into amino acids in the digestive tract; most of these are used elsewhere in the body, but some enter the brain. For example, the amino acid tryptophan is converted into serotonin. The name 5-HTP is short-hand for 5-hydroxytryptophan, a chemical in the body that is a close relative of tryptophan.

▶ How It Works

The body makes 5-HTP from tryptophan; and like tryptophan, 5-HTP is converted to serotonin in the brain. The supplement is derived from the seeds of an African tree.

▶ Health Claims

For decades European doctors have been prescribing 5-HTP to treat depression and insomnia (it is also being used for a wide variety of other ailments). The supplement is also being marketed for weight loss.

What we know. Some small studies suggest that 5-HTP may be as effective as standard antidepressants, but without the side effects of those medications. However, most of these studies were not well designed.

What we don't know. Nutritional neuroscience is only in its infancy. Thus far things remain murky, and there are few, if any, practical applications. Neurotransmitters are affected by many factors besides what foods we eat and what pills we take. Certain nutrients in foods may indeed affect mood, but the results are unpredictable and undoubtedly small. Certain supplements, such as 5-HTP, do seem to influence brain chemicals. But even though they may be "natural" (which is debatable), they can also have serious adverse effects, just like traditional antidepressants, as well as tryptophan or Redux.

For years people took tryptophan pills to treat insomnia and as a mood modifier, with some success. Then in 1989 an outbreak of a rare and incurable blood disease among thousands of people taking tryptophan led the FDA to ban all sales of the pills. At least 38 people died, and most of the other victims have remained crippled with painful nerve damage, severe joint pain, and scarring of internal organs. The epidemic was traced to a bad batch of tryptophan from one Japanese maker, which apparently introduced an impurity when it altered its manufacturing process.

There is still the worry of contamination with 5-HTP, even though its manufacture is very different from that of tryptophan. There have been a few reports, still unconfirmed, of symptoms similar to those caused by the contaminated tryptophan. And indeed researchers have identified one contaminant in 5-HTP. For these reasons, the potential dangers of using 5-HTP outweigh any possible benefits.

▶ Possible Side Effects

Reported side effects are generally mild and include nausea, constipation, gas, and drowsiness.

621

▶ Wellness Recommendation

Because of the possibility of contamination, it's best not to take 5-HTP. But if you do try it, the supplement should not be combined with other antidepressants, whether prescription or "herbal" (such as St. John's wort).

Fish Oil

▶ What It Is

Fish has been seen as a cardiovascular hero ever since it was observed years ago that Eskimos and Japanese people who eat lots of fish have a low rate of heart disease. The theory is that fish oil lowers cholesterol and triglycerides, makes blood less sticky, and perhaps even decreases blood pressure.

Beyond the heart benefits, it's claimed that fish oil can alleviate rheumatoid arthritis, psoriasis, and other auto-immune disorders. Even more health claims are made for fish oil capsules, which take up lots of shelf space in health-food stores and drugstores.

While population studies look at fish consumption, clinical studies almost always use fish oil capsules. It's generally assumed that the capsules provide the same health benefits as the fish itself. However, there may be other beneficial compounds in fish not found in capsules.

▶ How It Works

The fat in fish is rich in polyunsaturated fatty acids called omega-3s, the major marine types being eicosapentenoic acid (EPA) and docosahexenoic acid (DHA). Fatty fish are the richest sources. Like aspirin, these omega-3s make platelets in the blood less likely to stick together and may reduce inflammatory processes in blood vessels. Thus they reduce blood clotting, thereby lessening the chance of a heart attack.

▶ Health Claims

Among the claims are that fish oil lowers risk factors for heart disease, treats diabetes, and alleviates auto-immune disorders.

Cholesterol. According to some studies, fish oil lowers cholesterol, but according to other studies, it doesn't. If you *substitute* fish for meat (or for other sources of saturated fat), you will lower your blood cholesterol. But the same would happen if you replaced the meat with beans or other foods low in saturated fat. Thus, when researchers control for saturated fat intake, the effect of fish on cholesterol often turns out to be minimal, at best.

Triglycerides. Large amounts of fish oil are known to reduce triglycerides, the major type of fat that circulates in the blood. While some scientists believe that even moderately elevated triglycerides are an independent risk factor for heart disease, this is still unclear, as is what level should be considered "high."

High blood pressure. Once again, the studies have had contradictory results. If there is an effect, it would take large doses, and the effect would be small.

Heart disease. Most population studies find some beneficial effect, especially against heart attacks, but the results have been surprisingly inconsistent. Interestingly, some important studies—notably the Harvard Health Professionals Follow-up Study in 1995—have found that fish consumption doesn't reduce the risk of heart disease, but may reduce the risk of *dying* from it. A 1997 study that followed 1,800 men from the Chicago area for 30 years found that those who ate at least eight ounces of fish a week had a 40 percent lower risk of *fatal* heart attack than those who ate no fish (the study didn't look at nonfatal heart attacks).

Some research has also looked at fish's effect on the risk of sudden cardiac death. In 1998 the Physicians Health Study found that men who ate fish at least once a week had a 50 percent lower risk of sudden cardiac death, but at least three studies contradict this.

Much of the debate about fish oil is theoretical, not based on data from clinical studies. Perhaps if fish oil does protect the heart, it may not be by obvious means such as lowering blood cholesterol, triglycerides, or blood pressure. For instance, some studies suggest that omega-3s may be beneficial because they modulate electrical activity in the heart, thus making the heart less susceptible to dangerous, sometimes fatal, rhythm abnormalities.

In addition, in population studies that compare fish eaters to those who eat no fish, it's possible that the people who eat no fish have a less healthy life-style. Researchers adjust the data for such "confounding factors," but can't control for everything.

Diabetes. Some researchers are hopeful about fish oil being helpful in treating diabetes, but studies thus far have not found consistent benefits. In fact, some have shown that fish oil may actually impair blood sugar control in diabetics and perhaps also raise their blood cholesterol.

Rheumatoid arthritis and other inflammatory disorders. This may be where fish holds the most promise, though the research is preliminary. Fish oil may help relieve inflammatory symptoms of these auto-immune diseases by suppressing the immune response. More than a dozen studies have suggested that high doses of fish oil supplements taken long term and *with pain medica-*tion can reduce joint swelling, ease morning stiffness, and lessen fatigue in people with rheumatoid arthritis. There is also some preliminary evidence that fish oil may help reduce the itching and redness of psoriasis, another auto-immune disease.

▶ **Possible Side Effects**

Large doses of fish oil can cause nausea, diarrhea, belching, and a bad taste in the mouth. Also, large doses may suppress certain aspects of the immune system.

▶ **Precautions**

• The decreased ability of your blood to clot has a negative side, notably an increased risk of hemorrhagic stroke. People with bleeding disorders, those taking anticoagulants, or those with uncontrolled hypertension (who are already at high risk for a stroke) should *definitely not* take fish oil capsules.

• Like all fats, omega-3s are concentrated sources of calories: some recommended doses supply 200 calories a day.

• Fish oil in liquid or capsule form may contain pesticides or other contaminants. These are usually removed in the manufacturing process, but there's no guarantee.

• Cod liver oil is overly rich in vitamins A and D, which can be toxic in high doses. There's no reason to take it.

▶ **Wellness Recommendation**

We recommend fish, but not fish oil supplements. One exception: if you have rheumatoid arthritis or psoriasis, fish oil capsules may be worth a try, but consult your doctor. No one knows what is a safe and optimal dose of fish oil.

Fish itself is one of the best foods around.

623

Besides its oil, it is rich in protein, iron, B vitamins, and other nutrients, and it can take the place of meats that are high in saturated fat. Studies finding that fish enhances cardiovascular health suggest that two servings a week are enough. In fact, a higher intake of fish isn't necessarily better for your health.

Garlic

▶ What It Is

Garlic is a member of the onion family—closely related to scallions, leeks, shallots, chives, and onions. The onion family is not nutrient-dense (compared with, say, carrots or beans), but for thousands of years has enhanced the flavor of other foods. During much of that time, garlic has also been valued for its therapeutic potential. It's been used, internally and externally, to treat everything from headaches to tumors.

Today, garlic supplements are very popular, and modern science has taken the curative potential of garlic seriously. There have been hundreds of garlic studies in the past decade alone. But the results of this research have been inconsistent and hard to compare. In spite of heated claims, plus a deluge of advertising, wishful thinking, and misinformation, there's no clear evidence that garlic supplements have any health benefits.

▶ How It Works

The chemical that gives garlic its strong smell is allicin, an unstable compound that's formed only when the clove is bruised, chewed, or crushed. Allicin then breaks down into other sulfur-containing compounds. Some scientists argue that the allicin is what's beneficial in garlic; others think it's irrelevant. Allicin is not present in

cooked garlic or some garlic supplements. Thus, if it's the allicin that's helpful, you may need to eat your garlic raw.

Plain old garlic powder from the supermarket does contain some allicin, and the Center for Science in the Public Interest (CSPI) tested various supplements and ended up suggesting that people consume garlic powder instead of supplements, since the powder is much cheaper, and one-third teaspoon contains as much or more allicin than a range of bestselling supplements. CSPI was assuming, perhaps optimistically, that allicin has the proposed beneficial effects.

However, a study from the University of California at Irvine, published in the *Journal of Agricultural Food Chemistry,* showed that allicin is unlikely to survive in the digestive tract, and that it would be destroyed within minutes in the bloodstream. Thus it's highly improbable that it could reach your cells and accomplish anything. Of course, some compound other than allicin might have beneficial effects, but no one knows.

▶ Health Claims

Garlic promoters make countless claims, but here are four main areas of interest:

Lowers blood cholesterol. Two "meta-analyses," which combined and reanalyzed data from previous studies, seemed to indicate that eating a clove of garlic a day or its equivalent in garlic supplements reduces blood cholesterol by 9 percent in one analysis, and 12 percent in the other. If your blood cholesterol is 300, this could mean a drop to 274 (12 percent).

Yet not only was the quality of these meta-analyses poor, but the studies they used were flawed. Many had no control group, some were small, and most did not take into account other factors, such as fat in the diet, which also affects cholesterol levels. Some used pills, some used real garlic, and some didn't specify. In other studies, not included in the meta-analyses, garlic was found not to affect cholesterol levels at all.

More recently, a study appearing in *Archives of Internal Medicine* used a popular garlic powder tablet (Kwai); another study, in the *Journal of the American Medical Association,* used a garlic-oil preparation. Both involved people with elevated cholesterol levels, were placebo-controlled, and lasted 12 weeks. Neither found any effect on blood cholesterol.

Lowers blood pressure. Once again, studies are flawed and the results contradictory.

Prevents cancer. Some studies have suggested that people who eat garlic regularly reduce their risk of stomach and colon cancer, and possibly breast and prostate cancer as well, and this remains an interesting line of research. But two large, well-designed Dutch studies found no reduction in breast cancer risk among 2,100 women on garlic supplements, and no reduction in lung cancer risk among 3,600 men.

▶ Possible Side Effects

No serious side effects have been reported from taking garlic pills, but high doses can produce heartburn and stomach upset.

▶ Wellness Recommendation

Should you eat raw garlic? Cooked garlic? Take supplements with or without allicin?

In spite of heated claims, there is no clear evidence that garlic in any form has any health benefits. Nor is it known how long would you have to eat the garlic or take the supplements to get any benefits, or what the benefits, if any, would be. Like it or not, the only trustworthy evidence we have is for garlic as a wonderful flavoring agent in food for those who love the taste. If that applies to you, eat all you like.

Ginkgo Biloba

▶ What It Is

Ginkgo biloba is made from the leaves of the hardy ginkgo tree, a native of China that now grows everywhere, particularly in cities. An ancient Chinese herbal medicine, it is widely available in pill form in Western countries and has been actively promoted as a "brain booster" for healthy people. In 1998, a study of ginkgo biloba—as a possible treatment for Alzheimer's disease—was published in the *Journal of the American Medical Association (JAMA).* Ginkgo biloba appeared to help some patients to a limited extent. A cautionary statement from the Alzheimer's Association was all but drowned out. The ensuing fuss centered largely on whether taking the herb could help people remember.

▶ How It Works

Like all plant extracts, ginkgo biloba is full of chemicals—such as flavonoids and terpenoids, some apparently unique and as yet poorly understood. Some are antioxidants, though that does not necessarily mean they prevent disease. Ginkgo biloba bears an incidental resemblance to aspirin, in that it can keep blood clots from forming and may increase blood flow.

▶ Health Claims

This herb has been prescribed in France and Germany for years against vascular disease (circulation disorders) and "cerebral insufficiencies," which can mean anything from absent-mindedness and confusion to dementia. Though it has been studied in Europe, most of the studies have been small, poorly designed, or otherwise flawed.

What we know. Gingko biloba does show promise for some circulatory disorders, such as intermittent claudication (pain in the legs due to obstructed blood flow, which is usually caused by atherosclerosis) and possibly for improving memory in older people with mild dementia.

The *JAMA* study cited above was in reality not all that exciting. It was a yearlong trial of an extract of ginkgo biloba that began with more than 300 patients. All had been diagnosed with mild to moderate dementia—80 percent met the criteria for Alzheimer's. The dropout rate was high: only 137 of these people made it to the end. Some did not follow the treatment or thought it wasn't working, some were removed by their caregivers, and a few died. Improvements in mental function and behavior among those taking ginkgo biloba were small and of limited duration. About a third actually got worse.

Zaven Khachaturian, director of the Ronald and Nancy Reagan Alzheimer's Research Institute, called the study encouraging but cautioned against false hopes. He pointed out another problem: "Commercially available ginkgo products may not contain the same preparation of herbs as was used in this study, so there is no way to predict the effects, positive or negative."

Interestingly, tacrine, a not-very-successful prescription drug for Alzheimer's, has similar limited effects. It was approved by the FDA not because it's a cure or even a very effective treatment, but because it might help a few people temporarily. Tacrine can have side effects and is also much more expensive than ginkgo biloba. But at least tacrine has been extensively studied and standardized.

What we don't know. Many questions remain

unanswered about gingko biloba—how effective it is against one disorder or another, how long it should be used, what the proper dosage is. German and French doctors have never claimed miraculous powers for it.

There was no indication at all in the *JAMA* study that ginkgo biloba could be a "brain booster" for healthy people not suffering from dementia. That has hardly slowed down purveyors of ginkgo biloba, who did not need a study in the first place. Their products, unregulated and untested, are already everywhere, aimed not at Alzheimer's patients but at the general public—claiming that the herb sharpens mental focus, improves memory and concentration, and promotes circulation to the brain.

▶ **Possible Side Effects**

No serious side effects have been reported, except for two cases of bleeding after long-term use. But it's logical that ginkgo biloba might well interact with blood-thinning medications, such as aspirin and warfarin (Coumadin), to increase the risk of internal bleeding.

▶ **Wellness Recommendation**

If you're caring for an Alzheimer's patient, don't experiment with any kind of medication, herbal or otherwise, without professional advice.

If you're thinking of "crisping" your own mental powers, nobody knows whether ginkgo biloba would help or not (or even whether there is any ginkgo biloba in what's on the market).

Ginseng

▶ **What It Is**

Ginseng *(Panax)* has been used medicinally for

thousands of years. *Panax ginseng,* or Asian ginseng, is the most widely used form of the herb (and also the most extensively studied), but other forms are also available. In the United States alone, sales of ginseng run into hundreds of millions of dollars annually. One well-known Web site has advertised ginseng to treat 12 different ailments, from the common cold to HIV infection and Alzheimer's disease. Fruit shake bars all over the country will add ginseng to your smoothie. Deli refrigerators are full of ginseng-enriched teas and other soft drinks. Kids too young to buy beer can purchase ginseng elixirs laced with alcohol at convenience stores.

Thousands of books and papers on ginseng have been published, yet scientists are still largely in the dark about the medicinal benefits of ginseng.

▶ How It Works

The chemical properties have been studied thoroughly. The plant's active ingredients are called ginsenosides (among other terms), and 13 different types are known. But like most plants, ginseng contains many other compounds, too—volatile oils, sugar, fats, B vitamins, minerals, plant hormones, and a range of other active substances. It's not so simple to figure out which of these elements are the important ones.

What's actually in any product labeled ginseng depends on at least two things: first, what part of the plant it came from—leaves, roots, or stems, all of which have different chemical compounds—and second, which type of ginseng it is, since they have different biological properties. Asian ginseng, which is grown all over Asia, is also called Korean ginseng and other names as well. American ginseng *(Panax quinquefolius)* is on the endangered species list here, so intensively has it been cultivated and harvested as a cash crop.

A third type, Siberian ginseng *(Eleutherococcus senticosus),* contains still other chemicals and is not regarded as a true ginseng. In addition, ginseng comes in two general types, red and white, depending on how it was processed.

▶ Health Claims

Various researchers have claimed that ginseng boosts energy and athletic performance; that it prevents or reduces the risk of all kinds of cancer; that it fights emotional stress, enhances memory, boosts immunity, reduces blood sugar in diabetics, and promotes sexual potency and desire. It's often referred to as an "adaptogen," with claims that it promotes health, energy, and a sense of well-being, like the tonics of yore. But this is a meaningless term.

Since most studies have been of poor quality, we still don't know if ginseng works or how to use it. "Most of the literature in this area," according to Dr. Varro Tyler, the leading American expert on herbs and plant-based medicine, "is based more on superstition and subjective opinion than on objective, scientific evidence."

What we know. The few well-designed studies on the subject have not borne out claims that ginseng boosts athletic performance or energy. (You won't find this out from manufacturers' Web sites or catalogues.) Among other research, a well-designed study of 36 healthy men, published in the *Journal of the American Dietetic Association* in 1997, found that ginseng did not improve physical performance. There's preliminary evidence suggesting that the plant may help people with diabetes, but studies with purified extracts of ginseng have not found a benefit for them.

What we don't know. Obtaining authentic ginseng in standardized doses is difficult, and many studies do not specify what they used. The best

627

grades of ginseng are very expensive. And the herb is easily contaminated with other plant substances that may affect the outcome of trials.

That's also the problem with ginseng in the marketplace: a complete lack of quality control. You may pay for ginseng and not get any. Dr. Tyler has reported that of 54 commercial ginseng products analyzed by independent researchers, 60 percent contained little ginseng, and 25 percent had none at all.

Other studies have found that commercial ginseng products vary widely in the specific ginsenosides they contain, and some have none. As reported in *The Lancet* in 1994, one so-called ginseng product, sold by National Health Products in this country, actually contained ephedrine instead of ginseng. The Swedish athlete who used it ended up testing positive for "doping."

▶ Wellness Recommendation

There is no consistent evidence to support the use of ginseng. A thorough review in the *European Journal of Clinical Pharmacology* came to this conclusion, and called for more rigorous investigations with real, standardized ginseng. The herb contains many active ingredients, and it's hard to know which of these elements are important. And what's actually in any product labeled ginseng can vary greatly—some products contain no ginseng at all.

Glucosamine

▶ What It Is

Taken with another supplement, chondroitin sulfate, glucosamine has become a popular "cure" for osteoarthritis, the most common form of arthritis (see page 392).

▶ How It Works

Both glucosamine and chondroitin sulfate occur in the body and are vital to cartilage formation. It's the wearing down of cartilage that causes arthritis pain, which is why it has been easy for advertisers to convince people that swallowing these substances could help. But though glucosamine and chondroitin sulfate are marketed as "natural," the term is meaningless. The compounds are highly processed—extracted from crustacean shells and other animal by-products.

▶ Health Claims

A best-selling book has claimed that glucosamine and chondroitin sulfate cure osteoarthritis. There's an avalanche of other hype about them in the marketplace, too, so people in chronic pain can hardly be blamed for trying these supplements.

What we know. A few lab studies have shown that glucosamine stimulates the growth of cartilage and/or keeps it from degrading. Some studies have also shown that glucosamine relieves the pain and stiffness of osteoarthritis as effectively as aspirin or ibuprofen. But most studies have been short, and many have had flaws (for example, osteoarthritis was not always properly diagnosed). A more persuasive study, reported in 2001 in *The Lancet*, found that people with mild-to-moderate knee arthritis who took 1,500 milligrams of glucosamine daily for three years had 20 to 25 percent less pain and disability than those who took a placebo. The glucosamine group overall also showed less deterioration of cartilage.

What we don't know. There is still little known about the safety and effectiveness of glucosamine and chondroitin sulfate over the long term. Also, there is no evidence that the chondroitin you swallow is absorbed. More studies are underway. The Arthritis Foundation has called for further study, as has the American Academy of Orthopedic Surgeons. The National Institutes for Health is undertaking a long-term study that will answer the outstanding questions.

▶ Possible Side Effects

Reported side effects include headaches, abdominal pain, nausea, itching, and fatigue.

▶ Precautions

An earlier article in *The Lancet* pointed out that glucosamine, even in very low doses, can have adverse effects on blood sugar levels, possibly increasing insulin resistance. Many people with osteoarthritis are older and overweight, and have diabetes or are at risk for it. It's not known that the supplements actually harm people with diabetes or bring on diabetes, but they might.

▶ Wellness Recommendation

As an adjunct to proven treatments, glucosamine and chondroitin might help, and would probably do no harm. It takes about four weeks for the supplements' effects to be felt.

If you want to try them, let your physician know, particularly if you have diabetes. Also, remember that there is no standardization, and no guarantee you're getting what the labels say. Pregnant women should avoid these supplements.

Goldenseal

▶ What It Is

Goldenseal, a perennial plant with a yellow flower related to the buttercup, is one of the oldest herbal medicines. Varro Tyler, the American herb expert, calls goldenseal a "drug" and notes that it was a favorite remedy of the Cherokees, which then passed into wide use in patent medicines, such as "Dr. Pierce's Golden Medical Discovery." Folk herbalists in Indiana, he says, continue to recommend it as a remedy for cracked lips and canker sores.

▶ How It Works

The active ingredients in goldenseal, unlike those in many traditional folk remedies, have been identified—hydrastine and berberine. The latter is known to have effects against diarrhea.

▶ Health Claims

In addition to its antidiarrheal effects, goldenseal is also known as a cold remedy and a weak antiseptic, traditionally used as a wash to ease minor irritations of the mouth, lips, and eyes. It has also been promoted in health-food stores to "flush out" such drugs as marijuana, cocaine, and heroin, and thus prevent their detection in a urine test. Fortunately or unfortunately, this is wishful thinking.

What we know. As reported in the *Archives of Family Medicine*, two small clinical trials have shown berberine to be effective against diarrhea caused by such agents as *E. coli*, *Vibrio*, and *Giardia*. But there are drugs that work as well—and doctors don't often recommend goldenseal because of its unpredictable action and potential side effects.

What we don't know. While the pharmacology of the plant is understood, few clinical studies have been done. There is no scientific evidence for its use as an antiseptic.

▶ Possible Side Effects

According to the reference book *Herbal Medicines*, by three British herb experts, "excessive use of goldenseal should be avoided." This is because potential side effects include stomach upset, ner-

629

vous symptoms, depression, and (in large enough quantities) even death from respiratory failure.

▶ Precautions

Pregnant and nursing women should avoid goldenseal; so should children, as well as anyone with elevated blood pressure, heart disease, epilepsy, or blood clotting problems.

▶ Wellness Recommendation

We would caution against any use of goldenseal, since it is impossible in this country to get products with standardized doses. The product you buy may have little or no berberine or hydrastine—or a huge dose.

Grape Seed Extract

▶ What It Is

Marketers of this dietary supplement claim that it alleviates a host of problems and diseases, from cancer, arthritis, and diabetes to varicose veins and macular degeneration. There's no evidence it is effective against any of these disorders. It does, however, contain interesting compounds, which are being seriously studied and may have a bright future as more knowledge emerges.

▶ How It Works

What's special about grape seed extract is its high level of certain flavonoids, notably proanthocyanidins, also called procyanidins. These compounds are also found in green tea, red wine, and pine bark (the last is marketed as pycnogenol).

Test tube and animal studies have found that the special flavonoids in grape seed extract are potent antioxidants. There's very preliminary evidence that these compounds may help maintain

connective tissue (as in tendons, ligaments, and cartilage) and affect vascular disorders.

▶ Health Claims

Marketers claim that it treats everything from cancer, arthritis, and diabetes to varicose veins and macular degeneration. *However, scientists still understand little about the exact effects of these (and other) plant chemicals in the human body.* They don't know which grape species should be used or what doses taken.

▶ Wellness Recommendation

We cannot recommend that you take grape seed extract at this point. We can wholeheartedly recommend that you eat grapes, berries, and other fruits and vegetables rich in flavonoids and other phytochemicals. And drink tea, wine (in moderation), and grape juice, if you like them.

Guggulipid

▶ What It Is

Guggul is a gummy resin that oozes from a tree *(Commiphora mukul)* that grows in India. Used for centuries as a treatment for obesity, gout, and other disorders, an extract called guggulipid is approved as a cholesterol-lowering drug in India.

▶ How It Works

One component of guggulipid is guggulsterones, probably the active ingredient for lowering blood cholesterol. Similar plant extracts are known to have an effect on blood cholesterol—for example, the pine extracts in Benecol and the soy extracts in Take Control, two margarines allowed to make cholesterol-lowering claims.

▶ Health Claims

Guggulipid has had some promising results in lowering blood cholesterol. One good study conducted in India in 1994 showed that daily doses of 100 milligrams of guggulipid effectively reduced LDL ("bad") cholesterol and triglycerides. A clinical trial has been underway at the University of Pennsylvania

▶ Possible Side Effects

These include excessive menstrual bleeding. Digestive disorders, such as nausea, vomiting, and diarrhea, have also been reported.

▶ Precautions

Pregnant women and people with thyroid disorders, as well as those on medications such as calcium channel blockers, should not take guggulipid, nor should women with menstrual problems.

▶ Wellness Recommendation

If your cholesterol is high, you need medical advice and monitoring in order to lower it. The first line of defense is a diet low in saturated fat and cholesterol, plus regular exercise, and weight loss if necessary. Talk with your doctor about whether you also need medication. The recommended drugs at present are "statin" drugs (see page 203).

If you want to try guggulipid, be sure your physician knows about it and monitors its effects. As with most supplements in this country, you'll have no guarantee that what you buy is standardized—thus dosage is difficult to determine.

Melatonin

▶ What It Is

Discovered about 40 years ago, melatonin is a human hormone produced deep in the brain by the pineal gland, dubbed "the seat of the soul" by philosophers in ages past. Humans secrete melatonin throughout their lives, and while some have theorized that melatonin production declines with age, recent evidence indicates that melatonin levels may vary naturally in different groups; age, however, does not seem to be the factor. Different people have different levels, and levels vary according to time of day.

▶ How It Works

Melatonin has been called the "darkness" hormone. Production rises at night and falls by day. The hormone affects our internal body clock and sleep cycles, and one of its main functions is to help regulate cycles of sleep and wakefulness.

▶ Health Claims

Melatonin has been assumed, logically enough, to have some use as a sleeping aid. But in recent years, it has been marketed as a treatment for a variety of health concerns. Look on any Web site selling supplements or in any health-food catalogue, and you'll find melatonin recommended for jet lag, arthritis, stress, alcoholism, migraine, and the signs and symptoms of aging and menopause—along with assertions that it staves off heart disease and cancer. Some people recommend "melatonin replacement therapy" for all postmenopausal women.

What we know. Some research suggests that melatonin helps some people fall asleep faster, but it may not help them stay asleep. Like benzodiazepines (such as Valium or Halcion), often prescribed as sleeping pills, melatonin can produce a "hangover" and drowsiness the next day.

What we don't know. Long-term safety is still a question. It's true, as one researcher puts it, that

631

"no catastrophes have been related to its use" (such as the outbreak of severe illness caused by a similar "natural" substance, tryptophan, once sold as a sleeping pill). Melatonin is being heavily marketed as a sleeping pill, particularly for older people, but nobody knows if the products are pure or if the dosages listed on labels are accurate (or what dosages should be recommended, for that matter). Good clinical trials have never been done on melatonin treatment for insomnia.

As for jet lag, the benefits have never been clear. Various dosages of melatonin have been used in studies, making comparisons difficult. "Jet lag" itself is hard to measure. As reported recently in the *American Journal of Psychiatry*, a team of researchers devised a scale for measuring symptoms, and a group of Norwegian physicians flying between Oslo and New York were recruited as subjects. Melatonin showed no benefit against jet lag. It's possible that light exposure is more effective than melatonin (see page 359). Or maybe light works with the pills. Nobody knows.

A recent review of studies by researchers at Louisiana State University confirms that melatonin is indeed a powerful antioxidant, and so might offer protection against aging and chronic disease. But nobody knows what this means. Until we learn more, "the full potential benefits of melatonin must remain something of a mystery," these researchers concluded.

▶ Possible Side Effects

In addition to next-day drowsiness, other reported side effects include headache and stomach upset.

▶ Precautions

Adverse drug reactions have been reported in people taking common antidepressants (including SSRIs or MAO inhibitors) or steroid or sedative drugs. Melatonin can interact with other hormones, which is why, in part, pregnant women and children should never take it.

▶ Wellness Recommendation

If you are taking, or thinking of taking, melatonin, talk to a physician. Hormones are powerful substances that, even in small doses, can produce unexpected and unwanted results.

If you need a sleeping pill, your doctor can advise you. No known sleeping pill has proven safe and effective for more than short-term use.

Don't assume that because you are aging, your melatonin levels are declining and so need to be supplemented. If your body already produces enough melatonin, taking additional doses may not be advisable. No one knows what the long-term effect might be, but chronic use of melatonin supplements may suppress the body's own production of the hormone. It's also difficult to determine what "enough" is. Moreover, such drugs as aspirin, beta blockers, and tranquilizers can affect melatonin levels.

SAM-e

▶ What It Is

SAM-e has become one of the hottest supplements on the market. Not an herb, hormone, vitamin, or any kind of nutrient, SAM-e is a stabilized, synthetic form of S-adenosylmethionine (SAM), a chemical produced naturally in all animals. In supplement form, SAM-e is very expensive. A daily dose can cost anywhere from $2.50 to $18. You have to take it over the long term to get any results, it's said. All this is wonderful for the seller, but may be less so for you.

▶ How It Works

In the human body, SAM-e is known to be essential to at least 35 biochemical processes, including maintaining the structure of cell membranes and manufacturing substances vital to transmitting nerve impulses and influencing moods.

▶ Health Claims

SAM-e is said to be an effective, indeed magical, but also "natural" treatment for depression, arthritis, and liver disease, among other things.

What we know. Regardless of the hype, there may actually be something to the claims—or maybe there will be some day. Unlike much of what's on the market, SAM-e has been the subject of some scientific research. First tested as a treatment for schizophrenia, it proved ineffective. But in the 1970s some clinical trials in Italy, Germany, and other European countries did suggest that SAM-e might be an effective treatment for depression, with fewer side effects than antidepressant drugs.

Some research has shown that SAM-e provides relief from arthritis pain, without the stomach irritation caused by aspirin and similar drugs. And there are other possibilities, too. For instance, SAM-e may aid in joint repair. The possibilities are encouraging. Most studies so far have been small and brief (and some have used large intravenous doses), but since SAM is so important to life, SAM-e might have uses as a drug.

Contrary to rumor, SAM-e will not repair the liver damage caused by heavy drinking.

What we don't know. The problem is threefold: first of all, the possible benefits and risks of SAM-e remain unclear. In Europe it is sold as a prescription drug for arthritis, depression, and liver disease. At least that means a doctor is overseeing the treatment. Here, where SAM-e can be bought as easily as a multivitamin, people can simply dose themselves—which may be unwise when so much remains to be discovered.

Secondly, its promoters say SAM-e has no side effects, but anything that works like a drug has side effects of some kind, and may interact with medications or foods.

But the most important potential problem: SAM-e is converted into homocysteine in the body. High levels of homocysteine may raise the risk of heart disease. SAM-e is likely to promote higher levels, though no one knows how high.

Marketers of SAM-e generally say a "dose" is 400 milligrams daily, but there's no way to find a standardized dose in the current unregulated market. In addition, raw SAM-e is said to degrade quickly unless stored at proper temperatures, and you have no guarantee that the pills you buy have been properly handled.

▶ Possible Side Effects

Side effects have been reported, including stomach upset and other gastrointestinal problems.

▶ Wellness Recommendation

The real benefits and risks of SAM-e are still unclear. For healthy people, SAM-e has no value. Don't take it as a tonic or mood booster. It does not prevent any known disorder.

If you are suffering from depression, seek medical advice before trying this supplement. Depression is a treatable illness, requiring professional care. Don't try it on your own or combine it with antidepressant drugs. For those with bipolar disorder (manic depression), SAM-e may have unpredictable adverse effects.

If you have joint pain, talk to your doctor before taking SAM-e. Make sure it's actually arthritis that's causing the pain. Don't give up conven-

633

tional treatments in favor of SAM-e without at least telling your doctor of your decision.

If you do decide to try SAM-e, make certain your diet is rich in fruits and vegetables, and take a multivitamin. A high intake of three B vitamins (folic acid, B_6, and B_{12}) can lower homocysteine levels, in case SAM-e raises them.

Saw Palmetto

▶ What It Is

Phytotherapy (plant-derived substances used as drugs) for prostate problems is widely used in Europe and has attracted interest in the United States. Saw palmetto, derived from berries of the saw palm tree (*Serenoa repens, Serenoa serrulata,* and other species) is one such therapy that has become popular for treating symptoms of benign prostatic hyperplasia, or BPH (see page 178). This enlargement of the prostate is common in men over 40; half of all men over 60 have it to some degree.

▶ How It Works

Saw palmetto contains certain phytosterols, substances that seem to curb prostate cell growth. Its action in the body is probably similar to that of finasteride (Proscar) and other prescription drugs that are the first line of treatment for BPH. (Saw palmetto is much less expensive than the conventional drugs: a 90-day supply of finasteride costs about $200, compared with $10 to $50 for a 90-day supply of saw palmetto.)

▶ Health Claims

The chief claim for saw palmetto is that it shrinks the prostate, and may reduce symptoms of benign prostatic hyperplasia, such as more urgent and/or frequent urination or urinary leaking. But the evidence is pretty sparse.

What we know. A study in the *Journal of the American Medical Association* reviewed 18 clinical trials of saw palmetto, none of them first rate. For example, some were brief or small or limited in other ways. Only two used standardized doses. But they were deemed worthy of notice by these researchers. Compared with a placebo (a sham treatment), saw palmetto improved urinary tract symptoms, including nighttime urination, by about 25 percent. Men taking saw palmetto were twice as likely to report improvements as those taking a placebo. In Germany, other research studies have tended to support the effectiveness of saw palmetto.

However, another study of saw palmetto (supported by a supplement manufacturer and conducted at the University of Chicago Medical School) was not in any sense a scientific investigation, but a kind of loose "trial run" with 46 men and no control group. The researchers admitted that they hadn't proved anything, and that if their patients had improvements in urinary tract symptoms, which was questionable, it might simply have been a placebo effect.

What we don't know. There is still a lack of real scientific information based on well-designed clinical trials of saw palmetto. But clinical trials are enormously expensive and not likely to be conducted for a product that cannot be patented.

▶ Possible Side Effects

Fewer side effects (such as erectile dysfunction) are reported with saw palmetto than with drugs, at least in studies so far. Not much is known about the long-term effects of saw palmetto.

▶ Wellness Recommendation

If you want to try saw palmetto, do so only after seeing a doctor. You should not rely on a self-diagnosis of BPH; urinary symptoms may be caused by something more serious than BPH that needs immediate treatment.

Be aware that herbal remedies are not regulated or standardized: you may be getting what the label says, or you may not.

If you are taking saw palmetto or any other over-the-counter treatments, tell your doctor in advance of taking a PSA test, the screening test for prostate cancer (see page 80). Any drug, herbal or prescription, for BPH may alter the results of a PSA test and thus make prostate cancer more difficult to diagnose.

St. John's Wort

▶ What It Is

The yellow flowers of a plain old weed called St. John's wort (Latin name, *Hypericum perforatum*) have for centuries been used in teas and other preparations as a treatment for nervous disorders, and indeed for everything from anxiety and inflammation to insomnia and stomach ache. "Wort" comes from the Old English word for "plant," and this particular wort was named for St. John the Baptist, probably because the plant blooms around June 24, celebrated as the saint's birthday. St. John's wort is native to Europe but now grows throughout the United States and Canada. Unlike many herbal remedies, St. John's wort has been extensively studied; AIDS researchers, for example, are currently investigating it for antiviral activity.

Particularly in Germany, St. John's wort has long been used as an antidepressant. German physicians prescribed 66 million daily doses in tablet or capsule form in one year alone. In Germany, as in the United States and Canada, St. John's wort is sold over the counter. Books and articles, as well as word of mouth, have made it famous as a do-it-yourself antidepressant.

Currently, the most widely used prescription antidepressants include Prozac and the other so-called SSRIs—selective serotonin re-uptake inhibitors—as well as drugs that affect other brain chemicals. (Serotonin is the brain chemical that produces a "happy" feeling, and SSRIs help regulate serotonin.) But more than half the people taking such drugs experience side effects, sometimes severe ones. St. John's wort, according to some reports, may work as well as Prozac, at least for milder forms of depression, without serious side effects. Better treatments for depression would certainly be welcome.

635

▶ How It Works

Scientists aren't sure exactly how the herb works, but it is believed increase levels of serotonin. Like a prescription antidepressant, the herb must build up in your bloodstream over days or even weeks to have an effect.

▶ Health Claims

There has been no shortage of studies on St. John's wort, which have appeared in such respected publications as the *British Medical Journal* and *Journal of Geriatric Psychiatry and Neurology*. However, the evidence remains shaky.

What we know. A study in the *British Medical Journal* re-analyzed 23 studies of varying quality. In the studies that looked at an extract of St. John's wort standardized for hypericin (one of its active ingredients) versus a placebo (an inactive substance), half the patients on St. John's wort improved, as opposed to 22 percent on the placebo. In three studies comparing St. John's wort to standard antidepressants, it was somewhat more effective than the drugs. None of the studies lasted more than six weeks—not long enough to determine the duration of the effects or to detect any long-term side effects.

Commission E of the German Federal Health Agency, which oversees herbal remedies in that country, says the plant is not toxic. The Council of Europe lists the herb as a source of natural food flavoring, but limits the amount allowed.

What we don't know. There was no evidence that St. John's wort worked against serious, as opposed to mild, depression. In short, some results have been promising, but we still know fairly little as to whether the herb really works and, if so, how. The National Institutes of Health in this country has undertaken a large study of St. John's wort.

▶ Possible Side Effects

Minor side effects include gastrointestinal discomfort, fatigue, dry mouth, and dizziness. In addition, several recent studies have pointed out dangerous interactions between St. John's wort and other medications (see below).

▶ Precautions

St. John's wort contains at least ten compounds that can have pharmacological action. Consequently, a number of interactions with other medications have been observed. However, since the compounds in St. John's wort are not standardized, and people take such as wide range of dosages, the interactions are often unpredictable.

• The herb can reduce blood levels of an important HIV drug (indivir) by more than half. As a result, the body may clear the drug before it has

time to work fully. St. John's wort may also affect other HIV drugs that are similarly metabolized by the body.

• It reduces the effect of the anticoagulant warfarin (Coumadin) and of the heart drug digoxin.

• It reduces the effect of cyclosporin, which helps prevent organ rejection in people given transplants.

• If you are taking birth control pills, talk to your doctor if you want to take St. John's wort, since it can interact with some oral contraceptives (OCs) to cause breakthrough menstrual bleeding and may also reduce the effectiveness of OCs in preventing pregnancy.

• Older people taking prescription antidepressants (such as Prozac) and St. John's wort have suffered dizziness, confusion, anxiety, and headaches, according to one study. The elderly are particularly susceptible to this reaction, the symptoms of which are often misdiagnosed as worsening psychiatric symptoms or a neurologic disorder. But younger people also should not combine the herb with conventional antidepressants.

• Livestock that feed on the plant have developed sun sensitivity in the skin and eyes (it's unknown if this would occur in humans). If you are very sensitive to the sun or are taking the antibiotic tetracycline (which produces photosensitivity), you might be wise to avoid St. John's wort, or at least to discontinue it if such symptoms occur.

• Pregnant and lactating women should also avoid it.

• If you take St. John's wort and are going to receive anesthesia, make sure your anesthesiologist knows. The herb can intensify or prolong the effect of some anesthetic agents.

▶ Wellness Recommendation

Because St. John's wort has been extensively used in Europe, we see no reason not to try it for mild to moderate depression. But don't use it along with conventional antidepressants or if you are taking any of the other medications referred to previously because of a potential for adverse reactions. And don't make your own diagnosis. Instead, see a doctor or therapist, and at least let him/her know if you decide to try St. John's wort.

Valerian

▶ What It Is

Valerian, a popular herbal sleeping pill today, was known as a medicinal plant in Roman times. The dried roots of this plant *(Valerianae radix,* also known as heliotrope) can be brewed for tea, and valerian root is also sold as a tincture (combined with a small amount of alcohol), in tablets, and as capsules. Some people add it to bath water and apply it to their skin.

▶ How It Works

Nobody has yet discovered what element in the plant might produce the sedative effects, if any. Some component of valerian may have an action on the brain similar to that of tranquilizers like Valium or Halcion—but a milder effect less likely to produce habituation or dependency.

▶ Health Claims

Valerian is promoted as a "natural" sleep aid, inducing slumber without the unpleasant side effects of conventional drugs.

What we know. In some experiments, a dose of valerian before retiring seems to reduce the time it takes to fall asleep. But it has yet to be shown in a well-designed trial that, once you fall asleep, valerian improves the quality of sleep. Valerian has proven toxic in one animal study.

Dr. Varro Tyler, the American herbal expert, regards it as a "mild tranquilizer." Commission E, the agency that officially evaluates herbal remedies in Germany, regards valerian as safe and effective for treating "restlessness and sleeping disorders brought on by nervous conditions."

What we don't know. The U.S. Pharmacopeial Convention says there is inadequate scientific evidence to support valerian's use, though it recognizes its long history and calls for further research. No method has been developed for standardizing dosages of the herb.

▶ Possible Side Effects

Valerian can produce such side effects as headaches, palpitations, and nausea.

▶ Precautions

Pregnant and nursing women and children should avoid valerian. It's not a good idea to combine it with alcohol, tranquilizers, or barbiturates.

▶ Wellness Recommendation

If you suffer from severe insomnia, consider getting medical advice. If you want to try valerian, remember that it's unregulated and unstandardized, so the preparation you buy may supply more or fewer milligrams of valerian than it promises, or none at all. The tea or baths, by the way, are unlikely to have much effect. In any case, don't use valerian for more than two weeks.

637

Appendix

FOR MORE INFORMATION

Getting medical information once required either a trip to the library or contacting one of hundreds of organizations directly by phone or by mail. But millions of Americans now seek health and medical information online, and millions more join them every year. Most of them are venturing onto the Internet before seeing a doctor.

Like other forms of communication, the Internet has accomplished much and has enormous potential for good. It educates both doctors and the public and will surely become a powerful force for improving health care. But on almost any given medical topic, you will find hundreds of Web sites, and locating the most reliable and appropriate ones is challenging. How can you tell the experts from the misinformed, the charlatans, or the simply deluded? Many sites do not have recognized or reputable authorities standing behind the information they distribute—and many are in the business of selling products rather than increasing your understanding of a particular ailment.

Setting up a Web site is easy and cheap—anybody can sell anything or claim anything. There is no peer review, no guarantee that what you're reading is accurate and/or up-to-date. The Federal Trade Commission (FTC) has attempted to challenge some of the hundreds of Web sites that sell products of dubious value and push phony cures for everything from cancer to AIDS. The agency can force the sites to stop making claims, but it cannot shut them down or prevent them from doing business. As one company cleans up

its act, five more making unproven claims may spring up. For example, one "Pain Care Center" selling a fatty acid it claimed would cure arthritis and other disorders shut itself down before the FTC could even take it to court—not because the owners feared government action but because competitors making similar claims put it out of business.

THE POTENTIAL FOR CONFUSION

Even Web sites that aren't out to sell anything may contain inaccurate and even harmful information. Researchers writing for an issue of *Cancer,* published by the American Cancer Society, decided to test the Internet as a source of information about Ewing sarcoma, a rare tumor usually diagnosed in children. (They chose Ewing sarcoma because the number of sites was manageable, as opposed to more common cancers.) Using various search engines, they chose 400 Web site addresses, which led them to a huge welter of information, misinformation, and misleading statements. For example, the survival rate for Ewing sarcoma was reported to be anywhere from 5 percent to 85 percent. (It's actually thought to be 70 to 75 percent.) The researchers were concerned about the devastating effects misinformation might have on vulnerable patients, as well as the wedge it might drive between patients and doctors. They also found that locating the sites was "cumbersome and time-consuming." Many led only to dead ends.

Their conclusion was that it is vital for doctors to "maintain an open mind" about searches done by patients, and to take an active role in identifying and creating accurate Web sites. They also recommended that Internet skills be part of every physician's postgraduate education.

EVALUATING AND USING ONLINE INFORMATION

Here are tips to follow if you are using the Internet for researching your own (or your family's) health and medical concerns.

• *Don't rely solely on the Internet.* If you've been diagnosed with an illness and want more information, the Internet is a fine place to start. But share your findings with your health-care provider. Use the information as a basis for questions. Check a standard reference book.

• *Consider the authority of the source.* Reliable information is most likely to come from government organizations, major medical centers and university hospitals, professional associations, and major nonprofit organizations. On any site you turn to, experts should be identified by name, and their credentials and institutional affiliations clearly displayed.

• *Look for references.* Solidly based factual information will be accompanied by references to published reports in leading medical journals or from established organizations. An absence of references could mean that the "information" is based on opinion or anecdote, or is someone's personal interpretation of medical research. Be wary of testimonials; anybody can make up a story. And even true anecdotes don't constitute research.

• *Be suspicious of "medicalese."* Don't be taken in by text that disguises a lack of real information, that contains long lists of irrelevant articles from unheard-of journals, or that is built around words like "breakthrough," "secret ingredient," "miracle cure," "ancient remedy." Mysterious charts and scientific words like "ions" or "antioxidant" may or may not mean something.

• *Don't use the Web as your doctor.* Some Internet doctors offer online consultations, though it's very hard to know if their credentials are genuine. Use them as a source of information, if you wish, but don't accept a diagnosis from a doctor you have not seen personally and who does not have your medical records. Also, if you buy medications online, your own physician should do the prescribing, not some cyber-pharmacist—and there are many—who may be prescribing potentially dangerous drugs without ever seeing the patient. (And don't assume that you are getting bargain prices on-line. Some sites charge more than real drugstores.)

• *Pharmaceutical companies often have good sites.* Their sites are especially good at supplying full information about the drugs they sell and the conditions those drugs are meant to treat. But they won't tell you about similar drugs that are cheaper and may be just as effective.

• *Don't trust products claiming to cure everything—or the sites that sell them.* Likewise, pass up cyber-salesmen who claim that the government, medical profession, and scientific mainstream are in cahoots to suppress their products, or that doctors don't really want to cure cancer, heart disease, the common cold, and so forth.

RELIABLE SOURCES

For this book, more than 60 organizations and groups have been selected for a directory of providers of additional prevention and self-care information. This directory is intended to help provide background information. *If you have a specific medical problem, especially a serious one, you should consult a physician.*

The organizations listed offer a number of services, from providing online content to sending out literature on a specific ailment to making referrals to other information sources and to local physicians, hospitals, or support groups. Most of the organizations have toll-free phone numbers as well as Web sites and e-mail addresses. Many also have staff members available during normal working hours to assist you. Some of the government organizations will perform a computerized search of the latest medical studies and reports on a particular topic and send you the results. There is generally no charge for this information. Several federal government agencies also offer a 24-hour "fax-on-command" service that allows information to be sent to a fax number that you specify.

GOVERNMENT AGENCIES

Government agencies are primarily interested in disseminating information. The content they offer is consistently thorough, well reviewed, and objective. Many government sites also provide direct links to other reputable sites. The Department of Health and Human Services is the cabinet-level department of the federal government concerned with health and wellness. It accomplishes this through a number of divisions. Three of these are especially helpful to health consumers.

The Centers for Disease Control and Prevention (CDC)

1600 Clifton Road, NE
Atlanta, GA 30333
Switchboard: 404-639-3311
Office of Communications: 404-639-3286
Voice and Fax Information System: 888-232-3228
To send a fax: 888-237-3299
National Prevention Information Network (for AIDS, STDs, and TB): 800-458-5231
STD & AIDS Hotline: 800-342-2437
Office on Smoking and Health: 800-232-1311
Internet home page: www.cdc.gov

The Centers for Disease Control and Prevention is the federal agency charged with protecting the public health by providing leadership and direction in the prevention and control of communicable diseases and other preventable conditions and health emergencies. It develops and implements programs in chronic-disease prevention and control and programs to deal with environmental health problems, including responding to environmental, chemical, and radiation emergencies.

The Office of Communications responds to questions from the public on research conducted by the CDC in the areas of environmental health, infectious diseases, health promotion and education, prevention services, and occupational safety and health. Specific inquiries for assistance may also be referred to the appropriate CDC division or other federal, state, or private institutions.

Following are some of the CDC's major divisions. You can gain access to them through the CDC's Internet home page.

• *The National Center for Chronic Disease Prevention and Health Promotion* seeks to educate the public on the prevention of chronic disease and illness. It is the department most concerned with healthy lifestyle and wellness issues.

• *The National Center for Environmental Health* is primarily concerned with noninfectious, nonoccupational, and environmental illness, such as allergies and asthma.

• *The National Center for Infectious Diseases* maintains programs for preventing illness and death caused by infectious diseases in the United States and around the world.

• *The National Center for HIV, STD, and TB Prevention* provides information and recommendations for preventing and controlling human immunodeficiency virus (HIV) infection, sexually transmitted diseases (STDs) and tuberculosis (TB).

• **The National Center for Injury Prevention and Control** helps prevent death and disability from nonoccupational injuries, including those that are intentional and those that result from violence.

• **The National Institute for Occupational Safety and Health** is the primary federal agency engaged in research to eliminate on-the-job hazards to health and safety.

• **The National Center for Health Statistics** provides information on a wealth of health-related topics that is used to help guide government actions and policies to improve health.

U.S. Food and Drug Administration (FDA)

5600 Fishers Lane
Rockville, MD 20857-0001
General Information: 1-888-INFO-FDA (463-6332)
Internet home page: www.fda.gov

The aim of the Food and Drug Administration is to protect the public health from impure and unsafe foods, drugs, cosmetics, and other potential hazards. (See page 570 for more information on the FDA's role in approving drugs.)

Following are descriptions of some of the major departments within the administration. Each division has its own Internet site, which you can locate by going to the FDA Internet home page and clicking on the "Site Map," which contains links to all the FDA divisions. You can also reach the divisions by phone.

• **The Center for Biologics Evaluation and Research** (800-835-4709) oversees the regulation of biological products. Currently, it is the division of the FDA most concerned with AIDS-related activities, such as vaccine research.

• **The Center for Devices and Radiological Health** (301-827-3990) attempts to control unnecessary exposure to, and ensure the safe use of, potentially hazardous ionizing and nonionizing radiation. It also regulates medical devices.

• **The Center for Drug Evaluation and Research** (301-827-4573) develops policy with regard to the safety, effectiveness, and labeling of drug products.

• **The Center for Food Safety and Applied Nutrition** (800-723-3366) conducts research and develops standards on the composition, quality, and safety of foods, additives, and cosmetics.

The National Institutes of Health (NIH)

9000 Rockville Pike
Bethesda. MD 20892
General Inquiry: 301-496-1776
Internet home page: www.nih.gov

The National Institutes of Health is the principal medical research arm of the federal government. Its programs are oriented toward basic and applied scientific studies on the causes, diagnosis, prevention, treatment, and rehabilitation of disease and disability. It also fosters research into growth, development, and aging.

The NIH operates 25 separate Institutes and Centers as well as the National Library of Medicine, the nation's chief medical information source. The Institutes conduct and support research, perform clinical trials, make regulatory recommendations, and educate the public. Many of the Institutes also disseminate information and research data to the public through fact sheets, brochures, newsletters, and journals. The National Library of Medicine, while primarily for medical professionals and students, has some reference services for consumers.

You can reach the following Institutes and

643

Centers by phone or by going to the NIH Internet home page and clicking on "Institutes."

The National Cancer Institute
301-435-3848
The National Eye Institute
301-496-5248
The National Heart, Lung, and Blood Institute
301-496-4236
The National Human Genome Research Institute
301-402-0911
The National Institute on Aging
301-496-1752
The National Institute on Alcohol Abuse & Alcoholism
301-443-3860
The National Institute of Allergy and Infectious Diseases
301-496-5717
The National Institute of Arthritis and Musculoskeletal and Skin Diseases
301-496-8188
The National Institute of Child Health and Human Development
301-496-5133
The National Institute on Deafness and Other Communications Disorders
301-496-7243
The National Institute of Dental and Craniofacial Research
301-496-4261
The National Institute of Diabetes and Digestive and Kidney Diseases
301-496-3583
The National Institute on Drug Abuse
301-443-1124

The National Institute of Environmental Health Sciences
301-402-3378
The National Institute of General Medical Sciences
301-496-7301
The National Institute of Mental Health
301-443-4513
The National Institute of Neurological Disorders and Stroke
301-496-5751
The National Institute of Nursing Research
301-496-0207
National Center for Complementary & Alternative Medicine
301-496-1712
National Center for Research Resources
301-435-0888
The National Library of Medicine
301-496-6308

ADDITIONAL GENERAL SOURCES

If you cannot find an organization listed in these pages that covers your specific needs, or if you want to search for more than one topic, several general resources may prove helpful.

Medlineplus

www.nlm.nih.gov/medlineplus
This is the National Library of Medicine's consumer Web site. Medlineplus contains links to dozens of professional journals, allows you to perform detailed searches, and gives you access to a drug database with up-to-date information on more than 9,000 prescription and over-the-counter medications. It also links to many other good health-related Web sites.

Healthfinder

www.healthfinder.gov

Launched by the U.S. Department of Health and Human Services, Healthfinder links you to resources from the federal government, state and local agencies, nonprofit organizations, and universities. It is an excellent starting point for a general search of government-supported health information.

The Combined Health Information Database (CHID)

www.chid.gov

The online databases that make up CHID are sponsored by Federal health institutes and agencies. You can search through 18 separate databases that cover topics from Alzheimer's Disease to Weight Control. There is also a link to the NIH Health Information Index for links and referrals to federal agencies.

Medem

www.medem.com

This is a Web site that pools the online databases of several leading national medical societies, including the American Academy of Ophthalmology, American Academy of Pediatrics, American College of Allergy, Asthma & Immunology, American College of Obstetricians and Gynecologists, and the American Medical Association. The information—from basic overviews of ailments to recent clinical studies—is culled from professional journals and other peer-reviewed resources.

American Self-Help Clearinghouse

Northwest Covenant Medical Center
25 Pocono Road
Denville, NJ 07834
973-326-8853 or 973-326-6780
(call between 9 AM and 5 PM)
New Jersey residents can call 800-367-6274
Internet home page: www. selfhelpgroups.org
This nonprofit agency publishes a source book of several hundred national and international self-help groups that cover a wide range of illnesses, disabilities, addictions, and stressful life situations. The agency also provides information on how to start your own local self-help group.

ORGANIZATIONS AND SUPPORT GROUPS

This listing comprises voluntary, nonprofit, and professional organizations with fairly specific areas of interest. (These are the resources cited at the end of entries in the "Ailments and Disorders" section that begins on page 138.) Most of these organizations have a specific perspective on the issues relating to their areas of interest. This is especially true of support groups. If you don't feel at ease with one group, try contacting another. There are usually a number to choose from, and one is bound to be right for you.

American Academy of Allergy, Asthma & Immunology
611 East Wells Street
Milwaukee, WI 53202-3889
800-822-2762
www.aaaai.org

American Academy of Dermatology
930 North Meacham Road
Schaumburg, IL 60173
888-462- 3376/847-330-0230
www.aad.org

American Academy of Ophthalmology
PO Box 7424
San Francisco, CA 94120-7424
415-561-8500
www.eyenet.org

American Academy of Orthopaedic Surgeons
6300 North River Road
Rosemont, IL 60018-4262
800-346-2267/847-823-7186
www.aaos.org

American Academy of Otolaryngology-Head and Neck Surgery
One Prince Street
Alexandria, VA 22314-3357
703-836-4444
Fax: 703-683-5100
www.entnet.org

American Academy of Pediatrics
141 Northwest Point Boulevard
Elk Grove Village, IL 60007-1098
847-228-5005
www.aap.org

American Academy of Periodontology
737 N. Michigan Avenue
Suite 800
Chicago, IL 60611-2690
312-787-5518
Fax: 312/787-3670
www.perio.org

American Academy of Sleep Medicine
1610 14th Street, NW
Suite 300
Rochester, MN 55901
507-287-6006
Fax: 507-287-6008
www.asda.org

American Association for Chronic Fatigue Syndrome
c/o Harborview Medical Center
325 Ninth Avenue
Box 359780
Seattle, WA 98104
206-521-1932
Fax: 206-521-1930
www.aacfs.org

American Cancer Society
1599 Clifton Road, NE
Atlanta, GA 30329-4251
800-ACS-2345
www.cancer.org

American College of Cardiology
Heart House
9111 Old Georgetown Road
Bethesda, MD 20814-1699
800-253-4636
www.acc.org

American College of Obstetricians and Gynecologists
409 12th Street, SW
PO Box 96920
Washington, DC 20090-6920
www.acog.com

American College of Rheumatology
1800 Century Place, Suite 250
Atlanta, GA 30345
404-633-3777
Fax: 404-633-1870
www.rheumatology.org

American Council for Headache Education
19 Mantua Road
Mt. Royal, NJ 08061
856-423-0258
Fax: 856-423-0082
www.achenet.org

American Dental Association
Department of Public Education
and Information
211 East Chicago Avenue
Chicago, IL 60611
312-440-2500
www.ada.org

American Diabetes Association
1660 Duke Street
Alexandria, VA 22314
703-549-1500
www.diabetes.org

**American Foundation for
Urologic Disease**
300 West Pratt Street, Suite 401
Baltimore, MD 21201
800-242-2383
www.afud.org

**American Gastroenterological
Association**
7910 Woodmont Avenue
Seventh Floor
Bethesda, MD 20814
301-654-2055
Fax: 301-652-3890
www.gastro.org

American Hair Loss Council
401 North Michigan Avenue
Chicago, IL 60611
888-873-9719
www.ahlc.org

American Heart Association
7272 Greenville Avenue
Dallas, TX 75231-4596
800-242-8721/214-373-6300
www.americanheart.org

American Liver Foundation
75 Maiden Lane, Suite 603
New York, NY 10038
800-465-4837
www.liverfoundation.org

American Lung Association
1740 Broadway
New York, NY 10019
800-586-4872
www.lungusa.org

**American Lyme Disease
Foundation**
Mill Pond Offices
293 Route 100, Suite 204
Somers, NY 10589
800-876-5963
www.aldf.org

**American Optometric
Association**
243 North Lindbergh Boulevard
St. Louis, MO 63141
314-991-4100
www.aoanet.org

**American Orthopaedic Foot
and Ankle Society**
1216 Pine Street, Suite 201
Seattle, WA 98101
206-223-1120
Fax: 206-223 1178
www.aofas.org

**American Osteopathic
Association**
142 East Ontario Street
Chicago, IL 60611
800-621-1773/312-280-5800
Fax: 312-202-8200
www.am-osteo-assn.org

American Pain Foundation
111 South Calvert Street
Suite 2700
Baltimore, MD 21202
www.painfoundation.com

**American Podiatric Medical
Association**
9312 Old Georgetown Road
Bethesda, MD 20814-1698
800-366-8227/301-571-9200
www.apma.org

**American Psychological
Association**
750 First Street, NE
Washington, DC 20002-4242
800-374-2721/202-336-5500
www.apa.org

**American Sleep Apnea
Association**
1424 K Street, NW
Suite 302
Washington, DC 20005
2025 Pennsylvania Avenue, NW
202-293-3650
Fax: 202-293-3656
www.sleepapnea.org

**American Social Health
Association**
PO Box 13827
Research Triangle Park, NC
27709-3827
919-361-8400
Fax: 919-361-8425
800-230-6039
www.ashastd.org

**American Speech-Language-
Hearing Association**
10801 Rockville Pike
Rockville, Maryland 20852
800-498-2071
Recorded information:
888-321-2742
Fax-on-demand: 877-541-5035
www.asha.org

647

American Tinnitus Association
PO Box 5
Portland, OR 97207-0005
800-634-8978/503-248-9985
Fax: 503-248-0024
www.ata.org

American Urological Association
1120 North Charles Street
Baltimore, MD 21201
410-727-1100
Fax: 410-223-4370
www.auanet.org

Arthritis Foundation
1330 West Peachtree Street
Atlanta, GA 30309
800-283-7800/404-872-7100
www.arthritis.org

Asthma and Allergy Foundation of America
1125 15th Street, NW, Suite 502
Washington, DC 20005
800-727-8462
www.aafa.org

Back Pain Hotline
Texas Back Institute
6300 West Parker Road
Plano, TX 75093
800-247-2225
www.texasback.com

Better Hearing Institute
5021-B Backlick Road
Annandale, VA 22003
800-327-9355
www.betterhearing.org

CDC National Prevention Information Network
(Information on preventing HIV, STDs, and TB sponsored by the Centers for Disease Control and Prevention)
800-458-5231
www.cdcnpin.org

CDC National STD and AIDS Hotline
(sponsored by the Centers for Disease Control and Prevention)
800-227-8922

Celiac Disease Foundation
13251 Ventura Boulevard
Suite #1
Studio City, CA 91604
818-990-2354
Fax: 818-990-2379
www.celiac.org

Celiac Sprue Association/ USA Inc.
PO Box 31700
Omaha, NE 68131-0700
402-558-0600
Fax: 402-558-1347
www.csaceliacs.org

Chronic Fatigue and Immune Dysfunction Syndrome (CFIDS)
PO Box 220398
Charlotte, NC 28222-0398
Recorded information:
800-442-3437
Resource line: 704-365-2343
Fax: 704-365-9755
www.cfids.org

Fibromyalgia Network
P.O. Box 31750
Tucson, AZ 85751
800 853-2929
www.fmnetnews.com

Gastro-Intestinal Research Foundation (GIRF)
70 East Lake Street, Suite 1015
Chicago, IL 60601-5907
312-332-1350
www.girf.org

Glaucoma Research Foundation
200 Pine St.
Suite 200
San Francisco, CA 94104
800-826-6693/415-986-3162
Fax: 415-986-3763
www.glaucoma.org

International Foundation for Functional Gastrointestinal Disorders (IFFGD)
PO Box 17864
Milwaukee, WI 53217
888-964-2001/414-964-1799
www.iffgd.org

Intestinal Disease Foundation
1323 Forbes Avenue, Suite 200
Pittsburgh, PA 15219
412-261-5888
Fax: (412-471-2722

National Association for Continence
PO Box 8310
Spartanburg, SC 29305-8310
800-252-3337/864-579-7900
Fax: 864-579-7902
www.nafc.org

National Cancer Institute
Office of Cancer Communication
Bldg. 31, Rm. 10A24
Bethesda, MD 20892
800-422-6237
http://cancernet.nci.nih.gov

648

National Diabetes Information Clearinghouse
1 Information Way
Bethesda, MD 20892-3560
800-860-8747/301 654-3327
Fax: 301 907-8906
www.niddk.nih.gov/health/
diabetes/ndic.htm

National Digestive Diseases Information Clearinghouse
2 Information Way
Bethesda, MD 20892-3570
800-891-5389/301-654-3810
Fax: 301-654-3810
www.niddk.nih.gov/health/
digest/nddic.htm

National Eczema Association for Science and Education
1220 SW Morrison, Suite 433
Portland, OR 97205
800-818-7546
www.eczema-assn.org

National Headache Foundation
428 West St. James Place
Second Floor
Chicago, IL 60614-2750
800-843-2256
Fax: 773-525-7357
www.headaches.org

National Heart, Lung, and Blood Institute Information Center
PO Box 30105
Bethesda, MD 20824-0105
301-496-4236
www.nhlbi.nih.gov

National Institute of Allergy and Infectious Diseases
Building 31, Room 7A-50
31 Center Drive MSC 2520
Bethesda, MD 20892-2520
301-496-5717
www.niaid.nih.gov

National Institute of Arthritis and Musculoskeletal and Skin Diseases Information Clearinghouse
1 AMS Circle
Bethesda, MD 20892-3675
301-495-4484
www.nih.gov/niams

National Institute of Neurological Disorders and Stroke (NIH)
301-496-5751
www.ninds.nih.gov

National Jewish Medical and Research Center
1400 Jackson Street
Denver, CO 80206
800-222-5864 (LUNG)
303-388-4461
www.njc.org

National Kidney and Urologic Diseases Information Clearinghouse
3 Information Way
Bethesda, MD 20892-3580
301-654-4415
Fax: 301-907-8906
www.niddk.nih.gov/health/
kidney/nkudic.htm

National Mental Health Association
1021 Prince Street
Alexandria, VA 22314-2971
800-969-6642
703-684-7722
www.nmha.org

National Osteoporosis Foundation
1232 22nd Street, NW
Washington, DC 20037-1292
202-223-2226
www.nof.org

NIH Osteoporosis and Related Bone Diseases-National Resource Center
1232 22nd Street, NW
Washington, DC 20037-1292
800-624-2663/202-223-0344
www.osteo.org

National Psoriasis Foundation
6600 SW 92nd Avenue,
Suite 300
Portland, OR 97223-7195
800-723-9166/503-244-7404
Fax: 503-245-0626
www.psoriasis.org

National Sleep Foundation
1522 K Street, NW
Suite 500
Washington, DC 20005
Fax: 202-347-3472
www.sleepfoundation.org

Skin Cancer Foundation
PO Box 561
New York, NY 10156
800-754-6490/212-725-5176
www.skincancer.org

Simon Foundation for Incontinence
Box 835-F
Wilmette, IL 60091
800-237-4666
www.simonfoundation.org

649

GLOSSARY

For the definition of a term not contained in this glossary, consult the index. Medical specialties are defined on pages 86-87.

A

Achilles tendinitis. Inflammation of the Achilles tendon, which connects the calf muscles to the bones of the foot. This stress injury is most often due to tight calf muscles and is common among runners.

Aerobic exercise. Continuous rhythmic exercise using the large muscles of the body over an extended period of time. Aerobic exercise increases the body's demand for oxygen, thereby adding to the workload of the heart and lungs and elevating the heart rate.

Allergen. A substance that triggers an allergy. Common allergens include molds, pollens, ragweed, animal dander, feathers, cosmetics, and dust mites.

Analgesic. A substance that relieves pain. Analgesics are among the most common over-the-counter drugs. Examples include nonsteroidal anti-inflammatory drugs (NSAIDs), such as aspirin or ibuprofen, and other pain relievers such as acetaminophen.

Anaphylactic shock. An overreaction of the immune system that occurs in response to a substance that the person has been previously sensitized to, such as an insect sting from a bee or wasp or drugs like penicillin. This overreaction causes nausea, flushing, depressed blood pressure, irregular heartbeat, vomiting, and difficulty breathing, and it may lead to coma or death.

Anemia. A condition characterized by a decreased amount of hemoglobin in the blood. The most common type is iron-deficiency anemia (usually due to a diet low in iron), in which red blood cells are reduced in size and number and hemoglobin levels are low.

Angina. Chest pain resulting from lack of blood (and therefore oxygen) to the heart muscle. The correct medical term is angina pectoris.

Antibiotics. Drugs that kill or inhibit the growth of disease-causing bacteria and other infectious microbes. They are available in many forms, including pills, creams, and eye and ear drops, to treat a wide range of infections.

Antibodies. Substances produced by the immune system that recognize and neutralize specific invading microbes or foreign proteins (which may be introduced after an organ transplant), helping to ward off infection and disease. Also called immunoglobulins.

Antifungal. A drug that combats fungal infections, such as athlete's foot, jock itch, or nail fungus. Topical antifungal drugs are commonly available as creams or lotions to be applied externally to the skin or hair. There are also systemic antifungal drugs, which are taken orally.

Antioxidants. Chemical compounds that neutralize cell-damaging free radicals created when oxygen is utilized inside the body's cells. In combating free radicals, antioxidants may protect against cancer and possibly other diseases. The principal antioxidant nutrients are carotenoids (such as beta carotene), the mineral selenium, and vitamins C and E.

Astigmatism. A defect of the cornea or lens of the eye that causes blurred vision.

Atherosclerosis. A condition characterized by the accumulation of plaque within the arterial walls. This results in a narrowing of the arteries, which reduces blood and oxygen flow to the heart and brain, as well as to other parts of the body, and can lead to heart attack, stroke, and loss of function or death of other tissues.

B

Basal cell carcinoma. The most common form of skin cancer. Basal cell carcinoma usually grows slowly and rarely spreads and therefore is easily treated.primarily to treat high blood pressure and heart disease.

Biopsy. The removal of a small piece of living tissue for further diagnostic testing, which is commonly done to look for cancer.

Blood pressure. The force of the blood against the walls of the arteries. It is measured in two ways:

systolic pressure (the top number) and diastolic pressure (the bottom number).

Bursa. A small, fluid-filled sac beneath the tendons in such areas as the knees, elbows, or shoulders that helps to protect the joints.

C

Capillaries. The intricate network of tiny blood vessels that permeate most of the body's tissues. Capillaries serve as the juncture between the arterial and venous systems and help cells to maintain a proper exchange of oxygen and carbon dioxide.

Carcinogen. Any substance capable of causing cancer.

Cardiovascular. Pertaining to the heart and the blood vessels.

Carotenoids. Any of more than 600 yellow-orange pigments found in fruits and vegetables such as apricots, sweet potatoes, asparagus, carrots, cantaloupe, kale, tomatoes, and winter squash. Many of the carotenoids, which include beta carotene and lycopene, are thought to protect against heart disease and certain types of cancer.

Cartilage. Specialized fibrous connective tissue that forms an embryo's skeleton and much of an infant's skeleton. As the child grows, the cartilage becomes bone. In adults, cartilage is present in and around joints and makes up the primary skeletal structure in some parts of the body, such as the ears and the tip of the nose.

Collagen. The main supportive and connective tissue in the body. It forms the basic structure for tendons, ligaments, skin, and cartilage.

Coronary artery disease (CAD). Narrowing or blockage of the coronary arteries, which reduces the supply of blood, and therefore of oxygen, to the heart muscle.

Cryotherapy. The removal of unwanted tissue by freezing. Skin tags, for example, might be surgically removed by a dermatologist applying frozen liquid nitrogen. Also called cryosurgery.

Cyst. A membrane-enclosed sac containing fluid, pus, or other soft material that develops as an abnormal growth. Cysts can develop just under the skin (so-called epidermal cysts) or inside the body in organs such as the ovaries or kidneys.

D

Deciliter (dl). A metric unit of volume, equal to 1/10 of a liter. (A liter is slightly smaller than a quart.) Deciliters are commonly used in laboratory test measurements. Cholesterol test results, for example, are often given as grams of cholesterol per deciliter of blood (g/dl).

Dehydration. A depletion of body fluids that can hinder the body's ability to regulate its own temperature. During exercise, one can become dehydrated if the fluids lost through perspiration are not replaced.

Diastolic blood pressure. The lowest pressure in the arteries, which occurs when the heart is relaxed between beats. It is represented by the bottom number in the fraction of a blood-pressure reading.

Disk (intervertebral disk). A ring of cartilage and fibrous tissue with a pulpy or gel-like center located between the vertebrae of the spine. Disks act as shock absorbers and contribute to the spine's flexibility.

Diuretic. A substance that increases fluid output through urination. Caffeine, alcohol, and a number of medications act as diuretics and can cause the excretion of important vitamins and minerals.

Dysmenorrhea. The medical term for menstrual pain.

Dysplasia. Abnormal tissue development in a skin blemish (such as a mole) or in another area of the body that may develop into cancer if left untreated.

E

Electrocardiogram (ECG, EKG). A test to record the electrical processes originating within the heart, such as heartbeat, and to assess heart problems. The test involves electrodes, or leads, attached to the chest, neck, arms, and legs.

Electrolytes. Substances that conduct electricity in solution. Usually they are salts of minerals, such as

651

sodium and potassium, that are dissolved in blood and cellular fluids. Electrolytes are required for the proper functioning of many organs, including the heart.

Electrotherapy. The removal of unwanted tissue by burning. Skin blemishes, for example, might be removed by a dermatologist applying a directed electrical heat beam.

Endometrium. The lining of the uterus. If pregnancy does not occur, part of the endometrium sloughs off during menstruation each month.

Endorphins. Chemical substances produced by the central nervous system and other organs that suppress pain.

Enzymes. Proteins produced by the cells that are involved in every chemical reaction in the body. They initiate the reactions and control the rate at which they occur. There are thousands of enzymes. Each one has a specific function; for example, the digestive enzyme amylase acts on carbohydrates in foods to break them down.

Essential fatty acids. Fatty acids that the body cannot produce. They must be obtained from food.

Estrogen. One of the female sex hormones produced by the ovaries. Different forms of estrogen have been synthesized as drugs that may be used after menopause, when estrogen production declines, to counter the adverse effects of the low estrogen levels in the body.

F

Fats. Technically termed lipids, fats are the body's most concentrated source of energy. All fats are made up of carbon, hydrogen, and oxygen atoms that are arranged in combinations of glycerol and fatty acids. Fats found in foods are either in solid (butter) or liquid (oil) form. In the body, fat is part of all cell membranes, where it preserves the function of the cell and also serves as a stored form of energy, helps cushion organs, and helps create certain hormones.

Fatty acids. Chemical chains of carbon, hydrogen, and oxygen atoms that are part of a fat (lipid) and constitute the major component of triglycerides. Depend-

ing on the number and arrangement of these atoms, fatty acids are classified as either saturated, polyunsaturated, or monounsaturated.

Fiber. The indigestible part of plants. Fiber passes through much of the digestive tract virtually unaltered, absorbing water and helping to speed elimination. Some types of fiber are broken down by microorganisms in the large bowel into substances that can exert effects on the bowel wall or be absorbed by the body. These substances produce various physiological effects, such as inhibiting the production of cholesterol.

Folacin. An older term for the B vitamin folic acid or folate. Folacin plays an important role in cell reproduction and has a protective effect against a variety of disorders, especially birth defects.

Free radicals. Unstable molecules, usually containing oxygen, created by normal chemical processes in the body as well as by radiation (especially x-rays) and other environmental influences. The interaction of free radicals with DNA and other macromolecules leads to impaired functioning of the cells. Free radicals may be an important factor in the development of cancer and other diseases.

G

Gamma globulin. A protein formed in the blood that contains antibodies to diseases to which an individual is immune. Gamma globulin can be extracted from donated blood and is used in the prevention and treatment of certain diseases, such as hepatitis A and Rh-factor disorders. It is often given as an injection to individuals who may come into contact with a disease, but who are not immune to it.

Generic drug. An identical copy of a brand-name drug. A drug company that develops a drug can patent it and sell it exclusively for 17 years (This may be extended by five years in some cases); after that, any company can make and sell a chemically equivalent generic copy of that drug. Generics usually cost considerably less than brand-name drugs.

Glycogen. A compound produced by the liver from glucose and stored in the liver and muscles. It acts as an energy source for muscles and releases glucose from the liver to maintain blood sugar levels.

Gram. The metric unit of weight measurement equivalent to 1/1000 of a kilogram. One ounce is equal to 28.35 grams. A paper clip weighs about one gram.

H

HDL (High-density lipoprotein). A molecular package consisting of proteins and lipids that picks up cholesterol from the tissues and delivers it to the liver for reprocessing or excretion. Because it clears cholesterol out of the cardiovascular system, HDL has been called "good" cholesterol. There are several types of HDL.

Hemoglobin. The oxygen-carrying protein of the blood found in red cells.

Hormones. Chemical substances secreted by a variety of body organs that are carried by the bloodstream and usually influence cells some distance from the source of production. Hormones signal certain enzymes to perform their functions. In this way, hormones regulate such body functions as blood sugar levels, insulin levels, the menstrual cycle, and growth.

Hydrogenation. The process of adding hydrogen atoms to an unsaturated fat to make it more saturated and more resistant to chemical change. Manufacturers often hydrogenate fats to turn liquid fats into solids (as in margarine) or to give them a longer shelf life.

Hyperglycemia. A condition characterized by an abnormally high blood glucose level; it occurs in people with untreated or inadequately controlled diabetes.

Hypoglycemia. A condition characterized by an abnormally low blood glucose level. Severe hypoglycemia is rare and dangerous. It can be caused by medications such as insulin (those with diabetes mellitus are prone to hypoglycemia), severe physical exhaustion, and some illnesses.

I

Immunization. A procedure in which a dead or inactive bacteria, virus, or toxin is given orally or by injection to trigger an immune response to that specific disease.

Inflammation. The body's natural response to trauma, toxins, or infection, in which injured tissues release a variety of substances that increase blood flow to the area. White blood cells arrive to remove dead tissue and other debris. These and other vascular changes produce heat, swelling, and redness; pain or stiffness often ensue until healing occurs.

Insulin. A hormone secreted by the pancreas in response to elevated blood glucose levels. Insulin stimulates the liver, muscles, and fat cells to remove glucose from the blood for use or storage. People with diabetes mellitus either do not produce enough insulin or do not use it properly.

L

Lactose. The sugar found in milk. Lactose is a disaccharide composed of glucose and galactose.

LDL (Low-density lipoprotein). A protein and lipid molecule that is manufactured in the liver and transferred to the bloodstream. LDL delivers cholesterol to tissues and has been implicated in the accumulation of plaque within the arteries. It is often referred to as "bad" cholesterol.

Ligaments. Tough, fibrous bands of connective tissue that join bones together at joints and help support certain organs such as the liver, bladder, and uterus.

Lipids. The technical term for fats, waxes, and fatty compounds.

Lipoproteins. Packages of proteins, cholesterol, and triglycerides assembled by the intestine and liver that circulate in the bloodstream. One of their chief functions is to carry cholesterol.

Lumbar region. The five vertebrae in the lower spine that form the largest natural curve in the back.

Lymph. A pale fluid containing white blood cells and other substances that bathes cells throughout the body. Lymph is carried through the body by lymphatic vessels and plays an important role in transporting cells of the immune system. Some lymph flows back into the blood.

653

M

Macronutrients. The nutrients that are present in foods in large quantities—namely carbohydrates, proteins, and fats.

Magnetic resonance imaging (MRI). A diagnostic imaging technique that uses magnetic fields and radio waves to visualize internal structures.

Malignant tumor. An abnormal growth or tumor that can spread uncontrollably and in some cases prove fatal, as opposed to a benign growth.

Mammogram. A low-dose x-ray that is used to detect abnormalities of the breast.

Maximum heart rate (MHR). The highest heart rate you can achieve during your greatest effort exercising. MHR decreases with age and is determined by subtracting your age from 220. MHR is used to compute your target heart rate.

Megadose. A quantity of a vitamin or mineral that far exceeds the recommended level. In some cases, megadoses can be toxic and cause severe side effects.

Melanin. A dark pigment produced in the skin. Dark-skinned individuals produce more melanin. Melanin production increases in response to sunlight, causing the skin to become darker.

Melanoma. A malignant form of skin cancer that usually arises from a precancerous mole and can invade other parts of the body if not recognized early.

Metabolism. The sum of the chemical reactions in the body that are necessary to sustain life. All metabolic processes are driven by energy derived from the major nutrients in foods.

Microminerals. The minerals present in the body in small amounts (less than five grams). Also known as trace minerals, these include chromium, cobalt, copper, fluorine, iodine, iron, manganese, molybdenum, nickel, selenium, silicon, tin, vanadium, and zinc. The body must replenish these from foods.

Milligram. The metric unit of weight measurement that is equivalent to 1/1000 of a gram.

Minerals. Inorganic substances that are basic components of the earth's crust; they are also found in the human body. Humans constantly replenish their mineral supply with food and water. Minerals are crucial for a wide variety of bodily functions, including enzyme synthesis, regulation of the heart rhythm, bone formation, and digestion.

Monosaccharides. Sugars consisting of a single sugar molecule, such as glucose, fructose, or galactose.

Monounsaturated fatty acids. Fats consisting of a large percentage of unsaturated fatty acids that lack a single pair of hydrogen atoms. Olive, peanut, canola, and avocado oils are largely monounsaturated. These fats may be able to reduce total cholesterol by decreasing the amount of damaging LDL cholesterol in the blood without producing a reduction, or as much of a reduction, in heart-healthy HDL cholesterol.

N

Neurons. Active cells of the nervous system that transmit and receive messages.

Neuropathy. An abnormality of the nerves, which is caused by damage or pressure that can produce pain, numbness, tingling, or burning sensations. So-called peripheral neuropathies commonly occur in the arms, legs, hands, or feet.

Neurotransmitters. Chemicals in the brain and other nervous system tissues that aid in the transmission of nerve impulses. Various neurotransmitters are responsible for different functions such as controlling mood and muscle movement and inhibiting or causing the sensation of pain.

Non-REM sleep. The deepest stages of sleep, characterized by a general absence of body movement and slow, regular brain activity.

Norepinephrine. A hormone primarily secreted by the adrenal medulla gland in conjunction with epinephrine in response to threatening situations.

NSAIDs. An abbreviation for nonsteroidal anti-inflammatory drugs, which are used to treat mild to moderate pain and inflammation in such conditions as arthritis, tendinitis, backache, or sprains. Common over-the-counter NSAIDs include aspirin, ibuprofen (Advil, Motrin), naproxen sodium (Aleve), and ketoprofen (Orudis).

O

Obesity. A medical term that refers to the storage of excess fat in the body. A person is usually considered obese when his or her weight is 20 percent greater than the appropriate weight as determined by conventional height-weight tables.

Occult blood test. A diagnostic test performed on a stool sample for the presence of unseen (occult) blood, which may indicate colon cancer. Also called a fecal occult blood test.

Off-label use. The practice whereby a doctor prescribes a drug or combination of drugs for a condition that has not been specifically approved by the Food and Drug Administration (FDA). Once a drug has been approved for one purpose, doctors are generally free to prescribe it to treat any condition.

Omega-3 fatty acids. A unique group of polyunsaturated fatty acids found in fish oil and some seeds (such as in linseed oil). Omega-3s in fish oil significantly reduce blood clotting. They make platelets less likely to stick together and to blood vessels. Omega-3s may reduce the risk of heart attack or stroke.

Opiates. Narcotic pain relievers, such as morphine.

Orthotics. Foot supports that fit in shoes to correct for abnormal foot motion and alignment. Orthotics should be custom designed by a podiatrist or an orthopedist.

Over-the-counter (OTC). A designation for a drug that can be sold without a prescription. Common OTCs include laxatives, cough and cold medicines, pain relievers such as aspirin or ibuprofen, and antacids.

Oxalic acid. A substance that, when joined with calcium in the body, forms insoluble salts and hinders iron absorption from food. It is found in such vegetables as spinach, chard, and rhubarb.

P

Pap smear. A diagnostic test for detecting cervical cancer in which a sample of cervical cells is examined for cellular changes. The death rate from cervical cancer is almost zero among women who have regular Pap smears.

Placebo. A medication that contains no active ingredients. People may feel better after taking medication simply because they expect to. For this reason, placebos are commonly used in tests of new drugs to check whether the drug is actually having an effect.

Plaque (arterial). Deposits of fatty substances, such as cholesterol, in the inner lining of the artery walls. The buildup of these deposits can lead to atherosclerosis.

Plaque (dental). A thin film, composed of saliva, microscopic food particles, and bacteria that coats tooth and tongue surfaces. The sugars and starches you eat are digested by the bacteria, producing acid that attacks tooth enamel. This acid is the cause of tooth decay and, over the long term, of gum disease.

Polyunsaturated fatty acids. Fats consisting of a large percentage of unsaturated fatty acids lacking more than one pair of hydrogen atoms. Corn, safflower, and sesame oils are primarily polyunsaturated. These fats tend to lower LDL cholesterol, thus reducing the amount of artery-clogging cholesterol in the bloodstream.

Precancerous. A change in color, size, or shape in a skin blemish (such as a mole) or other abnormal growth anywhere on the body that may develop into cancer if left untreated.

Progesterone. A female sex hormone secreted by the ovaries. Progesterone and estrogen regulate changes that occur during the menstrual cycle.

Protein. Compounds containing hydrogen, oxygen, and nitrogen that are present in the body and in foods formed by complex combinations of amino acids. Protein is essential for life. Foods that supply the body with protein include meats, dairy products, eggs, and seafood, as well as grains, legumes, nuts, and vegetables.

PSA test. A test that measures blood levels of the prostate-specific antigen, a protein produced by the

655

prostate gland that may be elevated when cancer is present. The test has come into wide use as a screening device, especially for men over 50.

R

REM sleep. A phase of sleep during which the eyes move quickly (REM stands for "rapid eye movement"), heartbeat and metabolism speed up, and toes and fingers twitch. Dreaming takes place during REM sleep.

Resting heart rate (RHR). The number of heartbeats per minute while the body is at rest. It is most accurately measured by taking a pulse reading before rising in the morning.

Resting metabolic rate (RMR). The total amount of energy your body uses in a given period of time when at rest. RMR depends on body size, body composition, age, and other factors and can be temporarily affected by activity level and diet.

Retrovirus. A virus that has the ability to take over certain cells and interrupt their normal genetic function. Human Immunodeficiency Syndrome (HIV), the virus that causes Acquired Immune Deficiency Syndrome (AIDS), is one type of retrovirus.

Reye's syndrome. A rare but potentially fatal disorder affecting the liver and brain that has been linked to the use of aspirin in children and teenagers with chicken pox or flu (influenza). It is marked by vomiting, lethargy, seizures, and can even lead to coma and death. Because of the risk of Reye's syndrome, children 19 or younger should be given a medication other than aspirin (such as acetaminophen) to reduce fever or for pain relief.

Rhinoviruses. One of the main groups of viruses that causes colds.

RICE. An acronym for a recommended method of alleviating exercise-related injuries, both acute and overuse. RICE stands for Rest the injured body part; apply Ice; apply Compression; and Elevate the injured extremity above heart level.

S

Salmonella. A group of bacteria that causes intestinal infection. A frequent contaminator of foods, *Salmonella* is one of the most common causes of food poisoning.

Saturated fatty acids. Fats containing all the hydrogen atoms they can carry. Such fats, which are usually solid at room temperature, come mainly from animal sources (such as beef, butter, whole-milk dairy products, dark meat poultry, and poultry skin) as well as from tropical vegetable oils (coconut, palm, and palm kernel). Saturated fats in the diet are among the chief contributors to elevated blood-cholesterol levels.

Serotonin. A compound made from the amino acid tryptophan that serves as one of the brain's principal neurotransmitters. When a person eats a meal, the level of serotonin is raised or lowered—depending on the amounts of proteins, carbohydrates, and other substances consumed—and this level may affect mood.

Sexually transmitted disease (STD). An infection that is spread primarily through sexual contact. Common STDs include gonorrhea, syphilis, genital herpes, Acquired Immune Deficiency Syndrome (AIDS), chlamydia, and genital warts.

Sigmoidoscopy. A screening procedure to detect colon cancer and other abnormalities of the lower portion of the large intestine and of the rectum. The test is done by viewing the area with a long thin tube that is inserted into the rectum.

Soft tissue. Tissues other than bone, including muscles, tendons, ligaments, and cartilage. Most sports injuries involve damage to soft tissues.

SPF (Sun protection factor). A number that indicates the relative length of time that a sunscreen product will protect you from sunburn compared with using no sunscreen. A product with an SPF of 15, for example, would allow you to stay in the sun without burning 15 times longer than if you didn't apply sunscreen.

Stress fracture. A microscopic break in a bone caused by repeated impact. Stress fractures are common among aerobic dancers and long distance runners and usually affect the foot, shin, or thigh.

Stroke. A hemorrhage or a blockage in a blood vessel extending to the brain, resulting in insufficient delivery of blood (and therefore oxygen) to a portion of the brain. Many strokes can result in some degree of paralysis, but small strokes may occur without symptoms. Recurrent strokes can lead to mental deterioration.

Synapses. The connections between neurons.

Systemic. Having an effect on overall health or affecting a large area of the body. Systemic drugs, which can be taken orally or intravenously, are generally absorbed in the blood and distributed through much of the body.

Systolic blood pressure. The maximum pressure in the arteries when the heart is contracting. It is represented by the top number in the fraction of a blood-pressure reading.

T

Target heart rate (THR). A level of exercise intensity that enables one to gain the maximum training benefits from an aerobic workout. Also called training heart rate, THR is computed by taking 60 percent and 90 percent of one's maximum heart rate (MHR). During aerobic exercise, the number of heartbeats per minute should fall between these two figures.

Tendons. The strong, inelastic cords of connective tissue that anchor muscles to bones or, in some cases, to other tissues.

Testosterone. The principal male sex hormone that induces and maintains the changes that occur in males at puberty. In men, the testicles continue to produce testosterone throughout life, though there is some decline with age.

Topical. Designed to have an effect on a limited area of the body. Topical drugs, for example, include creams and lotions applied to the skin, eyes, ears, hair, or mucous membranes.

Toxicity. The potential ability of a substance to harm a living organism. Almost any substance in food, air, and water can become toxic if it is taken in a high enough concentration.

Trans fatty acids. Fats that are produced during the process of hydrogenation, which occurs when manufacturers add hydrogen to unsaturated fats to make them more solid or shelf stable. Studies have shown that trans fats act like saturated fatty acids, raising levels of total and LDL ("bad") cholesterol.

Triglycerides. Fats present in plants and animals. Triglycerides consist of three fatty acids (tri) attached to a molecule of glycerol. Most of the fat in foods is in the form of triglycerides, as is most of the fat stored in the human body. High levels of triglycerides in the bloodstream may be a risk factor for heart disease.

V

Vaccination. Administration of a vaccine—a preparation containing modified microbes (bacteria or viruses) or toxins that aren't strong enough to cause diseases yet can still stimulate the immune system to produce antibodies against diseases. The term is often used interchangeably with immunization.

Vascular. Pertaining to the blood vessels, such as arteries, veins, or capillaries, or to the vessels that conduct lymph fluid.

Vitamins. Organic substances (meaning they contain carbon) that the body requires to help regulate metabolic functions. For the most part, vitamins must be ingested; the body cannot manufacture them. Exceptions are vitamin D, which the body can synthesize, and to some extent vitamin K, which the body can produce from the bacteria that normally inhabit the intestines.

657

Chronic diseases. See also specific diseases
  in older adults, 563
  prevention of, 14
Chronic fatigue and immune dysfunction syndrome (CFIDS), 206–7
Chronic fatigue syndrome (CFS), 206–7
Chronic obstructive pulmonary disease (COPD), 39
Chrysanthemum flowers, dried, 430
Cigarette smoking. See Smoking
Circadian rhythms, 353, 358, 359, 428
Clenched fist injury, 107
Clotrimazole, 158, 360, 502
Cluster headaches, 307, 309, 311
Coal tar, 228, 417
Codeine, 222, 577
Coenzyme Q-10, 614–15
Coffee, 334, 477, 601
  for hangovers, 302
Colds, common, 208–12, 221, 441, 450, 575
  remedies, 209, 210, 575–80, 602
Cold sores, 185–87, 281
Colic, 213–14
Collagen implants, 485
Colloidal oatmeal, 126, 195, 249, 344, 439
Colon cancer, 16, 78–80, 556
Colonoscopy, 78, 79–80, 357, 554, 566, 593
Colorado tick fever, 135
Colorectal cancer screenings, 72, 78–80, 554, 566
Computers, 188, 189, 248, 310–11
Condoms, 57, 58–59, 282, 284, 291, 326, 341, 460, 489, 492, 493, 534, 537, 538
Conjunctivitis, 175, 215–16
Constipation, 217–19, 245, 260, 316, 495, 564
  hemorrhoids and, 321–23
Contact dermatitis, 172, 229, 230, 238
Contact lenses, 172, 175, 215, 216, 247, 248, 414, 582, 584
Contraception. See Birth control
Cooking foods, 243, 270, 272, 326, 402, 527
Coral stings, 132, 133
Corns, 220
Cornstarch powder, 158, 239, 360, 415, 457, 475

Coronary artery disease (CAD), 63–65
  cholesterol and, 16–17, 65
  diet and, 22, 64
  exercise and, 27, 64–65
  obesity and, 34
Coronary heart disease (CHD), 16–17, 64–65, 200, 550, 556
Corticoid lotions or creams, 149, 224
Cortisone ointments, 230
Cosmetics, 143, 172, 230, 424
  dermatitis and, 230, 231
  sensitive skin and, 231
  wrinkles and, 499–500
Cough drops, 222, 578–79
Cough medications, 209, 222, 265–66, 408, 575–80
Coughs (coughing), 154, 180, 221–23. See also Dry cough
  and flu, 265–66
  medications for, 575, 577–78
Coumadin (warfarin), 38, 66, 587, 599, 612, 636
COX-2 inhibitors, 396, 480, 598, 603
CPAP (continuous positive airway pressure) machine, 447
Crabs (pubic lice), 374–75
Cradle cap, 224–25, 434
Cramping, abdominal, 219, 240, 243, 244, 279
Cramps
  diarrhea and, 240, 243
  food poisoning and, 267–70
  menstrual, 384–85, 602
  muscle, 390–91
Cranberry juice, 487–88
Cross training, 318, 320
Croup, 226–27
Crunches, 163
Crutches, 152, 454
Crying, 226
  colic and, 213, 214
Cutaneous tags, 62
Cuts, 112–15
Cutting boards, 268
Cycling, 30, 165, 366, 367, 394, 454, 465, 526
Cyst, ganglion, 276
Cystic acne, 142
Cystitis, 486–88

Dairy products. See Lactose intolerance; Milk
Dandruff, 228

dandruff shampoos, 224, 228, 417, 434
Decongestant eyedrops, 175, 582, 584
Decongestants, 38, 146, 209, 252, 304, 441
  about, 574, 576–77, 579
Deer ticks, 376–78
DEET (N, N-deiethyltoluamide), 132, 136, 378, 608
Degenerative joint disease. See Osteoarthritis
Dehydration, 241–43, 279, 301, 518, 581
Dental appliances, 55
Dental care, 51–55, 518–19. See also Flossing teeth; Toothbrushing
Dental checkups, 53, 73, 168, 288, 547, 554, 566
Dental sealants, 51, 518–19
Dentin hypersensitivity, 435
Dentures, 168, 187
Depo-Provera, 535, 539
Depression
  fibromyalgia and, 254, 255, 257
  headaches and, 308
  postpartum, 545
  SAD and, 428–29
Dermatitis, 229–32
  contact, 172, 229, 230, 238
  seborrheic, 172, 224, 228, 229, 417, 434
Dermatologists, 86
Desmopressin, 170
Detached retina, 262, 263
Detergents, 229, 231, 239, 249
Development. See Growth and development
Deviated septum, 441, 448
DEXA (dual energy x-ray absorptiometry) test, 400
Dexfenfluramine, 38
Dextromethorphan, 180, 222, 266, 408, 577
DHEA (dehydroepiandrosterone), 615–17
Diabetes (diabetes mellitus), 233–37, 556. See also Type 2 diabetes
  cataracts and, 190
  fish oil and, 623
  hammer toe and, 299
  screening for, 82–83, 236, 554
  weight control and, 34, 234–36
Diabetic ketoacidosis, 233, 236

669

671

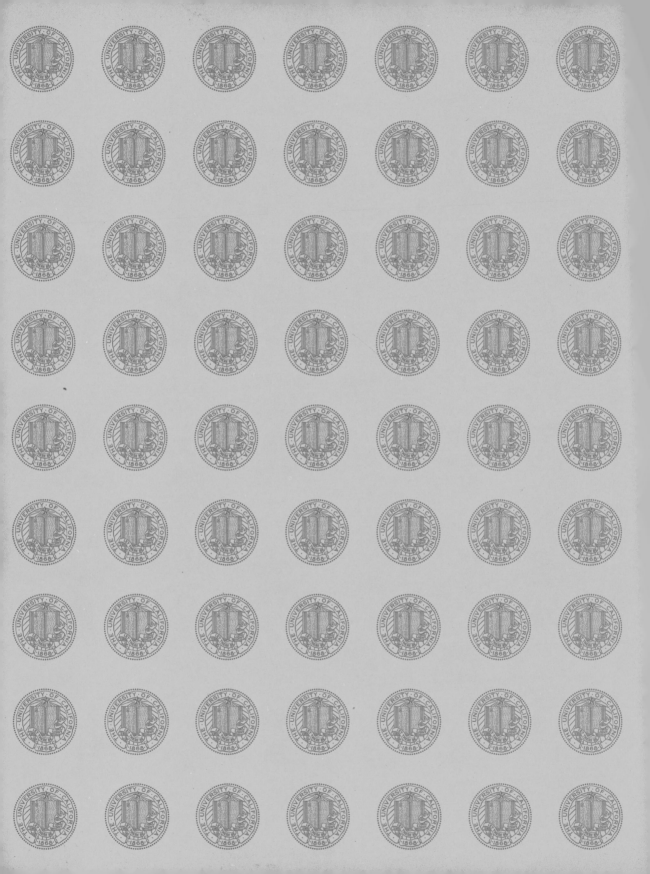